Hematology: Clinical Aspects and Applications

Hematology: Clinical Aspects and Applications

Edited by **Brian Jenkins**

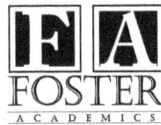

FA FOSTER ACADEMICS

New Jersey

Published by Foster Academics,
61 Van Reypen Street,
Jersey City, NJ 07306, USA
www.fosteracademics.com

Hematology: Clinical Aspects and Applications
Edited by Brian Jenkins

International Standard Book Number: 978-1-63242-447-1 (Hardback)

The publisher's policy is to use permanent paper from mills that operate a sustainable forestry policy. Furthermore, the publisher ensures that the text paper and cover boards used have met acceptable environmental accreditation standards.

Trademark Notice: Registered trademark of products or corporate names are used only for explanation and identification without intent to infringe.

Printed in the United States of America.

Contents

Preface

This book aims to highlight the current researches and provides a platform to further the scope of innovations in this area. This book is a product of the combined efforts of many researchers and scientists from different parts of the world. The objective of this book is to provide the readers with the latest information in the field.

Hematology deals with the study of blood and its components. It involves the cures and diagnosis of diseases related to blood. Such as hemophilia, anemia, general blood clots and blood cancer. Hematology although a separate discipline overlaps with oncology. This book provides significant information about the clinical aspects and applications of this field. From theories to research to practical applications, case studies related to all contemporary topics of relevance to this field have been included in this book. It consists of contributions made by international experts. Scientists and students actively engaged in this field will find this book full of crucial and unexplored concepts.

I would like to express my sincere thanks to the authors for their dedicated efforts in the completion of this book. I acknowledge the efforts of the publisher for providing constant support. Lastly, I would like to thank my family for their support in all academic endeavors.

Editor

The Epigenetic Landscape of Acute Myeloid Leukemia

Emma Conway O'Brien, Steven Prideaux, and Timothy Chevassut

Brighton and Sussex Medical School, University of Sussex, Falmer, Brighton BN1 9PS, UK

Correspondence should be addressed to Timothy Chevassut; t.chevassut@bsms.ac.uk

Academic Editor: Myriam Labopin

Acute myeloid leukemia (AML) is a genetically heterogeneous disease. Certain cytogenetic and molecular genetic mutations are recognized to have an impact on prognosis, leading to their inclusion in some prognostic stratification systems. Recently, the advent of high-throughput whole genome or exome sequencing has led to the identification of several novel recurrent mutations in AML, a number of which have been found to involve genes concerned with epigenetic regulation. These genes include in particular DNMT3A, TET2, and IDH1/2, involved with regulation of DNA methylation, and EZH2 and ASXL-1, which are implicated in regulation of histones. However, the precise mechanisms linking these genes to AML pathogenesis have yet to be fully elucidated as has their respective prognostic relevance. As massively parallel DNA sequencing becomes increasingly accessible for patients, there is a need for clarification of the clinical implications of these mutations. This review examines the literature surrounding the biology of these epigenetic modifying genes with regard to leukemogenesis and their clinical and prognostic relevance in AML when mutated.

1. Introduction

Acute myeloid leukemia (AML) is a genetically heterogeneous disease characterized by malignant clonal proliferation of immature myeloid cells in the bone marrow, peripheral blood, and occasionally other body tissues [1, 2]. It is the most common acute leukemia in adults and encompasses 15–20% of cases in children [2]. While the disease is most commonly found in individuals over 60 years, AML also occurs in younger people and occasionally may even be present at birth [1, 2]. Environmental factors that increase the risk of developing AML include smoking, benzene exposure, and chemotherapy or radiotherapy treatment [1, 2]. Preceding myelodysplastic syndrome (MDS) or myeloproliferative neoplasm (MPN) may also develop into AML [3]. Although highly variable, the outlook for most AML subtypes is dismal, with an overall 5-year survival rate of approximately 25% [1]. The genetic and epigenetic profile of the malignant cells influences the likelihood of achieving remission and risk of relapse [4]. A greater understanding of the underlying genetic and epigenetic processes may provide insight into the mechanism of leukemogenesis in AML, as well as offering prognostic information and potential therapeutic targets. The prognostic implications of many molecular mutations in AML are well reported [5]. However, the role of mutations in genes with epigenetic function is less clearly understood [6–8]. This literature review, therefore, aims to examine the pathological role and prognostic implications of mutations in epigenetic modifying genes.

2. Genetics and Risk Stratification in AML

Many patients with AML will have cytogenetic aberrations which can be detected through karyotyping or fluorescent in situ hybridization (FISH) [9–11]. Risk stratification—into low, intermediate, or high risk groups—can then be carried out according to the cytogenetic profile of the patient [9, 10]. However, there is variation between different cooperative groups as to the correct stratification of different mutations [1]. Furthermore, nearly half of the patients have cytogenetically normal (CN) AML and are ascribed to the intermediate risk category despite significant heterogeneity [5]. It is clear, therefore, that molecular mutational analysis has the potential to improve prognostication stratification systems. Currently, only a limited selection of genetic mutations is included in widely used prognostic stratification models—in the European LeukemiaNet (ELN) system, for example, NPM1, FLT3-ITD, and CEBPα are the only molecular mutations afforded prognostic significance [12]. The World Health Organization has included a provisional entity in its classification system which includes AML with NPM1 and CEBPα mutations [13]. Nonetheless, mutations which are not included in stratification systems may still impact on prognosis. In addition, increasing access to whole genome or exome mutational analysis techniques is yielding a bewildering array of novel mutations associated with AML. Newly diagnosed AML patients and their doctors are therefore likely to be faced with a complex combination of different mutations, with uncertain clinical significance, on genetic analysis.

3. The Two-Hit Hypothesis

For many years, the accepted model of leukemogenesis was the "two-hit hypothesis," which suggested that two different types of genetic mutation were required for malignant transformation of a myeloid precursor [8, 14]. Class I mutations were thought to lead to uncontrolled cellular proliferation and evasion of apoptosis and included mutations conferring constitutive activity to tyrosine kinases or dysregulation of downstream signaling molecules (in genes such as BCR-ABL, Flt-3, c-KIT, and RAS) [8, 14]. Class II mutations, such as the translocations associated with the core-binding factor (CBF) leukemias, were associated with inhibition of differentiation including key transcription factors, such as CBF and retinoic acid receptor alpha (RARα) [8, 14], and proteins that are involved in transcriptional regulation, such as p300, CBP, MOX, TIF2, and MLL [8, 14].

This hypothesis is supported by the observation that a single mutation alone does not appear to be adequate to engender acute leukemic transformation. Leukemia-associated genetic aberrations (such as CBF translocations) can be found in peripheral and cord blood in a proportion of healthy individuals [15, 16]. Similarly, induced CBF mutations in murine models are not sufficient to induce malignant transformation, despite resulting in increased self-renewal capacity and reduced differentiation [17]. Mice with CBF mutations have been found to only develop a leukemic syndrome when exposed to a further mutagen [18]. Additionally, rare familial leukemia syndromes, involving CEBPα and RUNX1 mutations, increase the risk of developing AML but do not guarantee it [1, 19]. The fact that many AML patients have more than one mutation in their leukemic cells also indicates that in many cases there must be more than one genetic "hit" required for leukemia to develop [20]. Kelly and Gilliland, in 2002, proposed that Class I mutations, occurring alone, would result in myeloproliferative diseases, such as chronic myeloid leukemia, while isolated Class II mutations may lead to the development of myelodysplastic syndromes [14]. It is likely, therefore, that the increased risk of development of AML in patients with either MPN or MDS is

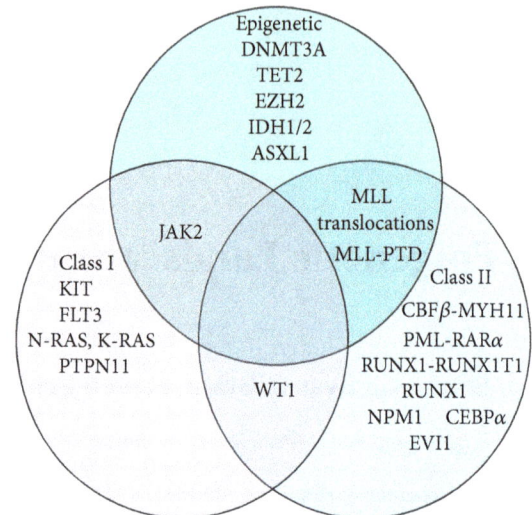

FIGURE 1: This Venn diagram highlights some of the key mutations found in AML and suggests classes to which these mutations could be ascribed.

related to the accrual of further mutations of a different class to those already present (see Figure 1).

Recent research highlighting the presence of epigenetic modifications to the AML genome suggests that Class I and II mutations are only one part of a more complex picture [8, 21]. Increasingly sophisticated methods of examining the human genome are highlighting mutations which previously remained undetected [8]. Novel mutations in genes that are related to epigenetic control of the genome, which encompasses DNA methylation (see Figures 2 and 3) and histone modification (see Figures 4 and 5), have been found in a significant proportion of AML patients [8]. Furthermore, modifications to the epigenome itself, such as localized CpG hypermethylation (see Figure 3) and global hypomethylation, are being examined in greater depth [1, 22–24]. Many of these mutations affecting epigenetic regulators are not regarded as belonging to Class I or Class II, suggesting that the "two-hit model" is no longer adequate [8]. The fact that some other mutations occurring in AML do not have a clear class (such as trisomy 22, which is well recognized in inv(16) leukemia yet has an uncertain role in leukemogenesis) further indicates that the "two-hit" theory is an oversimplification [8, 21]. Moreover, there is evidence that there is also a temporal component to leukemogenesis; mutations have to occur at a particular point in cell development, and in a particular order, to allow for leukemic transformation [16, 21, 25]. This has been reported, for example, in acute promyelocytic leukemia (APL). The PML-RARα fusion protein may occur at any point in the development of the myeloid cell but is only associated with leukemia if the translocation occurs at an early stage when there is sufficient neutrophil elastase levels (which reach a maximal point in promyelocytes) [25]. It is likely, therefore, that new models for the development of acute myeloid leukemia will become increasingly complex as novel mutations are detected and their role in leukemogenesis is evaluated.

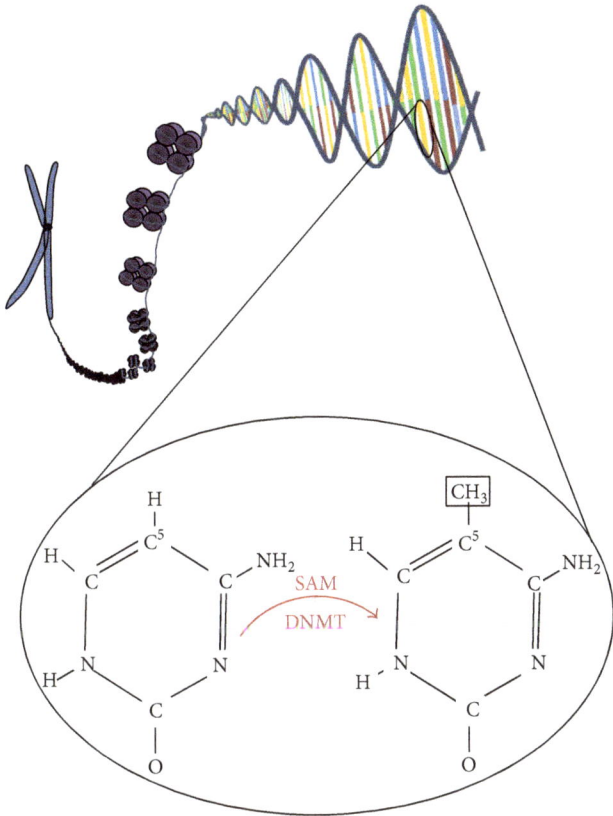

FIGURE 2: Figure showing methylation of cytosine residues at CpG sites. The addition of a methyl group to convert the DNA base cytosine to 5-methylcytosine is catalyzed by DNA methyltransferase (DNMT). The methyl group is transferred from S-adenosylmethionine (SAM) to the 5-carbon position of cytosine.

4. Epigenetic Regulation of the Genome

Epigenetic regulation refers to modulation of genetic transcription and expression which does not alter the genetic code [7]. Epigenetic modifications can be transient or physiologically irreversible and play key roles in developmental patterning in the embryo [7, 26]. Following embryogenesis, epigenetic changes continue throughout an organism's life [7]. The two main mechanisms of epigenetic regulation in the cell are posttranslational histone modifications (see Figure 4), discussed later, and DNA methylation and hydroxymethylation, discussed below [6, 7, 24, 27].

DNA methylation is one of the key epigenetic signaling methods that facilitate control of gene expression in eukaryotic cells. Methylation patterns are known to have crucial roles in embryonic patterning, X-inactivation, and genomic imprinting, as demonstrated by an early lethal effect in DNA methyltransferase- (DNMT-) null mice [22]. Control of gene expression is derived through methylation of cytosine residues in CpG sites—regions where a cytosine residue is adjacent to a guanine residue [8, 22]. Mammals, including humans, show global methylation patterns, that is, methylation of genomic, transposon, and intergenic sequences [23]. Regions with a high density of CpG sites are known as CpG

islands, and these are associated with the promoter regions of 50% of genes in humans [7, 22]. Cytosine methylation of promoter sites is associated with recruitment of corepressor complexes and reduced gene expression [28]. Methylation of genes associated with maintenance of stem cell status in hematopoietic cells, such as homeobox A9 (HOXA9) and meis homeobox 1 (MEIS1), increases as these cells differentiate, and demethylation occurs in genes concerned with differentiation of specific cell lines [26]. While non-CpG island methylation is reversible, methylation of CpG islands persists through mitosis and is only physiologically reversible in the embryo [7].

Hydroxylation of methylated cytosine residues is a mechanism by which non-CpG island methylation can be reversed and is catalyzed by the enzymes encoded by the genes TET1-3. Hydroxymethylated DNA is unable to bind to proteins that repress transcription, thus releasing the inhibitory effect of DNA methylation on the genome [29]. Leukemogenesis has been associated with both hypo- and hypermethylation of CpG islands at different loci and also with global methylation changes, although the pathological implications remain unclear.

5. DNA Methylation and AML

It is evident that methylation patterns play a role in altering expression of genes crucial to leukemogenesis (see Figures 2 and 3). Figueroa et al. carried out DNA methylation profiling of 344 AML samples and found that subjects could be separated into 16 subclasses according to methylation signatures [24]. These subclasses often reflected cytogenetic or molecular subgroups: PML-RARα, CBFβ-MYH11, and RUNX1-RUNX1T1 (AML1-ETO) were each associated with specific methylation signatures. Specific genetic lesions were enriched in further eight groups, while the remaining five groups did not appear to be associated with particular mutations. The finding that AML cases could be separated according to methylation signature, with some clusters highly enriched in specific mutations (t(8;21), inv(16), t(15;17), and 11q23), has been observed in a number of studies [24, 30, 31]. Figueroa et al. found that clinical outcomes could be predicted according to DNA methylation cluster, including the groups without specific mutations [24]. Moreover, cases in clusters enriched for a particular mutation, but not bearing it themselves, shared the prognostic implications of the group as a whole. This was seen in 9 patients classified into one of the CBF leukemia clusters [24]. The groups that were not associated with particular mutations may be reflecting a shared but as yet unknown genetic lesion, or there may be a number of mutations which result in the same epigenetic profile. It is apparent, therefore, that epigenetic changes in leukemic cells occur in a specific and distinct manner—methylation patterns may vary more between subclasses of AML than between AML and controls—and appear to be responsive to overlying genetic mutations [30].

The group also identified a group of 45 genes which were aberrantly methylated in the majority of AML cases compared to normal bone marrow cells. This may reflect

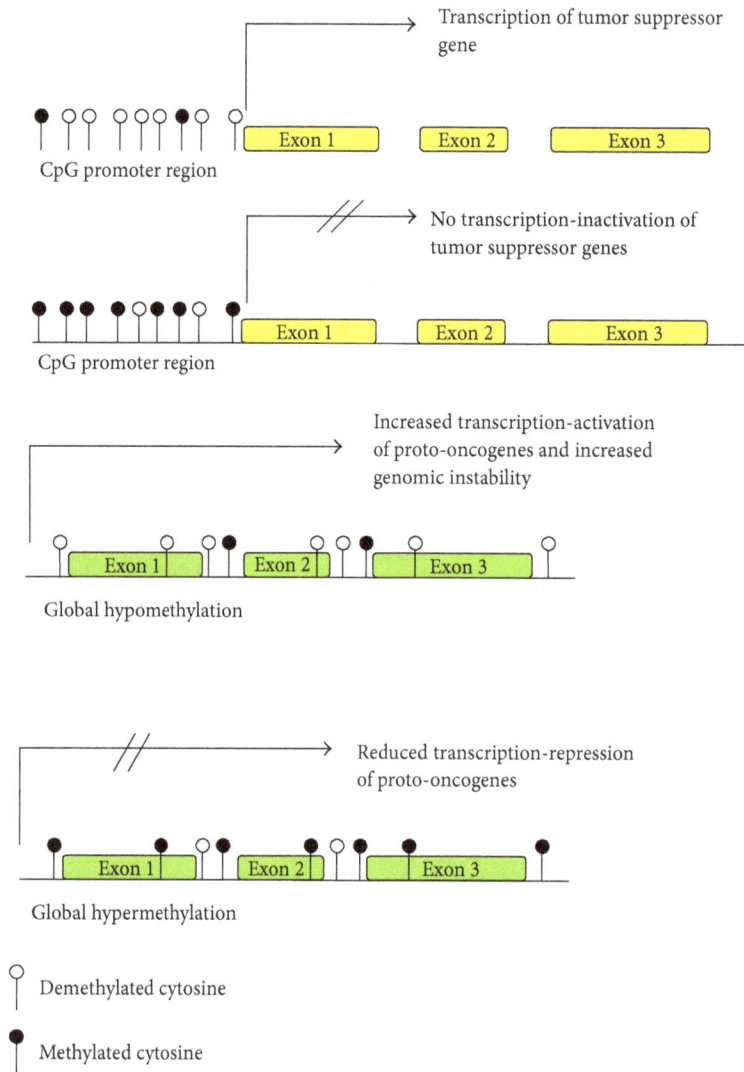

FIGURE 3: Methylation of CpG islands reduces gene transcription and is purported to play a role in malignancy through reduced expression of tumor suppressors and genes concerned with differentiation. Global hypomethylation is also frequently observed in malignant cells, and while it is likely that there is genetic instability and promotion of protooncogene expression, the exact role of global methylation patterns in the development of cancer is uncertain.

a shared epigenetic patterning process in leukemogenesis or the methylation profile of leukemia-permissive cells [24]. Genes coding for tumor suppressors, nuclear import proteins, transcription factors, factors associated with apoptosis, and a regulator of myeloid cytokines were included in the 45 genes aberrantly methylated in the AML cells [24]. This finding has been supported by evidence from other research groups who identified a core of hypermethylated genes which were present in all subclasses of AML analysed [24, 30, 31]. Downregulation of gene expression was associated with the hypermethylated genes identified in the majority of the AML cohort. These findings indicate that perturbation of these genes through DNA methylation is likely to be necessary, though probably not sufficient for leukemogenic transformation [24]. In addition to methylation of promoter CpG islands, Akalin et al. found evidence of specific and distinct DNA methylation patterns in coding and noncoding

CpG residues [30], while Saied et al. found the AML cells to be only 2.7% less globally methylated than controls [23]. Consequently, further research into DNA methylation, both global and localized, may highlight key leukemogenic pathways that have been overlooked by cytogenetic and molecular analysis.

5.1. DNMT3A. The finding of recurrent mutations in enzymes associated with DNA methylation in AML cells further indicates that aberrant epigenetic modulation of the genome has a pathological role in leukemogenesis. Mutations in DNMT3A (DNA methyltransferase 3A), an enzyme concerned with de novo methylation of CpG dinucleotides, are among the commonest somatic mutations, occurring in 15–25% of AML [8, 32, 33]. DNMT3A mutations have also been found in MDS and MPN and remain detectable after leukemic transformation suggesting that these mutations

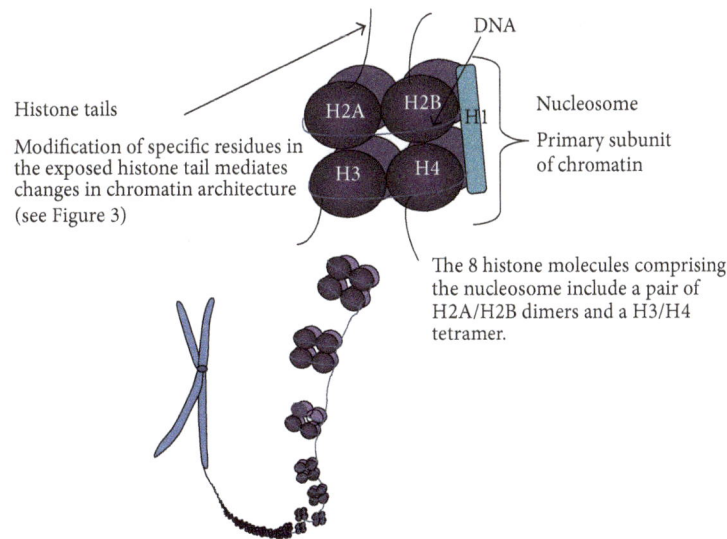

FIGURE 4: Histone tail modifications include methylation, acetylation, phosphorylation, ADP-ribosylation, and ubiquitination. Of these modifications, methylation and acetylation have the most influence on chromatin structure. Histone acetylases (HATs) catalyze acetylation of the histone tails, and histone deacetylases (HDACs) reverse acetylation. Histone methylation can involve mono-, di-, or trimethylation of arginine and lysine residues of one of the highly conserved histone units.

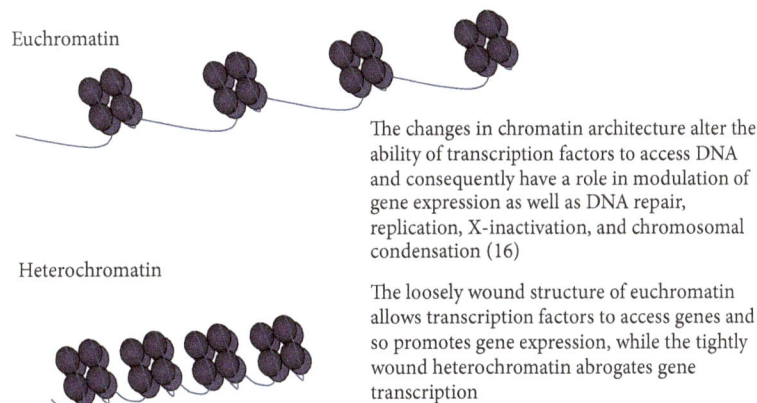

FIGURE 5: Transcriptionally active euchromatin has high levels of histone acetylation and enriched trimethylation of H3K4, H3K36, or H3K79 residues. Conversely, transcriptionally repressed heterochromatin is enriched in trimethylated H3K9, K3K27, and H4K20 and has reduced histone acetylation, mediated by HDAC activity. Heterochromatinization of euchromatin loci is induced by the binding of heterochromatin protein 1 (HP1) to methylated H3K9 and mediated by corepressor proteins such as retinoblastoma protein (pRb) and KAP1. Demethylation of specific histone residues is mediated by a number of histone demethylase enzymes, including LSD1 and Jumonji C-domain proteins (the latter mentioned above in relation to IDH mutations).

occur early in clonal evolution [34]. These mutations have also been found to be associated with M4/M5 FAB subtype, greater age, lower overall survival, and concurrent mutations including FLT3, NPM1, and IDH-1/IDH-2 [8, 32, 35, 36].

It is currently uncertain as to whether methylation or gene expression patterns are altered in DNMT3A^mutated AML. *In vitro*, missense mutations at R882 result in increased proliferation, and mutated DNMT3A has been found to have reduced methylation activity [37]. Murine models demonstrate both hyper- and hypomethylation of different loci, in addition to increased expression of genes involved in hematopoietic stem cell self-renewal [38]. Nonmalignant expansion of the stem cell compartment has been found in DNMT3A knockout mice [38]. However, the role of

DNMT3A mutations in human leukemogenesis is unclear. Ley et al. found that although DNMT3A expression, global methylation patterns, and overall levels of methylated cytosine were normal, hypomethylation at 182 loci indicated that there may be disruption of the expression of unknown genes in DNMT3A^mutated AML [32]. Yan et al. found that both gene expression and methylation patterns were altered, proposing that DNMT3A mutations gave rise to hypomethylation of HOX genes [39]. Conversely, Ribeiro et al. did not find a strong methylation signature, although they did identify one methylation cluster that was enriched for DNMT3A, FLT3-ITD, and NPM1 mutations and showed increased expression of various HOX genes [35]. This HOX overexpression may play a role in leukemic transformation [39]. HOX genes are known to be involved in normal hematopoiesis and also in leukemogenesis, with aberrant HOX expression being a well-recognized finding in leukemic cells [40]. It is apparent, therefore, that the role of DNMT3A mutations in the overexpression of certain genes, such as the HOX genes, is uncertain, and interactions with other somatic mutations such as NPM1 need further investigation.

While the evidence for a direct modulation of gene expression by mutated DNMT3A is currently lacking, there may be an indirect effect through aberrant methylation of nonpromoter sites. DNMT3A-mediated methylation of nonpromoter and nonproximal promoter regions was found, unexpectedly, to increase expression of genes associated with postnatal neurogenesis in mice, perhaps through opposition of polycomb repression [41]. It is evident, therefore, that the impact of DNMT3A mutations on methylation patterns and proximal and distant control of gene expression is complex and poorly understood.

While the exact mechanism remains obscure, it is likely that DNMT3A mutations play a significant role in the development of leukemogenesis. Krönke et al. analyzed 53 NPM-1^{mutated} AML cases at diagnosis and again at relapse. Of the 5 cases of NPM-1^{mutated} DNMT3A^{mutated} AML where the NPM-1 mutation was lost, the DNMT3A mutation remained detectable [42]. Sequencing demonstrated the same DNMT3A mutations at relapse as at first diagnosis, suggesting that the DNMT3A dominant clone gave rise to NPM-1^{mutated} and wildtype subclones (and that the latter was perhaps selected out by chemotherapy treatment) [42]. This finding called into question the proposed role of NPM-1 as a founder mutation, suggesting that DNMT3A mutations may precede NPM-1 mutations. Animal experiments have shown that DNMT3A knockout mice do not develop AML, however, demonstrating the necessity of subsequent mutations in the leukemogenic process [42]. Despite these findings, one case in the cohort lost a DNMT3A mutation but retained the NPM-1 mutation, indicating that the mutational sequence is probably not particularly strict [42]. The presence of these "founder mutations" and the requirement for secondary genetic hits are an intriguing insight into leukemogenesis and also suggest that total eradication of AML may be achieved through elimination of the preleukemic clones.

In addition to a putative role in the initiation of leukemogenesis, there is also evidence to suggest that mutations in genes concerned with DNA methylation and hydroxylation (DNMT3A, TET2, and IDH1/2) may play a role in promoting therapy resistance and relapse. Wakita et al. found that, unlike mutations considered to be "first hit" mutations, such as NPM1 and CEBPA, DNMT3A mutations were always still detectable at relapse [43]. Moreover, the early presence of DNMT3A mutations was associated with a higher incidence of FLT3-ITD positive clones at relapse [43]. It is possible that mutations in epigenetic modifiers result in genetic instability and promote both acquisition of novel FLT3-ITD mutations and the expansion of existing FLT3-ITD positive clones [43]. However, the role of DNMT3A mutations in genetic instability is also uncertain, as a number of studies have reported no increase in somatic mutations in DNMT3A^{mutated} disease

compared with DNMT3A$^{wild-type}$ disease [32]. This would challenge the theory that these mutations lead to significant genetic instability. It is nonetheless likely that DNMT3A mutations affect response to therapy, suggested by poorer outcomes in patients treated with conventional chemotherapy [43] and improved responses when treated with high-dose anthracycline induction [33].

The exact association between prognosis and DNMT3A mutations is a subject of some debate: Marcucci et al. found that non-R882 mutations were associated with an almost threefold increased risk of relapse or death ($P = 0.002$) once adjusted for mutations in NPM1, CEBPA, WT1, and FLT3-ITD in a multivariable analysis. However, R882 mutations had no prognostic impact on patients >60 years, with the inverse observed in younger patients [44]. This variation in prognostic significance according to age may reflect differences in concurrent mutations, such as changes in incidence of ameliorating mutations such as NPM1 [44]. Although variation in prognostic impact of mutation type in different age groups was not reported in other studies, perhaps due to noninclusion of older patient groups, Ley et al. and Thol et al. found that DNMT3A mutations heralded a poorer prognosis in NPM1^{wildtype}/FLT3-ITD^{mutated} CN-AML [32, 36]. Conversely, Ribeiro et al. found that DNMT3A mutations were a particularly poor prognostic indicator in NPM1^{wildtype}/FLT3^{wildtype} AML, and overall there was still an association with a worse outcome [35]. Gaidzik's large study of 1770 AML patients aged 18–60 and treated with regimens of a similar intensity found that DNMT3A mutations were associated with a poorer prognosis in the subgroup of patients with ELN unfavourable CN-AML [45]. An association with higher CCR rates across all classes of AML was likely to be related to the relative rarity of DNMT3A mutations in AML with unfavorable cytogenetics rather than a genuine association with DNMT3A mutations [45]. Thus, this study found that although DNMT3A had discernible prognostic significance in a subgroup of patients when the whole group was analyzed, the prognostic implications were masked, perhaps by cytogenetic status [45]. The evidence from this, the largest study to date, suggests that in young patients receiving intensive treatment there may be little role for DNMT3A as a prognostic marker, although other studies indicate that DNMT3A mutations could have prognostic relevance in specific patient groups [32, 35, 36]. It is likely that there is also a distinction between R882 and non-R882 mutations, both in terms of biological function and prognosis, which requires further investigation.

Interestingly, the recurrent favorable risk genetic translocations, t(8;21), inv(16), and t(15;17), are rarely, if ever, seen in conjunction with DNMT3A mutations [32]. The fact that these genetic lesions appear to be mutually exclusive with DNMT3A may suggest that they have similar roles in leukemogenesis, and so the occurrence of one is unnecessary if the other is already present. However, if this is the case, then it is unclear why the prognostic significance of the DNMT3A mutation is so much more adverse than the favorable risk translocations.

6. DNA Hydroxymethylation and AML

6.1. TET2. Other epigenetic modifiers that can be mutated in AML include TET2, IDH1, and IDH2. These mutations alter the epigenome through modulation of hydroxymethylation, and like DNMT3A, have been found to persist in AML from diagnosis to relapse [43]. TET 1-3 gene products are known to modulate hydroxymethylation by catalyzing the conversion of 5-methylcytosine to 5-hydroxymethylcytosine [29]. Mutations in TET2 have been detected in 7–23% of AML and in 10–20% of MPN/MDS [8, 33, 46–48]. TET2 and IDH mutations appear to be mutually exclusive. TET2 mutations have been found to occur in conjunction with other significant mutations such as NPM1, RARα, KIT, FLT3, RAS, MLL, and CEBPα, although there is no significant incidence-association [47–49]. Recent evidence also suggests that TET2 mutations occur more frequently in cytogenetically normal (CN) AML and are associated with older age, higher white blood cell counts, and lower platelet counts [48]. TET2 is found on chromosome 4q24, a breakpoint that has been associated with several leukemia-related translocations such as t(3;4), t(4;5), and t(4;7) [50]. TET2 mutations appear to convey loss of function, and the majority of cases are heterozygous for TET2 mutations [8]. This is supported by the finding that TET mutant proteins in myeloid malignancies are devoid of enzymatic function [51]. Furthermore, the mutual exclusivity of TET2 and IDH mutations supports the role of aberrant hydroxymethylation in leukemogenesis, as IDH gain-of-function mutations produce 2-hydroxyglutarate which inhibits TET2 catalytic activity [52].

It is thought that TET2 mutations are an early event in leukemogenesis and perhaps may even initiate the malignant process [29, 46, 53]. TET2 mutations may arise before or after JAK2 mutations are acquired in MPN and have also been found to occur for the first time in MPN undergoing leukemic transformation [47, 54]. Although the exact role of epigenetic changes resulting from TET2 mutations in leukemogenesis is uncertain, it is likely that TET2-mediated hydroxymethylation plays a pleiotropic role in modulation of self-renewal and differentiation [51, 52]. It has been observed that TET2 loss of function leads to increased replating activity *in vitro* and stem cell renewal in mice [55]. Murine models have also demonstrated that TET2 deletion results in progressive myeloproliferation, extramedullary hematopoiesis, and expansion of undifferentiated myeloid precursors occurring in a pattern highly reminiscent of human CMML [55]. Moreover, competitive reconstitution assays in lethally irradiated mice showed that the cells with induced deletion of TET2 had a proliferative advantage over wildtype cells [55]. *In vitro* and animal models, therefore, suggest that TET2 mutations result in a loss of control of cell renewal at many different points in hematopoietic differentiation [55]. This, along with the fact that TET2 mutations are seen in a wide spectrum of myeloid disorders in humans, suggests that loss of TET2 catalytic function may induce leukemogenesis by increasing the self-renewal capacity of cells and potentiating acquisition of further mutations [51, 52, 54, 55]. Cases of AML with TET2 mutations also appear to have their own gene expression signature, featuring deregulation of genes associated with stem cell self-renewal, cell cycle control, and cytokine and growth factor cell signaling [47]. Gaidzik et al. found that the gene expression signature identified in TET2^{mutated} AML was shared by a TET2^{wildtype} group, a large proportion of which was comprised of IDH^{mutated} AML [49]. This finding supports the theory that the two gene mutations share common pathological mechanism [49]. Interestingly, Metzeler et al. found altered gene expression signatures in TET2 mutated AML in the favorable risk group, but not in TET2 mutated AML in the intermediate risk group [47]. Both groups were also found to have differentially altered micro-RNA expression signatures which involved various micro-RNAs implicated in hematological malignancies and were nonoverlapping [47]. This finding indicates that TET2 has different implications for gene and micro-RNA expression according to AML subset.

The relationship between TET2 mutations and prognosis is unclear and different studies have shown conflicting results. It is likely that TET2 mutations do not affect MPN prognosis but may be a marker of better prognosis in MDS patients [53, 56]. Prognostic implications in AML are uncertain. Some studies, such as the relatively small study by Nibourel et al., have found no association between prognosis and TET2 mutation status [57]. Gaidzik et al. also detected no prognostic implications of TET2 in a large cohort of 783 subjects [49]. Conversely, other studies, for example, those by Abdel-Wahab et al. and Metzeler et al. both, concluded that TET2 was linked with poorer prognosis in AML [29, 46, 47, 57, 58]. Metzeler et al. found that as well as lower response rates and higher rates of relapse, TET2^{mutated} subjects had a median OS of 1.5 years, while TET2^{wildtype} subjects had a median OS of 3.8 years ($P = 0.001$). However, this observation was limited to ELN favorable risk category CN-AML and was not seen in ELN intermediate risk CN-AML [47]. These findings were echoed by Weissmann et al., who found that although OS was unchanged, EFS was reduced in TET2 mutated ELN favourable risk CN-AML alone [48]. The disparity between these findings may be related to differences in the cohorts studied; Metzeler et al., for example, enrolled older subjects (age range 18–83) and only included de novo AML [47]. By contrast, Gaidzik et al. analyzed data from younger patients (age range 18–60) with de novo and secondary AML [49]. The younger patient cohort is likely to include more patients receiving intensive chemotherapy, which may contribute to the disparate outcome data. However, this does not fully account for the disparity in results as Nibourel et al. studied an older cohort of AML patients yet identified no prognostic implications of TET2 mutations [57]. It is possible that age itself plays some role in the effect of TET2 mutations on survival, a suggestion perhaps supported by the findings of Weissman et al., who observed shorter EFS in TET2^{mutated} patients below 65 years but no effect on older individuals with a TET2 mutation [48]. The fact that many different mutations are observed in the TET2 gene may also contribute to the clinical variability seen in these studies—mutations in different regions of the gene may have varying effects on survival outcomes [48]. Thus, it is apparent that TET2 mutations interrupt normal DNA hydroxymethylation and have an as yet uncertain role in the development of leukemia. Although there is some debate concerning the prognostic implications of TET2 mutations in AML, there is reasonable evidence to suggest that TET2 mutations do have an adverse effect on prognosis in some AML subgroups. In the future, TET2 mutational status may have a role in contributing to prognostication, particularly in favorable risk CN-AML.

6.2. IDH1 and 2. The wildtype isocitrate dehydrogenases are a group of NADP$^+$ dependent enzymes which catalyze the conversion of isocitrate to α-ketoglutarate in the Krebs cycle and are thought to be involved in the prevention of oxidative damage within the cell [52, 59, 60]. IDH mutations, first identified in colorectal carcinoma and frequently found in brain tumors, arise in approximately 15–30% of de novo and secondary AML and around 5% MPN/MDS [52, 59, 60]. IDH mutations often occur in conjunction with NPM1 and are most common in patients with intermediate risk cytogenetics including CN-AML [61]. IDH1 and 2 mutations only occur together in around 0.3% of patients [52, 60, 62]. These mutations are typically heterozygous and occur at three particular arginine residues—R132 in IDH1 and R172 and R140 in IDH2. As yet, amino acid substitutions are the only type of mutation that has been detected in the IDH genes [59]. These mutations confer a neomorphic gain-of-function effect, catalyzing the conversion of α-ketoglutarate to 2-hydroxyglutarate (2-HG) [52, 63]. AML patients with IDH mutations frequently have markedly elevated 2-HG levels [59].

There are a number of mechanisms by which IDH mutations may contribute to leukemic transformation. TET2 catalytic activity is dependent on α-ketoglutarate, iron, and oxygen, meaning that IDH mutations result in loss of TET2 function [52]. IDH1 and 2 mutations are, as mentioned above, mutually exclusive with TET2 mutations [33, 52]. Figueroa et al. found that there was also significant overlap between the methylation signatures of IDH^{mutated} and TET2^{mutated} AML [52]. The methylation signature of IDH^{mutated} AML, featuring a globally hypermethylated pattern, is also distinct from other AML subtypes [52]. Many of the gene promoters aberrantly hypermethylated in IDH^{mutated} AML are thought to relate to transcription factors involved in myeloid differentiation and leukemogenesis, such as GATA 1/2 and EVI1 [52]. IDH mutations are likely to also affect a number of TET2-independent leukemogenic pathways, with histone demethylases numbering among other α-ketoglutarate-dependent enzymes [59]. Histone demethylase inhibition is thought to promote DNA methylation and so may contribute to the epigenetic derangement seen in leukemia [59]. Moreover, it is thought that high levels of the putative oncometabolite, α-ketoglutarate, may increase the production of reactive oxygen species and lead to increased DNA damage [59]. It is probable that any variance between the molecular and clinical characteristics of TET2^{mutated} AML and IDH^{mutated} AML is related to aberrancies in these additional pathways which are unaffected in TET2 mutation [8, 59].

The impact of IDH mutations on prognosis is uncertain, with some recent studies reporting an improved outcome [33, 64, 65], and others reporting an inferior outcome to IDH wildtype AML [65–67]. Other studies suggest that there is no impact on response to therapy or survival [64, 68]. A meta-analysis conducted by Feng et al., including 15 studies and data from a total of 8121 AML patients, concluded that IDH mutations are likely to have an adverse prognostic impact overall [69]. When the disease is stratified according to genotype, cytogenetics, and type of mutation, however, the implications of IDH mutations are unclear. Paschka et al. found in their study of 805 AML patients that IDH mutations predicted reduced relapse-free and overall survival in favorable risk NPM1^{mutated}/FLT3-ITD^{wildtype} AML (5-year OS was 41% compared with 65% in IDH^{wildtype} patients ($P = 0.03$)) [60], a finding replicated by Marcucci et al. [66]. Conversely, Patel et al. found that a favorable outcome associated with NPM1 mutations was only present when there were concurrent IDH mutations [33]. Furthermore, there may be differing prognostic implications according to the particular IDH mutation that is present—IDH2 R140 is thought to be associated with a good prognosis, while R172 is associated with a poor outcome [33, 70]. Differences between studies may reflect size of population studied, variation in therapeutic regimen, inclusion criteria (such as inclusion of de novo or secondary AML), and sensitivity of mutation detection techniques. There may also be difficulties analyzing data if there are variations in the prevalence of different mutational subtypes; for example, Thol et al. combined data for R140 and R172 mutations as only 3 subjects were found to bear the R172 mutation [68].

Finally, the fact that virtually all IDH mutations are detected at diagnosis, rather than arising later in the disease process, suggests that these mutations occur very early in leukemogenesis and are candidates as disease initiators [54, 71]. Increased acquisition of IDH mutations in advanced MPN and MDS and in secondary AML indicates that they may be involved in leukemic transformation [46, 54, 71]. Thus, IDH mutations appear to play a role in triggering leukemogenesis and may offer a useful biomarker of disease in the form of 2-hydroxyglutarate. Further research is required to reliably ascertain the impact of IDH mutations on prognosis.

7. Histone Modifications in AML

Histone tail modifications play a key role in epigenetic modulation of gene expression and may include methylation, acetylation, phosphorylation, ADP-ribosylation, and ubiquitination (see Figure 4) [27, 72]. Mechanisms of aberrant histone modification in AML include mutations in genes concerned with polycomb group complexes (PcG), widely considered to be the "bridge" between histone modification and DNA methylation [72, 73]. PcGs maintain stable and heritable transcriptional repression in specific target genes [72]. PcGs are related to body patterning, stem cell renewal, and they also may have pathogenic roles to play in oncogenesis [72, 73]. Genes coding for components of the PcG may be amplified or overexpressed, or the PcG may be "ectopically recruited" to nontarget genes in cancer development [72]. Mutations have been detected in a number of PcG components in myeloid disorders, with some, unexpectedly, conferring a loss of function [27, 73–76].

7.1. EZH2.

Enhancer of zeste homologue 2 (EZH2) mutations has been detected in approximately 7% of MDS, 3–13% MPN, and occasionally in AML [8, 75–77]. EZH2 is the catalytic component of PcG Repressor Complex 2 (PRC2), a highly conserved H3K27 methyltransferase [6, 8, 76]. Two further subunits, EED and SUZ12, comprise the PRC2 unit [6, 8]. Methylation of H3K27 leads to the recruitment of PRC1, followed by DNMT binding via EZH2 and consequent DNA methylation [75]. EZH2 can also interact with HDACs through EED and in this manner influences histone deacetylation and may exert further influence over the genome through interaction with noncoding RNA [75]. This results in promotion of chromatin condensation and suppression of genes concerned with cell fate decisions, thereby influencing stem cell renewal capacity [6].

Overexpression of EZH2 has been detected in various epithelial malignancies, and, more recently, activating mutations of EZH2 have been found in diffuse large B cell lymphoma [77]. It is likely that gain-of-function EZH2 mutations result in reduced expression of regulatory genes, such as BRCA-1 and p16, and increased activity of cellular pathways concerned with proliferation and invasion [75]. Overexpression of EZH2 bestows unlimited replicative potential on hematopoietic stem cells *in vitro* and prevents stem cell exhaustion following repeated serial transplants in irradiated mice [74]. Unexpectedly, missense, nonsense, and frameshift mutations have been found in MDS, MPN, and AML [6, 76, 77]. These mutations frequently result in a truncated SET domain, thought to be crucial to the catalytic activity of the protein [76]. These findings suggest that the loss-of-function mutations in EZH2 may contribute to myeloid neoplasm [6, 76, 77]. The oncogenic implications of both loss and gain of function of EZH2 implies dual, tissue-specific roles as both oncogene and tumor suppressor [6, 8, 77]. Mutations in EED and SUZ12 rarely occur in patients with MDS/MPN overlap disorders or PMF but may occur in conjunction with EZH2 [76].

EZH2 mutations have been detected in patients with refractory anemia, a relatively early stage of MDS, and have been found to remain constant as the disease progresses towards secondary AML [76]. It is likely, therefore, that this is an early event in myeloid disease and not an initiator of leukemic transformation. EZH2 is located on chromosome 7q, and loss of this chromosome in MDS has long been recognized as a poor prognostic indicator [76, 77]. Further research has found that it is likely that this poor prognosis in these patients is associated with loss of EZH2 [75, 78, 79]. The prognostic implications of EZH2 mutations in AML have been more elusive, largely due to the low incidence of these mutations in de novo disease. Wang et al. identified EZH2 mutations in 1.7% of 714 subjects with de novo AML, amounting to 13 patients, and were unable to identify any association with OS, EFS, or chance of CR [79]. The relevance of this observation to AML in general, however, is limited considering the small number of subjects bearing EZH2 mutations. The apparent role of the various EZH2 mutations in oncogenesis is an insight into the complex function of PRC2 as an epigenetic regulator.

7.2. ASXL-1.

Somatic nonsense, missense, frameshift, and point mutations of the additional sex combs-like gene (ASXL-1) are found in 10–25% MDS, 10–15% MPN, and 5–30% AML [6, 71, 80, 81]. These mutations are more frequently found in secondary than de novo AML and occur in about 45% of CMML [82]. The majority of mutations cause frameshift and mostly occur in the PHD domain, which is thought to be responsible for methylated lysine binding [73, 83]. It is unclear whether ASXL-1 mutations confer a loss or gain of function—however, evidence from Abdel-Wahab et al. suggests that a large proportion of these mutations results in reduced ASXL-1 expression [73]. It is thought that ASXL-1 exerts a modulatory effect on the epigenome through both activating and suppressive interactions with PcGs (particularly PRC2) and trithorax genes [73, 80]. Consequently, loss of ASXL-1 expression in myeloid neoplasm appears to result in reduced H3K27me3 concentrations at specific target loci, perhaps through inhibition of PRC2 recruitment, and consequent overexpression of leukemia-promoting genes [73]. Wildtype ASXL-1 may also interact with BAP-1 to form a deubiquitinase specific to H2AK119 which results in repression of gene transcription [80]. Mutations in ASXL-1 may also, therefore, affect epigenetic regulation through interruption of ubiquitin removal from specific histone lysine residues, although the relationship with leukemogenesis is unclear [84]. Furthermore, alteration of the epigenome through uncontrolled expression of posterior HOX genes is thought to be an additional consequence of ASXL-1 mutations [73, 84]. ASXL-1 appears to have a role in both repressing and promoting HOX gene expression in mice and flies [85]. Findings from murine knockout models have been controversial, with some researchers reporting only mild myeloerythroid lineage defects and others finding an MDS/MPN-like phenotype, particularly if there is concurrent RAS mutation [73, 85].

ASXL-1 mutations are frequently detected at diagnosis of MDS and MPN and remain constant throughout disease progression [46]. Despite one study which found increased mutation incidence in myelofibrosis secondary to other MPNs, evidence suggests that ASXL-1 mutations are early events which may precede JAK2 and TET2 mutations [46, 73]. ASXL-1 mutations—particularly frameshift—are associated with more aggressive disease, faster time to leukemic transformation and shorter overall survival in MPN and MDS [71, 81]. The prognostic implications of ASXL-1 mutations in AML are less clear. Some studies have found that, like TET2, ASXL-1 mutations confer a particularly poor prognosis in ELN favorable AML [97]. However, one large study by Shen et al. reported no association with outcome overall but reduced survival in the intermediate risk group [98]. Similarly, Pratcorona et al. found that there was a significant association with poorer survival and ASXL-1 mutations

TABLE 1: Key genetic mutations thought to have implications for prognosis in AML. The genetic mutations included in the table are reviewed below. Table compiled with information from [29, 32, 35, 39, 50, 52, 58, 61, 66, 67, 73, 76, 80, 86–96].

Gene	Mutation type	Mutation frequency	Consequence of mutation	Prognostic implications	Initiating lesion
DNMT3A	Mainly missense 60% at R882 Often heterozygous	15–25% AML	R882 mutations reduce binding affinity and catalytic activity—LOF	Likely poorer prognosis. Affected by R882/non-R882, CM, patient age Adverse prognosis in intermediate risk AML	Uncertain
TET2	46% frame shift Also missense, nonsense, and splice site variations Majority heterozygous	7–23% AML 10–20% MPN/MDS	Truncated protein and consequent reduction in hydroxymethylation—LOF*	Poorer prognosis in favorable risk CN-AML No effect in MPN, possibly improved prognosis in MDS	Early event, possibly initiating
IDH1 + 2	Amino acid substitutions R132 (IDH1) R172, and R140 (IDH2) Heterozygous	15–30% AML 5% MPN/MDS	Neomorphic gain of function Production of 2-HG, inhibition of TET2 function	Unclear—R140Q may have favorable effect on prognosis R132H/R172K may have no effect However some studies suggest IDH mutations have adverse impact on favorable CN-AML $NPM1^{mut}/IDH^{mut}$ AML has a favorable outcome	Early event, possibly initiating
ASXL1	Nonsense, missense, frame shift, and point mutations	10–15% MPN/AML 10–25% MDS	Uncertain if function lost or gained—research suggests reduced ASXL1 expression	Poor prognostic marker in AML and MPN	Very early, increased leukemic progression in MPN
EZH2	Missense, nonsense, and frame shift	Occasional in AML MDS 7% MPN 3–13%	Truncated SET domain—LOF Gain of function observed in other malignancies	Worse OS in MDS, CMML, and PMF (del)7q poor prognostic indicator in MDS—probably in part due to loss of EZH2	Very early event in MPN, probably not leukemic initiator

*LOF: loss of function.

which was particularly evident in the intermediate risk group but was also found overall [82]. Chou et al. found in a cytogenetically heterogeneous cohort that although ASXL-1 mutations were not significant predictors of prognosis in a multivariate analysis, they were associated with lower CR and OS [99]. Conversely, Schnittger et al. investigated intermediate risk patients and found that although there was a strong correlation between occurrence of ASXL-1^{mutated} and mutations with adverse prognostic implications (such as RUNX-1), ASXL-1 mutations remained an independent adverse risk factor [83]. The cytogenetically homogeneous nature of the study population supports the authors' finding that ASXL-1 is an adverse prognostic indicator in ELN intermediate risk AML. It is likely, therefore, that ASXL-1 mutations represent an independent risk factor for poor survival in particular genetic groups and perhaps in different age groups. The evidence suggests that ASXL-1 mutations have prognostic implications in MDS, MPN, and some categories of AML and perhaps in AML overall [80, 82, 99]. Although not yet fully understood, the apparent role of EZH2 and ASXL-1 mutations in leukemogenesis is indicative of

the significance of PRC2-mediated epigenetic modifications in normal and leukemic hematopoiesis.

8. Conclusion

Recent DNA sequencing studies have facilitated the identification of a hitherto unrecognized class of genetic mutations in AML—mutations in epigenetic modifying genes (see Table 1). The occurrence of mutations in epigenetic modifiers in AML highlights the inadequacy of the "two-hit model" as a mechanistic explanation of leukemogenesis. Mutations in genes concerned with regulation of the epigenome potentially offer a valuable insight into the process of leukemogenesis. These mutations also contribute to the existing body of knowledge that aids risk stratification of AML through molecular and cytogenetic analysis of leukemic cells. Mutations in genes such as TET2, DNMT3A, and ASXL-1 may be associated with a poor prognosis and as such may represent a novel subset of high risk AML which requires more aggressive treatment. The prognostic implications of IDH 1 and 2, and EZH2 mutations are unclear. There is considerable debate about the prognostic implications of various genetic mutations in AML, in part due to the fact that direct comparison between studies is difficult, if not impossible. Patient cohorts frequently vary according to age, type and intensity of therapy, and inclusion of different AML subtypes (e.g., all AML compared with CN-AML). Studies may also vary in their methodology, such as in differences in the subgroup analysis performed or the proportion of patients selected for analysis, which if low (e.g., Marcucci et al. and Ribeiro et al. only analysed 18% and 13% of their cohort resp.) [35, 44] has the potential to introduce an element of selection bias.

Identifying the prognostic implications of a single mutation holds many challenges for researchers. There are many factors which may alter prognosis in AML, and these factors may influence study results to different degrees. Grimwade et al. found that, as well as cytogenetic groups, the response to first course of chemotherapy was a significant prognostic indicator [1, 10]. There are a number of other indicators of prognosis, such as age, race, and performance status. White cell count, platelet count, LDH level, and bilirubin may also predict outcome [1, 4, 10]. It is likely that there is interplay between different prognostic factors; for example, Leith et al. found that elderly AML sufferers had increased expression of a multidrug resistance protein (MDR1) and high functional drug efflux, as well as a higher rate of unfavorable cytogenetics [100]. Thus, there are many variables which may alter outcome in AML other than genetic and cytogenetic mutations.

Nonetheless, clearer definition of unfavorable molecular profiles may help determine treatment; Patel et al. identified a subgroup of AML patients with particular mutations who benefited from an increased dose of daunorubicin [33]. While previously only favorable risk patients have been shown to benefit from intensified dose chemotherapy, individuals with unfavorable DNMT3A and MLL-PTD mutations (as well as the favorable NPM1) had improved responses [33]. These findings from Patel et al. suggest that incorporating data from more extensive mutational analyses can improve prognostic stratification [33]. Improved classification of AML based on molecular genetics as well as cytogenetics may also, therefore, yield improved outcomes.

Despite a rapidly growing base of knowledge concerning genetic mutations in AML, relatively few therapeutic options have arisen. This may change with a greater understanding of mutations in genes concerned with epigenetic modifications. The identification of novel mutations in AML may highlight putative drug targets; the neomorphic gain-of-function effect observed in IDH1 and 2 mutations is a potential target for enzyme inhibition, for example. Equally, the reversible nature of epigenetic modifications has led to hopes that treatments such as DNMT and histone deacetylase inhibitors may represent a valuable addition to the therapeutic arsenal in AML [6, 7]. These drugs have been used with some success in MDS and AML, particularly in elderly populations unable to undergo intensive chemotherapy regimens [101–105]. Further research into the role of epigenetic aberrations in leukemogenesis may inform the development of targeted histone deacetylase inhibitors and personalized treatment regimens. Furthermore, study of mutations occurring in epigenetic

modifying genes has identified potential biomarkers, such as 2-HG in IDH^{mutated} AML, which may reflect response to therapy and act as an early indicator of relapse [106].

Overall, therefore, the recent identification of mutations in genes with epigenetic function has added to the understanding of leukemia pathogenesis and identified potential therapeutic targets. Identification of mutations in other classes of genes, such as those concerned with cell adhesion and the spliceosome, in addition to elucidation of the role of micro-RNAs in AML, is likely to further inform prognostic and therapeutic decision making and understanding of the leukemogenic process. Indeed, it is clear from recent advances that whole genome or targeted exome sequencing has the potential to improve treatment strategies and thereby survival rates in AML, and in the future it may play an important role in the clinical workup of every patient with AML to facilitate more effective personalized therapy.

Conflict of Interests

The authors declare that there is no conflict of interests regarding the publication of this paper.

References

[1] F. Ferrara and C. A. Schiffer, "Acute myeloid Leukemia in adults," *The Lancet*, vol. 381, no. 9865, pp. 484–495, 2013.

[2] M. R. O'Donnell, C. N. Abboud, J. Altman et al., "Acute myeloid Leukemia," *Journal of the National Comprehensive Cancer Network*, vol. 10, no. 8, pp. 984–1021, 2012.

[3] Y. Koh, I. Kim, J.-Y. Bae et al., "Prognosis of secondary acute myeloid Leukemia is affected by the type of the preceding hematologic disorders and the presence of trisomy 8," *Japanese Journal of Clinical Oncology*, vol. 40, no. 11, pp. 1037–1045, 2010.

[4] E. H. Estey, "Acute myeloid Leukemia: 2013 update on risk-stratification and management," *American Journal of Hematology*, vol. 88, no. 4, pp. 318–327, 2013.

[5] T. L. Lin and B. D. Smith, "Prognostically important molecular markers in cytogenetically normal acute myeloid Leukemia," *American Journal of the Medical Sciences*, vol. 341, no. 5, pp. 404–408, 2011.

[6] O. Abdel-Wahab and A. T. Fathi, "Mutations in epigenetic modifiers in myeloid malignancies and the prospect of novel epigenetic-targeted therapy," *Advances in Hematology*, vol. 2012, Article ID 469592, 12 pages, 2012.

[7] Y. Oki and J. P. Issa, "Epigenetic mechanisms in AML—a target for therapy," *Cancer Treatment and Research*, vol. 145, pp. 19–40, 2010.

[8] A. H. Shih, O. Abdel-Wahab, J. P. Patel, and R. L. Levine, "The role of mutations in epigenetic regulators in myeloid malignancies," *Nature Reviews Cancer*, vol. 12, no. 9, pp. 599–612, 2012.

[9] D. Grimwade, H. Walker, G. Harrison et al., "The predictive value of hierarchical cytogenetic classification in older adults with acute myeloid Leukemia (AML): analysis of 1065 patients entered into the United Kingdom Medical Research Council AML11 trial," *Blood*, vol. 98, no. 5, pp. 1312–1320, 2001.

[10] D. Grimwade, H. Walker, F. Oliver et al., "The importance of diagnostic cytogenetics on outcome in AML: analysis of 1,612

patients entered into the MRC AML 10 trial," *Blood*, vol. 92, no. 7, pp. 2322–2333, 1998.

[11] W.-J. Hong and B. C. Medeiros, "Unfavorable-risk cytogenetics in acute myeloid Leukemia," *Expert Review of Hematology*, vol. 4, no. 2, pp. 173–184, 2011.

[12] H. Döhner, E. H. Estey, S. Amadori et al., "Diagnosis and management of acute myeloid Leukemia in adults: recommendations from an international expert panel, on behalf of the European LeukemiaNet," *Blood*, vol. 115, no. 3, pp. 453–474, 2010.

[13] J. W. Vardiman, J. Thiele, D. A. Arber et al., "The 2008 revision of the World Health Organization (WHO) classification of myeloid neoplasms and acute Leukemia: rationale and important changes," *Blood*, vol. 114, no. 5, pp. 937–951, 2009.

[14] L. M. Kelly and D. G. Gilliland, "Genetics of myeloid Leukemias," *Annual Review of Genomics and Human Genetics*, vol. 3, pp. 179–198, 2002.

[15] J. Basecke, L. Cepek, C. Mannhalter et al., "Transcription of AML1/ETO in bone marrow and cord blood of individuals without acute myelogenous Leukemia," *Blood*, vol. 100, no. 6, pp. 2267–2268, 2002.

[16] J. Song, D. Mercer, X. Hu, H. Liu, and M. M. Li, "Common Leukemia- and lymphoma-associated genetic aberrations in healthy individuals," *Journal of Molecular Diagnostics*, vol. 13, no. 2, pp. 213–219, 2011.

[17] J. R. Downing, "The core-binding factor Leukemias: lessons learned from murine models," *Current Opinion in Genetics and Development*, vol. 13, no. 1, pp. 48–54, 2003.

[18] M. Higuchi, D. O'Brien, P. Kumaravelu, N. Lenny, E.-J. Yeoh, and J. R. Downing, "Expression of a conditional AML1-ETO oncogene bypasses embryonic lethality and establishes a murine model of human t(8;21) acute myeloid Leukemia," *Cancer Cell*, vol. 1, no. 1, pp. 63–74, 2002.

[19] T. Pabst, M. Eyholzer, S. Haefliger, J. Schardt, and B. U. Mueller, "Somatic CEBPA mutations are a frequent second event in families with germline CEBPA mutations and familial acute myeloid Leukemia," *Journal of Clinical Oncology*, vol. 26, no. 31, pp. 5088–5093, 2008.

[20] J. S. Welch, T. J. Ley, D. C. Link et al., "The origin and evolution of mutations in acute myeloid Leukemia," *Cell*, vol. 150, no. 2, pp. 264–278, 2012.

[21] A. Murati, M. Brecqueville, R. Devillier, M. J. Mozziconacci, V. Gelsi-Boyer, and D. Birnbaum, "Myeloid malignancies: mutations, models and management," *BMC Cancer*, vol. 12, article 304, 2012.

[22] M. M. Suzuki and A. Bird, "DNA methylation landscapes: provocative insights from epigenomics," *Nature Reviews Genetics*, vol. 9, no. 6, pp. 465–476, 2008.

[23] M. H. Saied, J. Marzec, S. Khalid et al., "Genome wide analysis of acute myeloid Leukemia reveal Leukemia specific methylome and subtype specific hypomethylation of repeats," *PLoS ONE*, vol. 7, no. 3, Article ID e33213, 2012.

[24] M. E. Figueroa, S. Lugthart, Y. Li et al., "DNA methylation signatures identify biologically distinct subtypes in acute myeloid Leukemia," *Cancer Cell*, vol. 17, no. 1, pp. 13–27, 2010.

[25] J. T. Reilly, "Pathogenesis of acute myeloid leukaemia and inv(16)(p13;q22): a paradigm for understanding leukaemogenesis?" *British Journal of Haematology*, vol. 128, no. 1, pp. 18–34, 2005.

[26] J. Borgel, S. Guibert, Y. Li et al., "Targets and dynamics of promoter DNA methylation during early mouse development," *Nature Genetics*, vol. 42, no. 12, pp. 1093–1100, 2010.

[27] E. Bartova, J. Krejci, A. Harnicarova, G. Galiova, and S. Kozubek, "Histone modifications and nuclear architecture: a review," *Journal of Histochemistry & Cytochemistry*, vol. 56, no. 8, pp. 711–721, 2008.

[28] S. Takahashi, "Current findings for recurring mutations in acute myeloid Leukemia," *Journal of Hematology and Oncology*, vol. 4, article 36, 2011.

[29] O. Abdel-Wahab, A. Mullally, C. Hedvat et al., "Genetic characterization of TET1, TET2, and TET3 alterations in myeloid malignancies," *Blood*, vol. 114, no. 1, pp. 144–147, 2009.

[30] A. Akalin, F. E. Garrett-Bakelman, M. Kormaksson et al., "Base-pair resolution DNA methylation sequencing reveals profoundly divergent epigenetic landscapes in acute myeloid Leukemia," *PLOS Genetics*, vol. 8, no. 6, Article ID e1002781, 2012.

[31] L. Bullinger, M. Ehrich, K. Döhner et al., "Quantitative DNA methylation predicts survival in adult acute myeloid Leukemia," *Blood*, vol. 115, no. 3, pp. 636–642, 2010.

[32] T. J. Ley, L. Ding, M. J. Walter et al., "DNMT3A mutations in acute myeloid Leukemia," *The New England Journal of Medicine*, vol. 363, no. 25, pp. 2424–2433, 2010.

[33] J. P. Patel, M. Gonen, M. E. Figueroa et al., "Prognostic relevance of integrated genetic profiling in acute myeloid Leukemia," *The New England Journal of Medicine*, vol. 366, no. 12, pp. 1079–1089, 2012.

[34] I. Fried, C. Bodner, M. M. Pichler et al., "Frequency, onset and clinical impact of somatic DNMT3A mutations in therapy-related and secondary acute myeloid Leukemia," *Haematologica*, vol. 97, no. 2, pp. 246–250, 2012.

[35] A. F. Ribeiro, M. Pratcorona, C. Erpelinck-Verschueren et al., "Mutant DNMT3A: a marker of poor prognosis in acute myeloid Leukemia," *Blood*, vol. 119, no. 24, pp. 5824–5831, 2012.

[36] F. Thol, F. Damm, A. Lüdeking et al., "Incidence and prognostic influence of DNMT3A mutations in acute myeloid Leukemia," *Journal of Clinical Oncology*, vol. 29, no. 21, pp. 2889–2896, 2011.

[37] X.-J. Yan, J. Xu, Z.-H. Gu et al., "Exome sequencing identifies somatic mutations of DNA methyltransferase gene DNMT3A in acute monocytic Leukemia," *Nature Genetics*, vol. 43, no. 4, pp. 309–317, 2011.

[38] G. A. Challen, D. Sun, M. Jeong et al., "Dnmt3a is essential for hematopoietic stem cell differentiation," *Nature Genetics*, vol. 44, no. 1, pp. 23–31, 2012.

[39] X.-J. Yan, J. Xu, Z.-H. Gu et al., "Exome sequencing identifies somatic mutations of DNA methyltransferase gene DNMT3A in acute monocytic Leukemia," *Nature Genetics*, vol. 43, no. 4, pp. 309–315, 2011.

[40] E. A. Eklund, "The role of hox proteins in leukemogenesis: insights into key regulatory events in hematopoiesis," *Critical Reviews in Oncogenesis*, vol. 16, no. 1-2, pp. 65–76, 2011.

[41] H. Wu, V. Coskun, J. Tao et al., "Dnmt3a-dependent nonpromoter DNA methylation facilitates transcription of neurogenic genes," *Science*, vol. 329, no. 5990, pp. 444–447, 2010.

[42] J. Krönke, L. Bullinger, V. Teleanu et al., "Clonal evolution in relapsed NPM1-mutated acute myeloid Leukemia," *Blood*, vol. 122, no. 1, pp. 100–108, 2013.

[43] S. Wakita, H. Yamaguchi, I. Omori et al., "Mutations of the epigenetics-modifying gene (DNMT3a, TET2, IDH1/2) at diagnosis may induce FLT3-ITD at relapse in de novo acute myeloid Leukemia," *Leukemia*, vol. 27, no. 5, pp. 1044–1052, 2012.

[44] G. Marcucci, K. H. Metzeler, S. Schwind et al., "Age-related prognostic impact of different types of DNMT3A mutations in adults with primary cytogenetically normal acute myeloid Leukemia," *Journal of Clinical Oncology*, vol. 30, no. 7, pp. 742–750, 2012.

[45] V. I. Gaidzik, R. F. Schlenk, P. Paschka et al., "Clinical impact of DNMT3A mutations in younger adult patients with acute myeloid Leukemia: results of the AML Study Group (AMLSG)," *Blood*, vol. 121, no. 23, pp. 4769–4777, 2013.

[46] O. Abdel-Wahab, T. Manshouri, J. Patel et al., "Genetic analysis of transforming events that convert chronic myeloproliferative neoplasms to Leukemias," *Cancer Research*, vol. 70, no. 2, pp. 447–452, 2010.

[47] K. H. Metzeler, K. Maharry, M. D. Radmacher et al., "TET2 mutations improve the new European LeukemiaNet risk classification of acute myeloid Leukemia: a cancer and Leukemia group B study," *Journal of Clinical Oncology*, vol. 29, no. 10, pp. 1373–1381, 2011.

[48] S. Weissmann, T. Alpermann, V. Grossmann et al., "Landscape of TET2 mutations in acute myeloid Leukemia," *Leukemia*, vol. 26, pp. 934–942, 2011.

[49] V. I. Gaidzik, P. Paschka, D. Spath et al., "TET2 mutations in acute myeloid leukemia (AML): results from a comprehensive genetic and clinical analysis of the AML study group," *Journal of Clinical Oncology*, vol. 30, no. 12, pp. 1350–1357, 2012.

[50] F. Delhommeau, S. Dupont, V. Della Valle et al., "Mutation in TET2 in myeloid cancers," *The New England Journal of Medicine*, vol. 360, no. 22, pp. 2289–2301, 2009.

[51] M. Ko, Y. Huang, A. M. Jankowska et al., "Impaired hydroxylation of 5-methylcytosine in myeloid cancers with mutant TET2," *Nature*, vol. 468, no. 7325, pp. 839–843, 2010.

[52] M. E. Figueroa, O. Abdel-Wahab, C. Lu et al., "Leukemic IDH1 and IDH2 mutations result in a hypermethylation phenotype, disrupt TET2 function, and impair hematopoietic differentiation," *Cancer Cell*, vol. 18, no. 6, pp. 553–567, 2010.

[53] S. M. C. Langemeijer, R. P. Kuiper, M. Berends et al., "Acquired mutations in TET2 are common in myelodysplastic syndromes," *Nature Genetics*, vol. 41, no. 7, pp. 838–842, 2009.

[54] A. Tefferi, "Novel mutations and their functional and clinical relevance in myeloproliferative neoplasms: JAK2, MPL, TET2, ASXL1, CBL, IDH and IKZF1," *Leukemia*, vol. 24, no. 6, pp. 1128–1138, 2010.

[55] K. Moran-Crusio, L. Reavie, A. Shih et al., "Tet2 loss leads to increased hematopoietic stem cell self-renewal and myeloid transformation," *Cancer Cell*, vol. 20, no. 1, pp. 11–24, 2011.

[56] A. Tefferi, A. Pardanani, K.-H. Lim et al., "TET2 mutations and their clinical correlates in polycythemia vera, essential thrombocythemia and myelofibrosis," *Leukemia*, vol. 23, no. 5, pp. 905–911, 2009.

[57] O. Nibourel, O. Kosmider, M. Cheok et al., "Incidence and prognostic value of TET2 alterations in de novo acute myeloid Leukemia achieving complete remission," *Blood*, vol. 116, no. 7, pp. 1132–1135, 2010.

[58] W.-C. Chou, S.-C. Chou, C.-Y. Liu et al., "TET2 mutation is an unfavorable prognostic factor in acute myeloid Leukemia patients with intermediate-risk cytogenetics," *Blood*, vol. 118, no. 14, pp. 3803–3810, 2011.

[59] D. Rakheja, S. Konoplev, L. J. Medeiros, and W. Chen, "IDH mutations in acute myeloid Leukemia," *Human Pathology*, vol. 43, no. 10, pp. 1541–1551, 2012.

[60] P. Paschka, R. F. Schlenk, V. I. Gaidzik et al., "IDH1 and IDH2 mutations are frequent genetic alterations in acute myeloid Leukemia and confer adverse prognosis in cytogenetically normal acute myeloid Leukemia with NPM1 mutation without FLT3 internal tandem duplication," *Journal of Clinical Oncology*, vol. 28, no. 22, pp. 3636–3643, 2010.

[61] M. E. Figueroa, O. Abdel-Wahab, C. Lu et al., "Leukemic IDH1 and IDH2 mutations result in a hypermethylation phenotype, disrupt TET2 function, and impair hematopoietic differentiation," *Cancer Cell*, vol. 18, no. 6, pp. 553–567, 2010.

[62] S. Schnittger, C. Haferlach, M. Ulke, T. Alpermann, W. Kern, and T. Haferlach, "IDH1 mutations are detected in 6.6% of 1414 AML patients and are associated with intermediate risk karyotype and unfavorable prognosis in adults younger than 60 years and unmutated NPM1 status," *Blood*, vol. 116, no. 25, pp. 5486–5496, 2010.

[63] L. Dang, D. W. White, S. Gross et al., "Cancer-associated IDH1 mutations produce 2-hydroxyglutarate," *Nature*, vol. 462, no. 7274, pp. 739–744, 2009.

[64] K. Wagner, F. Damm, G. Göhring et al., "Impact of IDH1 R132 mutations and an IDH1 single nucleotide polymorphism in cytogenetically normal acute myeloid Leukemia: SNP rs11554137 is an adverse prognostic factor," *Journal of Clinical Oncology*, vol. 28, no. 14, pp. 2356–2364, 2010.

[65] W.-C. Chou, W.-C. Lei, B.-S. Ko et al., "The prognostic impact and stability of Isocitrate dehydrogenase 2 mutation in adult patients with acute myeloid Leukemia," *Leukemia*, vol. 25, no. 2, pp. 246–253, 2011.

[66] G. Marcucci, K. Maharry, Y.-Z. Wu et al., "IDH1 and IDH2 gene mutations identify novel molecular subsets within de novo cytogenetically normal acute myeloid Leukemia: a cancer and Leukemia group B study," *Journal of Clinical Oncology*, vol. 28, no. 14, pp. 2348–2355, 2010.

[67] S. Schnittger, C. Haferlach, M. Ulke, T. Alpermann, W. Kern, and T. Haferlach, "IDH1 mutations are detected in 6.6% of 1414 AML patients and are associated with intermediate risk karyotype and unfavorable prognosis in adults younger than 60 years and unmutated NPM1 status," *Blood*, vol. 116, no. 25, pp. 5486–5496, 2010.

[68] F. Thol, F. Damm, K. Wagner et al., "Prognostic impact of IDH2 mutations in cytogenetically normal acute myeloid Leukemia," *Blood*, vol. 116, no. 4, pp. 614–616, 2010.

[69] J. H. Feng, X. P. Guo, Y. Y. Chen, Z. J. Wang, Y. P. Cheng, and Y. M. Tang, "Prognostic significance of IDH1 mutations in acute myeloid Leukemia: a meta-analysis," *American Journal of Blood Research*, vol. 2, no. 4, pp. 254–264, 2012.

[70] C. L. Green, C. M. Evans, L. Zhao et al., "The prognostic significance of IDH2 mutations in AML depends on the location of the mutation," *Blood*, vol. 118, no. 2, pp. 409–412, 2011.

[71] M. Brecqueville, J. Rey, F. Bertucci et al., "Mutation analysis of ASXL1, CBL, DNMT3A, IDH1, IDH2, JAK2, MPL, NF1, SF3B1, SUZ12, and TET2 in myeloproliferative neoplasms," *Genes Chromosomes and Cancer*, vol. 51, no. 8, pp. 743–755, 2012.

[72] H. Boukarabila, A. J. Saurin, E. Batsché et al., "The PRC1 polycomb group complex interacts with PLZF/RARA to mediate leukemic transformation," *Genes and Development*, vol. 23, no. 10, pp. 1195–1206, 2009.

[73] O. Abdel-Wahab, M. Adli, L. M. LaFave et al., "ASXL1 mutations promote myeloid transformation through loss of PRC2-mediated gene repression," *Cancer Cell*, vol. 22, no. 2, pp. 180–193, 2012.

[74] L. M. Kamminga, L. V. Bystrykh, A. de Boer et al., "The Polycomb group gene Ezh2 prevents hematopoietic stem cell exhaustion," *Blood*, vol. 107, no. 5, pp. 2170–2179, 2006.

[75] F. Xu and X. Li, "The role of histone methyltransferase EZH2 in myelodysplastic syndromes," *Expert Review of Hematology*, vol. 5, no. 2, pp. 177–185, 2012.

[76] T. Ernst, A. J. Chase, J. Score et al., "Inactivating mutations of the histone methyltransferase gene EZH2 in myeloid disorders," *Nature Genetics*, vol. 42, no. 8, pp. 722–726, 2010.

[77] G. Nikoloski, S. M. C. Langemeijer, R. P. Kuiper et al., "Somatic mutations of the histone methyltransferase gene EZH2 in myelodysplastic syndromes," *Nature Genetics*, vol. 42, no. 8, pp. 665–667, 2010.

[78] O. Abdel-Wahab and A. T. Fathi, "Mutations in epigenetic modifiers in myeloid malignancies and the prospect of novel epigenetic-targeted therapy," *Advances in Hematology*, vol. 2012, Article ID 469592, 12 pages, 2012.

[79] X. Wang, H. Dai, Q. Wang et al., "EZH2 mutations are related to low blast percentage in bone marrow and -7/del(7q) in de novo acute myeloid Leukemia," *PLoS ONE*, vol. 8, no. 4, Article ID e61341, 2013.

[80] V. Gelsi-Boyer, M. Brecqueville, R. Devillier, A. Murati, M.-J. Mozziconacci, and D. Birnbaum, "Mutations in ASXL1 are associated with poor prognosis across the spectrum of malignant myeloid diseases," *Journal of Hematology & Oncology*, vol. 5, p. 12, 2012.

[81] F. Thol, I. Friesen, F. Damm et al., "Prognostic significance of ASXL1 mutations in patients with myelodysplastic syndromes," *Journal of Clinical Oncology*, vol. 29, no. 18, pp. 2499–2506, 2011.

[82] M. Pratcorona, S. Abbas, M. A. Sanders et al., "Acquired mutations in ASXL1 in acute myeloid Leukemia: prevalence and prognostic value," *Haematologica*, vol. 97, no. 3, pp. 388–392, 2012.

[83] S. Schnittger, C. Eder, S. Jeromin et al., "ASXL1 exon 12 mutations are frequent in AML with intermediate risk karyotype and are independently associated with an adverse outcome," *Leukemia*, vol. 27, no. 1, pp. 82–91, 2013.

[84] C. L. Fisher, I. Lee, S. Bloyer et al., "Additional sex combs-like 1 belongs to the enhancer of trithorax and polycomb group and genetically interacts with Cbx2 in mice," *Developmental Biology*, vol. 337, no. 1, pp. 9–15, 2010.

[85] C. L. Fisher, N. Pineault, C. Brookes et al., "Loss-of-function additional sex combs like 1 mutations disrupt hematopoiesis but do not cause severe myelodysplasia or Leukemia," *Blood*, vol. 115, no. 1, pp. 38–46, 2010.

[86] B. Falini, M. P. Martelli, N. Bolli et al., "Acute myeloid Leukemia with mutated nucleophosmin (NPM1): is it a distinct entity?" *Blood*, vol. 117, no. 4, pp. 1109–1120, 2011.

[87] H. Liu, E. H.-Y. Cheng, and J. J.-D. Hsieh, "MLL fusions: pathways to Leukemia," *Cancer Biology and Therapy*, vol. 8, no. 13, pp. 1204–1211, 2009.

[88] G. Nikoloski, S. M. C. Langemeijer, R. P. Kuiper et al., "Somatic mutations of the histone methyltransferase gene EZH2 in myelodysplastic syndromes," *Nature Genetics*, vol. 42, no. 8, pp. 665–667, 2010.

[89] R. Rau and P. Brown, "Nucleophosmin (NPM1) mutations in adult and childhood acute myeloid leukaemia: towards definition of a new leukaemia entity," *Hematological Oncology*, vol. 27, no. 4, pp. 171–181, 2009.

[90] Y. Zhang, A. Chen, X. M. Yan, and G. Huang, "Disordered epigenetic regulation in MLL-related Leukemia," *International Journal of Hematology*, vol. 96, no. 4, pp. 428–437, 2012.

[91] A. Dufour, F. Schneider, K. H. Metzeler et al., "Acute myeloid Leukemia with biallelic CEBPA gene mutations and normal karyotype represents a distinct genetic entity associated with a favorable clinical outcome," *Journal of Clinical Oncology*, vol. 28, no. 4, pp. 570–577, 2010.

[92] P. D. Kottaridis, R. E. Gale, M. E. Frew et al., "The presence of a FLT3 internal tandem duplication in patients with acute myeloid Leukemia (AML) adds important prognostic information to cytogenetic risk group and response to the first cycle of chemotherapy: analysis of 854 patients from the United Kingdom Medical Research Council AML 10 and 12 trials," *Blood*, vol. 98, no. 6, pp. 1752–1759, 2001.

[93] S. Schnittger, C. Schoch, W. Kern et al., "Nucleophosmin gene mutations are predictors of favorable prognosis in acute myelogenous Leukemia with a normal karyotype," *Blood*, vol. 106, no. 12, pp. 3733–3739, 2005.

[94] S. Schnittger, C. Schoch, M. Dugas et al., "Analysis of FLT3 length mutations in 1003 patients with acute myeloid Leukemia: correlation to cytogenetics, FAB subtype, and prognosis in the AMLCG study and usefulness as a marker for the detection of minimal residual disease," *Blood*, vol. 100, no. 1, pp. 59–66, 2002.

[95] C. Thiede, S. Koch, E. Creutzig et al., "Prevalence and prognostic impact of NPM1 mutations in 1485 adult patients with acute myeloid Leukemia (AML)," *Blood*, vol. 107, no. 10, pp. 4011–4020, 2006.

[96] D. Small, "FLT3 mutations: biology and treatment," *Hematology*, pp. 178–184, 2006.

[97] K. H. Metzeler, H. Becker, K. Maharry et al., "ASXL1 mutations identify a high-risk subgroup of older patients with primary cytogenetically normal AML within the ELN Favorable genetic category," *Blood*, vol. 118, no. 26, pp. 6920–6929, 2011.

[98] Y. Shen, Y.-M. Zhu, X. Fan et al., "Gene mutation patterns and their prognostic impact in a cohort of 1185 patients with acute myeloid Leukemia," *Blood*, vol. 118, no. 20, pp. 5593–5603, 2011.

[99] W.-C. Chou, H.-H. Huang, H.-A. Hou et al., "Distinct clinical and biological features of de novo acute myeloid Leukemia with additional sex comb-like 1 (ASXL1) mutations," *Blood*, vol. 116, no. 20, pp. 4086–4094, 2010.

[100] C. P. Leith, K. J. Kopecky, J. Godwin et al., "Acute myeloid Leukemia in the elderly: assessment of multidrug resistance (MDR1) and cytogenetics distinguishes biologic subgroups with remarkably distinct responses to standard chemotherapy. A Southwest Oncology Group Study," *Blood*, vol. 89, no. 9, pp. 3323–3329, 1997.

[101] D. Small, "Targeting FLT3 for the treatment of Leukemia," *Seminars in Hematology*, vol. 45, supplement 2, pp. S17–S21, 2008.

[102] M. Bornhäuser, T. Illmer, M. Schaich, S. Soucek, G. Ehninger, and C. Thiede, "Improved outcome after stem-cell transplantation in FLT3/ITD-positive AML," *Blood*, vol. 109, no. 5, pp. 2264–2265, 2007.

[103] R. E. Gale, R. Hills, P. D. Kottaridis et al., "No evidence that FLT3 status should be considered as an indicator for transplantation in acute myeloid Leukemia (AML): an analysis of 1135 patients, excluding acute promyelocytic Leukemia, from the UK MRCAML10 and 12 trials," *Blood*, vol. 106, no. 10, pp. 3658–3665, 2005.

[104] G. Marcucci, K. Maharry, M. D. Radmacher et al., "Prognostic significance of, and gene and MicroRNA expression signatures associated with, CEBPA mutations in cytogenetically normal acute myeloid Leukemia with high-risk molecular features: a cancer and Leukemia group B study," *Journal of Clinical Oncology*, vol. 26, no. 31, pp. 5078–5087, 2008.

[105] U. Bacher, C. Haferlach, W. Kern, T. Haferlach, and S. Schnittger, "Prognostic relevance of FLT3-TKD mutations in AML: the combination matters an analysis of 3082 patients," *Blood*, vol. 111, no. 5, pp. 2527–2537, 2008.

[106] U. Bacher, T. Haferlach, C. Schoch, W. Kern, and S. Schnittger, "Implications of NRAS mutations in AML: a study of 2502 patients," *Blood*, vol. 107, no. 10, pp. 3847–3853, 2006.

Variation of Red Blood Cell Distribution Width and Mean Platelet Volume after Moderate Endurance Exercise

Giuseppe Lippi,[1] Gian Luca Salvagno,[2] Elisa Danese,[2] Cantor Tarperi,[3] Gian Cesare Guidi,[2] and Federico Schena[3]

[1] *Laboratory of Clinical Chemistry and Hematology, Academic Hospital of Parma, Via Gramsci 14, 43126 Parma, Italy*
[2] *Laboratory of Clinical Biochemistry, Department of Life and Reproduction Sciences, University of Verona, Via delle Menegone, 37100 Verona, Italy*
[3] *Department of Neurological, Neuropsychological, Morphological and Movement Sciences, University of Verona, Via delle Menegone, 37100 Verona, Italy*

Correspondence should be addressed to Giuseppe Lippi; glippi@ao.pr.it

Academic Editor: Bashir A. Lwaleed

Although physical exercise strongly influences several laboratory parameters, data about the hematological changes after medium distance running are scarce. We studied 31 middle-trained athletes (mean training regimen 217 ± 32 min/week) who performed a 21.1 km, half-marathon run. Blood samples were collected before the run, at the end, and 3 and 20 hours thereafter. The complete blood count was performed on Advia 2120 and included red blood cell (RBC), reticulocyte, and platelet counts; hemoglobin; mean corpuscular volume (MCV); mean corpuscular hemoglobin (MCH); reticulocyte haemoglobin content (Ret CHR); RBC distribution width (RDW), mean platelet volume (MPV). No significant variations were observed for MCH and Ret CHR. The RBC, reticulocyte, and hemoglobin values modestly decreased after the run. The MCV significantly increased at the end of running but returned to baseline 3 hours thereafter. The RDW constantly increased, reaching a peak 20 hours after the run. The platelet count and MPV both increased after the run and returned to baseline 3 hours thereafter. These results may have implications for definition of reference ranges and antidoping testing, and may also contribute to explaining the relationship between endurance exercise and mortality, since previous studies reported that RDW and MPV may be significantly associated with cardiovascular disease.

1. Introduction

Physical exercise is an important preanalytical variable, which strongly influences several biological and metabolic pathways. These remarkable variations are often reflected by concomitant changes of a number of laboratory parameters [1]. The accurate identification of such paraphysiologic variations is pivotal in medicine and sports not only to prevent misinterpretation of data and hence to define the real state of health and fitness of the athletes but also to detect the potential use of unfair doping practices and to assist sport physicians in follow-up of athletic injuries [1].

Some previous studies have investigated the changes of red blood cell (RBC) and platelet biology that may be induced by endurance exercise [2–6], but the outcome of these trails was often controversial due to the heterogeneity of study populations (trained or untrained athletes), settings (sea level or altitude), types of sport (sprint, endurance, or mixed), and volumes and intensities of the physical effort (short, medium, or long term performance). Among the various sports disciplines, medium distance running (i.e., from 10 to 21 km) is the most practiced worldwide at both recreational or competitive levels [7], since it provides a good balance between time spent in running and job or personal life and does not require the level of fitness and training of marathon or ultramarathon running [8]. It has been reported, however, that the risk of cardiac complications after medium and long distance running is not meaningless, with an overall incidence of cardiac arrest of 0.37 and 0.19 per 100,000 runner hours in marathon runners and half-marathon runners, respectively [9].

Data about the hematological changes after medium distance running are scarce to the best of our knowledge.

Even more importantly, the changes in RBC distribution width (RDW) and mean platelet volume (MPV), which are two emerging biomarkers of cardiovascular disease and overall mortality [10, 11], are lacking. As such, we planned a prospective study to assess the changes of some parameters of the complete blood cell count (CBC) in athletes performing moderate endurance exercise in order to establish whether the increased cardiovascular problems that are occasionally observed after this kind of exercise may be mirrored by variation of either RDW or MPV.

2. Materials and Methods

The study population consisted in 31 middle-trained athletes (11 females and 20 males; mean age 44 ± 7 years), who performed a 21.1 km, half-marathon run. The athletes were recruited from a team of nonprofessional, amateur runners regularly involved in recreational running, with mean training regimen of 217 ± 32 min/week and maximal oxygen uptake of 51 ± 5 mL/kg/min. No exclusion criteria were applied. The distance was run on a hilly and demanding route in the town of Verona, Italy (197 m altitude gap, with inclines averaging 1.8% and peaks up to 7%), in a partially sunny day with temperatures between 14 and 17°C and humidity between 60 and 80%. Blood samples were collected in primary blood tubes containing K_2EDTA (Terumo Europe N.V., Leuven, Belgium) immediately before the run and at the end of the trial, as well as 3 and 20 hours thereafter. All samples were immediately transported to the clinical chemistry laboratory of the Academic Hospital of Verona under controlled conditions of temperature and humidity. The CBC was performed on Advia 2120 (Siemens Healthcare Diagnostics, Tarrytown NY, USA) and included RBC, reticulocyte, and platelet counts; hemoglobin; mean corpuscular volume (MCV); mean corpuscular hemoglobin (MCH); reticulocyte haemoglobin content (Ret CHR); RDW; MPV. Results of measurements were expressed as median and interquartile range (IQR) and differences were analyzed with Wilcoxon test for paired samples, using Analyse-it (Analyse-it Software Ltd, Leeds, UK). All subjects gave an informed consent for being enrolled in this study, which was approved by the local academic ethical committee and performed in accordance with the Helsinki Declaration of 1975.

3. Results

The results of this study are shown in Table 1. No significant variations were observed for MCH and Ret CHR throughout the study period. The number of RBC and the hemoglobin values decreased significantly immediately after the run and remained significantly decreased compared to the baseline up to 20 hours thereafter. A similar trend was observed for the absolute reticulocyte count. The MCV was found to be significantly increased at the end of the run, but values returned similar to the baseline 3 hours thereafter. The RDW exhibited a remarkable trend towards increased values, reaching the peak 20 hours after the end of the run (median increase, 2.2%; IQR, 0.8–3.3%). Both the platelet count and the MPV significantly increased after the end of the run (median increase of MPV, 5.7%; IQR, 0.6–9.3%), whereas the values of both parameters returned to values similar to the baseline 3 hours thereafter. The odds ratio (OR) for an increased RDW value (i.e., >13.8%) was 3.7 (95% CI, 1.03–13.4; $P = 0.044$) 20 hours after the end of the run. Similarly, the OR for an increased MPV value (i.e., >8.5 fL) was 10.4 (95% CI, 1.22–89.5; $P = 0.03$) 3 hours after the end of the half-marathon run.

4. Discussion

The results of this prospective study, which demonstrated for the first time that both RDW and MPV values may significantly vary in response to moderate endurance exercise, may have at least three meaningful implications. The first important issue is that the conventional reference ranges of some parameters of the CBC, including those of the RDW and MPV, may only be applicable in subjects at rest because all the other parameters tested in this study exhibited significant variations throughout the observational period. It is noteworthy that although the maximum percentage variation of the RDW remained lower than the within-subject biologic variation (i.e., 2.2% versus ±3.5%), the percentage increase of MPV largely exceeded the within-subject biologic variation (i.e., 5.7% versus ±4.3%) and should hence be considered clinically significant [12]. Interestingly, we also observed that the hemoglobin values marginally but significantly decreased immediately after the run, and persisted significantly reduced up to 20 hours thereafter. This is an original finding that was not observed in a previous similar investigation [13] but has minor clinical significance, since the maximum percentage variation observed in our study (i.e., −3.2%) was very close to the within-subject biologic variation (±3%) [12].

Another important issue is the potential impact of these variations on antidoping testing. The athlete biological passport (ABP) is a reliable strategy to monitor selected biological variables over time that indirectly reveal the effects of doping and includes a large number of hematological variables [14]. More specifically, the so-called "adaptative model" currently used by the World Anti-Doping Agency (WADA) is based on an algorithm integrating hemoglobin, RBC count, reticulocytes count, MCV, and MCH. According to our data, all these variables except MCH were variably modified by moderate endurance exercise, and this should hence be clearly acknowledged when interpreting results of both the hematological module and the abnormal blood profile score (ABPS) [15].

Some conclusions can also be made about the impact of a half-marathon run on the cardiovascular risk. Several lines of evidence now attest that a high RDW is associated with an increased risk of mortality and morbidity in patients with heart disease [16], as well as in the general population [17, 18]. Similarly, an increased MPV conventionally reflects platelet hyperreactivity [19], that is, a leading player in the complex pathogenesis of cardiovascular disorders [20]. This aspect has been confirmed in a recent meta-analysis showing that elevated MPV is associated with acute myocardial infarction, mortality following myocardial infarction, and restenosis after coronary angioplasty [21].

TABLE 1: Haematological changes in middle-trained athletes undergoing a half-marathon run.

	Baseline	Post run	After 3 h	After 20 h
RBC (10^{12}/L)	4.9 (4.6–5.1)	4.8[†] (4.5–5.1)	4.6[‡] (4.3–4.9)	4.7[‡] (4.4–4.9)
Hemoglobin (g/L)	149 (145–155)	148[†] (140–155)	142[‡] (136–148)	144[‡] (139–150)
MCV (fL)	94.9 (91.9–96.3)	95.3[†] (93.5–97.3)	94.1 (92.3–95.8)	94.9 (91.5–97.1)
MCH (pg)	31.0 (30.0–31.1)	31.5 (30.0–32.0)	31.0 (30.3–32.8)	30.5 (30.0–32.0)
RDW (%)	13.3 (13.1–13.5)	13.4[†] (13.1–13.6)	13.4[‡] (13.2–13.6)	13.5[‡] (13.3–13.8)
Reticulocytes (10^9/L)	60.5 (49.5–72.5)	60.4 (49.6–74.2)	58.0[‡] (46.7–69.3)	59.7[‡] (46.9–65.9)
Ret CHR (pg)	31.0 (31.0–32.0)	31.0 (31.0–32.0)	31.0 (31.0–32.0)	31.0 (31.0–32.0)
Platelets (10^9/L)	255 (216–298)	311[‡] (264–361)	263 (219–290)	255 (212–290)
MPV (fL)	9.2 (8.6–9.9)	9.5[‡] (9.1–10.2)	9.1 (8.1–9.4)	9.2 (8.7–9.7)

[†]$P < 0.05$ compared to baseline; [‡]$P < 0.01$ compared to baseline.
MCH: mean corpuscular hemoglobin; MCV: mean corpuscular volume; MPV: mean platelet volume; RBC: red blood cell; RDW: RBC distribution width; Ret CHR: reticulocyte hemoglobin concentration.

Although it has not been definitely elucidated whether anisocytosis and a larger platelet volume are risk factors or simple biomarkers of disease, the observation that RDW and especially MPV consistently increase after a moderate endurance effort reflects a clear perturbation of RBC and platelet biology. This is noteworthy considering that, according to recent statistics, the overall deaths per 100,000 marathon finishers were estimated at 0.75 (95% confidence interval [CI], 0.38–1.13) and, even more interestingly, myocardial infarction or atherosclerotic heart disease accounted for the vast majority of deaths (i.e., >90%) [22]. The results of this study should hence represent a reliable basis to further define whether anisocytosis and larger platelet volume may effectively contribute to explanation of the relationship between endurance exercise and mortality, especially in subjects at higher risk of cardiovascular disease.

Abbreviations

CBC: Complete blood cell count
IQR: Interquartile range
MCH: Mean corpuscular hemoglobin
MCV: Mean corpuscular volume
MPV: Mean platelet volume
RBC: Red blood cell
RDW: RBC distribution width
Ret CHR: Reticulocyte hemoglobin concentration.

Conflict of Interests

The authors declare that there is no conflict of interests regarding the publication of this paper.

References

[1] G. Lippi, G. Banfi, F. Botrè et al., "Laboratory medicine and sports: between Scylla and Charybdis," *Clinical Chemistry and Laboratory Medicine*, vol. 50, no. 8, pp. 1309–1316, 2012.

[2] C. L. Wells, J. R. Stern, and L. H. Hecht, "Hematological changes following a marathon race in male and female runners," *European Journal of Applied Physiology and Occupational Physiology*, vol. 48, no. 1, pp. 41–49, 1982.

[3] R. J. L. Davidson, J. D. Robertson, G. Galea, and R. J. Maughan, "Hematological changes associated with marathon running," *International Journal of Sports Medicine*, vol. 8, no. 1, pp. 19–25, 1987.

[4] K. E. Fallon, G. Sivyer, K. Sivyer, A. Dare, and E. J. Watts, "Changes in haematological parameters and iron metabolism associated with a 1600 kilometre ultramarathon," *The British Journal of Sports Medicine*, vol. 33, no. 1, pp. 27–31, 1999.

[5] G. Banfi, G. S. Roi, A. Dolci, and D. Susta, "Behaviour of haematological parameters in athletes performing marathons and ultramarathons in altitude ("skyrunners")," *Clinical and Laboratory Haematology*, vol. 26, no. 6, pp. 373–377, 2004.

[6] G. Lippi, G. Banfi, M. Montagnana, G. L. Salvagno, F. Schena, and G. C. Guidi, "Acute variation of leucocytes counts following a half-marathon run," *International Journal of Laboratory Hematology*, vol. 32, part 2, no. 1, pp. 117–121, 2010.

[7] S. Nettleton and M. Hardey, "Running away with health: the urban marathon and the construction of "charitable bodies"," *Health*, vol. 10, no. 4, pp. 441–460, 2006.

[8] M. Webb, "Raising the bar: sprints or marathons?" *Journal of Registry Management*, vol. 38, no. 2, pp. 105–106, 2011.

[9] L. Hart, "Marathon-related cardiac arrest," *Clinical Journal of Sport Medicine*, vol. 23, no. 5, pp. 409–410, 2013.

[10] G. Lippi and M. Plebani, "Red blood cell distribution width (RDW) and human pathology. One size fits all," *Clinical Chemistry and Laboratory Medicine*, vol. 52, no. 9, pp. 1247–1249, 2014.

[11] G. Sharma and J. S. Berger, "Platelet activity and cardiovascular risk in apparently healthy individuals: a review of the data," *Journal of Thrombosis and Thrombolysis*, vol. 32, no. 2, pp. 201–208, 2011.

[12] C. Ricós, V. Alvarez, F. Cava et al., "Current databases on biological variation: pros, cons and progress," *Scandinavian Journal of Clinical and Laboratory Investigation*, vol. 59, no. 7, pp. 491–500, 1999.

[13] M. Mohseni, S. Silvers, R. Mcneil et al., "Prevalence of hyponatremia, renal dysfunction, and other electrolyte abnormalities among runners before and after completing a marathon or half marathon," *Sports Health*, vol. 3, no. 2, pp. 145–151, 2011.

[14] G. Lippi, M. Plebani, F. Sanchis-Gomar, and G. Banfi, "Current limitations and future perspectives of the athlete blood passport," *European Journal of Applied Physiology*, vol. 112, no. 10, pp. 3693–3694, 2012.

[15] P. Sottas, N. Robinson, S. Giraud et al., "Statistical classification of abnormal blood profiles in athletes," *International Journal of Biostatistics*, vol. 2, no. 1, article 1, 2006.

[16] M. Tonelli, F. Sacks, M. Arnold, L. Moye, B. Davis, and M. Pfeffer, "Relation between red blood cell distribution width and cardiovascular event rate in people with coronary disease," *Circulation*, vol. 117, no. 2, pp. 163–168, 2008.

[17] T. S. Perlstein, J. Weuve, M. A. Pfeffer, and J. A. Beckman, "Red blood cell distribution width and mortality risk in a community-based prospective cohort," *Archives of Internal Medicine*, vol. 169, no. 6, pp. 588–594, 2009.

[18] K. V. Patel, L. Ferrucci, W. B. Ershler, D. L. Longo, and J. M. Gurainik, "Red blood cell distribution width and the risk of death in middle-aged and older adults," *Archives of Internal Medicine*, vol. 169, no. 5, pp. 515–523, 2009.

[19] A. Y. Gasparyan, L. Ayvazyan, D. P. Mikhailidis, and G. D. Kitas, "Mean platelet volume: a link between thrombosis and inflammation?" *Current Pharmaceutical Design*, vol. 17, no. 1, pp. 47–58, 2011.

[20] G. Lippi, M. Franchini, and G. Targher, "Arterial thrombus formation in cardiovascular disease," *Nature Reviews Cardiology*, vol. 8, no. 9, pp. 502–512, 2011.

[21] S. G. Chu, R. C. Becker, P. B. Berger et al., "Mean platelet volume as a predictor of cardiovascular risk: a systematic review and meta-analysis," *Journal of Thrombosis and Haemostasis*, vol. 8, no. 1, pp. 148–156, 2010.

[22] S. C. Mathews, D. L. Narotsky, D. L. Bernholt et al., "Mortality among marathon runners in the United States, 2000–2009," *The American Journal of Sports Medicine*, vol. 40, no. 7, pp. 1495–1500, 2012.

3

Influence of the Clinical Status on Stress Reticulocytes, CD 36 and CD 49d of SSFA$_2$ Homozygous Sickle Cell Patients Followed in Abidjan

Duni Sawadogo,[1,2] **Aïssata Tolo-Dilkébié,**[3] **Mahawa Sangaré,**[1,2] **Nelly Aguéhoundé,**[1]
Hermance Kassi,[4] **and Toussaint Latte**[4]

[1] *Department of Hematology, Faculty of Pharmacy, University Felix Houphouet Boigny, Cocody, BP 2308 Abidjan 08, Cote D'Ivoire*
[2] *Unit of Hematology, Central Laboratory, Teaching Hospital of Yopougon, BP 632 Abidjan 21, Cote D'Ivoire*
[3] *Clinic Hematology Service, Teaching Hospital of Yopougon, BP 632 Abidjan 21, Cote D'Ivoire*
[4] *AIDS Biological Unit, Central Laboratory, Teaching Hospital of Yopougon, BP 632 Abidjan 21, Cote D'Ivoire*

Correspondence should be addressed to Duni Sawadogo; dunisawadogo@yahoo.fr

Academic Editor: Aldo Roccaro

Background and Objectives. Interactions between sickle cells involving CD 49d, CD36, and the vascular endothelium may initiate vasoocclusion leading to acute painful episodes and multiple organ failure. *Materials and Methods.* We selected 60 SS patients who had never been treated by hydroxyurea. We performed a total blood count. We identified with immunophenotyping by flow cytometry total reticulocytes their distribution according to the degree of maturity (mature, intermediate, very immature) and CD 36$^+$ and CD 49d$^+$ antigens. Stress reticulocytes corresponded to the sum of intermediate and immature cells. *Results.* Subjects in crisis had more total reticulocytes and very immature reticulocytes than subjects in stationary phase ($P < 0.05$). During the crisis, total CD 36$^+$ reticulocytes ($214\,870 \pm 107\,584/\mu L$ versus $148\,878 \pm 115\,024/\mu L$; $P < 0.05$) and the very immature CD 36$^+$ reticulocytes ($28.9 \pm 7.9\%$ versus $23.0 \pm 6.4\%$; $P < 0.05$) increased. The clinical status had no impact on CD 49d$^+$ reticulocytes. *Conclusion.* The rates of stress reticulocytes in general and those expressing CD 49d and CD 36 were very high. The clinical status had an influence on CD 36$^+$ reticulocytes. The expression of adhesion molecules is only one of the parameters involved in sickle cell disease crisis.

1. Introduction

Sickle cell anemia (SCA) is a pathology characterized by acute pain and various organ failures, related to frequent vasoocclusive episodes. The mechanism that leads to these vasoocclusive events is not yet clearly defined. Vasoocclusion may be due to an interaction between sickle cells and the vascular endothelium. The result is a longer transit time of sickle cells in the capillary system [1–3]. Some of the molecules involved in these interactions have been identified for example CD 47, basal cell adhesion molecule-1/Lutheran (B-CAM-1/Lu), intercellular cell adhesion molecule 4 (ICAM-4) [3–5]. In this paper, we focused on α_4(CD 49d) β_1 (CD 29) integrin or very late activation antigen (VLA) 4 and CD 36 which are, exclusively present on stress reticulocytes [1–5].

Hydroxyurea (HU) is a cancer chemotherapy agent that decreases the frequency of SCA crises. HU may exert its therapeutic effect by generating nitric oxide (anti-inflammatory) and increasing the level of antisickling fetal hemoglobin (Hb F) [3, 5, 6]. Higher levels of Hb F result in clinically milder sickle cell disease [3, 6]. HU also led to a significant decrease in the expression of the CD 36, CD 49d, and CD 29 genes [7].

Lee et al. [8] and Trinh-Trang-Tan et al. [9] found that the presence or absence of CD 36 had no effect on the clinical manifestations of SCA. Browne and Hebbel [2] and Styles et al. [3] had a completely different point of view.

In Côte d'Ivoire, the frequency of Hb S hovers around 14% with 2% of major forms [10]. HU is not part of the armamentarium used for the treatment of sickle cell patients. Patients exclusively treated in Cote d'Ivoire have never received HU. Maintenance treatment is based on folic acid and vasodilators [10]. Crises are treated by nonsteroidal anti-inflammatory drugs, particularly ketoprofen [10, 11].

It is not common to find studies with a population composed only of SS patients clearly showing the results of the subjects in steady state or in crisis. This is why we set a goal to investigate whether the clinical status, namely, the crisis or the steady state, had an impact on total reticulocytes, stress reticulocytes, and the expression of adhesion molecules and CD 36 and CD 49 d in SS black African patients never treated by HU in Abidjan.

2. Materials and Methods

This was a cross-sectional study carried out in the central laboratory and in the Department of Clinical Hematology of the University Hospital of Yopougon in Abidjan. The study population consisted of 60 SCA (Hb SS) patients who provided their informed consent for participation; of these 30 were in steady state and 30 were in crisis. Steady state was defined by a period of at least 1 month since the patient's last crisis [8, 12]. Patients had been exclusively treated in Cote d'Ivoire. They never had received HU. We did not include subjects who were transfused in the three months preceding the investigation. If the samples were hemolyzed, if they contained clot or if the immunophenotyping tests were not perform within 48 h, the patients were not also selected [8, 12]. The samples were taken as soon as the patients in crisis were admitted, the first day of the hospitalization.

Blood was collected by venipuncture performed at the elbow in a tube containing an anticoagulant, the Ethylen-diaminetetraacetic acid (EDTA). We performed a complete blood count with Sysmex XT-2000i analyzer. The determination of the rate of reticulocytes and their degree of maturity was performed with immunophenotyping by flow cytometry with the FACSCalibur Flow Cytometer Becton Dickinson. We used the same device to demonstrate the CD 36 and CD 49d antigens on the surface of reticulocytes. At least 20 000 cells were analyzed on each samples. We used the following reagents: anti-CD 36 monoclonal antibodies coupled to fluorescein isothiocyanate (FITC), IgM isotype, kappa (FITC), anti-CD 49d monoclonal antibodies coupled to phycoerythrin (PE), IgG1 isotype, kappa (PE), Retic-Count or thiazole orange, saline phosphate, bovine serum albumin, and the fragment F (ab$'$) 2 IgG1 [3, 8].

The distribution of reticulocytes according to the degree of maturity with thiazole orange can be subdivided into mature reticulocytes (low fluorescence area or LFR), in retic-ulocytes of intermediate maturity (moderate fluorescence area or MFR) and in very immature reticulocytes (high fluorescence region or HFR). Stress reticulocytes correspond to the immature reticulocytes fraction (IRF) constituted by the sum of reticulocytes MFR and HFR [13]. The mean fluorescence intensity (MFI) was also measured.

VLA-4 is composed of CD 49d (α_4 integrin) and CD 29 (β_1 integrin). Both components were measured by Styles et al. [3] using flow cytometry. They found that that the expression

of CD 49d and CD 29 were virtually identical. On this basis, we only sought the expression of CD 49d [3].

Data were compared using Student's t-test or Chi-Square test. A P value <0.05 indicated a significant difference.

3. Results

60 SS patients (32 male and 28 female) were studied. The average age was 15.12 ± 10.57 (2–43 years). We separated patients according to clinical status: crisis or steady state (Table 1). Patients in crisis or in steady state had a similar distribution with regard to age, sex ratio, and the Hb fractions (Table 1). On the other hand, in terms of clinical history, subjects in crisis had had a longer length of hospital stay and a higher number of transfusions ($P < 0.05$) than subjects in steady state. Clinical status had an impact on most elements of the complete blood count (Table 1). Severe anemia and leukocytosis with neutrophilia were the highlights of the complete blood count (Table 1).

Subjects in crisis had statistically significantly more total reticulocytes (absolute and relative values) and very immature reticulocytes, HFR, than subjects in steady state (Table 2).

All patients (60/60) had expressed CD 49d on the reticulocytes. The distribution according to the degree of maturity was similar during the crisis or the steady state. Very immature cells predominated (Table 3).

80% (48/60) of patients expressed the CD 36. The mean fluorescence intensity (MFI) for the stress reticulocytes was 120 ± 10 whereas for the more mature reticulocytes MFI it was lower (35 ± 7). Stress reticulocytes were strongly stained. The relative and absolute rates of CD 36$^+$ reticulocytes were higher in crisis than in steady state (Table 4). Steady state was associated with an increase of CD 36$^+$ intermediate maturity reticulocytes. Immature reticulocytes value was higher for the SS patients in crisis (Table 4).

4. Comments

Data on age and sex were similar to the other studies carried out in Abidjan which stressed that sickle cell patients were mostly teenagers or young male adults [10, 11].

Clinical history showed that patients who were recruited when they were in crisis received more transfusions and were hospitalized longer (Table 1). The frequency of painful crises requiring hospitalization and the length of hospital stay are clinical criteria used to assess the severity of SCA. Platt et al. [14] showed that the number of painful episodes in a year is a measure of the clinical severity of the disease and that it is associated with early death especially in patients over 20 years.

Indeed, SCA is associated with an abnormal inflamma-tory reaction which is even more important during crises [4, 10, 12]. Since the work of Sangare et al. [10] that has demon-strated the beneficial effect of nonsteroidal anti-inflammatory drugs, ketoprofen is used for treating seizures in Abidjan. It is associated with a vasodilator, pentoxifylline. This anti-inflammatory drug shortened significantly and without any

TABLE 1: Influence of clinical status on epidemiological, clinical, and biological parameters.

Parameters	Painful crisis ($n = 30$) m ± sd (min–max)	Steady state ($n = 30$) m ± sd (min–max)	P
Age	13.9 ± 9 (2–37)	16.4 ± 11.9 (2–43)	0.364
Sex (M/F)	1.14	1.14	0.795
Number of crises/year	2.5 ± 1.01 (1–4)	2.3 ± 0.84 (1–4)	0.406
Hospitalization days/year	1.4 ± 1.01 (0–6)	0.47 ± 0.63 (0–2)	0.0002
Transfusions/year	0.93 ± 0.52 (0–2)	0.43 ± 0.5 (0-1)	0.0004
Hb S (%)	86.8 ± 5.7 (76–95)	86.1 ± 4.5 (73.6–93.6)	0.622
Hb F (%)	18.8 ± 5.1 (2.5–23.2)	11.5 ± 4.4 (3.9–23.6)	0.595
Hb A$_2$ (%)	2.3 ± 1.01 (1–4)	2.4 ± 0.6 (1.5–4.2)	0.599
Red blood cells/μL	2 011 000 ± 698 000	2 593 000 ± 605 000	0.001
Hemoglobin (g/dL)	5.64 ± 1.81	6.98 ± 1.47	0.0024
Hematocrit (%)	17.83 ± 5.12	21.01 ± 4.03	0.01
Mean cell volume (fL)	91.02 ± 10.94	82.42 ± 11.09	0.004
MCH (pg)	28.43 ± 3.15	27.32 ± 3.84	0.224
MCHC (%)	31.32 ± 2.22	33.15 ± 1.57	0.0005
Leukocytes/μL	23 778 ± 13 038	14 206 ± 11 515	0.004
Neutrophils/μL	13 046 ± 6 685	5 838 ± 3 013	10^{-6}
Platelets/μL	323 133 ± 159 263	407 867 ± 173 572	0.53

m ± sd (min–max): mean ± standard deviation (minimum–maximum).
MCV: mean cell volume.
MVH: mean cell hemoglobin.
MCHC: mean cell hemoglobin concentration.
P: Student's t-test.

TABLE 2: Distribution of reticulocytes according to their degree of maturity and to the clinical status.

Parameters	Painful crisis ($n = 30$) m ± sd	Steady state ($n = 30$) m ± sd	P
Total reticulocytes (%)	15.5 ± 10	8.4 ± 4.9	0.003
Total reticulocytes (/μL)	283 678 ± 153 711	200 721 ± 10 708	0.002
LFR	51.5 ± 15.9	56.6 ± 7.5	0.3
MFR	37.9 ± 10	36.7 ± 5.4	0.18
HFR (%)	10.7 ± 9.9	6.7 ± 3.5	0.012
IRF (%)	48.6 ± 15.9	43.4 ± 7.5	0.3

m ± sd: mean ± standard deviation.
P: Chi-Square test.
LFR: low fluorescence reticulocytes or mature reticulocytes.
MFR: medium fluorescence reticulocytes or semimature reticulocytes.
HFR: high fluorescence reticulocytes or immature reticulocytes.
IRF: index reticulocytes fraction or stress reticulocytes (MFR + HFR).

side effects the duration of sickle cell crisis and had an effect greater than that of a major opioid analgesic. Patients never had been treated by HU.

The clinical status, namely, the vasoocclusive crisis, had an impact on almost all parameters of the complete blood count except for the level of platelets (Table 1). The complete blood count has demonstrated abnormalities commonly described as severe anemia and leukocytosis [3, 8, 10, 15]. In the patients followed in the present study, a higher leukocyte count in the peripheral circulation and infections were shown. Infections related to the increase of white blood cells were often associated with the occurrence of vasoocclusive episodes. Sluggish flow, increased transit time, hypoxia, and

therefore sickling may be due to the probable interaction between sickle cells and leukocytes in the microcirculation [5]. A new multistep model for vasoocclusion in sickle disease is thus proposed. In this model, sickle cells or secondary inflammatory stimuli induced endothelial activation, leading to recruitment of adherent leukocytes. These leukocytes interacted with red blood sickle cells, thus hampering microvascular blood flow. In the end, sickle cells are trapped leading to vasoocclusion, as shown by Frenette [16].

The values of total reticulocytes (Table 2) were close to the results of other authors such as Styles et al. [3], Lee et al. [8], and Maier-Redelsperger et al. [15], which highlighted a hyperreticulocytosis ranging from 259 000/μL

TABLE 3: Profile of CD 49d$^+$ reticulocytes according to their degree of maturity and the clinical status.

Parameters	CD 49d$^+$ patients		P
	Painful crisis ($n = 30$)	Steady state ($n = 30$)	
	m ± sd	m ± sd	
Total reticulocytes (%)	44.1 ± 17.7	40.9 ± 7.7	0.13
Total reticulocytes (/μL)	134 604 ± 108 223	83 782 ± 54 222	0.06
LFR	9.9 ± 19.6	5.8 ± 2.1	0.91
MFR	26.4 ± 8.5	28.4 ± 6.5	0.8
HFR (%)	63.7 ± 18.1	65.8 ± 7.6	0.19
IRF (%)	90.1 ± 19.6	94.2 ± 2.1	0.65

m ± sd: mean ± standard deviation.
P: Chi-Square test.
LFR: low fluorescence reticulocytes or mature reticulocytes.
MFR: medium fluorescence reticulocytes or semimature reticulocytes.
HFR: high fluorescence reticulocytes or immature reticulocytes.
IRF: index reticulocytes fraction or stress reticulocytes (MFR + HFR).

TABLE 4: Distribution of CD 36$^+$ reticulocytes according to their degree of maturity and the clinical status.

Parameters	CD 36$^+$ patients		P
	Painful crisis ($n = 23$)	Steady state ($n = 25$)	
	m ± sd	m ± sd	
Total reticulocytes (%)	53.4 ± 14.3	46.1 ± 11.4	0.006
Total reticulocytes (/μL)	214 870 ± 107 584	144 878 ± 115 024	10^{-5}
LFR	9.2 ± 7.4	8.9 ± 6.4	0.32
MFR	61.9 ± 8.9	68.1 ± 6.2	0.001
HFR (%)	28.9 ± 7.9	23 ± 6.4	0.002
IRF (%)	90.8 ± 7.4	91.2 ± 6.4	0.3

m ± sd: mean ± standard deviation.
P: Chi-Square test.
LFR: low fluorescence reticulocytes or mature reticulocytes.
MFR: medium fluorescence reticulocytes or semimature reticulocytes.
HFR: high fluorescence reticulocytes or immature reticulocytes.
IRF: index reticulocytes fraction or stress reticulocytes (MFR + HFR).

[8] to 320 000/μL [3, 15]. Crisis resulted in a statistically significant increase in relative and absolute values of total reticulocytes (Table 2). On the other hand the clinical status had no effect on the rate of stress reticulocytes (IFR) which was high. This result was surprising but it could be possible that some biological alterations still persisted at one month after the crisis even if the patients were in steady state.

Among the stress reticulocytes, the fraction of very immature cells was higher during crises than during steady state (10.7 ± 9.9% versus 6.7 ± 3.5%; $P = 0.04$). These values were lower than those of Maier-Redelsperger et al. [15] who found a frequency of 13% for very immature reticulocytes in SS patients [15]. Hebbel [1] was the first to show in 1980 that the red blood cells of SS patients had pathological adhesion to vascular endothelium. J. L. Wautier and M. P. Wautier [17] also noted that the adhesion was more important if the blood was collected in the vaso-occlusive crisis. According to Trinh-Trang-Tan et al. [9] reticulocytes which are more abundant and express more adhesion molecules may contribute to the hyperadhesiveness.

We only sought the expression of CD 49d which was positive for all patients (Table 2). The percentage of reticulocytes expressing CD 49d was 44.1 ± 17.7% for the painful crisis and 40.9 ± 7.7% for the steady state (Table 3). The difference was not significant ($P = 0.37$). Styles et al. [3] also found that the crisis or stationary phase did not influence the relative value of CD 49d$^+$ reticulocytes. However, our results were higher than those of Styles et al. [3] and Lee et al. [8]. Styles et al. [3] had found that the percentage of reticulocytes expressing CD 49d was 29.0 ± 5.9%, that is, 129 000 ± 39 000/μL. Lee et al. [8] showed that 22 ± 2% reticulocytes carried CD 49d. These high rates could be explained by the fact that the subjects we selected were much more anemic.

For CD 36$^+$ subjects, the level of total reticulocytes was 53.4 ± 14.3% for subjects in crisis and 46.1 ± 11.4% for subjects in steady state (Table 4). These results differed from those of Lee et al. [8] who only found 24% ± 8.1% CD 36$^+$ reticulocytes. They were close to those of Styles et al. [3] with 55.3 ± 6.4% CD 36$^+$ reticulocytes before HU treatment. Browne and Hebbel [2] obtained 39.8 ± 21.9% for the total reticulocytes of CD 36$^+$ patients. This value was lower than the results of Lee [8] but higher than the percentage given by Styles et al. [3].

We investigated SCA patients who never received HU. We compared the results with authors [3, 8] who had worked on SS patients treated by HU. It is well documented that HU decreases CD 49d and CD 36 expression even after months [3, 8]. In fact, Lee et al. [8] collected the samples before the introduction of HU treatment. Styles et al. [3] followed the SCA patients from the onset of therapy with HU.

According to Styles et al. [3], we found that CD 36 expression on reticulocytes was higher than that of CD 49d. Nevertheless, these authors emphasized that adhesion mediated by VLA-4 or α_4 (CD 49d) β_1 (CD 29) integrin would be more tenacious than that involving the CD 36 [3].

The contribution of CD 36 has been called into question with the finding that sickle cell patients who have a CD 36 deficiency of reticulocytes and mature red blood cells can have a normal clinical course [8, 9]. Trinh-Trang-Tan et al. [9] showed that there is dissociation between adhesiveness and adhesion molecules. It is therefore conceivable that CD 36, although in reduced amounts, might be activated by abnormal constitutive phosphorylation [9].

Blood flow is compromised in sickle microcirculation. Under low flow, sickle cell adherence to endothelium increased with contact time in the absence of endothelial activation or adhesive protein addition. Contact time between sickle cells and endothelium seemed a more important determinant of adherence than high-affinity receptor-ligand interactions [18].

The signalization cascade leading to receptor activation rather than the expression level only of adhesion molecules should also play an important role in the adhesion of sickle cells to the blood vessels [4].

5. Conclusion

In SCA, the clinical status—crisis or steady state—had an impact on the clinical history, namely, the number of hospital days and the number of transfusions. Anemia, leukocytosis, and total and immature reticulocytes were higher in patients in crisis than those in steady state. There was no difference between subjects in crisis and those in steady state for CD 49d$^+$ reticulocytes. Concerning the CD 36$^+$ subjects, the crisis had resulted in an increase in total reticulocytes and very immature reticulocytes.

SCA is the result of complex mechanism involving adhesion molecules such as CD 49d and CD 36. There is a correlation between the adhesion systems and the stress reticulocytes. However these facts are not sufficient to predict the occurrence and severity of sickle cell crisis.

Conflict of Interests

The authors declare that there is no conflict of interests regarding the publication of this paper.

References

[1] R. P. Hebbel, M. A. B. Boogaerts, J. W. Eaton, and M. H. Steinberg, "Erythrocyte adherence to endothelium in sickle-cell anemia. A possible determinant of disease severity," *The New England Journal of Medicine*, vol. 302, no. 18, pp. 992–995, 1980.

[2] P. V. Browne and R. P. Hebbel, "CD36-positive stress reticulocytosis in sickle cell anemia," *Journal of Laboratory and Clinical Medicine*, vol. 127, no. 4, pp. 340–347, 1996.

[3] L. A. Styles, B. Lubin, E. Vichinsky et al., "Decrease of very late activation antigen-4 and CD36 on reticulocytes in sickle cell patients treated with hydroxyurea," *Blood*, vol. 89, no. 7, pp. 2554–2559, 1997.

[4] J.-P. Cartron and J. Elion, "Erythroid adhesion molecules in sickle cell disease: effect of hydroxyurea," *Transfusion Clinique et Biologique*, vol. 15, no. 1-2, pp. 39–50, 2008.

[5] D. K. Kau, E. Finnegan, and G. A. Barabino, "Sickle red cell-endothelium interactions," *Microcirculation*, vol. 16, no. 1, pp. 97–111, 2009.

[6] S. Charache, M. L. Terrin, R. D. Moore et al., "Effect of hydroxyurea on the frequency of painful crises in Sickle cell anemia," *The New England Journal of Medicine*, vol. 332, no. 20, pp. 1317–1322, 1995.

[7] S. Gambero, A. A. Canalli, F. Traina et al., "Therapy with hydroxyurea is associated with reduced adhesion molecule gene and protein expression in sickle red cells with a concomitant reduction in adhesive properties," *European Journal of Haematology*, vol. 78, no. 2, pp. 144–151, 2007.

[8] K. Lee, P. Gane, F. Roudot-Thoraval et al., "The nonexpression of CD36 on reticulocytes and mature red blood cells does not modify the clinical course of patients with sickle cell anemia," *Blood*, vol. 98, no. 4, pp. 966–971, 2001.

[9] M.-M. Trinh-Trang-Tan, C. Vilela-Lamego, J. Picot, M.-P. Wautier, and J.-P. Cartron, "Intercellular adhesion molecule-4 and CD36 are implicated in the abnormal adhesiveness of sickle cell SAD mouse erythrocytes to endothelium," *Haematologica*, vol. 95, no. 5, pp. 730–737, 2010.

[10] A. Sangare, K. G. Koffi, O. Allangba et al., "Etude comparative du Ketoprofène et de la Buprenorphine dans le traitement des crises douloureuses drepanocytaires," *Medecine d'Afrique Noire*, vol. 44, pp. 138–143, 1998.

[11] A. Tolo-Diebkile, K. G. Koffi, D. C. Nanho et al., "Drepanocytose homozygote chez l'adulte ivoirien de plus de 21 ans," *Cahiers d'Études et de Recherches Francophones/Santé*, vol. 20, pp. 63–67, 2010.

[12] A. A. Solovey, A. N. Solovey, J. Harkness, and R. P. Hebbel, "Modulation of endothelial cell activation in sickle cell disease: a pilot study," *Blood*, vol. 97, no. 7, pp. 1937–1941, 2001.

[13] B. H. Davis, M. DiCorato, N. C. Bigelow, and M. H. Langweiler, "Proposal for standardization of flow cytometric reticulocyte maturity index (RMI) measurements," *Cytometry*, vol. 14, no. 3, pp. 318–326, 1993.

[14] O. S. Platt, B. D. Thorington, D. J. Brambilla et al., "Pain in sickle cell disease—rates and risk factors," *The New England Journal of Medicine*, vol. 325, no. 1, pp. 11–16, 1991.

[15] M. Maier-Redelsperger, A. Flahault, M. G. Neonato, R. Girot, and D. Labie, "Automated analysis of mature red blood cells and reticulocytes in SS and SC disease," *Blood Cells, Molecules, and Diseases*, vol. 33, no. 1, pp. 15–24, 2004.

[16] P. S. Frenette, "Sickle cell vaso-occlusion: multistep and multicellular paradigm," *Current Opinion in Hematology*, vol. 9, no. 2, pp. 101–106, 2002.

[17] J. L. Wautier and M. P. Wautier, "Molecular basis of erythrocyte adhesion to endothelial cells in diseases," *Clinical Hemorheology and Microcirculation*, vol. 53, pp. 11–21, 2013.

[18] R. A. O. Montes, J. R. Eckman, L. L. Hsu, and T. M. Wick, "Sickle erythrocyte adherence to endothelium at low shear: role of shear stress in propagation of vaso-occlusion," *American Journal of Hematology*, vol. 70, no. 3, pp. 216–227, 2002.

4

Decitabine Compared with Low-Dose Cytarabine for the Treatment of Older Patients with Newly Diagnosed Acute Myeloid Leukemia: A Pilot Study of Safety, Efficacy, and Cost-Effectiveness

Linu A. Jacob, S. Aparna, K. C. Lakshmaiah, D. Lokanatha, Govind Babu, Suresh Babu, and Sandhya Appachu

Department of Medical Oncology, Kidwai Memorial Institute of Oncology, Dr. M. H. Mari Gowda Road, Hombegowda Nagar, Bangalore, Karnataka 560030, India

Correspondence should be addressed to S. Aparna; aparnasmurthy25@gmail.com

Academic Editor: Shaji Kumar

Introduction. The incidence of Acute Myeloid Leukemia (AML) increases progressively with age and its treatment is challenging. This prospective case control study was undertaken to compare the safety, efficacy, and cost-effectiveness of decitabine with those of cytarabine in older patients with newly diagnosed AML who are not fit for intensive chemotherapy. *Materials and Methods.* 30 eligible patients above 60 years old with newly diagnosed AML were assigned to receive decitabine or cytarabine. The primary end point was overall survival (OS). The secondary objective was to compare adverse events and cost-effectiveness of therapy in the two study groups. *Results.* In this study, 15 patients received decitabine and 15 patients received cytarabine. The median OS was 5.5 months for each of the treatment groups. The hazard ratio between the treatment groups was 0.811 with 95% CI of 0.390 to 1.687. Toxicity profile was similar in both groups. Cost per cycle of chemotherapy in INR was 24,200 for decitabine and 1,600 for low-dose cytarabine group. Median of simplified cost-effectiveness ratio was 0.00022 for decitabine group and 0.0034 for low-dose cytarabine group. *Conclusions.* For elderly patients with AML, decitabine and low-dose cytarabine should be chosen based on the patient's choice and affordability. Our study has shown that both of these agents have similar OS and toxicity. Low-dose cytarabine scores over decitabine in developing countries as it is more cost-effective.

1. Introduction

The incidence of Acute Myeloid Leukemia (AML) increases progressively with age, from approximately 1 per 100,000 at age 40 to more than 15 per 100,000 at age 75 and older [1]. Unlike younger adults with AML in whom the treatment is straightforward and the goal is cure with intensive chemotherapy, treatment decisions in elderly patients with AML are difficult. Aggressive treatment necessitates hospitalization and separation from family and home, has toxic and potentially fatal side effects, and is often ineffective. The optimal treatment decision for older adults with AML remains highly controversial and is a major challenge for clinicians treating these patients. The clinician has to choose from at least four different approaches: supportive care only, less intensive chemotherapy, standard intensive chemotherapy (IC), or enrolment into a controlled clinical trial. In a developing country like ours, the clinician has to consider the fact that our patients have a higher frequency of poverty, illiteracy, malnutrition, and chronic infectious diseases. Hence, there is a need to explore a treatment strategy which is feasible, affordable, acceptable, accessible, and, more importantly, effective. This study was undertaken to compare the efficacy, safety, and cost-effectiveness of decitabine with those of cytarabine in older patients with newly diagnosed AML.

2. Materials and Methods

This was a prospective case control study conducted according to the Declaration of Helsinki after approval by the Institutional Ethics Committee. Between June 2011 and December 2014, patients attending our outpatient department were screened for inclusion in the study. Eligible patients were ≥60 years old with newly diagnosed, histologically confirmed de novo or secondary AML (>20% blasts) who were not fit for intensive chemotherapy with 3 + 7 induction. Exclusion criteria included acute promyelocytic leukemia, inaspirable bone marrow, and HIV infection. Patients must not have had previous chemotherapy (except hydroxyurea) or used experimental drugs for 4 weeks prior to recruitment.

Informed written consent was obtained from all patients prior to protocol entry. A thorough history and physical examination, complete blood count, biochemical profile, chest X-ray, bone marrow aspiration, biopsy, flow cytometry, and cytogenetics were performed at baseline. Patients were assigned to decitabine or low-dose cytarabine depending on the patient's affordability and patient choice guided by the physician. Patients assigned to receive decitabine received 1-hour IV infusion of decitabine 20 mg/m^2 once a day for five consecutive days every 4 weeks. Patients either were hospitalized or received chemotherapy infusion in daycare department. Patients who opted for cytarabine received 20 mg/m^2 of cytarabine once a day subcutaneously for 10 consecutive days every 4 weeks. Subcutaneous injections were administered by the primary care physicians in patients' household or patients attenders were trained to give subcutaneous injections. Treatment was continued until death, unacceptable toxicity, lack of clinical benefit, intercurrent illness preventing treatment, or patient request/physician decision to stop. Treatment was delayed at the discretion of the investigator for febrile neutropenia (38.5°C, absolute neutrophil count [ANC] <1,000/μL), clinical and/or microbiologic evidence of infection with grade 3 to 4 neutropenia (ANC <1,000/L), or hemorrhage with grade 4 thrombocytopenia (<25,000 platelets/L). If renal or hepatic dysfunction occurred, treatment was stopped until resolution.

Bone marrow aspiration for response assessment was done only if blood counts normalized with no blasts in the peripheral smear. The primary end point of the study was overall survival (OS). OS was defined as the time from recruitment until death from any cause or last follow-up. The secondary objective was to compare adverse events (AEs) and cost-effectiveness of therapy in the two study groups. All the adverse events during treatment were recorded and graded according to National Cancer Institute Common Toxicity Criteria for Adverse Events (version 3.0) with investigators determining the relationship to the study drug. A simplified cost-effectiveness ratio was calculated in which OS was divided by the cost of the chemotherapy (cost including medicines and daycare charges) multiplied by the number of cycles received.

2.1. Statistical Analysis. The patient demographics and baseline clinical characteristics were reported using median and range. Median and range were used to compare number of

Table 1: Patient demographics and baseline clinical characteristics.

Patient characteristics	Decitabine ($N = 15$)	Low-dose cytarabine ($N = 15$)
Age in years (median)	65	62
Sex		
Male, N (%)	12 (80)	12 (80)
Female, N (%)	3 (20)	3 (20)
Duration of symptoms (in months) (median)	2	1
Type of AML		
De novo, N (%)	13 (86.67)	15 (100)
Secondary, N (%)	2 (13.33)	0 (0)
Performance score (ECOG), N (%)		
1	8 (53.3)	5 (33.3)
2	7 (46.7)	10 (66.7)
Bone marrow blasts, N (%)		
20–30%	2 (13.33)	8 (53.3)
30–50%	9 (60)	3 (20)
	4 (26.7)	4 (26.7)
Cytogenetics		
Unsatisfactory	7 (46.7)	8 (53.3)
Normal karyotype	5 (33.3)	6 (40)
Inv(16)	0 (0)	1 (6.7)
Abnormality of chromosome 8	2 (13.3)	0 (0)
Abnormality of chromosome 7	1 (6.7)	0 (0)

cycles received and OS. The Kaplan-Meier method was used to describe OS. Analysis of OS was done by log-rank test. Hazard ratios (HRs) and 95% confidence interval (CI) were calculated by using a Cox regression model. The comparison of toxicity between treatments was reported using count (N) and percentage (%).

3. Results

30 patients were considered for analysis with 15 patients receiving decitabine and 15 patients receiving cytarabine (Table 1). The study observed 12 male patients and 3 female patients in each of the treatment regimes. The mean age was 65, with range of 60–80 years in decitabine group. Similarly, the mean age was 62, with range of 60–73 years in cytarabine group. 86.67% of patients in the decitabine group had de novo AML whereas all the patients in the cytarabine group were de novo in type. Patient demographics and baseline clinical characteristics were well balanced in the two study groups (Table 1). This was a high-risk population as 56% of the patients had ECOG PS 2 and the median blast count in the bone marrow was 40% at baseline.

The patients in both study groups received a median of 4 treatment cycles (Table 2). The median OS was 5.5 for each of the treatment groups. Based on Kaplan-Meier estimates, the mean OS was 5.38 months and 6.27 months, respectively, for

TABLE 2: Comparison of outcomes in the study groups.

Outcome	Decitabine ($N = 15$)	Low-dose cytarabine ($N = 15$)
Number of cycles received		
Median	4	4
Range	(1–7)	(1–14)
Overall survival (in months)		
Median	5.5	5.5
Range	(0.5–13)	(0.5–17.10)
Mean survival time	5.38	6.27
Testing equality of survival distribution		
Log-rank test, P value	0.5586	
Hazard ratio (95% Wald confidence interval)	0.811 (0.390–1.687)	
Toxicity, N (%)		
Febrile neutropenia	5 (33.33)	5 (33.33)
Anemia	8 (53.33)	7 (46.67)
Neutropenia	7 (46.67)	8 (53.33)
Thrombocytopenia	8 (53.33)	8 (53.33)
Mucositis	4 (26.67)	4 (26.67)
Hypocalcemia	3 (20.00)	2 (13.33)
Hypokalemia	2 (13.33)	2 (13.33)
Fatigue	4 (26.67)	5 (33.33)

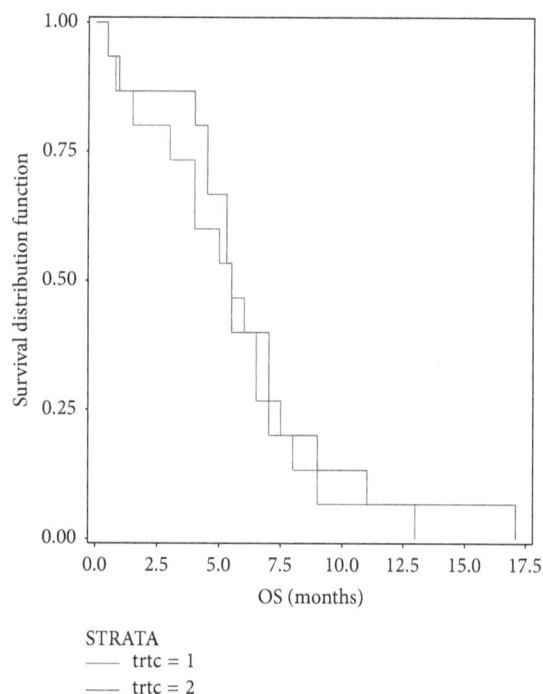

FIGURE 1: Kaplan-Meier survival curve. Treatment 1: decitabine. Treatment 2: low-dose cytarabine.

decitabine and cytarabine group. The comparison of survival distribution between treatment groups showed no significant difference at 5% level (Figure 1). The hazard ratio between the treatment groups was 0.811 with 95% CI of 0.390 to 1.687.

It was observed that 2 deaths in each arm were induction mortality. Median OS was 6.0 months and 5.5 months, respectively, for decitabine and cytarabine group after excluding induction mortality patients (Table 3). The comparison of survival distribution after excluding induction mortality patients between treatment groups observed no significant difference at 5% level. The hazard ratio between the treatments was observed as 0.786 with 95% CI of 0.357 to 1.731 excluding induction mortality patients.

Myelosuppression was the most common toxicity observed in both study groups (Table 2). The most common grade 3 and 4 treatment-related AEs with decitabine and cytarabine were thrombocytopenia (decitabine, 53%; cytarabine, 53%), neutropenia (decitabine, 47%; cytarabine, 53%), and anemia (decitabine, 53%; cytarabine, 46%). Febrile neutropenia occurred in 33% of patients in both study groups. Incidence of mucositis, hypokalemia, and hypocalcemia was similar in both study groups.

Cost per cycle of chemotherapy in INR was 24,200 for decitabine and 1,600 for low-dose cytarabine group (Table 5). Median of total cost of therapy was 96,800 and 6,400 for decitabine and low-dose cytarabine group, respectively. Median of simplified cost-effectiveness ratio was 0.00022 for decitabine group and 0.0034 for low-dose cytarabine group.

4. Discussion

AML is a common disease of the adult age with a peak incidence between 65 and 70 years. Elderly AML is a clinical entity distinct from the AML in younger adults or children. According to recent epidemiological data, ≥75% of patients with AML are ≥60 years old [2].

TABLE 3: Comparison of outcome, excluding induction mortality subjects.

Outcome	Decitabine ($N = 13$)	Low-dose cytarabine ($N = 13$)
Overall survival (in months), excluding induction mortality subjects		
Median	6	5.5
Range	(1.5–13)	(4.0–17.10)
Mean survival time	6.12	7.13
Testing equality of survival distribution		
Log-rank test, P value		0.5311
Hazard ratio (95% Wald confidence interval)		0.786 (0.357–1.731)

TABLE 4: Different dosage and schedules of low-dose cytarabine.

	Baccarani and Tura [10]	Moloney and Rosenthal [11]	Weh et al. [17]	Kantarjian et al. [13]	Bashir et al. [14]	Present study
Dose of cytarabine	$10\,mg/m^2$ 12 hourly for 21 days	$10\,mg/m^2$ 12 hourly for 15 days	$10\,mg/m^2$ 12 hourly for 14–28 days	$20\,mg/m^2$ once a day for 10 days	$20\,mg/m^2$ 12 hourly for 4 days/week	$20\,mg/m^2$ once a day for 10 days
Overall survival (range)				5 months	18 months (3–24 months)	5.5 months (0.5–17.1 months)

TABLE 5: Cost-effectiveness analysis of chemotherapy in the study groups.

	Decitabine	Low-dose cytarabine
Cost per cycle of chemotherapy (INR)	24,200	1,600
Total cost of therapy (median) (INR)	96,800	6,400
Total cost of therapy (mean) (INR)	95,186	7146
Simplified cost-effectiveness ratio (median)	0.00022	0.0034
Simplified cost-effectiveness ratio (mean)	0.00023	0.0039

In patients above 60 years old, AML is an incurable disease with less than 10% of patients being alive at 2 years [3]. Such a dismal outcome has been traditionally explained by the concurrence of comorbidities and biologically poor-risk AML features. In spite of the above facts, population-based studies have demonstrated that IC prolongs survival and ameliorates quality of life in all age groups, as compared to palliative therapy [4]. Nevertheless, only about one-third of elderly patients receive IC [5].

Cytarabine arabinoside is a pyrimidine analogue which acts by false incorporation into DNA causing reiteration of DNA segments. It also inhibits glycoprotein and glycolipid synthesis, thereby altering membrane structure and antigenicity and thus making tumour cells more prone to natural immune mechanisms. Cytarabine induces synthesis of ceramides and transcriptional factors like junfos and junjun and thus helps apoptosis [6–9]. Cytarabine acts at multiple levels which makes it an essential part of all AML treatment regimens, albeit at different dosages and schedule. It has many advantages like subcutaneous route of administration which eliminates the need for hospitalization and is inexpensive. Low-dose cytarabine has been studied by various authors like Baccarani and Tura [10], Moloney and Rosenthal [11], Housset et al. [12], Kantarjian et al. [13], and Bashir et al. [14] for the treatment of AML (Table 4). Bashir et al. [14] used $20\,mg/m^2$ of cytarabine subcutaneously in two divided doses 12 hours apart for 4 days every week for 4 weeks which constituted induction, followed by reassessment. A repeat cycle was administered whenever needed and after attainment of remission, complete or partial. Low-dose cytarabine was continued for 2 days/week as maintenance. 20% of patients achieved complete remission, 30% patients achieved partial remission, and mean duration of survival was 18 months. We chose once-a-day schedule to improve patient compliance and duration of 10 days as used by Kantarjian et al. [13]. In our study, subcutaneous injections of cytarabine were administered by either their primary care physicians or trained attenders of patients. This was convenient for the patients and most patients were compliant with the schedule.

Methylation is involved in silencing the tumor suppressor CCAAT/enhancer binding protein in AML pathogenesis [15]. Decitabine (5-aza-20-deoxycytidine) is a hypomethylating agent with a dual mechanism of action: reactivation of silenced genes and differentiation at low doses and cytotoxicity at high doses. At low "epigenetic" doses, decitabine acts as a hypomethylating agent and inhibits DNA methyltransferase, which appears to have direct cytotoxic effects and/or affect cellular differentiation and apoptosis. In a multicenter, randomized, phase III trial, Kantarjian et al. [13] compared the efficacy and safety of decitabine with treatment choice (TC) in older patients with newly diagnosed AML and poor- or intermediate-risk cytogenetics. Patients ($N = 485$) aged ≥65 years were randomly assigned 1:1 to receive decitabine $20\,mg/m^2$ per day as a 1-hour intravenous infusion for five consecutive days every 4 weeks or TC (supportive care or cytarabine 20 mg/m^2 per day as a subcutaneous injection for 10 consecutive days every 4 weeks). The primary analysis with 396 deaths (81.6%) showed a nonsignificant increase in median OS with decitabine (7.7 months; 95% CI, 6.2 to 9.2) versus TC (5.0 months; 95% CI, 4.3 to 6.3; P = 0.108; hazard ratio [HR], 0.85; 95% CI, 0.69 to 1.04). Our results are similar to this study with both study groups having a similar OS with no statistically significant difference. Though decitabine is useful in the management of elderly patients with AML, it has many disadvantages like intravenous infusions requiring hospitalization and is very expensive.

"Pharmacoeconomics" is an important topic concerning cancer therapy in the developing countries. Pharmacoeconomics is a scientific discipline that compares the difference in the value of one pharmaceutical drug or drug therapy compared to another for their benefit in a particular health condition [16]. It is a branch of health economics which considers the cost (expressed in monetary terms) and effects (expressed in terms of monetary value, efficacy, or enhanced quality of life) of a pharmaceutical product and estimates the cost : benefit ratio of the drug. Pharmacoeconomic studies are helpful in optimal healthcare resource allocation in resource limited settings. A large number of patients suffering from cancer in India belong to low socioeconomic group. These patients present with advanced stage disease and delay treatment due to the high costs involved. The challenge for resource poor countries like India is to devise treatment strategies which will enable a large number of patients to avail themselves of treatment at affordable costs and obtain a substantial benefit.

From the perspective of a developing country, cytarabine scores over decitabine in terms of its cost-effectiveness, given the equal OS benefit and toxicity profile. Moreover, the induction mortality was also similar in both study groups.

Our study is not without limitations. First, being a nonrandomized study, it is prone to selection bias. Second, the sample size is small and a study with a bigger sample size can only substantiate our observations. Third, response assessment was not done at the end of the first cycle of chemotherapy and remission rates were not documented. Also, as we did bone marrow examination for reassessment only if peripheral blood counts normalized, we could have missed many CRi (complete remission with incomplete blood count recovery). Fourth, quality of life of patients was not considered. Fifth, cytogenetic risk stratification was not done. We are planning a further randomized controlled study keeping the above limitations in mind.

To conclude, our study has demonstrated that, in older patients with newly diagnosed AML who are not fit for aggressive chemotherapy, decitabine and low-dose cytarabine are equally efficacious and have similar toxicity profile. Low-dose cytarabine, being inexpensive and easy to administer as outpatient basis, is more cost-effective and appropriate for resource poor settings. Our study has shown that cytarabine given 20 mg/m^2/day for 10-day schedule gives acceptable OS and toxicity profile. Low-dose cytarabine could be a safe, acceptable, accessible, and feasible treatment option for elderly AML patients in developing countries.

5. Conclusions

Management of AML in older patients is a therapeutic challenge. For patients not eligible for intensive chemotherapy, decitabine and low-dose cytarabine should be chosen based on the patient's choice and affordability. Our study has shown that both of these agents have similar OS rates and toxicity profile. Low-dose cytarabine scores over decitabine in developing countries as it is much less expensive and more cost-effective.

Conflict of Interests

The authors declare that there is no conflict of interests regarding the publication of this paper.

References

[1] National Cancer Institute, "Surveillance, Epidemiology, and End Results. SEER Cancer Statistics Review 1975–2005," February 2009, http://seer.cancer.gov/csr/1975_2005/index.html.

[2] G. Juliusson, P. Antunovic, Å. Derolf et al., "Age and acute myeloid leukemia: real world data on decision to treat and outcomes from the Swedish Acute Leukemia Registry," Blood, vol. 113, no. 18, pp. 4179–4187, 2009.

[3] F. R. Appelbaum, H. Gundacker, D. R. Head et al., "Age and acute myeloid leukemia," Blood, vol. 107, no. 9, pp. 3481–3485, 2006.

[4] S. M. Luger, "Treating the elderly patient with acute myelogenous leukemia," ASH Education Book, vol. 2010, no. 1, pp. 62–69, 2010.

[5] J. M. Rowe, "Closer to the truth in AML," Blood, vol. 113, no. 18, pp. 4129–4130, 2009.

[6] G. L. Bianchi Scarrà, M. Romani, D. A. Coviello et al., "Terminal erythroid differentiation in the K-562 cell line by 1-beta-D-arabinofuranosylcytosine: accompaniment by c-myc messenger RNA decrease," Cancer Research, vol. 46, no. 12, pp. 6327–6332, 1986.

[7] G. Juliusson, M. Höglund, K. Karlsson et al., "Increased remissions from one course for intermediate-dose cytosine arabinoside and idarubicin in elderly acute myeloid leukaemia when combined with cladribine. A Randomized Population-Based Phase II Study," British Journal of Haematology, vol. 123, no. 5, pp. 810–818, 2003.

[8] G. Juliusson, P. Antunovic, Å. Derolf et al., "Age and acute myeloid leukemia: real world data on decision to treat and outcomes from the Swedish acute leukemia registry," Blood, vol. 113, no. 18, pp. 4179–4187, 2009.

[9] H. K. Al-Ali, N. Jaekel, and D. Niederwieser, "The role of hypomethylating agents in the treatment of elderly patients with AML," Journal of Geriatric Oncology, vol. 5, no. 1, pp. 89–105, 2014.

[10] M. Baccarani and S. Tura, "Differentiation of myeloid leukaemic cells: new possibilities for therapy," British Journal of Haematology, vol. 42, no. 3, pp. 485–487, 1979.

[11] W. C. Moloney and D. S. Rosenthal, "Treatment of early acute nonlymphoblastic leukemia with low-dose cytosine arabinoside," in Modern Trends in Human Leukemia Cells IV, R. Neth, R. C. Gallo, T. Graf, K. Mannweiler, and K. Winker, Eds., pp. 59–62, Springer, Berlin, Germany, 1981.

[12] M. Housset, M. T. Daniel, and L. Degos, "Small doses of ARA-C in the treatment of acute myeloid leukaemia: differentiation of myeloid leukaemia cells?" *British Journal of Haematology*, vol. 51, no. 1, pp. 125–129, 1982.

[13] H. M. Kantarjian, X. G. Thomas, A. Dmoszynska et al., "Multicenter, randomized, open-label, phase III trial of decitabine versus patient choice, with physician advice, of either supportive care or low-dose cytarabine for the treatment of older patients with newly diagnosed acute myeloid leukemia," *Journal of Clinical Oncology*, vol. 30, no. 21, pp. 2670–2677, 2012.

[14] Y. Bashir, S. Geelani, N. Bashir et al., "Role of low dose cytarabine in elderly patients with acute myeloid leukemia: an experience," *South Asian Journal of Cancer*, vol. 4, no. 1, pp. 4–6, 2015.

[15] S. Agrawal, W.-K. Hofmann, N. Tidow et al., "The C/EBPδ tumor suppressor is silenced by hypermethylation in acute myeloid leukemia," *Blood*, vol. 109, no. 9, pp. 3895–3905, 2007.

[16] R. J. G. Arnold and S. Ekins, "Time for cooperation in health economics among the modelling community," *PharmacoEconomics*, vol. 28, no. 8, pp. 609–613, 2010.

[17] H. J. Weh, R. Zschaber, A. von Paleske, and D. K. Hossfeld, "Treatment of acute myeloid leukemia and myelodysplastic syndrome by low dose cytosine arabinoside," *Haematology and Blood Transfusion*, vol. 29, pp. 60–62, 1985.

5

H. pylori May Not Be Associated with Iron Deficiency Anemia in Patients with Normal Gastrointestinal Tract Endoscopy Results

Tayyibe Saler,[1] Şakir Özgür Keşkek,[2] Sibel Kırk,[1] Süleyman Ahbab,[3] and Gülay Ortoğlu[2]

[1]*Department of Internal Medicine, Umraniye Training and Research Hospital, 34767 Istanbul, Turkey*
[2]*Department of Internal Medicine, Numune Training and Research Hospital, Yüreğir, 01240 Adana, Turkey*
[3]*Department of Internal Medicine, Haseki Training and Research Hospital, 34087 Istanbul, Turkey*

Correspondence should be addressed to Şakir Özgür Keşkek; drkeskek@yahoo.com

Academic Editor: Andreas Neubauer

Background. The aim of this study was to investigate the association between iron deficiency anemia and *H. pylori* in patients with normal gastrointestinal tract endoscopy results. *Materials and Methods.* A total of 117 male patients with normal gastrointestinal tract endoscopy results were included in this retrospective study. The study and control groups included 69 and 48 patients with and without iron deficiency anemia, respectively. The prevalence of *H. pylori*, the number of RBCs, and the levels of HGB, HTC, MCV, iron, and ferritin were calculated and compared. *Results.* There was no statistically significant difference found between the groups according to the prevalence of *H. pylori* (65.2% versus 64.6%, $P = 0.896$). Additionally, the levels of RBCs, HGB, HTC, MCV, iron, and ferritin in the patients in the study group were lower than those in the control group ($P < 0.05$). Finally, there was no association between iron deficiency anemia and *H. pylori* (OR 1.02, Cl 95% 0.47–2.22, and $P = 0.943$). *Conclusion.* *H. pylori* is not associated with iron deficiency anemia in male patients with normal gastrointestinal tract endoscopy results.

1. Introduction

Anemia is the most common disorder of the blood and is characterized by a decrease in the number of red blood cells or a less-than-normal quantity of hemoglobin in the blood. The hemoglobin value below which anemia is defined varies, although the World Health Organization (WHO) hemoglobin thresholds of less than 13 g/dL for men and less than 12 g/dL for women [1] are the most common definitions used for anemia.

Iron deficiency anemia is the most common form of anemia worldwide. It is a global public health problem affecting both developing and developed countries, with major consequences for human health as well as social and economic development. The causes of iron deficiency anemia include inadequate iron intake, chronic blood loss, and impaired iron absorption. Blood loss from the gastrointestinal tract is the most common cause in men and postmenopausal women [2, 3].

Helicobacter pylori is a Gram-negative bacterium that colonizes human gastric mucosa, leading to chronic antral gastritis and peptic ulcer disease. It is also associated with serious diseases, including gastric cancer and gastric mucosa-associated lymphoid tissue lymphoma. *H. pylori* remains one of the most common infections in the world, with an estimated 50% of the world's population being carriers of the bacterium [4, 5].

Previous studies have shown that *H. pylori* colonization of the gastric mucosa may impair iron uptake and increase iron loss, potentially leading to iron deficiency anemia [6, 7]. There have been no studies performed in patients with intact gastric mucosa. Therefore, in this study we aimed to investigate the association between *H. pylori* and iron deficiency anemia in patients with normal gastrointestinal tract endoscopy results.

2. Materials and Methods

For this study, a total of 1251 patient files were analysed. There were 906 patients with sufficient data for this study, but patients with chronic diseases, under 18 years old, diagnosed

TABLE 1: Characteristics of the study and control groups.

	Study group (N = 69)	Control group (N = 48)	P
Age (years)	37.4 ± 10.4	40.2 ± 10.0	0.143
H. pylori N (%)	45 (65.2%)	31 (64.6%)	0.896
RBC (4.2–5.1 × 10⁶/uL)	3.84 ± 0.36	4.69 ± 0.38	<0.001
Hemoglobin (12–15 gr/dL)	9.6 ± 1.3	13.4 ± 0.97	<0.001
HTC (%)	31.9 ± 3.3	40.5 ± 2.7	<0.001
MCV (80–96 fl)	71.5 ± 5.8	85.9 ± 6.2	<0.001
Iron (37–145 μg/dL)	26.1 ± 12	74 ± 27	<0.001
Ferritin (13–150 ng/mL)	5.4 ± 2.8	66.7 ± 51.9	<0.001

TABLE 2: Measurements of patients in study group according to the *Helicobacter pylori* infection.

	H. pylori (+) (N = 45)	H. pylori (−) (N = 24)	P
RBC (4.2–5.1 × 10⁶/uL)	3.89 ± 0.37	4.00 ± 0.35	0.234
Hemoglobin (12–15 gr/dL)	9.5 ± 1.4	9.8 ± 1.2	0.466
HTC (%)	31.5 ± 3.4	32.5 ± 3.0	0.261
MCV (80–96 fl)	71.2 ± 6.1	72.1 ± 5.2	0.546
Iron (37–145 μg/dL)	26.6 ± 13.7	25.0 ± 8.2	0.584
Ferritin (13–150 ng/mL)	5.5 ± 2.5	5.2 ± 3.2	0.439

with anemia other than iron deficiency anemia, abnormal gastrointestinal tract endoscopy results, malignancies, parasitosis, positive fecal occult blood tests, and those taking medications that affect H. pylori, blood levels, or iron levels, as well as females, were excluded. Finally, 117 male patients with normal gastrointestinal tract endoscopy results were included in this study. The study group consisted of 69 patients with iron deficiency anemia, and the control group consisted of 48 patients without anemia. Females were excluded due to a high prevalence of anemia due to other causes, such as menstruation.

Iron deficiency anemia was defined according to the World Health Organization (WHO) criteria [1], which define anemia as a hemoglobin level of <13 g/dL in men and <12 g/dL in women. The definition of iron deficiency anemia was accepted as being when the serum iron was <37 μg/dL and ferritin was <13 ng/mL. The complete blood counts, serum iron levels, and ferritin concentrations of all of the patients were reported, and the peripheral blood samples were evaluated. Additionally, the complete blood counts were measured using the Sysmex XE 2100i (Japan) by fluorescence flow cytometry. The serum iron levels and ferritin concentrations were measured with the Roche C-601 analyser tract (Japan) using an electrochemiluminescence immunoassay at the institute. A Fujinon EG-590 WR HD (Saitama, Japan) model device was used for the gastrointestinal tract endoscopy procedures (esophagogastroduodenoscopy and colonoscopy) in those years at the institute.

Biopsy samples taken from the antrum during the operation were evaluated after being stained with PAS-AB or modified Giemsa by an experienced pathologist. According to the patient files, we reported that the analyses of H. pylori were made via histological examination and the rapid urease test (CLO test: Campylobacter-like organism test). According to the CLO test (Delta West Bentley, WA, Australia), the change in the colour of the test from yellow to red was accepted as a positive result [8]. The prevalence of H. pylori infections, the number of RBCs, and the levels of HGB, HTC, MCV, iron, and ferritin were calculated and compared in both groups.

MedCalc 12.7 software program (MedCalc Belgium) was used for statistical analysis. Categorical measurements were

reported as number and percentage. Quantitative measurements were reported as the mean ± SD (Standard Deviation). Kolmogorov-Smirnov test was used to show the normal distribution of quantitative measurements. Chi square test was used to compare categorical measures and frequency of metabolic syndrome between the groups. t-test or Mann-Whitney U tests were used for comparison of quantitative measurements between the two groups. An odds ratio was used to analyse the degree of association between H. pylori and iron deficiency anemia. The level of statistical significance was set as 0.05 in all tests.

3. Results

The characteristics of the groups are shown in Table 1, and the mean ages are comparable in both groups: 37.4 ± 10.4 and 40.2 ± 10.0 in the study and control groups, respectively (P = 0.143). There was no statistically significant difference between the groups according to the prevalence of H. pylori (65.2% versus 64.6%, resp.; P = 0.896). Not surprisingly, the RBC, HGB, HTC, MCV, iron, and ferritin levels of the patients in the study group were lower than those in the control group. There were no statistically significant differences between the RBC, HGB, HTC, MCV, iron, and ferritin levels in the patients with or without H. pylori infections according to the presence or absence of iron deficiency anemia (P > 0.05; Tables 2 and 3). When we mixed the patients (anemic and nonanemic) and divided them according to the H. pylori infections, we saw that there was no statistically significant difference (P > 0.05; Table 4). Finally, there was no association between iron deficiency anemia and H. pylori (OR 1.02, Cl 95% 0.47–2.22, P = 0.943).

4. Discussion

In this study, we have shown that H. pylori is not associated with iron deficiency anemia in men with normal gastrointestinal tract endoscopy results. Iron deficiency anemia is a common health problem in the general population [1, 2]. Similarly, H. pylori is a common gastrointestinal tract infection that affects a majority of the population. Guidelines on iron deficiency anemia have confirmed the etiological role of H. pylori, but the relationship remains controversial. Some previous studies have reported that H. pylori is associated

TABLE 3: Measurements of patients in control group according to the *Helicobacter pylori* infection.

	H. pylori (+) N = 31	H. pylori (−) N = 17	P
RBC (4.2–5.1 × 10⁶/uL)	4.7 ± 0.35	4.59 ± 0.44	0.351
Hemoglobin (12–15 gr/dL)	13.5 ± 0.97	13.3 ± 0.97	0.402
HTC (%)	40.7 ± 2.6	40.2 ± 2.9	0.535
MCV (80–96 fl)	86.0 ± 6.6	85.9 ± 5.7	0.959
Iron (37–145 μg/dL)	73.9 ± 30.5	75.7 ± 22.5	0.830
Ferritin (13–150 ng/mL)	59.7 ± 43.7	79.4 ± 63.8	0.213

TABLE 4: Measurements of patients according to the *Helicobacter pylori* infection.

	H. pylori (+) N = 76	H. pylori (−) N = 41	P
RBC (4.2–5.1 × 10⁶/uL)	4.2 ± 0.54	4.2 ± 0.46	0.803
Hemoglobin (12–15 gr/dL)	11.1 ± 2.3	11.2 ± 2.0	0.863
HTC (%)	35.3 ± 5.5	35.7 ± 4.8	0.695
MCV (80–96 fL)	77.2 ± 9.6	77.8 ± 8.7	0.747
Iron (37–145 μg/dL)	45.9 ± 32.1	46.0 ± 29.7	0.788
Ferritin (13–150 ng/mL)	27.6 ± 38.5	36.0 ± 54.8	0.949

with iron deficiency anemia; since *H. pylori* colonization in the gastric mucosa may disturb some functions of the mucosa, it leads to a decrease in iron absorption and increases iron loss [6, 7]. This is an excellent description for the results reported in these studies; however, these results may be acceptable only for patients with abnormal gastrointestinal tract endoscopy.

According to our opinion, iron deficiency anemia and *H. pylori* infections may be a coincidence because both of the diseases are highly prevalent. Moreover, there are many causes that lead to iron deficiency anemia, such as malnutrition, vitamin deficiencies, chronic disorders, infections, and conditions associated with chronic blood loss [9, 10]. Therefore, we planned our study in patients with normal gastrointestinal tract endoscopy results and found no association. Furthermore, we have shown no difference between the RBC, HGB, HTC, MCV, iron, and ferritin levels in the patients with or without *H. pylori* infections in both groups. To our knowledge, this is the first study that investigates the association between iron deficiency anemia and *H. pylori* in patients with normal gastrointestinal tract endoscopy. Male gender in this study may constitute a bias; however, we planned this study with males because women have greater risks for iron deficiency anemia and the majority of them are due to menstruation bleeding. Consequently, we could develop incorrect results if we included women in this study.

According to the literature, there are some studies which have shown the benefits of *H. pylori* treatment on iron deficiency anemia. For example, improved iron deficiency was reported after the eradication of *H. pylori* [11, 12]. In Malik et al.'s study, they have shown that the eradication of *H. pylori* resulted in a significantly better response to oral iron supplementation among *H. pylori* infected pregnant women with iron deficiency anemia [11]. Nevertheless, gastrointestinal endoscopy was not performed in this study; additionally, antiulcer treatment was given to the patients in the study group. In another study, Huang et al. reported that *H. pylori* eradication therapy combined with iron administration is more effective than iron administration alone for the treatment of iron deficiency anemia [12]. They also stated that bismuth based triple therapy has a better response in terms of increased hemoglobin and serum ferritin concentrations

than proton pump inhibitor based triple therapy. It is understood that all patients in their study had gastrointestinal problems because they were given bismuth or a proton pump inhibitor based triple therapy. In such cases, iron deficiency anemia is an expected condition due to the impaired mucosa, but in our study all patients had intact mucosa.

Hsiang-Yao et al. studied 882 patients in Taiwan and showed no significant association between chronic *H. pylori* infections and anemia. The sample size of their study was larger, but they did not exclude most of the concomitant conditions. Moreover, gastrointestinal system endoscopy was not performed for all of the patients [13]. Qu et al. performed a meta-analysis of observational studies and randomized controlled trials, and they concluded that iron deficiency anemia could not specifically be related to *H. pylori* infections. Moreover, they did not recommend a strategy of population-based screening and treatment for *H. pylori* infections to prevent iron deficiency anemia [14].

In the present study, iron deficiency in patients with normal gastrointestinal system endoscopy results may be associated with lifestyle, for example, inadequate or improper nutrition and excessive drinking of tea and/or coffee.

The small sample size is a limitation in this study; however, a total of 1251 patient files were analysed at the baseline. We excluded most of the patients due to the wide exclusion criteria, although the wide exclusion criteria may be a strong point for this study.

In conclusion, we can say that *H. pylori* is not associated with iron deficiency anemia in men with normal gastrointestinal tract endoscopy results. However, *H. pylori* may be associated with iron deficiency anemia in patients with impaired gastrointestinal mucosa.

Conflict of Interests

The authors declare that there is no conflict of interests regarding the publication of this paper.

Authors' Contribution

Tayyibe Saler A, B, D, Şakir Özgür Keşkek C, E, D, F, Sibel Kırk B, Süleyman Ahbab B, Gülay Ortoğlu D.

References

[1] World Health Organization, *Worldwide Prevalence of Anemia 1993–2005: WHO Global Database on Anemia*, World Health Organization, Geneva, Switzerland, 2008.

[2] U. D. Bayraktar and S. Bayraktar, "Treatment of iron deficiency anemia associated with gastrointestinal tract diseases," *World Journal of Gastroenterology*, vol. 16, no. 22, pp. 2720–2725, 2010.

[3] N. D. Goldberg, "Iron deficiency anemia in patients with inflammatory bowel disease," *Clinical and Experimental Gastroenterology*, vol. 6, pp. 61–70, 2013.

[4] J. G. Kusters, A. H. M. Van Vliet, and E. J. Kuipers, "Pathogenesis of Helicobacter pylori infection," *Clinical Microbiology Reviews*, vol. 19, no. 3, pp. 449–490, 2006.

[5] A. Sethi, M. Chaudhuri, L. Kelly, and W. Hopman, "Prevalence of *Helicobacter pylori* in a first nations population in Northwestern Ontario," *Canadian Family Physician*, vol. 59, no. 4, pp. e182–e187, 2013.

[6] H. Monzón, M. Forné, M. Esteve et al., "*Helicobacter pylori* infection as a cause of iron deficiency anaemia of unknown origin," *World Journal of Gastroenterology*, vol. 19, no. 26, pp. 4166–4171, 2013.

[7] K. Muhsen and D. Cohen, "Helicobacter pylori infection and iron stores: a systematic review and meta-analysis," *Helicobacter*, vol. 13, no. 5, pp. 323–340, 2008.

[8] L. A. Laine, R. A. Nathwani, and W. Naritoku, "The effect of GI bleeding on *Helicobacter pylori* diagnostic testing: a prospective study at the time of bleeding and 1 month later," *Gastrointestinal Endoscopy*, vol. 62, no. 6, pp. 853–859, 2005.

[9] L. E. Damon, C. Andreadis, and C. A. Linker, *Blood Disorders: Current Medical Diagnosis and Treatment*, McGraw-Hill, New York, NY, USA, 52nd edition, 2014.

[10] J. W. Adamson, "Iron deficiency and other hypoproliferative anemias," in *Harrison's Principles of Internal Medicine*, D. L. Longo, A. S. Fauci, D. L. Kasper, S. L. Hauser, J. L. Jameson, and J. Loscalzo, Eds., pp. 844–851, McGraw-Hill, New York, NY, USA, 18th edition, 2012.

[11] R. Malik, K. Guleria, I. Kaur, M. Sikka, and G. Radhakrishnan, "Effect of Helicobacter pylori eradication therapy in iron deficiency anaemia of pregnancy—a pilot study," *Indian Journal of Medical Research*, vol. 134, no. 8, pp. 224–231, 2011.

[12] X. Huang, X. Qu, W. Yan et al., "Iron deficiency anaemia can be improved after eradication of *Helicobacter pylori*," *Postgraduate Medical Journal*, vol. 86, no. 1015, pp. 272–278, 2010.

[13] S. Hsiang-Yao, K. Fu-Chen, S. Sophie et al., "*Helicobacter pylori* infection and anemia in Taiwanese adults," *Gastroenterology Research and Practice*, vol. 2013, Article ID 390967, 4 pages, 2013.

[14] X.-H. Qu, X.-L. Huang, P. Xiong et al., "Does Helicobacter pylori infection play a role in iron deficiency anemia? A meta-analysis," *World Journal of Gastroenterology*, vol. 16, no. 7, pp. 886–896, 2010.

6

Plasmablastic Lymphoma: A Review of Current Knowledge and Future Directions

Ghaleb Elyamany,[1,2] Eman Al Mussaed,[3] and Ali Matar Alzahrani[4]

[1]Department of Pathology and Blood Bank, Prince Sultan Military Medical City, P.O. Box 7897, Riyadh 11159, Saudi Arabia
[2]Department of Hematology, Theodor Bilharz Research Institute, Egypt
[3]Hematopathology Division, Department of Basic Science, College of Medicine, Princess Nourah Bint Abdulrahman University, Riyadh, Saudi Arabia
[4]Department of Oncology, Prince Sultan Military Medical City, Saudi Arabia

Correspondence should be addressed to Ghaleb Elyamany; ghalebelyamany@yahoo.com

Academic Editor: Elvira Grandone

Plasmablastic lymphoma (PBL) is an aggressive subtype of non-Hodgkin's lymphoma (NHL), which frequently arises in the oral cavity of human immunodeficiency virus (HIV) infected patients. PBL shows diffuse proliferation of large neoplastic cells resembling B-immunoblasts/plasmablasts, or with plasmacytic features and an immunophenotype of plasma cells. PBL remains a diagnostic challenge due to its peculiar morphology and an immunohistochemical profile similar to plasma cell myeloma (PCM). PBL is also a therapeutic challenge with a clinical course characterized by a high rate of relapse and death. There is no standard chemotherapy protocol for treatment of PBL. Cyclophosphamide, doxorubicin, vincristine, and prednisone (CHOP) or CHOP-like regimens have been the backbone while more intensive regimens such as cyclophosphamide, vincristine, doxorubicin, high-dose methotrexate/ifosfamide, etoposide, high-dose cytarabine (CODOX-M/IVAC), or dose-adjusted etoposide, prednisone, vincristine, cyclophosphamide, and doxorubicin (DA-EPOCH) are possible options. Recently, a few studies have reported the potential value of the proteasome inhibitor bortezomib and thalidomide in PBL patients. The introduction of genes encoding artificial receptors called chimeric antigen receptors (CARs) and CAR-modified T cells targeted to the B cell-specific CD19 antigen have demonstrated promising results in multiple early clinical trials. The aim of this paper is to review the recent advances in epidemiology; pathophysiology; clinical, pathologic, and molecular characteristics; therapy; and outcome in patients with PBL.

1. Introduction

Plasmablastic lymphoma (PBL) is a rare lymphoma associated with immunosuppression. It is strongly associated with human immunodeficiency virus (HIV) infection and often occurs within the oral cavity. PBL is also seen in elderly patients with age-associated immunosuppression and other patients receiving immunosuppressive therapy; however, despite its predisposition for the immunocompromised patients, PBL has been diagnosed in immunocompetent patients [1, 2].

This lymphoma is now considered a separate diagnostic entity, distinct from diffuse large B-cell lymphoma (DLBCL), not otherwise specified, in the 2008 World Health Organization (WHO) classification of lymphoid neoplasms [3].

HIV-related lymphomas are frequently associated with EBV. Dual infection with EBV and human herpesvirus 8 (HHV8) has been demonstrated in PBL [4]. Cases of PBL occurring in immunocompetent patients have been documented and increasingly described particularly in HIV-negative patients [5–7].

Since the initial reports of PBL [1], it has been described in several other sites, including the gastrointestinal tract, omentum, lung, nasal and paranasal regions, testes, bones, soft tissue, lymph nodes, bone marrow, skin, and CNS [8–13]. PBL has also been documented to arise from long-standing sacrococcygeal cysts in HIV-positive persons [14].

Although the clinical and pathologic features of this lymphoma are well characterized, its molecular pathogenesis remains poorly understood, partly owing to its rarity [15, 16].

The diagnosis of PBL remains a diagnostic challenge given its rarity, peculiar morphology, and an immunohistochemical profile similar to PCM. Additionally, there is a wide differential diagnosis within the subgroup of DLBCL and PCM with plasmablastic morphology that is still a common problem because of the lack of a distinctive phenotype [17]. Distinction between extramedullary plasmablastic neoplasms remains critical for patient management, and correlation with clinical findings is essential [18].

Currently, very little is known about the molecular characteristics of PBL. Array comparative genomic hybridization (aCGH) involving 16 PBLs demonstrated that the genomic aberration pattern of PBL is more similar to DLBCL than to PCM [19], despite the high degree of immunophenotypical similarity between PBL and PCM [20].

The clinical course of PBL is characteristically aggressive. It is generally associated with early dissemination and poor response to therapy and has a reported median overall survival (OS) time of 15 months [16]. Currently, treatment responses are usually partial and temporary; however, prolonged and durable responses to chemotherapy [14, 21, 22] have been reported.

The main goal of this paper is to systematically review the most recent advances in epidemiology; pathophysiology; clinical, pathologic, and molecular characteristics; therapy; and prognosis in patients with PBL.

2. Epidemiology

PBL is primarily a disease of adults, affecting men more often than women. The M/F ratio is 5.7 : 1 for the oral type and 4 : 1 for the extraoral type [15]. It is strongly associated with HIV infection and, in the setting of HIV infection, the most frequent site of involvement is the oral cavity. It can also affect other extranodal sites with a predilection for mucosal tissues.

PBL has also been reported in HIV-negative persons, particularly those who have immunosuppression. In the last decade, several case reports and series have been published, accounting for 590 cases [23]. PBL involving extraoral sites have been reported in several immunocompetent individuals [24–30].

PBL is a rare entity, thought to account for approximately 2.6% of all AIDS-related lymphomas (ARLs) [31, 32]. It is unclear if the actual incidence of PBL has increased in recent years. The apparent increase in published case reports and series could be a reflection of an increased awareness of PBL among clinicians and pathologists [33]. Furthermore, the actual incidence of PBL not associated with HIV infection has not yet been determined. In a literature review of 228 patients with PBL, 157 patients (69%) were HIV-positive and 71 (31%) were HIV-negative [26]; among HIV-negative patients, 33% of the patients have some form of immunosuppression, most often solid organ transplantation or steroid therapy [15]. The remainder of the HIV-negative patients are apparently immunocompetent. In a recent case series from Korea, none of the patients reported showed evidence of immunosuppression [28].

The majority of patients with PBL are middle-aged adults with a mean age at presentation of 39 years in HIV-positive patients and 58 years in HIV-negative patients [16]. Although the majority of patients are adults, PBL has also been reported in the pediatric age group [24, 34–40]; however, a literature review identified only 17 cases. It is unclear if there is a racial or ethnic predominance in PBL patients. However, cases have been reported in populations from different continents [6]. The median age was 10 years (range 2–17), >80% with advanced stage at presentation and jaw/oral cavity as the most common site of initial disease [41]; however, extranodal locations have also been reported. Prognosis is usually poor, with two reported long-term survivors [41, 42].

The actual prevalence of human herpesvirus 8 (HHV8) infection in PBL is more controversial, possibly depending on the sensitivity of the techniques used. On the basis of available literature HHV8 testing was reported in 27 out of 68 cases, and results were positive in only 4 (14.81%) [43].

3. Pathogenesis

The pathogenesis of PBL is poorly understood and likely determined by the complexity of biological interplays between HIV-related immunodeficiency, molecular events, coinfecting oncogenic viruses, and chronic immune activation [33].

It has been proposed that ARLs may develop along four pathogenetic pathways involving EBV and HHV8 infection, as well as c-MYC, p53, and BCL-6 gene aberrations [44].

The contribution of HIV to PBL pathogenesis might develop through four main mechanisms, the duration and the degree of immunodeficiency or immunosuppression; chronic B-cell proliferation/exhaustion due to chronic antigenic stimulation; loss of immune control of oncogenic herpesvirus as EBV; and an incomplete immune reconstitution or factors unrelated to immune dysfunction [45–50]. Similar to other ARLs, such as Burkitt lymphoma (BL) and immunoblastic and primary effusion lymphoma (PEL), PBL has a strong association with Epstein-Barr virus (EBV) infection, and EBV infection is associated with prevention of apoptosis in B-cells by several mechanisms related to EBV antigens [23, 24].

In HIV-associated PBL, 74% of the cases showed the presence of EBV within the tumor cells [16]. EBV infection has been demonstrated based on the expression of EBV-encoded RNA (EBER) [26]. The association between PBL and HHV8 at this time is unclear.

It has been proposed that Kaposi sarcoma-associated HHV8 may play a relevant role in the pathogenesis of PBL. A few studies have demonstrated expression of HHV8-associated proteins in PBL [51, 52]; however, other studies do not support such an association [30, 53]. Furthermore, it is unclear if these HHV8-associated PBL cases originated from multicentric Castleman disease, which should place them in a different category [54].

Based on immunohistochemical, molecular, and genetic studies, PBL probably develops from postgerminal center, terminally differentiated, active B-cells in transition from immunoblasts to plasma cells [23]. In these processes, there are chromosomal aberrations likely associated with the development of malignancy. A recent study has shown recurring rearrangements involving *MYC* and the immunoglobulin

(a)

(b)

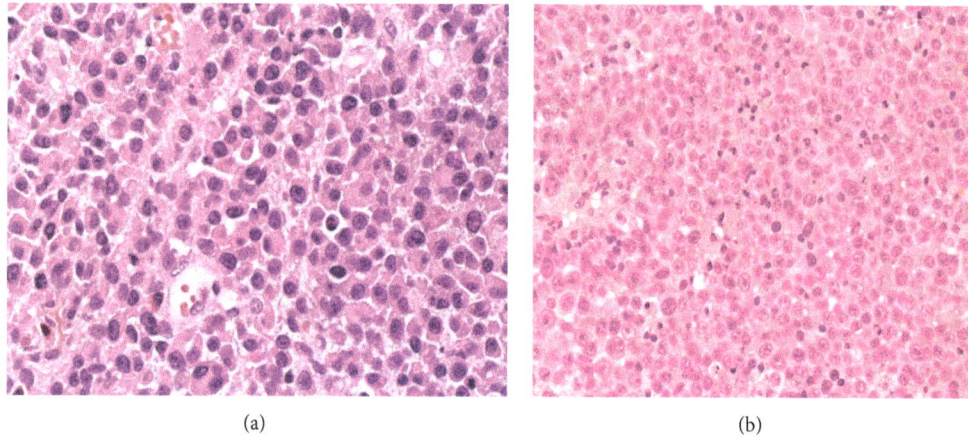

Figure 1: Histopathologic features of PBL: (a) H&E stain shows sheets of large atypical lymphoid cells with plasmacytic differentiation with abundant cytoplasm, paranuclear hof, and large nuclei; (b) it displays large cells with an immunoblastic appearance, with central oval nuclei with prominent nucleoli and moderately abundant cytoplasm.

gene [55]; *MYC* gene rearrangements involving the κ and λ light chain genes and other non-Ig genes have also been described [23]; however, it is not sufficient to cause lymphoma, because low levels of t(8; 14)(q24; q32) have been detected in healthy individuals by using highly sensitive polymerase chain reaction [56]. It has been suggested that aberration of the genes involved in cell cycle regulation may contribute to PBL oncogenesis. Hypermethylation of the *p16* gene has been reported [57], and *MYC* upregulation by translocation between the *MYC* gene and immunoglobulin heavy chain gene (*MYC/IgH*) was reported recently in 3 separate case reports [58].

4. Clinical Features

PBL is characterized for its predilection of involving the oral cavity of HIV-positive individuals as originally described [1]. Following the first report, a number of cases have been reported in extraoral sites, in HIV-positive cases. The most commonly affected sites are the GI tract, lymph nodes, and skin [11, 16]. A similar pattern is seen in patients with HIV-negative PBL, with the oral cavity and GI tract being the most commonly involved sites [39].

The frequency of oral involvement is higher in HIV-positive (58%) than in HIV-negative patients (16%) [26]. Other less common extraoral sites include the CNS [59, 60], paranasal sinus [27, 60], mediastinum, lungs [8, 27, 61], liver [61], and testes [11]. Bone marrow involvement has been reported at 30% in both HIV-positive and HIV-negative patients [26].

No significant differences in age and gender have been reported between oral and extraoral PBL. The peak of incidence for the oral and extraoral types occurs at 41 years (range 7–86 years) and 46 years (range 11–86 years), respectively, and both are more common in males [15].

In both HIV-positive and HIV-negative patients, most present with rapid growing, sometimes destructive, disease

in advanced clinical stage (Ann Arbor stage 3 or 4), with elevated LDH and B symptoms at diagnosis [26, 62].

5. Pathologic Features

5.1. Histologic Findings. The histopathological features are frequently ambiguous, thus rendering the correct diagnosis quite difficult. Diagnosis requires a properly evaluated tissue biopsy of mass lesion or lymph node. Excisional biopsy is the gold standard; however, when the site of the disease is difficult to access, core needle biopsy and fine needle aspiration (FNA) may be performed in conjunction with appropriate ancillary techniques for the diagnosis and differential diagnosis. This type of lymphoma is apparently observed more frequently in the immunodeficiency associated cases.

PBL was first described as a specific clinicopathologic entity by Delecluse and colleagues [1] as an aggressive B-cell lymphoma occurring in the oral cavity arising in the context of HIV infection characterized by sheets of plasmablasts without intermingled plasma cells. The presence of a spectrum of plasmacellular differentiation has been introduced in the following years and is a frequent feature of plasmablastic lymphomas outside the oral cavity [63].

The minimum morphological criteria required to diagnose PBL are monomorphic cellular proliferation of plasmablasts, with either centrally or eccentrically placed nuclei with high nuclear-cytoplasmic ratio, a moderate amount of eosinophilic cytoplasm, a high mitotic index, and the absence of neoplastic plasma cells in the background [33, 64].

Overall, PBL is characterized by cellular proliferation of large atypical cells with immunoblastic, plasmablastic, or plasmacytic features, including eccentric nuclei with a vesicular chromatin, either prominent central nucleolus or peripheral nucleoli, abundant eosinophilic cytoplasm, and a perinuclear hof, in a diffuse sheet-like and cohesive growth pattern (Figure 1). Apoptotic bodies and mitotic figures are frequent, and tingible-body macrophages are easily detectable leading to a starry-sky appearance. Smaller neoplastic cells with

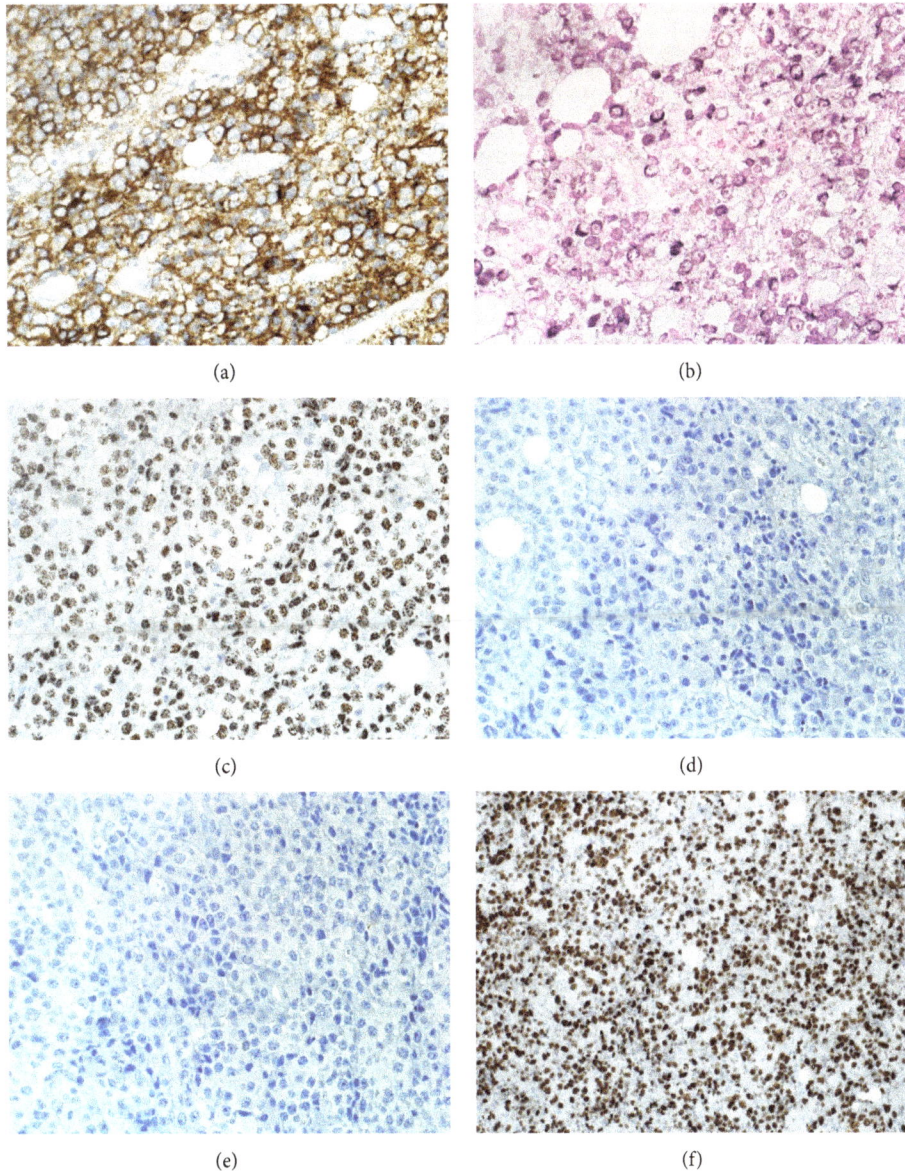

FIGURE 2: Selected immunophenotype of PBL: the PBL cells demonstrate immunoreactivity to CD138 (a), lambda light chain, *ISH* (b), and HHV8 (c) and negativity for CD20 (d) and CD56 (e). Proliferation index is high (f).

obvious plasmacytic differentiation may also be present. Areas of necrosis are occasionally identified [1, 3].

However, these histologic features may be seen in other disorders, such as plasmablastic PCM, BL, DLBCL with plasmacytoid differentiation, PEL, and anaplastic lymphoma kinase- (ALK-) positive DLBCL which make the correct diagnosis challenging [62].

6. Immunophenotype

PBL is a high-grade B-cell lymphoma that arises from postgerminal center B-cell. The hallmark immunohistochemical staining pattern of PBL is that of terminally differentiated B-cell. PBL demonstrates little to no expression of leukocyte common antigen (LCA) or the B-cell markers CD20, CD79a, and PAX5. However, the plasma cell markers VS38c, CD38, multiple myeloma oncogene-1 (MUM1), and CD138 (syndecan-1) seem to be almost universally expressed [3, 16, 32]. PBL is characterized by a high proliferation index reflected by Ki67 expression, usually >80% (Figure 2).

Cytoplasmic immunoglobulins are expressed in near 70% of cases. PBL is also variably positive for CD30, epithelial and endothelial markers such EMA and CD31, posing some problems in differential diagnosis with poorly differentiated solid tumors [65]. PBL usually does not express CD56, distinguishing it from true plasma cell neoplasms. Recently, an immunohistochemistry stain for BLIMP1 and XBP1, markers of terminal B-cell differentiation has been proposed to identify PBL; however this finding remains investigational [45] and these markers are often not routinely available.

7. Genomic Profile

Currently, very little is known about the molecular genetic basis that drives PBL. One study showed that up to 47% of EBV-positive AIDS-related PBLs are marked by C-MYC translocations, which have previously been associated with other ARLs [55, 64].

MYC gene rearrangement is the first recurrent cytogenetic abnormality detected in PBL [55, 62], occurring in approximately 50% of cases. The most common partner for the MYC oncogene is the immunoglobulin gene with translocations most often occurring in the context of complex karyotypes. MYC rearrangements were more often seen in EBV-positive compared to EBV-negative tumors [55].

Chang et al., studied the genomic profile of 16 cases of PBL, 13 cases of AIDS-related DLBCL, 13 cases of non-AIDS-related DLBCL, and eight cases of PCM [19]. Their findings revealed that the genomic aberration pattern of PBL was more closely related to DLBCL than PCM. These findings suggest that PBL is best classified as a DLBCL based on genomic expression criteria despite the high degree of immunophenotypical similarity between PBL and PCM [19].

In contrast, in a series of four PBL patients showed complex cytogenetic changes that were more closely related to PCM [39]. These findings likely represent the molecularly heterogeneous nature of PBL [6]. Interestingly, two different studies reported single cases showing a concomitant IgH and T cell receptor gene rearrangement [57, 66].

8. Differential Diagnosis

The clinical and histopathological features are usually ambiguous, thus rendering the correct diagnosis quite difficult in the absence of an exhaustive integration of clinical, morphological, phenotypic, and molecular features. The diagnosis of such neoplasms could be even more challenging in the setting of extraoral localizations and in immunocompetent patients.

Differential diagnosis with the activated B-cell-like (ABC-like) subgroup of DLBCL and PCM with plasmablastic morphology is still a common problem because of the lack of a distinctive phenotype.

The differential diagnosis includes immunoblastic DLBCL and other lymphoid neoplasms with plasmacytic features such as ALK-positive DLBCL, PEL both classic (body cavity-based) and solid (extracavitary) variants, BL with plasmacytoid differentiation, and plasmablastic plasmacytoma/myeloma (Table 1) [67].

Immunoblastic DLBCL and BL can be excluded on the basis of the characteristic immunophenotypic pattern of PBL with CD20 negativity in combination with positive markers of postgerminal center B-cells and plasma cells, such as CD138/syndecan [1, 9]. CD20 and LCA immunoreactivity is uniformly present with DLBCL and BL and generally absent but may be present in a small proportion of malignant cells in PBL. PBL is distinguished from ALK-positive DLBCL by its lack of expression of the ALK protein, and absence of HHV8 coinfection distinguishes PBL from PEL.

Differentiation from plasmacytoma/myeloma particularly with anaplastic/plasmablastic morphology is the most difficult issue in the differential diagnosis and morphologic distinction is not always possible. In practice, the distinction between PBL and plasmablastic PCM frequently depends on clinical correlation [19]. Detection of paraproteinemia in blood and/or excess light chains (Bence Jones proteins) in urine, lytic bone lesions, and hypercalcemia or anemia favors the diagnosis of PCM over PBL. Immunosuppression, especially HIV-related, is much more frequently associated with PBL as well as the presence of EBV [11]. Of note, PCM and plasmacytoma may occasionally occur in the setting of AIDS [68, 69]. The identification of a *MYC* gene rearrangement can help to distinguish PBL from plasmacytoma as the *MYC* rearrangement is rare in the latter disorder. In addition to lymphoid neoplasms, the diagnosis of PBL can be complicated by its morphologic resemblance to myeloid malignancies particularly extramedullary myeloid tumor which can be excluded by immunohistochemical studies of myeloid markers.

In brief, although there are wide ranging differential diagnoses, the main differential diagnosis considered is extramedullary plasmablastic myeloma. Though difficult, it is clinically important and critical to differentiate between these two entities, as the treatment for the two diseases is significantly different [19].

9. Prognosis

PBL generally has a poor prognosis with most patients dying within 2 years from initial presentation, and long-term survivors are very few. The average survival time reported by Delecluse et al. was a few months, and half of the original 16 patients died within 1 year [1]; however, more recent reports have reported improved survival when treatment with both HAART and appropriate chemotherapy is used, similar to outcomes of HIV-infected patients with other NHLs [21, 22, 40, 70].

Several prognostic factors have been identified in HIV-associated lymphomas. These factors include the International Prognostic Index (IPI) score and CD4$^+$ cell count. Data on prognostic factors in PBL are lacking and these analyses are unlikely to be performed prospectively given the rarity of this malignancy [71]. The identification of prognostic factors in this population may allow a better understanding of the biology of this disease.

A large literature review of treated cases of PBL shows an overall response rate (ORR) to chemotherapy of 77%, with 46% of patients achieving a complete response (CR) and 31% a partial response (PR) [72, 73]. Despite a good ORR to chemotherapy, the median OS is 14 months with a 5-year OS rate of 31% [16]. Of note, these survival data represent a variety of therapeutic approaches in a heterogeneous patient population.

However, in a recent literature review, more intensive regimens have not been shown to confer a survival advantage when compared to CHOP/CHOP-like regimens [72, 73].

Patients carrying MYC/IgH gene rearrangement have been shown to have a very poor median OS of only 3 months. The association of MYC with poor prognosis has been suggested by additional studies [55], but based on the small sample size, it should be considered preliminary.

TABLE 1: The main differential diagnosis of PBL.

Clinical presentation	Frequently oral cavity	Often extranodal (jaws and orbits)	Wide variety of presentations	Involves body cavity	Wide variety of presentations	BM (extramedullary in plasmacytoma)	BM (extramedullary in plasmacytoma)
Immunocompetency	+/−	++	+++	+/−	+	++	++
Association with HIV	+++	++	++	+++	−	−	−
Association with HHV8	+/− (usually −)	−	−	+	−	−	−
LCA	+/−	+	+	+/−	+/−	+/−	+/−
B-cell markers							
CD20	−	+	+	+/−	−	−	−
CD79a	+/− (usually −)	+	+	−	−	+/− (usually −)	+/− (usually −)
CD138	+	−	−	+	−	+	+
CD56	+/− (usually −)	Rare +	Rare +	Rare +	+/−	Usually +	Usually +
Ki67	High >70%	High >90%	High <90%	High >80%	High >80%	Low	High >70%
Other	BLIMP1+	CD10 +	BCL-6 Usually +	CD30 Usually +	ALK+	Serum M-spike CRAB	Serum M-spike CRAB

CRAB: hypercalcemia, kidney disease, anemia, and bone lytic lesions [67].

The use of HAART showed a trend towards statistical significance for a better survival in patients with HIV-associated PBL [73].

It is currently unclear if HIV status alone confers a better prognosis in patients with PBL. In a recent review of the literature, patients with PBL and HIV infection were found to have an OS of 14 months compared to 9 months in HIV-negative patients [26]. A potential explanation for this finding is that the use of HAART may restore immune surveillance to combat the tumor more efficiently. Additionally, other factors, such as extent of disease and performance status, may have also played a role in this difference.

10. Therapy

PBL is a therapeutic challenge with a clinical course characterized by a high rate of relapse and death. A standard therapy has not yet been established. Treatment usually consists of chemotherapy with or without consolidation radiation and hematopoietic stem cell transplantation [74]. Various chemotherapy regimens including cyclophosphamide, doxorubicin, vincristine, and prednisone (CHOP), R-CHOP, and cyclophosphamide, vincristine, doxorubicin, high-dose methotrexate/ifosfamide, etoposide, and high-dose cytarabine (CODOX-M/IVAC) are also possible options [73, 75]. Patients with PBL who were not treated with chemotherapy invariably died with a median survival of 3 months [26]. The presence of MYC translocations in a proportion of patients with PBL justifies a more thorough assessment of more intensive regimens.

Due to the lack of CD20 expression, the use of the anti-CD20 monoclonal antibody rituximab is of uncertain utility and unlikely to be of benefit; however it could be considered if partial expression of CD20 is detected within the malignant cells [33]. Although CHOP therapy is often given to treat PBL [16, 23], standard CHOP seems an inadequate treatment [76].

Intensification of induction chemotherapy with autologous hematopoietic stem cell transplantation (auto-HSCT), thought to be a good option in HIV-negative patients with chemosensitive disease, has also been shown to be feasible in HIV+ patients [77, 78].

In the HIV-infected population, the addition of highly active antiretroviral therapy (HAART) also improves prognosis. In a recent study of 70 patients with HIV-positive PBL treated with chemotherapy, the use of HAART was associated with a statistical trend towards improved survival [73]. Interestingly, HAART without chemotherapy has been associated with spontaneous remissions in a few cases [79, 80].

Due to disappointing response and survival rates, the NCCN guidelines recommend against CHOP in favor of more intensive regimens, such as infusional EPOCH, hyper-CVAD, or CODOX-M/IVAC [75]. However, Castillo and colleagues evaluated treatment outcomes in patients receiving CHOP, CHOP-like, and more intense regimens. They reported no statistical difference in the overall survival between the less and more intensive treatment regimens, although only a quarter of the patients reported in the literature have been treated with more intensive regimens than CHOP [73].

11. New Drugs and Future Directions

Due to the rarity of PBL, there is no current consensual standard therapy available. Lack of standard treatment for PBL and its poor therapeutic outcome suggest that new therapeutic approaches are needed. Novel agents used in myeloma therapy are currently applied to PBL considering that PBL shares many morphologic and immunophenotypic characters with plasmablastic myelomas.

One of the newly emerged therapeutic options for PBL is bortezomib, which is a proteasome inhibitor and a cornerstone in myeloma therapy and relapsed or refractory mantle cell lymphoma [81]. Some studies have reported that the proteasome inhibitor bortezomib alone or in combination with chemotherapy may have an antitumor effect in PBL or overcoming the typical chemoresistance of this disease. For the same reason, the use of lenalidomide has been reported in PBL [33]. In recently published cases, bortezomib has shown promising results in PBL [7, 81–85]. Although most of these responses were not sustained, bortezomib represents a new therapeutic option for PBL. Bibas and colleagues have used bortezomib alone or in combination with chemotherapy in patients with PBL and they reported that the results were promising but failed to show any survival advantage over standard chemotherapy [86]. Despite initial promising results, the drugs were used at case report level and the response with the new agents was transient and should be further explored in larger clinical trials [7, 86, 87].

Owing to improved gene transfer technology, novel adoptive cellular therapies have been developed. Adoptive transfer of tumor-reactive T cells into cancer patients with the intent of inducing a cytotoxic antitumor effector response and durable immunity has long been proposed as a novel therapy for a broad range of malignancies [88, 89] The introduction of genes, adoptive cellular therapy, involves the encoding of artificial receptors known as chimeric antigen receptors (CARs). These CARs are recombinant receptors that comprise an extracellular antigen-targeting domain in conjunction with one or more intracellular T cell signaling domains that can be introduced into T cells by genetic modification to redirect the specificity and function of immune effectors. CAR-modified T cells targeted to the B-cell-specific CD19 antigen have demonstrated promising results in multiple early clinical trials, supporting further investigation in patients with B-cell cancers. Recent preclinical studies support additional genetic modifications of CAR-modified T cells to achieve optimal clinical efficacy using this novel adoptive cellular therapy. However, its use had limited clinical application in the treatment of hematological malignancies. This approach is further limited by complications including a lack of efficient cloned TCR expression [90]. An ongoing study is evaluating the therapeutic value of autologous EBV-specific CAR T cells with CD30 as the target. Potentially, CAR T cells can be directed against EBV antigens in patients with EBV-associated lymphomas including PBL [23].

As reported before approximately 30% of PBL cases express the activation marker CD30 [32, 55] and a recent report showed response to brentuximab vedotin in a patient with CD30-expressing relapsed PBL [91]. More recently, a case series of 3 previously untreated patients with PBL, 2 of them HIV-positive, has shown efficacy with the combination of bortezomib and dose-adjusted EPOCH [92].

12. CNS Prophylaxis

Considering the high risk of progression during the treatment or recurrence during the remission, the use of intrathecal prophylaxis is considered a mandatory part of the systemic treatment [93]. Controlled studies on this field are not available, so the standard procedure has not been defined. However, intrathecal methotrexate or cytarabine are administered at each cycle of chemotherapy, based upon institutional preference [94].

13. Refractory or Relapsed Patients

Treatment in patients with refractory or relapsed HIV-associated PBL is considered palliative although some cases of long-term survival have been described. In general, a more intensive chemotherapy is planned for relapsed patients, and for fit patients intensification of chemotherapy with autologous HSCT may be an option [33].

As the outcome of patients with relapsed or refractory PBL is very poor [73] and the outcome is significantly superior in patients with relapsed NHL who received autologous HSCT compared with those who did not, it seems rational to explore the use of autologous HSCT earlier in the course of disease: at least in the patients with high-risk disease to improve the overall survival (OS) rate [93]. Due to the dismal outcome of salvage chemotherapy, autologous HSCT appears to be feasible and possibly beneficial compared with multiagent chemotherapy in the setting of relapsed and refractory disease [77, 95]. Effectiveness of such therapy was not significantly different between HIV-positive and HIV-negative patients, in terms of treatment-related mortality, opportunistic infections, immune recovery, and OS; however, allogeneic BMT is a more limited option in HIV-positive relapsed PBL [77, 78].

14. Conclusion

PBL has a predilection for immunocompromised individuals based on its prevalence in both HIV-positive patients and in those undergoing solid organ transplantation. PBL is best classified as a form of DLBCL. However, based on immunohistochemical data, PBL is much more similar to PCM. Clinically, it has a predilection for oral cavity involvement, a feature not typically seen in other lymphoid malignancies. Recent studies have shown a high prevalence of MYC translocations that may contribute to its aggressive nature. The pathogenesis has not clearly been defined but is thought to involve dysregulation of terminal B-cell differentiation and apoptosis, potentially via the effects of MYC translocation and EBV infection. Treatment has been centered on CHOP chemotherapy with good response, but poor survival; however, more intensive therapies are recommended. Recent case reports of a good clinical response to bortezomib are encouraging and may provide clues to the underlying pathophysiology of PBL. Finally, it is worthwhile to highlight that no prospective therapeutic trials have been done specifically in patients with PBL.

Conflict of Interests

The authors declare that they have no competing interests.

Acknowledgment

The authors thank Mr. Jon Johnston, Principal Clinical Scientist from Histopathology Lab, for editing this review article.

References

[1] H. J. Delecluse, I. Anagnostopoulos, F. Dallenbach et al., "Plasmablastic lymphomas of the oral cavity: a new entity associated with the human immunodeficiency virus infection," *Blood*, vol. 89, no. 4, pp. 1413–1420, 1997.

[2] N. Medel and A. Hamao-Sakamoto, "A case of oral plasmablastic lymphoma and review of current trends in oral manifestations associated with human immunodeficiency virus infection," *Journal of Oral and Maxillofacial Surgery*, vol. 72, no. 9, pp. 1729–1735, 2014.

[3] H. Stein, N. L. Harris, and E. Campo, "Plasmablastic lymphoma," in *WHO Classification of Tumours of Haematopoietic and Lymphoid Tissues*, S. H. Swerdlow, E. Campo, N. L. Harris et al., Eds., pp. 256–257, IARC Press, Lyon, France, 4th edition, 2008.

[4] O.-J. Lee, K.-W. Kim, and G. K. Lee, "Epstein-Barr virus and human immunodeficiency virus-negative oral plasmablastic lymphoma," *Journal of Oral Pathology & Medicine*, vol. 35, no. 6, pp. 382–384, 2006.

[5] J. J. Liu, L. Zhang, E. Ayala et al., "Human immunodeficiency virus (HIV)-negative plasmablastic lymphoma: a single institutional experience and literature review," *Leukemia Research*, vol. 35, no. 12, pp. 1571–1577, 2011.

[6] J. J. Castillo and J. L. Reagan, "Plasmablastic lymphoma: a systematic review," *TheScientificWorldJournal*, vol. 11, pp. 687–696, 2011.

[7] N. S. Saba, D. Dang, J. Saba et al., "Bortezomib in plasmablastic lymphoma: a case report and review of the literature," *Onkologie*, vol. 36, no. 5, pp. 287–291, 2013.

[8] Y. Lin, G. D. Rodrigues, J. F. Turner, and M. A. Vasef, "Plasmablastic lymphoma of the lung: report of a unique case and review of the literature," *Archives of Pathology and Laboratory Medicine*, vol. 125, no. 2, pp. 282–285, 2001.

[9] R. Chetty, N. Hlatswayo, R. Muc, R. Sabaratnam, and K. Gatter, "Plasmablastic lymphoma in HIV+ patients: an expanding spectrum," *Histopathology*, vol. 42, no. 6, pp. 605–609, 2003.

[10] S. A. Schichman, R. McClure, R. F. Schaefer, and P. Mehta, "HIV and plasmablastic lymphoma manifesting in sinus, testicles, and bones: a further expansion of the disease spectrum," *American Journal of Hematology*, vol. 77, no. 3, pp. 291–295, 2004.

[11] H. Y. Dong, D. T. Scadden, L. de Leval, Z. Tang, P. G. Isaacson, and N. L. Harris, "Plasmablastic lymphoma in HIV-positive patients: an aggressive Epstein-Barr virus-associated extramedullary plasmacytic neoplasm," *The American Journal of Surgical Pathology*, vol. 29, no. 12, pp. 1633–1641, 2005.

[12] L. B. Jordan, A. M. Lessells, and J. R. Goodlad, "Plasmablastic lymphoma arising at a cutaneous site," *Histopathology*, vol. 46, no. 1, pp. 113–115, 2005.

[13] J.-P. Dales, A. Harket, D. Bagnères et al., "Plasmablastic lymphoma in a patient with HIV infection: an unusual case located in the skin," *Annales de Pathologie*, vol. 25, no. 1, pp. 45–49, 2005 (French).

[14] J. Ojanguren, J. Collazos, C. Martínez, J. Alvarez, and J. Mayo, "Epstein-Barr virus-related plasmablastic lymphomas arising from long-standing sacrococcygeal cysts in immunosuppressed patients," *AIDS*, vol. 17, no. 10, pp. 1582–1584, 2003.

[15] P. R. Raviele, G. Pruneri, and E. Maiorano, "Plasmablastic lymphoma: a review," *Oral Diseases*, vol. 15, no. 1, pp. 38–45, 2009.

[16] J. Castillo, L. Pantanowitz, and B. J. Dezube, "HIV-associated plasmablastic lymphoma: lessons learned from 112 published cases," *American Journal of Hematology*, vol. 83, no. 10, pp. 804–809, 2008.

[17] S. A. Jaffar, G. Pihan, B. J. Dezube, and L. Pantanowitz, "Differentiating HIV-associated lymphomas that exhibit plasmacellular differentiation," *HIV and AIDS Review*, vol. 4, no. 3, pp. 43–49, 2005.

[18] C. Thakral, L. Thomas, A. Gajra, R. E. Hutchison, G. C. Ravizzini, and N. Vajpayee, "Plasmablastic lymphoma in an immunocompetent patient," *Journal of Clinical Oncology*, vol. 27, no. 25, pp. e78–e81, 2009.

[19] C.-C. Chang, X. Zhou, J. J. Taylor et al., "Genomic profiling of plasmablastic lymphoma using array comparative genomic hybridization (aCGH): revealing significant overlapping genomic lesions with diffuse large B-cell lymphoma," *Journal of Hematology and Oncology*, vol. 2, article 47, 2009.

[20] F. Vega, C. C. Chang, L. J. Medeiros et al., "Plasmablastic lymphomas and plasmablastic plasma cell myelomas have nearly identical immunophenotypic profiles," *Modern Pathology*, vol. 18, no. 6, pp. 806–815, 2005.

[21] R. Lester, C. H. Li, P. Phillips et al., "Improved outcome of human immunodeficiency virus-associated plasmablastic lymphoma of the oral cavity in the era of highly active antiretroviral therapy: a report of two cases," *Leukemia and Lymphoma*, vol. 45, no. 9, pp. 1881–1885, 2004.

[22] G. Panos, E. A. Karveli, O. Nikolatou, and M. E. Falagas, "Prolonged survival of an HIV-infected patient with plasmablastic lymphoma of the oral cavity," *The American Journal of Hematology*, vol. 82, no. 8, pp. 761–765, 2007.

[23] J. J. Castillo, M. Bibas, and R. N. Miranda, "The biology and treatment of plasmablastic lymphoma," *Blood*, vol. 125, no. 15, pp. 2323–2330, 2015.

[24] J. Morscio, D. Dierickx, J. Nijs et al., "Clinicopathologic comparison of plasmablastic lymphoma in HIV-positive, immunocompetent, and posttransplant patients: single-center series of 25 cases and meta-analysis of 277 reported cases," *The American Journal of Surgical Pathology*, vol. 38, no. 7, pp. 875–886, 2014.

[25] K. G. Babu, M. C. S. Babu, L. J. Abraham et al., "Plasmablastic lymphoma: does prognosis differ with HIV status and site of disease?" *Oncology, Gastroenterology and Hepatology Reports*, vol. 3, no. 2, pp. 25–29, 2014.

[26] J. J. Castillo, E. S. Winer, D. Stachurski et al., "Clinical and pathological differences between human immunodeficiency virus-positive and human immunodeficiency virus-negative patients with plasmablastic lymphoma," *Leukemia and Lymphoma*, vol. 51, no. 11, pp. 2047–2053, 2010.

[27] L. Colomo, F. Loong, S. Rives et al., "Diffuse large B-cell lymphomas with plasmablastic differentiation represent a heterogeneous group of disease entities," *American Journal of Surgical Pathology*, vol. 28, no. 6, pp. 736–747, 2004.

[28] J. E. Kim, Y. A. Kim, W. Y. Kim et al., "Human immunodeficiency virus-negative plasmablastic lymphoma in Korea," *Leukemia and Lymphoma*, vol. 50, no. 4, pp. 582–587, 2009.

[29] M. A. Scheper, N. G. Nikitakis, R. Fernandes, C. D. Gocke, R. A. Ord, and J. J. Sauk, "Oral plasmablastic lymphoma in an HIV-negative patient: a case report and review of the literature," *Oral Surgery, Oral Medicine, Oral Pathology, Oral Radiology and Endodontology*, vol. 100, no. 2, pp. 198–206, 2005.

[30] J. Teruya-Feldstein, E. Chiao, D. A. Filippa et al., "CD20-negative large-cell lymphoma with plasmablastic features: a clinically heterogenous spectrum in both HIV-positive and -negative patients," *Annals of Oncology*, vol. 15, no. 11, pp. 1673–1679, 2004.

[31] A. Carbone and A. Gloghini, "Plasmablastic lymphoma: one or more entities?" *American Journal of Hematology*, vol. 83, no. 10, pp. 763–764, 2008.

[32] G. S. Folk, S. L. Abbondanzo, E. L. Childers, and R. D. Foss, "Plasmablastic lymphoma: a clinicopathologic correlation," *Annals of Diagnostic Pathology*, vol. 10, no. 1, pp. 8–12, 2006.

[33] M. Bibas and J. J. Castillo, "Current knowledge on HIV-associated plasmablastic lymphoma," *Mediterranean Journal of Hematology and Infectious Diseases*, vol. 6, no. 1, Article ID e2014064, 2014.

[34] S. Apichai, A. Rogalska, I. Tzvetanov, Z. Asma, E. Benedetti, and S. Gaitonde, "Multifocal cutaneous and systemic plasmablastic lymphoma in an infant with combined living donor small bowel and liver transplant," *Pediatric Transplantation*, vol. 13, no. 5, pp. 628–631, 2009.

[35] P. Chabay, E. De Matteo, M. Lorenzetti et al., "Vulvar plasmablastic lymphoma in a HIV-positive child: a novel extraoral localisation," *Journal of Clinical Pathology*, vol. 62, no. 7, pp. 644–646, 2009.

[36] A. Gogia and S. Bakhshi, "Plasmablastic lymphoma of oral cavity in a HIV-negative child," *Pediatric Blood & Cancer*, vol. 55, no. 2, pp. 390–391, 2010.

[37] C. Hernandez, A. S. Cetner, and E. L. Wiley, "Cutaneous presentation of plasmablastic post-transplant lymphoproliferative disorder in a 14-month-old," *Pediatric Dermatology*, vol. 26, no. 6, pp. 713–716, 2009.

[38] R. Radhakrishnan, S. Suhas, R. V. Kumar, G. Krishnanand, R. Srinivasan, and N. N. Rao, "Plasmablastic lymphoma of the oral cavity in an HIV-positive child," *Oral Surgery, Oral Medicine, Oral Pathology, Oral Radiology and Endodontology*, vol. 100, no. 6, pp. 725–731, 2005.

[39] J. J. Castillo, E. S. Winer, D. Stachurski et al., "HIV-negative plasmablastic lymphoma: not in the mouth," *Clinical Lymphoma, Myeloma and Leukemia*, vol. 11, no. 2, pp. 185–189, 2011.

[40] A. Sharma, T. V. S. V. G. K. Tilak, R. Lodha, M. C. Sharma, and D. Dabkara, "Long-term survivor of human immunodeficiency virus-associated plasmablastic lymphoma," *Indian Journal of Medical and Paediatric Oncology*, vol. 34, no. 2, pp. 96–98, 2013.

[41] J. I. Vaubell, Y. Sing, A. Ramburan et al., "Pediatric plasmablastic lymphoma: a clinicopathologic study," *International Journal of Surgical Pathology*, vol. 22, no. 7, pp. 607–616, 2014.

[42] S. Pather, D. MacKinnon, and R. S. Padayachee, "Plasmablastic lymphoma in pediatric patients: clinicopathologic study of three cases," *Annals of Diagnostic Pathology*, vol. 17, no. 1, pp. 80–84, 2013.

[43] S. C. Sarode, G. S. Sarode, and A. Patil, "Plasmablastic lymphoma of the oral cavity: a review," *Oral Oncology*, vol. 46, no. 3, pp. 146–153, 2010.

[44] A. Carbone, "Emerging pathways in the development of AIDS-related lymphomas," *The Lancet Oncology*, vol. 4, no. 1, pp. 22–29, 2003.

[45] S. Montes-Moreno, A.-R. Gonzalez-Medina, S.-M. Rodriguez-Pinilla et al., "Aggressive large B-cell lymphoma with plasma cell differentiation: immunohistochemical characterization of plasmablastic lymphoma and diffuse large B-cell lymphoma with partial plasmablastic phenotype," *Haematologica*, vol. 95, no. 8, pp. 1342–1349, 2010.

[46] M. Bibas and A. Antinori, "EBV and HIV-related lymphoma," *Mediterranean Journal of Hematology and Infectious Diseases*, vol. 1, no. 2, Article ID e2009032, 2009.

[47] S. C. Boy, M. B. van Heerden, C. Babb, W. F. van Heerden, and P. Willem, "Dominant genetic aberrations and coexistent EBV infection in HIV-related oral plasmablastic lymphomas," *Oral Oncology*, vol. 47, no. 9, pp. 883–887, 2011.

[48] J. J. Castillo, M. Furman, B. E. Beltrán et al., "Human immunodeficiency virus-associated plasmablastic lymphoma: poor prognosis in the era of highly active antiretroviral therapy," *Cancer*, vol. 118, no. 21, pp. 5270–5277, 2012.

[49] A. Carbone, E. Cesarman, M. Spina, A. Gloghini, and T. F. Schulz, "HIV-associated lymphomas and gamma-herpesviruses," *Blood*, vol. 113, no. 6, pp. 1213–1224, 2009.

[50] A. Carbone and A. Gloghini, "KSHV/HHV8-associated lymphomas," *British Journal of Haematology*, vol. 140, no. 1, pp. 13–24, 2008.

[51] A. M. Cioc, C. Allen, J. R. Kalmar, S. Suster, R. Baiocchi, and G. J. Nuovo, "Oral plasmablastic lymphomas in AIDS patients are associated with human herpesvirus 8," *The American Journal of Surgical Pathology*, vol. 28, no. 1, pp. 41–46, 2004.

[52] S. Verma, G. J. Nuovo, P. Porcu, R. A. Baiocchi, A. N. Crowson, and C. M. Magro, "Epstein-Barr virus- and human herpesvirus 8-associated primary cutaneous plasmablastic lymphoma in the setting of renal transplantation," *Journal of Cutaneous Pathology*, vol. 32, no. 1, pp. 35–39, 2005.

[53] R. S. D. Brown, D. A. Power, H. F. Spittle, and K. J. Lankester, "Absence of immunohistochemical evidence for human herpesvirus 8 (HHV8) in oral cavity plasmablastic lymphoma in an HIV-positive man," *Clinical Oncology*, vol. 12, article 194, 2000.

[54] P. G. Isaacson, E. Campo, and N. L. Harris, "Large B-cell lymphoma arising in HHV8-associated multicentric Castleman disease," in *WHO Classification of Tumours of Haematopoietic and Lymphoid Tissues*, S. H. Swerdlow, E. Campo, N. L. Harris et al., Eds., IARC Press, Lyon, France, 4th edition, 2008.

[55] A. Valera, O. Balagué, L. Colomo et al., "IG/MYC rearrangements are the main cytogenetic alteration in plasmablastic lymphomas," *The American Journal of Surgical Pathology*, vol. 34, no. 11, pp. 1686–1694, 2010.

[56] S. Janz, M. Potter, and C. S. Rabkin, "Lymphoma- and leukemia-associated chromosomal translocations in healthy individuals," *Genes Chromosomes and Cancer*, vol. 36, no. 3, pp. 211–223, 2003.

[57] J. L. Arbiser, K. P. Mann, E. M. Losken et al., "Presence of p16 hypermethylation and Epstein-Barr virus infection in transplant-associated hematolymphoid neoplasm of the skin," *Journal of the American Academy of Dermatology*, vol. 55, no. 5, pp. 794–798, 2006.

[58] A. Hassan, F. Kreisel, L. Gardner, J. S. Lewis Jr., and S. K. El-Mofty, "Plasmablastic lymphoma of head and neck: report of two new cases and correlation with c-myc and IgVH gene mutation status," *Head and Neck Pathology*, vol. 1, no. 2, pp. 150–155, 2007.

[59] S. Shuangshoti, T. Assanasen, S. Lerdlum, T. Srikijvilaikul, T. Intragumtornchai, and P. S. Thorner, "Primary central nervous system plasmablastic lymphoma in AIDS," *Neuropathology and Applied Neurobiology*, vol. 34, no. 2, pp. 245–247, 2008.

[60] C. Ustun, M. Reid-Nicholson, A. Nayak-Kapoor et al., "Plasmablastic lymphoma: CNS involvement, coexistence of other malignancies, possible viral etiology, and dismal outcome," *Annals of Hematology*, vol. 88, no. 4, pp. 351–358, 2009.

[61] S. C. Sarode, G. A. Zarkar, R. S. Desai, V. S. Sabane, and M. A. Kulkarni, "Plasmablastic lymphoma of the oral cavity in an HIV-positive patient: a case report and review of literature,"

International Journal of Oral and Maxillofacial Surgery, vol. 38, no. 9, pp. 993–999, 2009.

[62] A. M. Bogusz, A. C. Seegmiller, R. Garcia, P. Shang, R. Ashfaq, and W. Chen, "Plasmablastic lymphomas with MYC/IgH rearrangement: report of three cases and review of the literature," *American Journal of Clinical Pathology*, vol. 132, no. 4, pp. 597–605, 2009.

[63] D. Hansra, N. Montague, A. Stefanovic et al., "Oral and extraoral plasmablastic lymphoma: similarities and differences in clinicopathologic characteristics," *The American Journal of Clinical Pathology*, vol. 134, no. 5, pp. 710–719, 2010.

[64] S. Kane, A. Khurana, G. Parulkar et al., "Minimum diagnostic criteria for plasmablastic lymphoma of oral/sinonasal region encountered in a tertiary cancer hospital of a developing country," *Journal of Oral Pathology and Medicine*, vol. 38, no. 1, pp. 138–144, 2009.

[65] A. Carbone, E. Vaccher, A. Gloghini et al., "Diagnosis and management of lymphomas and other cancers in HIV-infected patients," *Nature Reviews Clinical Oncology*, vol. 11, no. 4, pp. 223–238, 2014.

[66] A. Tzankov, T. Brunhuber, A. Gschwendtner, and A. Brunner, "Incidental oral plasmablastic lymphoma with aberrant expression of CD4 in an elderly HIV-negative patient: how a gingival polyp can cause confusion," *Histopathology*, vol. 46, no. 3, pp. 348–350, 2005.

[67] G. Elyamany, A. M. Alzahrani, M. Aljuboury et al., "Clinicopathologic features of plasmablastic lymphoma: single-center series of 8 cases from Saudi Arabia," *Diagnostic Pathology*, vol. 10, no. 1, article 78, 2015.

[68] A. S. Fiorino and B. Atac, "Paraproteinemia, plasmacytoma, myeloma and HIV infection," *Leukemia*, vol. 11, no. 12, pp. 2150–2156, 1997.

[69] S. Kumar, D. Kumar, V. J. Schnadig, P. Selvanayagam, and D. P. Slaughter, "Plasma cell myeloma in patients who are HIV-positive," *American Journal of Clinical Pathology*, vol. 102, no. 5, pp. 633–639, 1994.

[70] S. D. Nasta, G. M. Carrum, I. Shahab, N. A. Hanania, and M. M. Udden, "Regression of a plasmablastic lymphoma in a patient with HIV on highly active antiretroviral therapy," *Leukemia & Lymphoma*, vol. 43, no. 2, pp. 423–426, 2002.

[71] N. Mounier, M. Spina, J. Gabarre et al., "AIDS-related non-Hodgkin lymphoma: final analysis of 485 patients treated with risk-adapted intensive chemotherapy," *Blood*, vol. 107, no. 10, pp. 3832–3840, 2006.

[72] J. J. Castillo, "Plasmablastic lymphoma: are more intensive regimens needed?" *Leukemia Research*, vol. 35, no. 12, pp. 1547–1548, 2011.

[73] J. J. Castillo, E. S. Winer, D. Stachurski et al., "Prognostic factors in chemotherapy-treated patients with HIV-associated plasmablastic lymphoma," *The Oncologist*, vol. 15, no. 3, pp. 293–299, 2010.

[74] C. Saraceni, N. Agostino, D. B. Cornfield, and R. Gupta, "Plasmablastic lymphoma of the maxillary sinus in an HIV-negative patient: a case report and literature review," *SpringerPlus*, vol. 2, no. 1, article 142, 2013.

[75] NCCN Practice Guidelines in Oncology, AIDS-related B-cell lymphomas (AIDS-2), November 2010, http://www.nccn.org/professionals/physician_gls/PDF/nhl.pdf.

[76] National Comprehensive Cancer Network guidelines in Oncology NHL version 2, 2014, http://www.nccn.org/professionals/physician_gls/pdf/nhl.pdf.

[77] M. M. Al-Malki, J. J. Castillo, J. M. Sloan, and A. Re, "Hematopoietic cell transplantation for plasmablastic lymphoma: a review," *Biology of Blood and Marrow Transplantation*, vol. 20, no. 12, pp. 1877–1884, 2014.

[78] K. Dunleavy and W. H. Wilson, "How I treat HIV-associated lymphoma," *Blood*, vol. 119, no. 14, pp. 3245–3255, 2012.

[79] R. Armstrong, J. Bradrick, and Y.-C. Liu, "Spontaneous regression of an HIV-associated plasmablastic lymphoma in the oral cavity: a case report," *Journal of Oral and Maxillofacial Surgery*, vol. 65, no. 7, pp. 1361–1364, 2007.

[80] M. Gilaberte, F. Gallardo, B. Bellosillo et al., "Recurrent and self-healing cutaneous monoclonal plasmablastic infiltrates in a patient with AIDS and Kaposi sarcoma," *British Journal of Dermatology*, vol. 153, no. 4, pp. 828–832, 2005.

[81] C. Cao, T. Liu, H. Zhu, L. Wang, S. Kai, and B. Xiang, "Bortezomib-contained chemotherapy and thalidomide combined with CHOP (Cyclophosphamide, Doxorubicin, Vincristine, and Prednisone) play promising roles in plasmablastic lymphoma: a case report and literature review," *Clinical Lymphoma Myeloma and Leukemia*, vol. 14, no. 5, pp. e145–e150, 2014.

[82] M. Yan, Z. Dong, F. Zhao et al., "CD20-positive plasmablastic lymphoma with excellent response to bortezomib combined with rituximab," *European Journal of Haematology*, vol. 93, no. 1, pp. 77–80, 2014.

[83] C. A. Dasanu, F. Bauer, I. Codreanu, P. Padmanabhan, and M. Rampurwala, "Plasmablastic haemato-lymphoid neoplasm with a complex genetic signature of Burkitt lymphoma responding to bortezomib," *Hematological Oncology*, vol. 31, no. 3, pp. 164–166, 2013.

[84] M. Lipstein, O. O'Connor, F. Montanari, L. Paoluzzi, D. Bongero, and G. Bhagat, "Bortezomib-induced tumor lysis syndrome in a patient with HIV-negative plasmablastic lymphoma," *Clinical Lymphoma, Myeloma & Leukemia*, vol. 10, no. 5, pp. E43–E46, 2010.

[85] P. Bose, C. Thompson, D. Gandhi, B. Ghabach, and H. Ozer, "AIDS-related plasmablastic lymphoma with dramatic, early response to bortezomib," *European Journal of Haematology*, vol. 82, no. 6, pp. 490–492, 2009.

[86] M. Bibas, S. Grisetti, L. Alba, G. Picchi, F. Del Nonno, and A. Antinori, "Patient with HIV-associated plasmablastic lymphoma responding to bortezomib alone and in combination with dexamethasone, gemcitabine, oxaliplatin, cytarabine, and pegfilgrastim chemotherapy and lenalidomide alone," *Journal of Clinical Oncology*, vol. 28, no. 34, pp. e704–e708, 2010.

[87] P. H. Wiernik, I. S. Lossos, J. M. Tuscano et al., "Lenalidomide monotherapy in relapsed or refractory aggressive non-Hodgkin's lymphoma," *Journal of Clinical Oncology*, vol. 26, no. 30, pp. 4952–4957, 2008.

[88] R. J. Brentjens and K. J. Curran, "Novel cellular therapies for leukemia: CAR-modified T cells targeted to the CD19 antigen," *Hematology*, vol. 2012, no. 1, pp. 143–151, 2012.

[89] C. J. Turtle, "Chimeric antigen receptor modified T cell therapy for B cell malignancies," *International Journal of Hematology*, vol. 99, no. 2, pp. 132–140, 2014.

[90] A. Jorritsma, R. Schotte, M. Coccoris, M. A. de Witte, and T. N. M. Schumacher, "Prospects and limitations of T cell receptor gene therapy," *Current Gene Therapy*, vol. 11, no. 4, pp. 276–287, 2011.

[91] B. M. Holderness, S. Malhotra, N. B. Levy, and A. V. Danilov, "Brentuximab vedotin demonstrates activity in a patient with

plasmablastic lymphoma arising from a background of chronic lymphocytic leukemia," *Journal of Clinical Oncology*, vol. 31, no. 12, pp. e197–e199, 2013.

[92] J. J. Castillo, J. L. Reagan, W. M. Sikov, and E. S. Winer, "Bortezomib in combination with infusional dose-adjusted EPOCH for the treatment of plasmablastic lymphoma," *British Journal of Haematology*, vol. 169, no. 3, pp. 352–355, 2015.

[93] M. Spina, E. Chimienti, F. Martellotta et al., "Phase 2 study of intrathecal, long-acting liposomal cytarabine in the prophylaxis of lymphomatous meningitis in human immunodeficiency virus-related non-Hodgkin lymphoma," *Cancer*, vol. 116, no. 6, pp. 1495–1501, 2010.

[94] A. Re, M. Michieli, S. Casari et al., "High-dose therapy and autologous peripheral blood stem cell transplantation as salvage treatment for AIDS-related lymphoma: long-term results of the Italian Cooperative Group on AIDS and Tumors (GICAT) study with analysis of prognostic factors," *Blood*, vol. 114, no. 7, pp. 1306–1313, 2009.

[95] C. Cattaneo, H. Finel, G. McQuaker, E. Vandenberghe, G. Rossi, and P. Dreger, "Autologous hematopoietic stem cell transplantation for plasmablastic lymphoma: the European society for blood and marrow transplantation experience," *Biology of Blood and Marrow Transplantation*, vol. 21, no. 6, pp. 1146–1147, 2015.

7

Evaluation of Ferric and Ferrous Iron Therapies in Women with Iron Deficiency Anaemia

Ilhami Berber,[1] **Halit Diri,**[2] **Mehmet Ali Erkurt,**[1] **Ismet Aydogdu,**[1] **Emin Kaya,**[1] **and Irfan Kuku**[1]

[1] *Division of Hematology, Department of Hematology, Faculty of Medicine, Medical School, Inonu University, 44280 Malatya, Turkey*
[2] *Department of Internal Medicine, Medical School, Inonu University, 44280 Malatya, Turkey*

Correspondence should be addressed to Ilhami Berber; drilhamiberber@gmail.com

Academic Editor: Meral Beksac

Introduction. Different ferric and ferrous iron preparations can be used as oral iron supplements. Our aim was to compare the effects of oral ferric and ferrous iron therapies in women with iron deficiency anaemia. *Methods.* The present study included 104 women diagnosed with iron deficiency anaemia after evaluation. In the evaluations performed to detect the aetiology underlying the iron deficiency anaemia, it was found and treated. After the detection of the iron deficiency anaemia aetiology and treatment of the underlying aetiology, the ferric group consisted of 30 patients treated with oral ferric protein succinylate tablets (2×40 mg elemental iron/day), and the second group consisted of 34 patients treated with oral ferrous glycine sulphate tablets (2×40 mg elemental iron/day) for three months. In all patients, the following laboratory evaluations were performed before beginning treatment and after treatment. *Results.* The mean haemoglobin and haematocrit increases were 0.95 g/dL and 2.62% in the ferric group, while they were 2.25 g/dL and 5.91% in the ferrous group, respectively. A significant difference was found between the groups regarding the increase in haemoglobin and haematocrit values ($P < 0.05$). *Conclusion.* Data are submitted on the good tolerability, higher efficacy, and lower cost of the ferrous preparation used in our study.

1. Introduction

Iron deficiency is defined as the state in which the body iron is lower than the amount that is sufficient to maintain normal haemoglobin production and normal functions of iron-containing enzymes. Iron deficiency anaemia (IDA) is an important public health concern worldwide, particularly in developing countries in which nutritional problems are more common. Since this is the most frequent reason for anaemia, it should be kept in mind in the differential diagnosis of patients with anaemia. The cause of IDA is the failure of iron intake from food to meet the iron requirements of the body, and it is most commonly seen in women. Menstrual bleeding, pregnancy, abortion, and curettage are the most commonly encountered etiological causes of iron deficiency in women [1–3].

The reduced form (ferrous) is required for iron absorption, and the effects of reduced substances, such as ascorbate or succinate, on the iron valance (reduction of ferric iron) improve iron absorption. Phytates in cereals, tannins in tea, polyphenols in wine, antacids in milk, oxalate, and some antibiotics (tetracycline, e.g.) can form complexes with iron which do not resolve in water and can impede iron absorption [4, 5]. Achlorhydria, malabsorption states, and bypass through a gastrojejunostomy can cause iron deficiencies [6, 7].

To maintain the iron balance, 1.0–1.5 mg of iron absorption is required daily for men. However, an average of 60 mL/month of iron loss occurs in women during their menstrual cycles, and there is 0.4 mg of iron per millilitre of blood. Thus, women require an additional iron supplementation of approximately 30 mg per month. There is a tendency towards a decrease in iron storage during pregnancy, due to the increased maternal blood volume and the additional iron requirement for fetal haemoglobin synthesis. Therefore, the daily iron requirement increases to 5-6 mg/day during pregnancy. The most common cause of IDA is blood loss for both men and women, and the most frequent reasons for blood loss are gastrointestinal bleeding in men and menstrual bleeding in women. In menopausal women, the cause of IDA is the gastrointestinal system, unless proven otherwise. The gastrointestinal system should be evaluated in patients with IDA, even in the absence of a positive stool guaiac test or melena. IDA can be the first finding in right colon tumours or other occult cancers of the colon [8, 9].

For IDA treatment, the goals are to treat the underlying cause, correct the anaemia, and fill the iron stores. For this purpose, oral agents are generally preferred because of their ease of usage, low rate of adverse effects, and effectiveness. The routine approach in IDA management is to restore haemoglobin and haematocrit values by using full doses of oral agents over 3 months, followed by half doses over additional 3 months in order to replace the stored iron. Ferrous (Fe^{+2}) and ferric (Fe^{+3}) iron preparations are both used as oral agents [8–10]. However, Raja et al. and Jacobs reported that the absorption of Fe^{+2} iron from the intestine is 3 times higher than that of Fe^{+3} iron [4, 5].

Dose-dependent adverse effects, such as nausea, vomiting, abdominal pain, diarrhea, and constipation, can occur during the treatment of IDA by oral agents; however, these adverse events are rarely severe enough to discontinue the supplements. Symptomatic treatment, dose reduction, or ingestion after meals can generally relieve these adverse effects [10].

Iron therapy generally relieves fatigue and weakness within the first week, but reticulocytosis does not occur until 7–10 days after therapy begins. No elevation is seen in the haemoglobin level until 2 to 2.5 weeks after therapy, and a few months are needed to achieve normal haemoglobin values. Ferritin levels should be measured after the reconstruction of iron storages [11].

The aim of the present study was to evaluate Fe^{+3} and Fe^{+2} iron therapies in IDA treatment in women with regard to adverse events and efficiency. Using more effective and less expensive agents in IDA management will lead to rapid recovery and decreased costs.

2. Materials and Methods

The present study included 104 women who presented at the Haematology Outpatient Clinic of Inonu University School of Medicine and were diagnosed with iron deficiency anaemia after evaluation. The Fe^{+3} group ($n = 54$) received an oral Fe^{+3} protein succinylate flacon, while the second group ($n = 50$) received oral Fe^{+2} glycine sulphate tablets to be taken for 3 months.

In all patients, the following iron laboratory evaluations were performed before treatment began: complete blood count (CBC), serum iron level, total iron binding capacity (TIBC), transferrin saturation, serum ferritin level, and stool guaiac test, as well as parasite evaluations if necessary. Transferrin saturation was estimated by using the following formula: serum iron level/TIBC × 100.

In our study, the serum iron levels and TIBCs were measured via the colorimetric method by Olympus device (Germany), using an OSR6186 kit, and the serum ferritin levels were measured via the nephelometric method using the BNII device (Dade Behring, Germany). The CBCs were performed by using an LH750-ANA device (Beckman Coulter, USA). All analyses were performed on the same day by using blood samples drawn in the morning, after one night of fasting.

The following criteria were used to diagnose IDA in our female patients: haemoglobin < 12 g/dL, haematocrit < 35%, serum iron level < 50 μg/dL, transferrin saturation < 10%, and serum ferritin level < 10 ng/dL. It was ensured that all criteria were met by our study patients.

The inclusion criteria were as follows: women aged 19–60 years who were diagnosed with IDA, the detection of the IDA aetiology and treatment of the underlying aetiology before iron therapy, absence of pregnancy, lack of comorbid disease (chronic disease anaemia, thalassemia, other haematological diseases, chronic renal failure, hypothyroidism, Addison's disease, malignancy, alcoholism, or gastrointestinal disease with impaired iron absorption), no acute or chronic infection, and no therapy with an iron preparation or blood product within 6 months prior to the investigation.

Before treatment, all patients were informed about the general principles of the study and the potential adverse effects of the iron preparations. All patients gave written informed consent. Because the diagnosis and treatment of the underlying aetiology are important for the success of treatment in iron deficiency anaemia, anamnesis (history, comorbid disease, hypermenorrhea, internal haemorrhoid, gastrointestinal bleeding, and nutritional characteristics), physical examination, and laboratory evaluations (stool guaiac test and parasite evaluations) were performed in all patients. Endoscopy and colonoscopy were performed in all postmenopausal women, even in the presence of a negative stool guaiac test, and therapies directed toward the underlying aetiology were completed before iron therapy. Since the cause of IDA was hypermenorrhea in most of the patients, hypermenorrhea therapy was arranged by the Obstetrics and Gynaecology Department of the Inonu University Medical School. The treatment of internal haemorrhoids was arranged according to the degree of the disease. Moreover, all patients were informed about the beverages and drugs which impair iron absorption.

The patients included were randomly assigned into 2 groups receiving either Fe^{+2} or Fe^{+3}. Oral Fe^{+3} protein succinylate (40 mg elemental iron, twice daily) was initiated in Fe^{+3} group ($n = 54$), and Fe^{+2} glycine sulphate tablets (40 mg elemental iron, twice daily) were given to the second group ($n = 50$). It was recommended that the patients take the drugs before meals in each group for better absorption. The above-mentioned recommendations were in agreement with the pharmacological information of the drugs.

There were no adjuncts other than proteinaceous compounds, such as folic acid, ascorbic acid, and citric acid, in either preparation used. Protein succinylate and glycol sulphate, bound to the iron for better absorption, are two compounds with a similar protein structure. Additionally, there are 2 other preparations with identical elemental iron contents, which have adjuncts with similar protein structures but without adjuncts such as folic acid, ascorbic acid, or citric acid; however, they are not present in the drug market for comparison.

Patients were phoned and asked for using suitable form and dose of drug once a month. At the control visits (after 3 months), anamneses regarding the treatment period, adverse effects, additional drugs, and nutritional status were taken, and a physical examination was performed in all patients. Some patients attended a "control visit" before the 3-month control visit because of adverse effects, or for other reasons. At the end of the therapy, routine blood analyses (CBC, serum iron level, total iron binding capacity (TIBC), and serum ferritin level) were performed to compare the baseline values.

The exclusion criteria included missed control visits, non-compliance with the drugs due to any reason, development of comorbid disease during therapy, use of additional drugs or beverages which impair the absorption of the study drugs, treatment with erythrocyte suspension or iron preparation, development of severe bleeding or haemolysis, and detection of failure in the treatment of the underlying aetiology.

3. Statistics

In our study, statistical analyses were performed by using SPSS for Windows. Continuous variables were expressed as a mean ± standard deviation. Categorical variables were expressed as the number and percent. Normality for the continuous variables in the groups was determined using the Shapiro-Wilk test. The variables showed a normal distribution ($P > 0.05$); therefore, the paired and unpaired t-tests were used for intragroup and intergroup comparisons of the haematological parameters. The Pearson Chi square test was used to detect the aetiology underlying the IDA. Fisher's exact test was used to detect the groups regarding adverse drug effects, and $P > 0.05$ was considered to be statistically significant.

4. Results

Overall, 104 patients began this study, 54 patients in the first group receiving Fe^{+3} protein succinylate and 50 patients in the second group receiving Fe^{+2} glycine sulphate. Total 40 patients were excluded in agreement with various criteria (Table 1). Thus, 64 patients overall (30 patients in the Fe^{+3} group and 34 patients in the Fe^{+2} group) were included in the analyses.

In the Fe^{+3} group, the mean age was 40.7 ± 7.3 years. In the Fe^{+2} group, the mean age was 39.1 ± 6.4 years. No significant difference was found between the groups with regard to age ($P > 0.05$). In the evaluations performed to detect the aetiology underlying the IDA, it was found that, of the 30 patients, 20 had hypermenorrhea (66%), 6 had malnutrition (20%), and 4 had internal haemorrhoids (14%) in the Fe^{+3} group. In the Fe^{+2} group, it was found that, of the 34 patients, 23 had hypermenorrhea (67%), 7 had

TABLE 1: Total 40 patients were excluded in agreement with above-mentioned criteria.

Adverse effect	Fe^{+3} group	Fe^{+2} group
Epigastric pain	2	1
Constipation	0	1
Hypermenorrhea	9	6
Erythrocyte suspension	2	2
Not attending control visit	11	6
Total number of patients	24	16

malnutrition (20%), and 4 had internal haemorrhoids (13%). No significant differences were found between the two groups regarding aetiology ($P > 0.05$).

In the Fe^{+3} group and Fe^{+2} group, haemoglobin (Hg), haematocrit (Htc), red blue cell (RBC), mean corpuscular volume (MCV), mean corpuscular haemoglobin (MCH), mean corpuscular haemoglobin concentration (MCHC), iron (Fe), TIBC, transferrin saturation, and ferritin levels were shown in Tables 2(a) and 2(b).

In the analysis which was the primary argument of our study, we compared the pre- and posttreatment laboratory values between the two groups in Table 3. Hg, Htc, and TIBC showed a significant increase in the Fe^{+2} group when compared to that in the Fe^{+3} group ($P < 0.05$). There were differences between the two groups regarding the increase in Ferritin, RBC, MCV, MCH, and MCHC values, and it was found that the Fe^{+2} group had a better response regarding the increase in MCV, MCH, and MCHC values but no significant differences ($P > 0.05$). No differences were found between groups regarding the other parameters.

The study groups were compared regarding adverse effects during therapy. Two patients refused to continue therapy due to epigastric pain in the Fe^{+3} group, while 2 patients in the Fe^{+2} group discontinued therapy due to epigastric pain ($n = 1$) and constipation ($n = 1$). These patients were excluded from the study. Two patients reported constipation after the initiation of the drug in the Fe^{+3} group. It was recommended to continue therapy and add a laxative agent in two patients who presented with constipation during therapy. In the Fe^{+2} group, 2 of the 34 patients reported adverse effects, including epigastric pain in one and constipation in the other, and symptomatic treatment was prescribed to these patients. Patients reporting adverse effects during therapy were cited that their symptoms were relieved by symptomatic therapy without causing noncompliance to the iron treatment. In conclusion, drug-related adverse effects developed in 4 (7.4%) of the 54 patients receiving Fe^{+3} and 4 (8.0%) of the 50 patients receiving Fe^{+2}. No significant differences were found between the groups regarding adverse effects ($P > 0.05$).

5. Discussion

The therapeutic value of oral iron preparations is determined by the intestinal bioavailability and gastrointestinal tolerability of the iron content [12]; therefore, many studies have been conducted regarding the absorption and bioavailability of

TABLE 2: (a) A general analysis of 54 patients receiving Fe^{+3}, 24 patients from the study, and the remaining 30 patients. (b) A general analysis of 50 patients receiving Fe^{+2}, 16 patients from the study, and the remaining 34 patients.

(a)

Parameters	Before treatment	After treatment	P
Hg (g/dL)	11.2	12.4	S**
Htc (%)	34.2	36.8	S
RBC ($\times 10^{12}$/L)	4.3	4.6	S
MCV (fL)	79.8	82.4	S
MCH (pg/cell)	26.4	27.61	S
MCHC (g/dL)	33.3	33.3	NS*
Fe (μg/dL)	18.3	68.2	S
TIBC (μg/dL)	333	352.5	NS
Trans. sat. (%)	5.5	19.5	S
Ferritin (ng/dL)	9	12.3	S

*NS: not statistically significant; **S: statistically significant.

(b)

Parameters	Before treatment	After treatment	P
Hg (g/dL)	10.3	12.6	S
Htc (%)	32.07	37.9	S
RBC ($\times 10^{12}$/L)	4.37	4.70	S
MCV (fL)	72.5	82.1	S
MCH (pg/cell)	23	27	S
MCHC (g/dL)	31.5	33.2	S
Fe (μg/dL)	22.7	61.9	S
TIBC (μg/dL)	366.4	329.6	S
Trans. sat. (%)	6.2	18.52	S
Ferritin (ng/dL)	8.2	12.2	S

TABLE 3: Pre- and posttreatment laboratory values between the groups.

Parameter	Fe^{+3} group	Fe^{+2} group	P
Hg (g/dL)	0.95 ± 0.74	2.25 ± 0.94	S
Htc (%)	2.62 ± 2.07	5.9 ± 2.3	S
RBC ($\times 10^{12}$/L)	0.24 ± 0.14	0.32 ± 0.33	NS
Ferritin (ng/dL)	4.13 ± 7.5	4.05 ± 10.2	NS
TIBC	19.5 ± 53.3	36.8 ± 71.9	S

oral iron preparations. Widely accepted opinion suggests that the absorption of Fe^{+2} iron from the intestine is 3-fold higher than that of Fe^{+3} iron [4, 5]. Thus, World Health Organization recommends Fe^{+2} iron in the treatment of IDA [9, 13]. There are conflicting results in the studies comparing oral Fe^{+2} and Fe^{+3} preparations regarding the rate of success in the restoration of anaemia [14, 15]. In 1992, Glassman compared oral Fe^{+3} and Fe^{+2} iron preparations with distinct combinations (Fe^{+2} fumarate and polysaccharide-iron complex) regarding changes in haematological parameters, but the authors found no significant differences [16].

In 1993, Jacobs et al. found no significant differences regarding the increase in haemoglobin and haematocrit values between groups receiving 60 mg (daily) Fe^{+2} sulphate and 100 mg (twice daily) Fe^{+3} polymaltose complex. Less improvement was seen in anaemia in the group receiving the 100 mg (daily) Fe^{+3} polymaltose complex when compared to the other groups [17]. In 1994, Nielsen et al. compared Fe^{+2} sulphate and the ferric-polymaltose complex and found that there was no significant change in the mean haemoglobin value in the group receiving the ferric-polymaltose. However, a significantly increased mean haemoglobin value was detected in the group receiving Fe^{+2} sulphate over 4 weeks [18].

In a study in 1996, Casparis et al. compared 4 groups, including pregnant and postpartum women. The first group received 75 mg (twice daily, orally) of liquid Fe^{+2} gluconate, and the second group received 80 mg (daily, orally) of solid Fe^{+2} gluconate. The third group received 105 mg (daily, orally) of solid Fe^{+2} sulphate, and the fourth group received 80 mg (twice daily, orally) of liquid Fe^{+3} protein succinylate. After 30 days of therapy, no significant differences were observed among the groups regarding an increase in RBC, haemoglobin, haematocrit, and serum iron values [19].

In a study (in 2004) from Taiwan, in which Fe^{+2} fumarate and Fe^{+3} polysaccharide preparations were compared, Saha et al. found that Fe^{+2} fumarate was more effective after 12 weeks of therapy regarding improvements in the haematological parameters [20]. In a study from India, Saha et al. assigned 100 pregnant women into 2 groups to receive 120 mg of Fe^{+2} sulphate and 100 mg of Fe^{+3} polymaltose complex. They recommended the Fe^{+3} polymaltose complex for pregnant women, although there was no significant difference between the groups regarding improvements in haematological parameters after 8 weeks of therapy [21].

Ruiz-Argüelles et al., in a study from Mexico, reported that iron hydroxide polymaltose therapy failed in the treatment of IDA [22]. Aycicek et al. reported a new study to compare the total oxidant and antioxidant effects of different oral iron preparations in children with IDA. A total of 65 children with IDA were randomized to receive 5 mg Fe/kg/day of iron (II) sulphate (Fe^{+2} group, $n = 33$) or iron (III-) hydroxide polymaltose complex (Fe^{+3} group, $n = 32$). Healthy controls ($n = 28$) were also included in this study. The study concluded that Fe^{+2} sulphate (Fe^{+2}) had a faster effect than Fe^{+3} polymaltose (Fe^{+3}) on increasing the oxidant status in children with IDA [23].

In the treatment of IDA, gastrointestinal tolerability and the incidence of adverse side events are as important as bioavailability and efficiency when comparing the drugs used. There are several studies in the literature regarding gastrointestinal intolerance to oral iron preparations. Harvey et al. compared oral Fe^{+3} and Fe^{+2} iron preparations and found no significant differences between the groups regarding adverse effects [19]. In the study by Reddy et al., liquid Fe^{+2} gluconate was considered to be the safest supplement with regard to adverse effects [24]. Kavaklı et al. reported that both drugs were safe with regard to adverse effects and well tolerated, although the rate of gastrointestinal adverse effects was slightly higher in the group receiving Fe^{+2} fumarate. The authors noted that the inability to compare pure Fe^{+2} and Fe^{+3} iron preparations which did not include adjuncts, such as ascorbic acid, folic acid, or polysaccharide compounds, was an important limitation [20].

Saha et al. found that gastrointestinal adverse events were more common with Fe^{+2} sulphate therapy [21]. In a study in 2001, Harvey et al. suggested that gastrointestinal adverse effects were more frequently observed with Fe^{+2} iron when compared to Fe^{+3} iron, which could result from the production of more hydroxyl free radicals in the gastrointestinal mucosa. The authors recruited 23 patients (15 patients with inflammatory colon disease) with an intolerance to Fe^{+2} iron preparations and gave the patients Fe^{+3} trimaltol iron therapy. No adverse effects were detected in any of the patients, and significant increases were achieved in the haemoglobin and haematocrit levels with 3 months of therapy [24]. In another study, Kavaklı et al. evaluated the development of gastrointestinal adverse effects with the Fe^{+3} polymaltose complex and Fe^{+2} fumarate treatments in 100 women and reported that the Fe^{+3} polymaltose caused less adverse effects [25]. In 2004, Kavaklı et al. evaluated the development of oxidation-related toxicity and adverse effects in 2 groups of patients receiving either Fe^{+3} or Fe^{+2} iron. The authors found no significant differences between the groups [26].

When studies comparing oral Fe^{+3} and Fe^{+2} iron preparations were evaluated, with regard to the development of gastrointestinal intolerance, no definitive conclusion could be made about the superiority of any preparations. It was seen that Fe^{+3} iron preparations in the same form (solid-liquid) did not cause more adverse effects than Fe^{+2} iron preparations; however, it was also seen that they caused less intolerance in some studies.

In our study, 40 mg (twice daily; 0.5 hours before meals) oral Fe^{+3} protein succinylate flacons and 40 mg (twice daily; 0.5 hours before meals) oral Fe^{+2} glycine sulphate tablets were used; however, no significant difference was found regarding the adverse effects, and both preparations were found to be safe.

In evaluations regarding anaemia, haemoglobin and haematocrit are more valuable than RBC, MCV, MCH, and MCHC. Thus, we valued the increases in the haemoglobin and haematocrit levels, rather than those of the RBC, MCV, MCH, MCHC, serum iron, TIBC, transferrin saturation, and ferritin levels after 3 months of therapy, when compared to the baseline levels.

In our study, Fe^{+2} iron preparations were found to be superior to oral Fe^{+3} protein succinylate and Fe^{+2} glycol sulphate containing the same amounts of elemental iron. However, there are several oral Fe^{+3} and Fe^{+2} iron preparations with various forms. Given the different forms of preparations in the literature, it is difficult to make suggestions, such as "all Fe^{+2} iron preparations lead to better improvements in anaemia when compared to all Fe^{+3} iron preparations," based on the comparison of the preparations used in our study.

The limitations of our study included a relatively small sample size (64 patients overall) at the end of a 6-month study period and an assessment of the patients only at the end of month 3. Larger and more comprehensive studies are required with more frequent controls (e.g., at months 0, 1, 3, and 6), which could include a greater number of patients and compare more preparations.

One interesting finding of our study was regarding cost. According to the 2013 year prices, the Fe^{+3} iron preparation was found to be more expensive than the Fe^{+2} iron preparation when the costs of 3 months of therapy were compared.

6. Conclusion

In conclusion, it was found that the Fe^{+2} and Fe^{+3} preparations used in our study were safe with regard to gastrointestinal intolerance; however, the Fe^{+2} was more effective and less expensive. Using more effective and less expensive agents in IDA management leads to a rapid recovery with decreased costs. Larger, multicentre studies should be performed on the absorption, adverse effects, and efficiency of oral iron preparations by evaluating scientific concerns before cost.

Abbreviations

IDA:	Iron deficiency anaemia
Hg:	Haemoglobin
Htc:	Haematocrit
TIBC:	Total iron binding capacity
Fe^{+3}:	Ferric
Fe^{+2}:	Ferrous
RBC:	Red blue cell
Fe:	Iron
MCV:	Mean corpuscular volume
MCH:	Mean corpuscular haemoglobin
MCHC:	Mean corpuscular haemoglobin concentration.

Ethical Approval

This study was approved by the Inonu University Medical Faculty Ethics Committee.

Disclaimer

This report reflects the opinion of the authors and does not represent the official position of any institution or sponsor.

Conflict of Interests

The authors declare that they have no conflict of interests.

Authors' Contribution

Ilhami Berber was responsible for reviewing previous research, the journal searches, and drafting the report. Halit Diri and Mehmet Ali Erkurt contributed to the final draft of the paper and the analysis of the relevant data. Ismet Aydogdu was responsible for project coordination. All authors read and approved the final paper.

Acknowledgment

This study was financed by the Inonu University Medical Faculty Research Project Coordination Department.

References

[1] E. Beutler, "The common anemias," *The Journal of the American Medical Association*, vol. 259, no. 16, pp. 2433–2437, 1988.

[2] C. Hershko, "Storage iron regulation," *Progress in Hematology*, vol. 10, pp. 105–148, 1977.

[3] A. Deiss, "Iron metabolism in reticuloendothelial cells," *Seminars in Hematology*, vol. 20, no. 2, pp. 81–90, 1983.

[4] K. B. Raja, S. E. Jafri, D. Dickson et al., "Involvement of iron (ferric) reduction in the iron absorption mechanism of a trivalent iron-protein complex (iron protein succinylate)," *Pharmacology and Toxicology*, vol. 87, no. 3, pp. 108–115, 2000.

[5] P. Jacobs, "Equivalent bioavailability of iron from ferrous salts and a ferric polymaltose complex. Clinical and experimental studies," *Arzneimittel-Forschung*, vol. 37, no. 1, pp. 113–116, 1987.

[6] P. Jacobs, T. Bothwell, and R. W. Charlton, "Role of hydrochloric acid and iron absorption," *Journal of Applied Physiology*, vol. 19, pp. 187–188, 1964.

[7] J. D. Cook and E. R. Monsen, "Food iron absorption in human subjects. III. Comparison of the effect of animal proteins on nonheme iron absorption," *The American Journal of Clinical Nutrition*, vol. 29, no. 8, pp. 859–867, 1976.

[8] E. Pollitt, "Iron deficiency and educational deficiency," *Nutrition Reviews*, vol. 55, no. 4, pp. 133–141, 1997.

[9] W. B. Freire, "Strategies of the pan American health organization/world health organization for the control of iron deficiency in Latin America," *Nutrition Reviews*, vol. 55, no. 6, pp. 183–188, 1997.

[10] V. Polin, R. Coriat, G. Perkins et al., "Iron deficiency: from diagnosis to treatment," *Digestive and Liver Disease*, vol. 45, no. 10, pp. 803–809, 2013.

[11] C. A. Finch, V. Bellotti, S. Stray et al., "Plasma ferritin determination as a diagnostic tool," *Western Journal of Medicine*, vol. 145, no. 5, pp. 657–663, 1986.

[12] G. Sas, E. Nemesanszky, H. Brauer, and K. Scheffer, "On the therapeutic effects of trivalent and divalent iron in iron deficiency anaemia," *Arzneimittel-Forschung*, vol. 34, no. 11, pp. 1575–1579, 1984.

[13] E. M. de Maeyer, P. Dallman, J. M. Gurney et al., *Preventing and Controlling Iron Deficiency Anaemia Through Primary Healthcare: A Guide for Health Administrators and Programme Managers*, World Health Organization, Geneva, Switzerland, 1989.

[14] S. M. Kelsey, R. C. Hider, J. R. Bloor, D. R. Blake, C. N. Gutterridge, and A. C. Newland, "Absorption of low and therapeutic doses of ferric maltol, a novel ferric iron compound, in iron deficient subjects using a single dose iron absorption test," *Journal of Clinical Pharmacy and Therapeutics*, vol. 16, no. 2, pp. 117–122, 1991.

[15] D. M. Reffitt, T. J. Burden, P. T. Seed, J. Wood, R. P. H. Thompson, and J. J. Powell, "Assessment of iron absorption from ferric trimaltol," *Annals of Clinical Biochemistry*, vol. 37, no. 4, pp. 457–466, 2000.

[16] E. Glassman, "Oral iron therapy with ferrous fumarate and polysaccharide iron complex," *The American Nephrology Nurses' Association*, vol. 19, no. 3, pp. 277–323, 1992.

[17] P. Jacobs, D. Fransman, and P. Coghlan, "Comparative bioavailability of ferric polymaltose and ferrous sulphate in iron-deficient blood donors," *Journal of Clinical Apheresis*, vol. 8, no. 2, pp. 89–95, 1993.

[18] P. Nielsen, E. E. Gabbe, R. Fischer, and H. C. Heinrich, "Bioavailability of iron from oral ferric polymaltose in humans," *Arzneimittel-Forschung*, vol. 44, no. 6, pp. 743–748, 1994.

[19] D. Casparis, P. Del Carlo, F. Branconi, A. Grossi, D. Merante, and L. Gafforio, "Effectiveness and tolerance of oral doses of liquid ferrous gluconate in iron-deficiency anaemia during pregnancy and in the immediate post-natal period: comparison with other liquid or solid formulations containing bivalent or trivalent iron," *Minerva Ginecologica*, vol. 48, no. 11, pp. 511–518, 1996.

[20] T.-C. Liu, S.-F. Lin, C.-S. Chang, W.-C. Yang, and T.-P. Chen, "Comparison of a combination ferrous fumarate product and a polysaccharide iron complex as oral treatments of iron deficiency anemia: a Taiwanese study," *International Journal of Hematology*, vol. 80, no. 5, pp. 416–420, 2004.

[21] L. Saha, P. Pandhi, S. Gopalan, S. Malhotra, and P. K. Saha, "Comparison of efficacy, tolerability, and cost of iron polymaltose complex with ferrous sulphate in the treatment of iron deficiency anemia in pregnant women," *Medscape General Medicine*, vol. 9, no. 1, article 1, 2007.

[22] G. J. Ruiz-Argüelles, A. Díaz-Hernández, C. Manzano, and G. J. Ruiz-Delgado, "Ineffectiveness of oral iron hydroxide polymaltose in iron-deficiency anemia," *Hematology*, vol. 12, no. 3, pp. 255–256, 2007.

[23] A. Aycicek, A. Koc, Y. Oymak, S. Selek, C. Kaya, and B. Guzel, "Ferrous sulfate (Fe^{2+}) had a faster effect than did ferric polymaltose (Fe^{3+}) on increased oxidant status in children with iron-deficiency anemia," *Journal of Pediatric Hematology/Oncology*, vol. 36, no. 1, pp. 57–61, 2014.

[24] P. S. N. Reddy, B. B. Adsul, K. Gandewar, K. M. Korde, and A. Desai, "Evaluation of efficacy and safety of iron polymaltose complex and folic acid (Mumfer) versus iron formulation (ferrous fumarate) in female patients with anaemia," *Journal of the Indian Medical Association*, vol. 99, no. 3, pp. 154–155, 2001.

[25] R. S. J. Harvey, D. M. Reffitt, L. A. Doig et al., "Ferric trimaltol corrects iron deficiency anaemia in patients intolerant of iron," *Alimentary Pharmacology and Therapeutics*, vol. 12, no. 9, pp. 845–848, 1998.

[26] K. Kavaklı, D. Yılmaz, B. Çetinkaya et al., "Safety profiles of Fe^{+2} and Fe^{+3} oral preparations in the treatment of iron deficiency anaemia in children," *Pediatric Hematology-Oncology*, vol. 21, no. 5, pp. 403–410, 2004.

8

Eculizumab Therapy Leads to Rapid Resolution of Thrombocytopenia in Atypical Hemolytic Uremic Syndrome

Han-Mou Tsai[1] and Elizabeth Kuo[2]

[1] iMAH Hematology Associates, New Hyde Park, NY 11040, USA
[2] Department of Medicine, University of Texas Southwestern School of Medicine, Dallas, TX 75235, USA

Correspondence should be addressed to Han-Mou Tsai; hmtsai@gmail.com

Academic Editor: Estella M. Matutes

Eculizumab is highly effective in controlling complement activation in patients with the atypical hemolytic uremic syndrome (aHUS). However, the course of responses to the treatment is not well understood. We reviewed the responses to eculizumab therapy for aHUS. The results show that, in patients with aHUS, eculizumab therapy, when not accompanied with concurrent plasma exchange therapy, led to steady increase in the platelet count and improvement in extra-renal complications within 3 days. By day 7, the platelet count was normal in 15 of 17 cases. The resolution of hemolytic anemia and improvement in renal function were less predictable and were not apparent for weeks to months in two patients. The swift response in the platelet counts was only observed in one of five cases who received concurrent plasma exchange therapy and was not observed in a case of TMA due to gemcitabine/carboplatin. In summary, eculizumab leads to rapid increase in the platelet counts and resolution of extrarenal symptoms in patients with aHUS. Concurrent plasma exchange greatly impedes the response of aHUS to eculizumab therapy. Eculizumab is ineffective for gemcitabine/carboplatin associated TMA.

1. Introduction

Many patients with the diagnosis of atypical hemolytic uremic syndrome (aHUS) are found to have defective regulation of the alternative complement system [1]. This discovery leads to the use of a humanized monoclonal antibody of complement C5, eculizumab, for aHUS [2]. However, presently available laboratory tests do not identify all patients with defective complement regulation. The tests also have very lengthy turnaround times. Consequently, clinicians have to initiate eculizumab therapy based on a presumptive diagnosis of aHUS. A positive response to eculizumab therapy helps confirm the diagnosis of aHUS. However, there is little data to determine how long the treatment should be continued before a patient's disorder is considered unresponsive to eculizumab therapy.

Mechanistically the complications of aHUS belong to four groups: renal dysfunction and hypertension due to ischemic or membrane attack complex- (MAC-) mediated glomerular injury; thrombocytopenia due to platelet consumption in thrombosis; microangiopathic hemolytic anemia (MAHA) due to abnormal shear stress created by thrombosis or intimal swelling; and extrarenal complications such as edema of the brain, lung, or the digestive organs due to abnormal vascular permeability mediated by anaphylatoxins C3a and C5a [3].

We hypothesize that thrombocytopenia and extrarenal symptoms should begin to resolve soon after complement activation is suppressed by eculizumab, when no new thrombosis occurs and no additional anaphylatoxins are released. In contrast, improvement in renal function depends on the reversibility of glomerular injury and the resolution of arteriolar stenosis. In TMA, arteriolar stenosis results from a variable mix of endothelial swelling, which is expected to resolve quickly when complement activation ceases; and thrombosis, which is dissolved by the fibrinolytic system at slower paces. Consequently, improvement in the renal function in response to anticomplement therapy is likely to be quite variable. Similarly, remission of MAHA, also depending on the resolution of arteriolar stenosis, is expected to be variable. In patients with arteriolar stenosis predominated by endothelial swelling, MAHA should resolve quickly. On the other hand, in patients with extensive arteriolar thrombosis or subendothelial fibrosis, resolution of MAHA may take weeks to months. To explore the merits of this hypothesis, we have reviewed the records of patients who were treated with eculizumab for aHUS.

2. Methods

The records of patients who were treated with eculizumab for presumptive diagnosis of aHUS were reviewed. Patients presenting with MAHA, thrombocytopenia, and renal failure were considered to have aHUS if the plasma ADAMTS13 activity was greater than 10% and other causes of the syndrome of MAHA and thrombocytopenia such as DIC, systemic autoimmune disorders, lupus anticoagulants, metastatic neoplasms, Shiga toxin, or neuraminidase associated HUS were excluded. Molecular analysis was performed (Molecular Otolaryngology and Renal Research Laboratories, University of Iowa) to detect mutations of *complement factor H* (*CFH*), *membrane cofactor protein* (*MCP*), *complement factor I, complement factor B, C3,* and *thrombomodulin*; copy numbers of *complement factor H-related protein 1* (*CFHR1*); and antibodies of CFH. Plasma ADAMTS13 activity levels were performed (the Blood Center of Wisconsin, Milwaukee, WI) to exclude the diagnosis of TTP. The diagnosis of aHUS was considered confirmed if one or more genetic alterations or CFH antibodies affecting the regulation of the alternative complement pathway were detected or the patient showed a clear response to eculizumab therapy.

We also reviewed case records in the literature via search of PubMed using the terms of atypical hemolytic uremic syndrome and eculizumab and included cases with platelet counts within the first 7 days for assessment.

3. Results

During a period of three years, the authors encountered 7 cases of presumed or confirmed aHUS, of which 5 were treated with eculizumab and were further analyzed for this report. For comparison, 10 cases of acquired TTP, 2 cases of hereditary TTP, and one case of MAHA and thrombocytopenia presumably due to lupus vasculitis which had resolved by the time of evaluation were encountered during the same period.

The demographics, comorbid conditions, presenting features, pathological findings of kidney biopsy, and results of molecular testing are summarized in Table 1. Case 1 presented with bloody diarrhea and was initially suspected to have Shiga toxin associated HUS. However, her stools were negative for Shiga toxins. Case 2, previously reported [4], presented three months after undergoing autologous hematopoietic stem cell therapy (HSCT) for advanced multiple myeloma. Case 3, also previously reported [4], had recurrent episodes of severe hypertension accompanied with mild renal insufficiency and MAHA for four and a half years before he was found to have aHUS and treated with eculizumab. Case 4 presented at 22 weeks of her third pregnancy and was initially assumed

to have preeclampsia; however, her disease persisted after termination of pregnancy. This patient was retreated for relapse 3 months after eculizumab therapy was discontinued. Case 5 had kidney biopsy performed for renal failure at 3 weeks after her seventh triweekly course of chemotherapy with gemcitabine and carboplatin for metastatic cholangiocarcinoma.

Four patients (Cases 1–4) presented with abdominal symptoms of pain, nausea, vomiting, and/or diarrhea. All five patients had altered mental status (confusion or somnolence). One had visual scotoma. Two patients had severe albeit brittle hypertension as high as 220/146 and 221/159 mmHg, respectively.

Kidney biopsy, performed in 3 patients (Cases 3–5), revealed the changes of thrombotic microangiopathy (TMA). Molecular testing detected complement factor H antibodies in the case after autologous HSCT (Case 2). This patient also had heterozygous genomic deletion of CFHR3 and CFHR1 and an uncommon nucleic acid sequence alteration (c.1697A >C, p.Glu566Ala) of complement factor B of undetermined significance. A rare alteration (c.3607C>T [rs145347741], p.Arg1203Trp) of CFH was detected in the case with onset during pregnancy (Case 4).

As expected, the laboratory tests revealed anemia with elevated LDH and thrombocytopenia (Table 2). In none of the patients was the platelet count less 50×10^9/L. The serum creatinine concentration was 2.51–5.52 mg/dL at presentation, rising to higher levels in each case after admission. Dialysis was required in Cases 2 and 5.

The plasma ADAMTS13 activity was normal or slightly decreased in all cases. Four patients were treated with 5–17 sessions of plasma exchange before the treatment was switched to eculizumab. With plasma exchange, the platelet count increased in 3 patients and LDH decreased in all five patients. However, in none of the patients was the platelet count normalized or altered mental status or visual symptoms completely resolved (Table 3).

The responses to eculizumab therapy, also summarized in Table 3, are notable for the normalization of the platelet count by day 7 in each of the 5 courses of eculizumab therapy in Cases 1–4. The platelet count did not increase in the case of gemcitabine/carboplatin associated TMA. In that case, the platelet count was never normalized after 4 doses of eculizumab.

The responses in serum creatinine and LDH were variable, with none normalizing by day 7. Improvement of renal function by one stage was observed by day 14 during both courses of treatment in Case 4; by day 63 in Case 3; and by day 378 in Case 2. In Case 2, further improvement by one stage occurred by day 483. The LDH normalized by day 14 in Cases 3 and 4 and by day 70 in Case 2; it did not normalize by day 21 in Case 3 and by day 84 in Case 5.

The courses depicted in Figure 1 show that the platelet count began to exhibit steady increase within 3 days in each of the 5 courses in Cases 1–4. No increase in the platelet count occurred in Case 5 while she was being treated with eculizumab (Figure 2).

From the literature, we identified 15 and 17 cases, respectively, in 9 reports with data available for analysis of the

TABLE 1: Characteristics of the patients.

Case	Age, y	Gender	Comorbidity	Presenting features	Pathology	Molecular defects
1	61	F	None	Abdominal pain, diarrhea, and confusion	None available	None detected
2	57	F	3 months after auto-HCT for advanced multiple myeloma; MM in remission	Abdominal pain, diarrhea, vomiting, and confusion	None available	Anti-CFH, CFHR1-CFHR3 +/−, and CFB c.1697A>C, p.Glu566Ala*
3	50	M	None	Abdominal pain, nausea, vomiting, headache, gross hematuria, confusion, and hypertension (highest blood pressures 220/146 mmHg)	Kidney biopsy: TMA	None detected
4-1	22	F	Gestation at 22 weeks	Anorexia, anasarca, scotoma, and hypertension (highest blood pressures 205/134 mmHg)	Kidney biopsy: TMA	CFH c.3607C>T, p.Arg1203Trp**
4-2			3 months after discontinuing eculizumab	Nausea, vomiting, dyspnea, and hypertension (highest blood pressures 221/159 mmHg)		
5	66	F	Gemcitabine/carboplatin and cholangiocarcinoma	Fatigue, somnolence, and confusion	Kidney biopsy: TMA	None detected

* An uncommon variant that is found in chimpanzee's CFB, which is 99% identical to human CFB.
** A rare variant (prevalence of CT genotype, 0.001) in the CFH SCR-20 domain of uncertain consequence.
Abbreviations: CFH: complement factor H; HCT: hematopoietic stem cell therapy; MM: multiple myeloma; TMA: thrombotic microangiopathy.

TABLE 2: Laboratory findings at presentation.

Case	WBC ×10⁹/L	Hb g/L	Platelet ×10⁹/L	LDH U/L	BUN mg/dL	Cr mg/dL	Cr$_{max}$ mg/dL	ADAMTS13 %	Plasma exchange Number of sessions
1	10.1	125	52	3,330	76	2.6	6.5 on day 3	86	17 for 19 days
2*	12.5	85	99	1,271	39	3.37	—	55	15 for 18 days
3	10.48	95	96	1,471	55	4.84	5.99 on day 32	79	1 for 1 day
4-1	13.59	71	65	910	28	2.51	4.02 on day 17	85	6 for 6 days
4-2	5.07	84	63	770	46	5.52	6.86 on day 2	—	0
5**	2.69	111	57	892	71	5.43	5.53 on day 2	74	5 for 6 days

*The patient was on hemodialysis at the time of transfer.
**The patient received her last dose of gemcitabine and carboplatin 3 weeks before presentation.
Normal ADAMTS13 activity, >67%; Cr$_{max}$: maximal serum creatinine.

TABLE 3: Responses to eculizumab therapy.

Case	Day	Hb g/L	Platelet ×10⁹/L	LDH U/L	Cr mg/dL	Extrarenal complications	Days to normal values* Platelet	LDH	Days to CKD ↓ 1 stage
1	0	83	134	884	1.13	Intermittent confusion, and anasarca	≤7	>21	>21
	7	85	186	965	1.18	Resolved			
2	0	98	81	902	3.47	Somnolence, confusion, and vomiting	≤7	70	378, 483
	7	91	162	859	4.45	Resolved			
3	0	86	131	1,235	5.12	Headache, confusion, abdominal pain, nausea, and vomiting	≤7	14	63
	7	92	303	672	4.41	Resolved and HTN stabilized			
4-1	0	71	105	250	3.79	Anasarca, headache, and visual scotoma	3	14	14
	7	71	198	NA	2.66	Resolved			
4-2	0	84	63	770	5.52	Nausea, vomiting, and dyspnea	6	14	14
	6	83	230	321	NA	Resolved			
5	0	98	65	693	3.99	Somnolence and intermittent confusion	>84	>84	>84
	7	85	42	818	4.06	No improvement			

*Since the tests were not performed daily, the actual days may be less than the given values.
CKD: chronic kidney disease.

platelet count responses and its normalization by day 7 after the first dose of eculizumab therapy for aHUS (Table 4) [5–13]. Among the patients who were not receiving concurrent plasma exchange therapy, the platelet count began to show steady increase within 3 days in each of the 10 cases and was normalized by day 7 in 10 of 12 cases. In contrast, among the 5 patients with concurrent plasma exchange, only one showed immediate and steady increase in the platelet count, and none had normalized platelet counts by day 7. The difference in the platelet count response between the groups with and without concurrent plasma exchange was highly significant ($P \leq 0.001$ by Fisher's exact test).

4. Discussion

For patients presenting with the syndrome of MAHA, thrombocytopenia, and renal failure but no comorbid conditions, aHUS is the likely diagnosis once the diagnosis of TTP is excluded. Other causes of idiopathic TMA such as mutations of *diacylglycerol kinase epsilon* (DGKE) and cobalamin C disease are very rare or have not been described in adults [4, 14–16]. An association between aHUS and plasminogen mutations has been suggested but remains to be confirmed [17].

The diagnosis of aHUS is much less straightforward for patients with comorbid conditions such as HSCT, autoimmune disorders, pregnancy, or various drugs. In such cases,

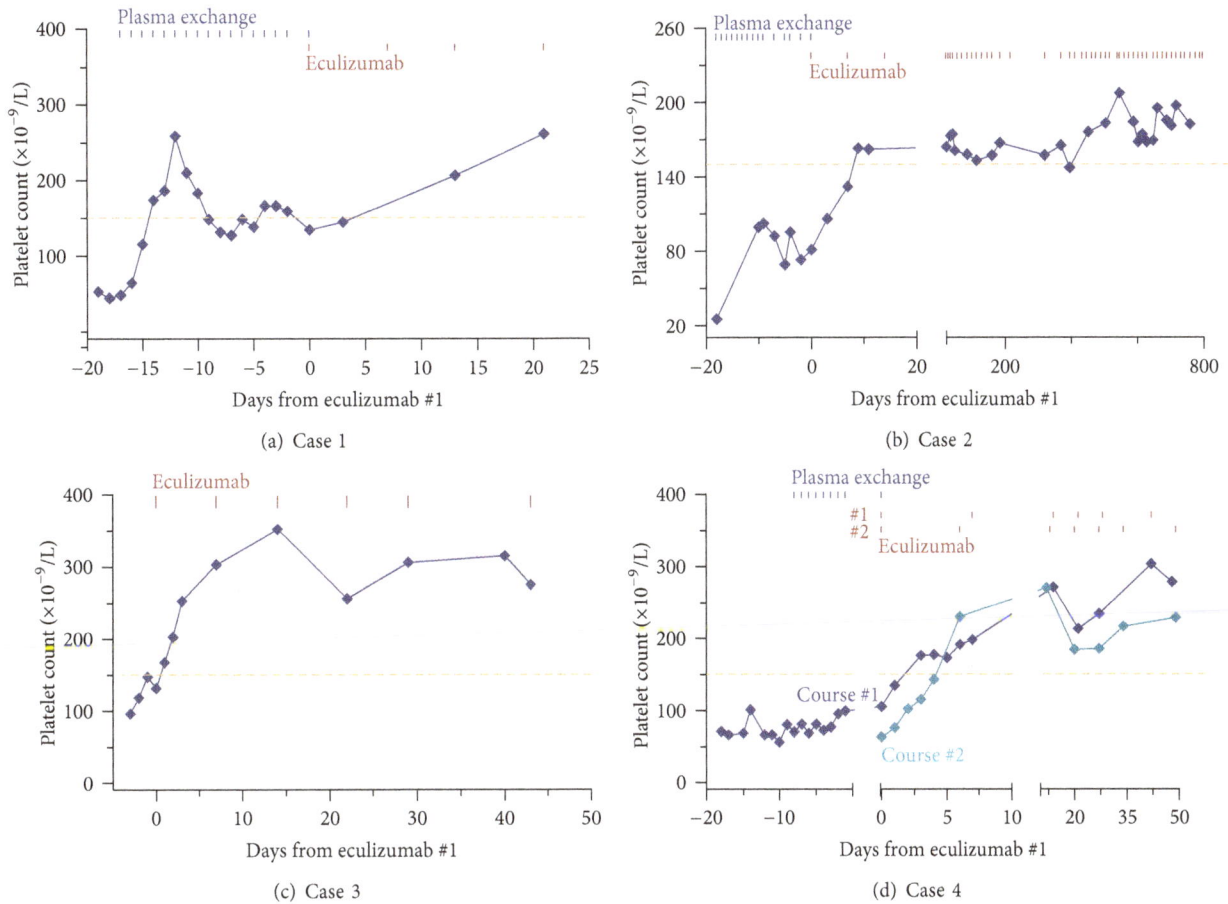

FIGURE 1: Rapid resolution of thrombocytopenia with eculizumab therapy for aHUS. In Cases 1–4 of aHUS (panels a–d), the platelet counts began to steadily increase within 3 days, normalizing by day 7 following initiation of eculizumab therapy. Such rapid and steady increase in the platelet count did not occur in three cases when they were treated with plasma exchange. The dashed lines mark the lower limit of normal platelet counts.

even the finding of TMA in kidney biopsy does not necessarily constitute the diagnosis of aHUS, because TMA may result via other mechanisms of endothelial injury [3]. In addition to Shiga toxins, microbial neuraminidases, and drugs such as bevacizumab that disrupts the vascular endothelial growth factor (VEGF) signaling pathway, TMA may occur in association with drugs such as gemcitabine and other chemotherapeutic agents via as yet known mechanisms.

For patients with a suspected diagnosis of aHUS, a trial of anticomplement therapy is warranted to prove or refute a role of defective complement regulation. Nevertheless, clinicians are often reluctant to institute the therapy because eculizumab is costly and associated with a small but definite risk of fulminant meningococcal infection. Once the therapy is started, clinicians are often confronted with the question of how to assess the response of aHUS to eculizumab. Should one expect simultaneous improvement in all the complications of aHUS, including thrombocytopenia, MAHA, renal failure, hypertension, and extrarenal complications? When is it safe to discontinue the therapy for lack of response?

In this study, we find eculizumab therapy leads to rapid resolution of thrombocytopenia and extrarenal symptoms

of aHUS. Evidence of improvement in both is obvious by day 7, before the second dose of eculizumab. Lack of rapid resolution in thrombocytopenia or extrarenal complications may be taken as evidence against continuing eculizumab therapy beyond the first dose. In this regard, the lack of response in Case 5 after one dose of eculizumab suggests that gemcitabine/carboplatin associated TMA is not due to uncontrolled complement activation.

Our review of the literature identifies 12 additional cases with platelet count responses within 7 days of treatment that support our findings. Importantly, it also shows that concurrent plasma exchange greatly impedes the response of aHUS to eculizumab therapy. Since plasma exchange removes the infused medication, the delay in response is not unexpected. Historically, aHUS has been treated like TTP with plasma exchange. The response of aHUS to plasma exchange is variable and unpredictable. In 3 of our cases of aHUS, plasma exchange therapy resulted in partial improvement. However, the platelet counts did not normalize and the extrarenal symptoms persisted. Clinical trials have demonstrated that anticomplement therapy with eculizumab is superior to plasma exchange for the treatment of aHUS

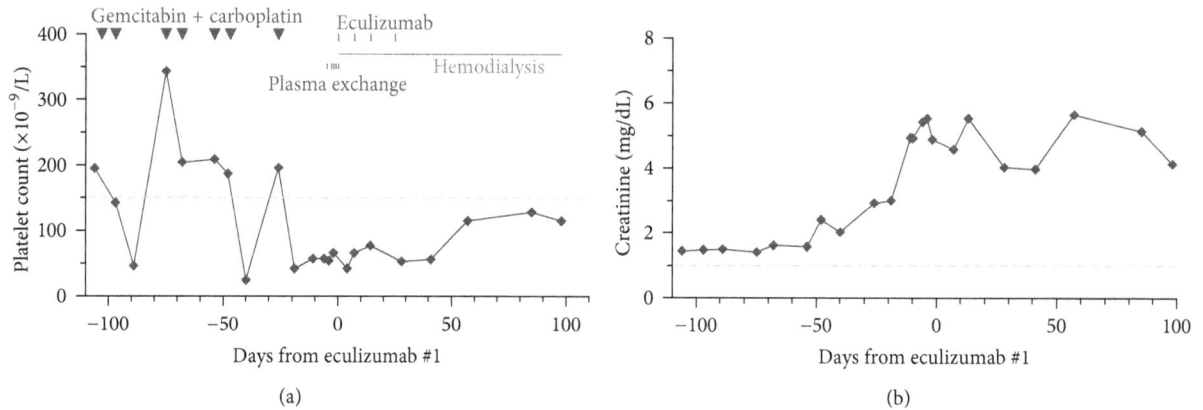

FIGURE 2: Development of thrombocytopenia and renal failure in a patient of metastatic cholangiocarcinoma treated with gemcitabine and carboplatin and the lack of response to eculizumab therapy. Neither plasma exchange nor eculizumab therapy increased the platelet counts or improved the renal function of this case. The thrombocytopenia induced by chemotherapy was transient before renal failure occurred. Thus, the lack of platelet response to eculizumab therapy was not due to bone marrow suppression by chemotherapy. The dashed lines mark the lower limit of normal platelet count and the upper limit of serum creatinine, respectively.

TABLE 4: Resolution of thrombocytopenia following initiation of eculizumab therapy for aHUS.

	Without concurrent plasma exchange		With concurrent plasma exchange	
Source	Steady increase by day 3	Normalized in ≤7 days	Steady increase by day 3	Normal in ≤7 days
Literature	10/10	10/12	1/5	0/5
This series	5/5	5/5	0	—
Total	15/15	15/17	1/5*	0/5*

Numerator indicates the number of cases with response; denominator is the number of cases with available data.
*$P = 0.001$ and 0.0008, respectively, versus its counter group without plasma exchange (Fisher's exact test).

[2]. The responses in our cases of aHUS are consistent with this finding. Therefore, plasma exchange is now only used for the treatment of aHUS when eculizumab is not available or TTP is not yet excluded. For patients with aHUS or presumed aHUS, TTP should have been excluded and there is no reason to continue plasma exchange therapy when eculizumab therapy is initiated.

The resolution of MAHA and renal failure is less predictable and may not be apparent for several weeks. Our data shows that normalization of LDH may take at least 10 weeks in some cases. Improvement of renal function by one stage may take one year. The slowness of renal function recovery has important clinical implications. Patients with advanced renal failure due to aHUS should not be rushed to kidney transplantation within one year (or even longer) of eculizumab treatment. On the other hand, if a patient has stable renal function and no thrombocytopenia, MAHA, or extrarenal complications, eculizumab therapy is unlikely to help confirm or refute the presumptive diagnosis of aHUS. For asymptomatic stable patients whose diagnosis of aHUS is not yet confirmed, it is prudent to withhold immediate eculizumab therapy and wait for the results of molecular testing. Nevertheless, the patients should be closely monitored for any change that would require immediate therapeutic intervention.

Case 5, who developed TMA after 7 courses of chemotherapy with gemcitabine and carboplatin, did not respond to eculizumab therapy. Before the onset of her renal dysfunction, her chemotherapy typically suppressed her platelet count to a nadir by days 7-8, recovering in time for her next scheduled chemotherapy at week 3. Therefore, the lack of increase in the platelet count following eculizumab therapy was not due to bone marrow suppression by her chemotherapy. Together with the lack of improvement in her mental status and renal function, it was very unlikely that the TMA of Case 5 was due to uncontrolled complement activation.

In summary, eculizumab therapy leads to rapid resolution of thrombocytopenia and extrarenal symptoms after the first dose. The resolution of MAHA and improvement of renal function is less predictable and may not occur for weeks to months. Concurrent plasma exchange impedes the response to eculizumab and should be avoided unless there is a compelling reason for continuation. Anticomplement therapy is ineffective for gemcitabine/carboplatin associated TMA.

Conflict of Interests

Han-Mou Tsai received lecture honoraria from Alexion.

References

[1] M. Noris, J. Caprioli, E. Bresin et al., "Relative role of genetic complement abnormalities in sporadic and familial aHUS and their impact on clinical phenotype," *Clinical Journal of the American Society of Nephrology*, vol. 5, no. 10, pp. 1844–1859, 2010.

[2] C. M. Legendre, C. Licht, P. Muus et al., "Terminal complement inhibitor eculizumab in atypical hemolytic-uremic syndrome," *The New England Journal of Medicine*, vol. 368, no. 23, pp. 2169–2181, 2013.

[3] H.-M. Tsai, "A mechanistic approach to the diagnosis and management of atypical hemolytic uremic syndrome," *Transfusion Medicine Reviews*, 2014.

[4] H.-M. Tsai, "Thrombotic thrombocytopenic purpura and the atypical hemolytic uremic syndrome. An update," *Hematology/Oncology Clinics of North America*, vol. 27, no. 3, pp. 565–584, 2013.

[5] R. A. Gruppo and R. P. Rother, "Eculizumab for congenital atypical hemolytic-uremic syndrome," *The New England Journal of Medicine*, vol. 360, no. 5, pp. 544–546, 2009.

[6] C. J. Mache, B. Acham-Roschitz, V. Frémeaux-Bacchi et al., "Complement inhibitor eculizumab in atypical hemolytic uremic syndrome," *Clinical Journal of the American Society of Nephrology*, vol. 4, no. 8, pp. 1312–1316, 2009.

[7] J. Nürnberger, O. Witzke, A. O. Saez et al., "Eculizumab for atypical hemolytic-uremic syndrome," *The New England Journal of Medicine*, vol. 360, no. 5, pp. 542–544, 2009.

[8] C. F.-D. Larrea, F. Cofan, F. Oppenheimer, J. M. Campistol, G. Escolar, and M. Lozano, "Efficacy of eculizumab in the treatment of recurrent atypical hemolytic-uremic syndrome after renal transplantation," *Transplantation*, vol. 89, no. 7, pp. 903–904, 2010.

[9] H. C. Prescott, H. M. Wu, S. R. Cataland, and R. A. Baiocchi, "Eculizumab therapy in an adult with plasma exchange-refractory atypical hemolytic uremic syndrome," *The American Journal of Hematology*, vol. 85, no. 12, pp. 976–977, 2010.

[10] G. Ardissino, M. W. Ossola, G. M. Baffero, A. Rigotti, and M. Cugno, "Eculizumab for atypical hemolytic uremic syndrome in pregnancy," *Obstetrics and Gynecology*, vol. 122, no. 2, part 2, pp. 487–489, 2013.

[11] R. D. Gilbert, D. J. Fowler, E. Angus, S. A. Hardy, L. Stanley, and T. H. Goodship, "Eculizumab therapy for atypical haemolytic uraemic syndrome due to a gain-of-function mutation of complement factor B," *Pediatric Nephrology*, vol. 28, no. 8, pp. 1315–1318, 2013.

[12] B. Thajudeen, A. Sussman, and E. Bracamonte, "A case of atypical hemolytic uremic syndrome successfully treated with eculizumab," *Case Reports in Nephrology and Urology*, vol. 3, no. 2, pp. 139–146, 2013.

[13] F. Fakhouri, Y. Delmas, F. Provot et al., "Insights from the use in clinical practice of eculizumab in adult patients with atypical hemolytic uremic syndrome affecting the native kidneys: an analysis of 19 cases," *The American Journal of Kidney Diseases*, vol. 63, no. 1, pp. 40–48, 2014.

[14] M. Lemaire, V. Frémeaux-Bacchi, F. Schaefer et al., "Recessive mutations in DGKE cause atypical hemolytic-uremic syndrome," *Nature Genetics*, vol. 45, no. 5, pp. 531–536, 2013.

[15] E. Cornec-le Gall, Y. Delmas, L. de Parscau et al., "Adult-onset eculizumab-resistant hemolytic uremic syndrome associated with cobalamin C deficiency," *American Journal of Kidney Diseases*, vol. 63, no. 1, pp. 119–123, 2014.

[16] S. M. Brunelli, K. E. C. Meyers, M. Guttenberg, P. Kaplan, and B. S. Kaplan, "Cobalamin C deficiency complicated by an atypical glomerulopathy," *Pediatric Nephrology*, vol. 17, no. 10, pp. 800–803, 2002.

[17] F. Bu, T. Maga, N. C. Meyer et al., "Comprehensive genetic analysis of complement and coagulation genes in atypical hemolytic uremic syndrome," *Journal of the American Society of Nephrology*, vol. 25, no. 1, pp. 55–64, 2014.

9

Determining Risk Factors of Bleeding in Patients on Warfarin Treatment

Evren Uygungül,[1] **Cuneyt Ayrik,**[2] **Huseyin Narci,**[2] **Semra Erdoğan,**[3] **İbrahim Toker,**[4] **Filiz Demir,**[5] **and Ulas Karaaslan**[6]

[1] *Department of Emergency Medicine, Silifke State Hospital, Mersin, Turkey*
[2] *Department of Emergency Medicine, Faculty of Medicine, Mersin University, Mersin, Turkey*
[3] *Department of Biostatistics, Faculty of Medicine, Mersin University, Mersin, Turkey*
[4] *Department of Emergency Medicine, Tepecik Research Hospital, İzmir, Turkey*
[5] *Department of Emergency Medicine, State Hospital, Niğde, Turkey*
[6] *Department of Emergency Medicine, State Hospital, Balıkesir, Turkey*

Correspondence should be addressed to Huseyin Narci; hsnnarci@gmail.com

Academic Editor: Elvira Grandone

Background. Warfarin is a commonly used oral anticoagulant agent. The most common adverse effects of warfarin are bleeding complications. *Methods.* We performed a 1-year retrospective chart review of emergency department patients using warfarin. A total of 65 patients with bleeding disorder (study group) and 63 patients without bleeding (control group) were included, making up a total of 128 subjects. Demographic data, frequency of international normalized ratio (INR) checks, and routine blood results were extracted. Logistic regression analysis was used to determine which factors were most closely associated with bleeding complications. *Results.* Median age was 62.0 ± 14.4 and 61.9 ± 14.5 for study group and control group, respectively. Educational status and frequency of INR checks were similar in both groups ($P = 0.101$ and $P = 0.483$, resp.). INR levels were higher in the study group (5.45 ± 3.98 versus 2.63 ± 1.71, $P < 0.001$). Creatinine levels were also higher in the study group (1.14 ± 0.57 mg/dL versus 0.94 ± 0.38 mg/dL, $P = 0.042$). Acetylsalicylic acid use was more frequent in the study group and was associated with a 9-fold increase in bleeding complications ($P < 0.001$). *Conclusions.* High INR levels, high creatinine levels, and acetylsalicylic acid use were associated with bleeding complications in ED patients using warfarin.

1. Introduction

The oral anticoagulant agent warfarin is used for treatment and prophylaxis of various thromboembolic diseases such as deep vein thrombosis, pulmonary embolism, stroke, heart valve replacement, and atrial fibrillation [1]. The most common parameter used to monitor its effect on the clotting system during follow-up of patients is the international normalized ratio (INR). Usually, the dose of warfarin is frequently adjusted to maintain the INR level between 2 and 3.5 based on the underlying disease. Because of its narrow therapeutic index, patients using warfarin may have minor and major bleeding, especially in those with poor medication compliance [2, 3].

Patient-related risk factors for bleeding while using warfarin include age, INR, creatinine level, genetic characteristics (*VKORC1* and *CYP2C9* mutations), duration of warfarin use, and concomitant acetylsalicylic acid use. Conflicting results were attained from studies assessing the relationship between age and bleeding [4, 5]. High INR levels are an important risk factor for bleeding [6]. Renal failure and concomitant use of warfarin and acetylsalicylic acid are also risk factors for bleeding [7, 8]. The associations of bleeding with chronic diseases, liver function, and infectious diseases are still not well defined.

In this study, we aimed to determine the risk factors for bleeding in our emergency department (ED) in patients taking warfarin.

TABLE 1: Demographic data (age, gender, and education level), concomitant use of acetylsalicylic acid, and INR sampling frequency in 128 patients using warfarin with bleeding-related (SG) and non-bleeding-related (CG) reasons for their emergency department visit.

	CG		SG		P
	n	%	n	%	
Gender					
Female	33	52.4	38	58.5	0.489
Male	30	47.6	27	41.5	
Highest level of education					
Unschooled	10	15.9	15	23.1	
Primary school	33	52.4	39	60.0	0.101
High school	13	20.6	4	6.2	
University	7	11.1	7	10.8	
Time between INR checks					
Unscheduled	4	6.3	11	16.9	
<30 days	15	23.8	10	15.4	0.483
30–90 days	42	66.6	43	66.2	
>90 days	2	3.3	1	1.5	
Acetylsalicylic acid use					
Yes	54	85.7	25	38.5	**<0.001**
No	9	14.3	40	61.5	

2. Materials and Methods

A 1-year retrospective charts of adult patients (age $\geq$ 17 years) presenting to the emergency department of our tertiary care university hospital were examined. Charts of those taking warfarin were then examined further to extract demographic and clinical data for analysis. Patients were divided into two groups: study group (SG) consisting of 65 patients on warfarin use who were admitted to our emergency service for major or minor bleeding episodes and control group (CG) consisting of 63 patients on warfarin treatment who were admitted to our emergency service for various reasons without bleeding.

Patients sent to our ED from another healthcare facility for purposes of vitamin K, plasma, or blood administration were excluded from the analysis.

Demographic data such as age, gender, educational status, INR control intervals, and blood analysis data such as INR, hemoglobin, platelet count, AST, ALT, creatinine, and CRP levels were recorded into questionnaire. Lab values: hemoglobin (nl 11.7–16 g/dL), platelet count (nl 150–400 $\times$ $10^3/\mu$L), CRP (nl 0–5 mg/dL), creatinine (nl 0–0.9 mg/dL), AST (nl 0–32 U/L), ALT (nl 0–55 U/L), and INR. Hemoglobin and platelet count were determined using an electronic cell counter (Sysmex XT 2000). Serum AST and ALT levels were measured by enzymatic kinetic methods (COBAS INTEGRA 800). Serum creatinine levels were measured by enzymatic calorimetric methods (COBAS INTEGRA 800). Serum CRP levels were measured by turbidimetric methods (COBAS INTEGRA 800).

3. Statistical Methods

SPSS version 11.5 (statistical package for the social sciences windows) was used for statistical analysis. The Shapiro-Wilk test was used to determine if the continuous variables had a normal distribution. Student's t-test was used to assess the difference of mean age values and Mann-Whitney U test was used to assess the difference of biochemical parameters such as INR, AST, ALT, drug dose, and duration of drug use. Pearson chi-square and likelihood chi-square tests were used to assess differences between categorical variables. Descriptive statistics (minimum, maximum, mean, standard deviation, and median and 25th–75th quartiles) for continuous variables and the number and percentages for categorical variables are given. Logistic regression analysis was performed to evaluate risk factors. Comparisons with a P value of less than 0.05 were considered statistically significant.

4. Results

During the study period, 128 patients who presented to the ED using warfarin were included. Indications for warfarin use were deep vein thrombosis (7%), pulmonary embolism (8%), atrial fibrillation (25%), prosthetic heart valve (38%), cerebrovascular disease prophylaxis (20%), and coronary artery bypass surgery (2%). Of these patients, 65 were determined to have bleeding as a cause of presentation to the ED (SG), and 63 patients had no bleeding (CG).

Comparisons between the two groups (SG and CG) regarding age, gender, level of education, and acetylsalicylic acid use are listed in Table 1. While differences in age (mean age of 62 years in both groups) and gender were not different between groups, acetylsalicylic acid use was much more common (61%) in the study group compared to the control group (14%, $P < 0.001$). The level of education was lower in the study group, but this comparison did not reach statistical significance ($P = 0.101$).

Comparison between the two groups, regarding warfarin dose, duration of warfarin use, INR sampling frequency, and laboratory results is displayed in Table 2.

TABLE 2: Dose and duration of warfarin use and laboratory results of 128 patients using warfarin with bleeding-related (SG) and non-bleeding-related (CG) reasons for their emergency department visits.

	CG			SG			P
	Min–max	Mean ± SD	Median [25–75% quartiles]	Min–max	Mean ± SD	Median [25–75% quartiles]	
Age (years)	23–88	61.9 ± 14.5	—	23–91	62.0 ± 14.4	—	0.970
Dose (mg/week)	17.5–42.5	25.36 ± 8.24	22.5 [17.5–35.0]	8.75–70.0	30.17 ± 13.42	35 [17.5–35.0]	0.053
Duration (months)	1–276	49 ± 59	24 [10–72]	1–288	53 ± 60	24 [12–72]	0.583
INR	0.88–11.00	2.63 ± 1.71	2.19 [1.64–3.03]	1.08–18.30	5.45 ± 3.98	4.46 [2.38–6.70]	**<0.001**
Hemoglobin (g/dL)	7.4–16.4	12.46 ± 2.12	12.60 [10.90–14.2]	4.9–17.1	11.10 ± 2.68	11.1 [9.05–13.40]	**0.005**
Platelet count ($10^3/\mu$L)	109–489	246 ± 80	229 [188–306]	81–585	266 ± 96	247 [204–309]	0.231
AST (U/L)	10.3–71.6	29.3 ± 14.6	23.9 [19.1–36.4]	9.2–149.0	33.0 ± 24.2	25.3 [19.9–35.4]	0.710
ALT (U/L)	5.3–94.0	22.4 ± 14.5	17.8 [13.7–25.3]	3.7–136.0	23.4 ± 21.2	17.5 [14.0–23.4]	0.598
Creatinine (mg/dL)	0.5–2.7	0.9 ± 0.4	0.8 [0.7–1.1]	0.5–3.1	1.1 ± 0.6	1.0 [0.7–1.4]	**0.042**
BUN (mg/dL)	13.2–132.1	37.6 ± 21.8	32.3 [26.4–40.1]	12.9–199.2	50.3 ± 33.8	39.1 [28.7–58.3]	**0.009**
CRP (mg/dL)	0.09–271.97	15.46 ± 38.38	4 [1.5–12.8]	0.07–369.90	39.83 ± 66.31	13.50 [2.70–57.20]	**0.002**

Warfarin dose, duration of warfarin use, and platelet counts were not significantly different in the two groups ($P = 0.53$, $P = 0.58$, and $P = 0.23$, resp.). Mean INR levels were significantly higher in SG (5.45±3.98) than in CG (2.63±1.71) ($P < 0.001$). Mean CRP levels were significantly higher in SG (39.8 ± 66.3 mg/dL) than in CG (15.5 ± 38.4 mg/dL) ($P = 0.002$).

Mean creatinine and BUN levels were also significantly higher in the SG patients ($P = 0.042$ and $P = 0.009$, resp.).

When significant parameters such as INR, hemoglobin, creatinine, BUN, CRP, and concomitant use of acetylsalicylic acid were examined by logistic regression analysis, INR (1.42-fold increase) and concomitant acetylsalicylic acid use (9.25-fold increase) were significantly associated with a higher risk of bleeding. Odds ratios with confidence intervals for various parameters are listed in Table 3.

5. Discussion

The oral anticoagulant warfarin is commonly used in the prophylaxis and treatment of several thromboembolic diseases. It is also ranked among the medications with the highest adverse effects due to its narrow therapeutic index, variation in effectiveness with dietary changes, and noncompliance with INR monitoring. Minor and major bleeding episodes (sometimes fatal) are not uncommon.

Regarding the level of education in patients with bleeding-related ED visits, 83% of our SG patients had primary school level education or less. This very high percentage should lead clinicians to strongly consider giving more education about warfarin's risks and arranging closer follow-up of patients with little education.

TABLE 3: Odds ratios (ORs), 95% confidence intervals (CIs), and P values when comparing laboratory values and acetylsalicylic acid use between patients using warfarin with bleeding-related (SG) and non-bleeding-related (CG) reasons for their emergency department visits.

	OR [95% CI]	P
INR	1.417 [1.149–1.748]	**0.001**
Hemoglobin	0.812 [0.656–1.005]	0.055
Creatinine	1.041 [0.173–6.273]	0.965
BUN	0.994 [0.964–1.026]	0.722
CRP	1.008 [0.998–1.018]	0.103
Acetylsalicylic acid	9.255 [3.062–27.968]	**<0.001**

In the studies of warfarin users that assessed the relationship of age to bleeding episodes, the risk was lower in younger patients, especially those who had stable INR levels over the long term [3]. In these patients, the authors suggested extending the duration between INR checks from every 3-4 weeks to 8–12 weeks. In a study of 102 cardiac patients on warfarin, INR levels were higher in older patients compared to younger patients taking the same warfarin dose [4]. The authors concluded that age is an important risk factor for bleeding in patients using warfarin. While Fang et al. found increased bleeding rates (including intracranial hemorrhage) in patients over 80 years, in their study of over 13,000 atrial fibrillation patients, these rates were similar in those taking and not taking warfarin [5]. Concomitant acetylsalicylic acid use was not an important contributor to bleeding risk in their study. They concluded that warfarin is reasonably safe to use in elderly atrial fibrillation patients if they are carefully monitored. Our patients on warfarin who presented with bleeding to the ED were not significantly older than those who had no bleeding complaint.

Other factors that might influence the risk of bleeding are frequency of INR checks, dose of warfarin, and genetic variants. Most of our patients had regular INR check-ups, every 30–90 days; the intervals in both groups were not significantly different from each other. The *VKORC1* and *CYP2C9* gene mutations are associated with higher bleeding risk in patients on warfarin, thus dosages should be modified when these mutations are found [7, 8].

Without careful monitoring, bleeding risks increase with the duration of warfarin use. Hylek et al. found that bleeding risk increased significantly in patients over 80 years who had an INR level over 4 and who had been using warfarin for more than 90 days [9]. Similarly, in a study of 184 warfarin-using patients younger than 12 years, INR levels were higher in those using warfarin for an extended duration [10]. However, Aspinall et al. found that the duration of warfarin use was not an independent risk factor for increased bleeding risk in patients followed up in an anticoagulation clinic [11].

Those with moderate to severe renal failure on warfarin have higher INR levels and risk of bleeding compared to those with normal kidney function [12, 13]. We found that our patients using warfarin who presented due to bleeding (SG) had higher creatinine levels than CG patients. Careful adjustment of warfarin dose and frequent monitoring of INR may help prevent bleeding episodes in these patients.

Many drugs affect the metabolism of warfarin, increasing or decreasing its levels and activity [1, 14]. Acetylsalicylic acid is probably the most problematic agent, as it is commonly used and its platelet-inhibiting properties act synergistically with those of warfarin to enhance any bleeding that might occur. The risk of clinically important minor and major bleeding increases 1.5–2-fold when acetylsalicylic acid and warfarin are used together [15]. As seen in Table 3, the use of aspirin was much more frequent in our patients with bleeding than in those without bleeding complaints.

Gando et al. found that coagulation pathways were triggered in cases of severe infections; therefore, one might expect an increased bleeding risk in patients using warfarin who have severe infections [16]. In our study, we found higher CRP levels in our SG patients than in our CG patients. However, most patients had no symptoms or signs of clinical infection; thus, it is difficult to associate the higher CRP levels with a specific infection or inflammatory response. Further studies should be done to clarify this relationship.

6. Limitations

This was a small, retrospective study. Bleeding scores and creatinine clearance were not calculated. To increase the success rate of data prediction, it was aimed to reach at least 30% of patients on warfarin treatment who were admitted to emergency service. After analyzing computer data retrospectively, 50% of patients on warfarin use were considered as reachable.

7. Conclusion

In emergency department patients using warfarin, increased INR level, high creatinine, and concomitant use of acetylsalicylic acid are strongly associated with a bleeding-related visit. These results will be useful in our practice here, as this is the first study in Turkey of warfarin-using patients in the emergency department and their clinical and laboratory findings. In the future, studies of genetic variations among emergency department patients using warfarin who have bleeding-related complaints should be performed.

Conflict of Interests

The authors have no conflict of interests.

Authors' Contribution

Study concept and design were done by Evren Uygungül, Cuneyt Ayrik, Huseyin Narci, and Filiz Demir. Analysis and interpretation of data were done by Evren Uygungül, Cuneyt Ayrik, and Semra Erdoğan. Drafting of the paper was made by Evren Uygungül, Cuneyt Ayrik, İbrahim Toker, Filiz Demir, and Ulas Karaaslan. Critical revision of the paper for important intellectual content was done by Evren Uygungül, Cuneyt Ayrik, Huseyin Narci, and Semra Erdoğan.

References

[1] K. R. Olson, "Warfarin and superwarfarin toxicity," 2013, http://emedicine.medscape.com/article/821038-overview.

[2] S. Schulman, S. Granqvist, M. Holmström et al., "The duration of oral anticoagulant therapy after a second episode of venous thromboembolism," *The New England Journal of Medicine*, vol. 336, no. 6, pp. 393–398, 1997.

[3] D. M. Witt, T. Delate, N. P. Clark et al., "Outcomes and predictors of very stable INR control during chronic anticoagulation therapy," *Blood*, vol. 114, no. 5, pp. 952–956, 2009.

[4] T. Miura, T. Nishinaka, T. Terada, and K. Yonezawa, "Relationship between aging and dosage of warfarin: the current status of warfarin anticoagulant therapy for Japanese outpatients in a department of cardiovascular medicine," *Journal of Cardiology*, vol. 53, no. 3, pp. 355–360, 2009.

[5] M. C. Fang, A. S. Go, E. M. Hylek et al., "Age and the risk of warfarin-associated hemorrhage: the anticoagulation and risk factors in atrial fibrillation study," *Journal of the American Geriatrics Society*, vol. 54, no. 8, pp. 1231–1236, 2006.

[6] D. A. Garcia, S. Regan, M. Crowther, and E. M. Hylek, "The risk of hemorrhage among patients with warfarin-associated coagulopathy," *Journal of the American College of Cardiology*, vol. 47, no. 4, pp. 804–808, 2006.

[7] R. S. Epstein, T. P. Moyer, R. E. Aubert et al., "Warfarin genotyping reduces hospitalization rates. Results from the MM-WES (Medco-Mayo Warfarin Effectiveness Study)," *Journal of the American College of Cardiology*, vol. 55, no. 25, pp. 2804–2812, 2010.

[8] M. Wadelius, L. Y. Chen, K. Downes et al., "Common *VKORC1* and *GGCX* polymorphisms associated with warfarin dose," *Pharmacogenomics Journal*, vol. 5, no. 4, pp. 262–270, 2005.

[9] E. M. Hylek, C. Evans-Molina, C. Shea, L. E. Henault, and S. Regan, "Major hemorrhage and tolerability of warfarin in the first year of therapy among elderly patients with atrial fibrillation," *Circulation*, vol. 115, no. 21, pp. 2689–2696, 2007.

[10] B. S. Moffett, M. Ung, and L. Bomgaars, "Risk factors for elevated INR values during warfarin therapy in hospitalized pediatric patients," *Pediatric Blood and Cancer*, vol. 58, no. 6, pp. 941–944, 2012.

[11] S. L. Aspinall, B. E. DeSanzo, L. E. Trilli, and C. B. Good, "Bleeding risk index in an anticoagulation clinic," *Journal of General Internal Medicine*, vol. 20, no. 11, pp. 1008–1013, 2005.

[12] N. A. Limdi, T. M. Beasley, M. F. Baird et al., "Kidney function influences warfarin responsiveness and hemorrhagic complications," *Journal of the American Society of Nephrology*, vol. 20, no. 4, pp. 912–921, 2009.

[13] N. A. Limdi, M. A. Limdi, L. Cavallari et al., "Warfarin dosing in patients with impaired kidney function," *Journal of Nephrology*, vol. 23, pp. 648–652, 2010.

[14] L. E. Hines, D. Ceron-Cabrera, K. Romero et al., "Evaluation of warfarin drug interaction listings in US product information for warfarin and interacting drugs," *Clinical Therapeutics*, vol. 33, no. 1, pp. 36–45, 2011.

[15] K. M. Galatro, P. C. Adams, M. Cohen, R. McBride, and H. Blanke, "Bleeding complications and INR control of combined warfarin and low-dose aspirin therapy in patients with unstable angina and Non-Q-Wave myocardial infarction," *Journal of Thrombosis and Thrombolysis*, vol. 5, no. 3, pp. 249–255, 1998.

[16] S. Gando, S. Nanzaki, S. Sasaki, and O. Kemmotsu, "Significant correlations between tissue factor and thrombin markers in trauma and septic patients with disseminated intravascular coagulation," *Thrombosis and Haemostasis*, vol. 79, no. 6, pp. 1111–1115, 1998.

10

Erythrocyte Catalase Activity in More Frequent Microcytic Hypochromic Anemia: Beta-Thalassemia Trait and Iron Deficiency Anemia

Sandra Stella Lazarte,[1] María Eugenia Mónaco,[1,2] Cecilia Laura Jimenez,[1] Miryam Emilse Ledesma Achem,[1] Magdalena María Terán,[1] and Blanca Alicia Issé[1]

[1]*Instituto de Bioquímica Aplicada, Facultad de Bioquímica, Química y Farmacia, Universidad Nacional de Tucumán (UNT), Balcarce 747, San Miguel de Tucumán, 4000 Tucumán, Argentina*
[2]*Instituto de Biología, Facultad de Bioquímica, Química y Farmacia, Universidad Nacional de Tucumán, Chacabuco 461, San Miguel de Tucumán, 4000 Tucumán, Argentina*

Correspondence should be addressed to Sandra Stella Lazarte; slazarte@fbqf.unt.edu.ar

Academic Editor: Elvira Grandone

Most common microcytic hypochromic anemias are iron deficiency anemia (IDA) and β-thalassemia trait (BTT), in which oxidative stress (OxS) has an essential role. Catalase causes detoxification of H_2O_2 in cells, and it is an indispensable antioxidant enzyme. The study was designed to measure erythrocyte catalase activity (ECAT) in patients with IDA (10) or BTT (21), to relate it with thalassemia mutation type (β^0 or β^+) and to compare it with normal subjects (67). Ninety-eight individuals were analyzed since September 2013 to June 2014 in Tucumán, Argentina. Total blood count, hemoglobin electrophoresis at alkaline pH, HbA_2, catalase, and iron status were performed. β-thalassemic mutations were determined by real-time PCR. Normal range for ECAT was 70,0–130,0 MU/L. ECAT was increased in 14% (3/21) of BTT subjects and decreased in 40% (4/10) of those with IDA. No significant difference ($p = 0,245$) was shown between normal and BTT groups, while between IDA and normal groups the difference was proved to be significant ($p = 0,000$). In β^0 and β^+ groups, no significant difference ($p = 0,359$) was observed. An altered ECAT was detected in IDA and BTT. These results will help to clarify how the catalase activity works in these anemia types.

1. Introduction

Normal erythrocytes are protected against potentially dangerous combination of oxygen and iron (hemichromes and heme associated iron) for extremely efficient endogenous mechanisms, such as superoxide dismutase (SOD), catalase, glutathione peroxidase (GPx), reduced glutathione, and vitamin E. Microcytosis is the physiological consequence of reduced hemoglobin content in the red blood cell (RBC) due to a synthesis defect of globin chains or heme [1]. Experimental data in mice showed that the mitotic events during differentiation are associated with a substantial reduction in the mean corpuscular volume (MCV) [2]. In addition to morphological, biochemical, and metabolic changes, small cell erythrocytes are characterized by shorter survival, being the oxidative damage to RBC membrane, one of the underlying mechanisms responsible [3].

Microcytosis is defined by MCV lower than 80 fL and hypochromia through mean corpuscular hemoglobin lower than 27 pg. Hypochromic microcytic anemia may result from an iron deficiency (iron deficiency anemia), a defect in the globin genes (hemoglobinopathies or thalassemia), a defect in heme synthesis (sideroblastic anemia), or a defect in iron availability and acquisition by erythroblast (anemia of chronic disease).

According to World Health Organization (WHO), the primary cause of anemia is iron deficiency, especially in pregnant women and children [4]. Regarding hemoglobinopathies, at present, about 5% of world population is carrier of a potentially pathological hemoglobin gene.

Beta- (β-) thalassemia is the most common hemoglobinopathy in the Mediterranean basin, the Middle East, and Asia [5]. Accordingly, in Argentina, β-thalassemia is the most common inherited anemia [6–8]. Therefore, the most frequent hypochromic microcytic anemias are iron deficiency anemia and β-thalassemia.

There are two molecular forms of β-thalassemia, β^+ thalassemia in which a small amount of β-globin chains are detectable and β^0 thalassemia, in which they are undetectable. Till this day there are over 200 gene mutations capable of producing thalassemia phenotypes [9]. Clinically, β-thalassemia is classified as minor (asymptomatic) or major (severe anemia), depending on the mutation responsible for this alteration is present in heterozygous or homozygous state. There is also a moderate clinical features syndrome known as thalassemia intermedia (homozygous or double heterozygous). In β-thalassemia, as a result of β-chains decrease, a relative alpha- (α-) chains excess occurs [10]. Free α-chains are unable to form viable tetramers and precipitate in RBC precursors in bone marrow forming inclusion bodies called hemichromes. They are responsible for the large intramedullary destruction of erythroblasts and therefore for ineffective erythropoiesis in β-thalassemia [11]. Hemichromes also precipitate in membrane of mature RBC and cause changes in its structure which induce lipid peroxidation and exposure of anionic phospholipids, which together leads to premature clearance by the spleen [12]. In both, erythroid precursors and mature RBCs, free iron resulting from heme denaturation produces damage to lipids membrane, cellular proteins, or DNA. Free iron is toxic because it triggers Fenton reaction in which free radicals are formed, increasing cellular oxidative stress (OxS) due to reactive oxygen species (ROS) production, such as superoxide, hydrogen peroxide (H_2O_2), and hydroxyl radicals [13].

Several studies have evaluated the oxidant and antioxidant status in thalassemia major and intermedia [14, 15], and in severe β-thalassemia it is difficult to evaluate the role played by the antioxidant enzymes because of the relevant proportion of normal red cells due to multiple transfusions. Furthermore little is known about the oxidative status in β-thalassemia trait (BTT) subjects and its relation with different β-thalassemia mutations. Such assessment is important due to the large genotypic and phenotypic heterogeneity of different populations.

The antioxidant system has been proposed as a biomarker of OxS through measuring detoxifying enzymes such as catalase [16]. The enzyme was first discovered by Louis Jacques Thenard in 1818. It is an intracellular enzyme constituted by four polypeptide chains with four heme-porphyrin groups. The human catalase gene (CAT, NCBI Gene ID: 847) is localized on the short arm of chromosome 11 (11p13) NM 001752.3 and NP 001743.1. Catalase is responsible for detoxification of H_2O_2 in cells [15]. Decreased activity of catalase may lead to increased H_2O_2 concentration and damage of oxidation sensitive tissues that may contribute to the manifestation of various diseases such as diabetes mellitus and anemia [17].

Iron deficiency affects activity of many iron-dependent enzymes (like catalase), and in iron deficiency anemia (IDA) RBCs are more susceptible to oxidation. RBCs from IDA subjects lyse more readily than normal cells on *in vitro* exposure to H_2O_2 [18], suggesting some defect in the protection mechanism of iron-deficient RBCs against oxidant damage. Increased hemoglobin autoxidation and subsequent generation of ROS can account for the shorter RBC lifespan and other pathological changes associated with IDA [19]. The literature offers contradictory and limited data on oxidative stress and antioxidant defense in patients with IDA, and increased [20] and decreased catalase activity [21] have been reported.

The present study was designed to measure catalase activity in individuals suffering from some of the most common microcytic hypochromic anemia, that is, IDA or BTT, and to compare it with normal subjects. It was also proposed to relate the type of β-thalassemia mutation with the catalase activity.

2. Materials and Methods

Design. A descriptive cross-sectional study was conducted.

Subjects. The sample consisted of 31 patients who attended *Instituto de Bioquímica Aplicada* (Tucumán, Argentina), for the diagnosis of hereditary anemia during the period of September 2013 up to June 2014. Sixty-seven normal individuals, whose participation was voluntary, were also included. Blood was drawn and placed in two different tubes, one containing K_2-EDTA anticoagulant and the other without anticoagulant with the purpose of obtaining serum.

Inclusion Criteria. Patients diagnosed with β-thalassemia minor or iron deficiency anemia and normal subjects that needed to be older than 1 year old were included.

Exclusion Criteria. People under vitamin intake, people who smoke, with diabetes, coronary heart disease, rheumatoid arthritis, dyslipidemia, hypertension, malignancy, chronic liver disease, and renal dysfunction, and patients under iron therapy during 21 days prior to analysis or who have received transfusions in the last three months were excluded.

Hematological Studies. Total blood count was performed in hematology analyzer Sysmex KX-21N (Kobe, Japan). The diagnosis of the β-thalassemia trait was performed by cellulose acetate hemoglobin (Hb) electrophoresis at alkaline pH and HbA_2 quantification by microcolumn chromatography (BioSystems, Barcelona, Spain). IDA diagnosis was made by determining serum iron, total iron binding capacity (TIBC), and transferrin saturation (SAT) through colorimetric method (Wiener Lab, Rosario, Argentina). SAT lower than 16% was considered diagnostic of IDA.

Erythrocyte Catalase Activity (ECAT). The enzyme was analyzed in K_2-EDTA anticoagulated whole blood using Góth technique [22]. Absorbance (A) of the yellow complex of molybdate and hydrogen peroxide was measured at 405 nm against blank 3. Sample contained 1,0 mL substrate (65 μmol/mL H_2O_2 in 60 mmol/L sodium-potassium buffer pH 7,4) and 30 μL hemolysate, and after 60 seconds the enzymatic reaction was stopped by adding 1,0 mL of 32,4 mmol/L ammonium molybdate. Blank 1 contained 1,0 mL substrate, 1,0 mL molybdate, and 30 μL hemolysate; blank 2 contained 1,0 mL substrate, 1,0 mL molybdate, and 30 μL buffer; blank 3 contained 1,0 mL buffer, 1.0 mL molybdate, and 30 μL buffer. One unit of catalase decomposes 1 μmol of H_2O_2 in 1 minute under these conditions and it is related to 1 L of whole blood. Catalase activity was expressed in Mega Units/L (MU/L) and was calculated with the following formula:

Erythrocyte catalase activity [MU/L]

$$= \frac{[A \text{ (blank 1)} - A \text{ (sample)}] \times 4,26 \times 100}{A \text{ (blank 2)} - A \text{ (blank 3)}}. \quad (1)$$

Molecular Analysis. Characterization of β-thalassemic mutations was realized by real-time PCR. Genomic DNA isolation was performed with High Pure PCR Template Preparation Kit (Roche Diagnostics). PCR, dissociation curves, and subsequent analysis were executed on the LightCycler 2.0 (Roche) equipment, simultaneously measuring signals from two different fluorophores. Primers were designed to amplify a 587 bp region of β-globin gene: Forward Primer, 5′-gctgtcatc act acctca tag-3′; Reverse Primer, 5′-gct gcaagt-caccactca g-3′. Two combinations of hybridization probes labeled with different fluorophores were used [23].

Statistical Analysis. Results were analyzed using SPSS 21.0 statistical program. The results were reported as Media ± Standard Deviation. For comparison Student t-Test and ANOVA were used. A significance level of $p < 0.05$ was adopted. The influence of iron serum on catalase values, independent of the group (normal, IDA, or BTT), was evaluated by simple regression analysis.

3. Results

Ninety-eight individuals were studied of which 67 were normal (N group), 21 with β-thalassemia trait (BTT group), and 10 with iron deficiency anemia (IDA group). Table 1 shows the results for catalase activity, hematological parameters, and iron status in all BTT and IDA patients. Subjects were divided according to age: children (≤12 years), adolescents (13–18 years), adults (19–59 years), and older adults (≥60 years). ANOVA detected no significant differences ($p = 0,187$) in ECAT between the stated groups.

Five individuals, who were more than 60 years old, were normal (5/67, 7.5%), 2 β-thalassemia carriers (2/21, 9.5%), and 2 IDA (2/10, 20%). Only one of these subjects, which belonged to the normal group, showed increased catalase activity (139 MU/L). Apparently, age has no influence in the ECAT of this population.

In order to establish the normal range of catalase activity, 5th and 95th percentiles of N group results were determined. A range from 70,0 to 130,0 MU/L was obtained.

Increased catalase activity in 14% (3/21) of BTT subjects was observed. No significant differences ($p = 0,245$) were observed when N and BTT groups were compared.

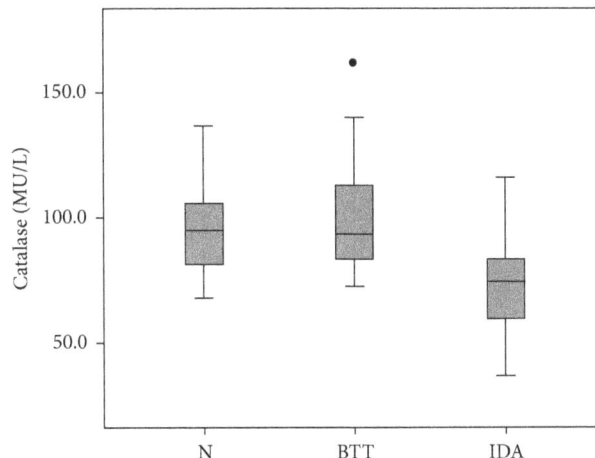

FIGURE 1: Erythrocyte catalase activity in β-thalassemia minor, iron deficiency anemia, and normal subjects. $p < 0,05$ between IDA and N groups. N, normal; IDA, iron deficiency anemia; BTT, β-thalassemia trait.

Four IDA individuals (40%) showed decreased catalase activity. No significant differences between men and women were detected in all groups. When N and IDA groups were compared, significant difference ($p = 0,000$) was observed, since the IDA subjects had lower values than N group (Figure 1).

Table 2 shows the results in N, BTT, and IDA groups according to sex. Female IDA subjects have significant differences ($p < 0,05$) with normal group in all parameters, except TIBC. Catalase in male IDA patients did not demonstrate significant differences ($p > 0,05$) when compared with normal and BTT groups.

The β-thalassemia mutations detected in order of frequency were codon 39 (C → T) (5 subjects), IVS-I-110 (G → A) (5 subjects), IVS-I-1 (G → A) (4 subjects), and IVS-I-6 (T → C) (2 subjects), and in 5 cases the mutation could not be assigned. The small number of patients for each group prevented the comparative study between them. Therefore differences between β^0 (9 subjects; ECAT = 104,6 ± 31,6 MU/L) and β^+ (7 subjects; ECAT = 91,8 ± 17,4 MU/L) groups were studied, which were not significant ($p = 0,359$).

There was no influence of iron levels on catalase values ($r^2 = 0,153$) in these samples.

4. Discussion

Oxidative stress is defined as the interruption of balance between oxidants and reductants within the body, due to the excess production of peroxides and free radicals. During the course of metabolism, superoxide anion is converted to H_2O_2 by ubiquitous enzyme SOD. Normally H_2O_2 is converted to innocuous compounds by the action of catalase and peroxidase. But if free iron is available, it reacts with H_2O_2 to form hydroxyl radicals which are extremely reactive species leading to depolymerisation of polysaccharide, DNA strand breakage, inactivation of functional proteins, and other events [24]. Therefore, this imbalance will cause

TABLE 1: Laboratory data of β-thalassemia trait and iron deficiency anemia patients.

Groups	Age [years]	HTO [L/L]	HB [g/L]	ECAT [MU/L]	Fe [μg/dL]	TIBC [μg/dL]	SAT [%]
IDA group							
Female (6)							
P1	3	0,26	64	116,2	13	262	5
P2	14	0,34	103	54,3	25	444	6
P3	76	0,37	118	61,0	33	293	11
P4	44	0,35	101	59,8	29	313	9
P5	43	0,38	117	81,3	43	358	12
P6	15	0,17	38	37,0	31	397	8
Male (4)							
P1	1	0,33	97	90,4	15	352	4
P2	1	0,31	89	83,4	18	323	6
P3	11	0,31	79	71,7	25	216	12
P4	63	0,40	115	77,0	32	403	8
BTT group							
Female (15)							
P1	12	0,35	106	95,3	78	297	26
P2	10	0,33	100	87,3	75	380	20
P3	57	0,37	107	113,9	34	233	15
P4	48	0,39	121	88,8	80	247	32
P5	33	0,37	108	87,9	90	285	31
P6	33	0,36	103	83,5	63	203	31
P7	34	0,34	104	83,6	50	180	28
P8	38	0,38	115	106,2	176	341	52
P9	63	0,38	110	73,0	81	238	34
P10	56	0,36	106	79,8	100	220	45
P11	11	0,35	105	75,2	103	322	32
P12	32	0,37	111	127,9	80	228	35
P13	22	0,35	104	86,5	104	332	31
P14	28	0,37	114	162,2	71	258	28
P15	26	0,34	101	140,1	83	283	29
Male (6)							
P1	45	0,39	115	135,4	259	266	97
P2	1	0,32	93	74,4	29	347	8
P3	12	0,38	112	93,4	66	244	27
P4	65	0,47	142	107,3	144	318	45
P5	21	0,40	121	113,3	127	208	61
P6	16	0,41	126	100,0	58	247	23

HTO, hematocrit; HB, hemoglobin; ECAT, erythrocyte catalase activity; Fe, serum iron; TIBC, total iron binding capacity; SAT, transferrin saturation; IDA, iron deficiency anemia; BTT, β-thalassemia trait; P, patient.

damage to cellular components and tissues in the body leading to OxS, and catalase has a role in it.

Kósa et al. [25] revealed a significant decrease in catalase activity of 43 β-thalassemia carriers and attributed it to catalase protein damage by increased free radicals and H_2O_2. Another study reported increased levels of antioxidant enzymes like SOD, catalase, and GPx in RBCs of β-thalassemia minor individuals and near normal values of these enzymes in RBCs of β-thalassemia major patients [26]. They concluded that β-thalassemia minor RBCs react to increased OxS rising activities of antioxidant enzymes, while in β-thalassemia major normal antioxidant enzyme levels are due to the presence of normal RBCs from multiple blood transfusions. However, Boudrahem-Addour et al. [27] observed a significant increase ($p < 0,05$) of catalase activity in β-thalassemia major and intermedia. The present results,

TABLE 2: Hematological parameters, iron status, and catalase according to pathology and sex (Media ± Standard Deviation).

Pathology Sex	Age [years]	HTO [L/L]	HB [g/L]	ECAT [MU/L]	Fe [μg/dL]	TIBC [μg/dL]	SAT [%]
IDA group							
Female (6)	20 ± 19	0,31 ± 0,08*‡	90 ± 32*‡	68,3 ± 27,4*‡	29 ± 10*‡	344 ± 68‡	8 ± 3*‡
Male (4)	19 ± 30	0,34 ± 0,04*	95 ± 15*	80,6 ± 8,1	22 ± 8*	324 ± 79	7 ± 3*
BTT group							
Female (15)	34 ± 17	0,36 ± 0,02†	108 ± 6†	99,4 ± 25,9	84 ± 32	270 ± 56	31 ± 9
Male (6)	27 ± 6	0,39 ± 0,05†	118 ± 16†	104,0 ± 20,4	114 ± 83	272 ± 52	44 ± 32
N group							
Female (39)	36 ± 13	0,41 ± 0,02	137 ± 10	96,8 ± 17,5	81 ± 18	301 ± 54	28 ± 11
Male (28)	37 ± 15	0,44 ± 0,02	147 ± 9	93,1 ± 15,4	94 ± 28	282 ± 38	34 ± 11

* $p < 0,05$ between IDA and N groups by sex; † $p < 0,05$ between BTT and N groups by sex; ‡ $p < 0,05$ between IDA and BTT women.
IDA, iron deficiency anemia; BTT, β-thalassemia trait; N, normal; HTO, hematocrit; HB, hemoglobin; ECAT, erythrocyte catalase activity; Fe, iron; TIBC, total iron binding capacity; SAT, transferrin saturation.

in concordance with Gerli et al. [26], showed that some BTT subjects had increased catalase activity.

Several authors reported increased antioxidant capacity in BTT individuals, but they do not measured catalase activity [28, 29]. Instead, they used a novel automated measurement method and Trolox equivalent antioxidant capacity.

In the catalase activity comparison between β^0 and β^+ thalassemia traits, the results were not significant. Also, Kósa et al. [25] did not find significant differences and concluded that catalase activity was not related to specific β-thalassemia mutations. Furthermore, Labib et al. [30] reported no differences in total antioxidant capacity of β^0 and β^+ thalassemia traits.

The normal range of erythrocyte catalase activity was slightly lower than the one reported by another authors [31], which was 80,3 to 146,3 MU/L. Difference may be due to the racial characteristics of the population, methodological differences, and because they used 2,5th and 97,5th percentiles to establish normal range. Men and women have no significant differences in what catalase activity concerns. Instead, Vitai and Góth [31] found slightly higher values in male subjects.

In this study, like Ondei et al. [29], there was no relationship between ECAT and iron serum. In β-thalassemia major and intermedia, iron excess can lead to organ damage, especially in liver and heart, and to endocrine dysfunction [32]. Recent studies have shown the importance of other markers such as non-transferrin bound iron (NTBI) and labile plasma iron (LPI) to detect iron excess in thalassemia patients due to the direct correlation of these markers with the formation of free radicals [33].

Decreasing serum iron concentration causes insufficient Hb synthesis with subsequent reduction of erythrocytes proliferation. Iron deficiency also affects the production of other iron-containing proteins, such as cytochrome, myoglobin, catalase, and peroxidase. Therefore, a decreased catalase activity could be anticipated in iron deficiency and has been corroborated in this study, in agreement with other works [21, 34, 35]. However, Madhikarmi and Murthy [20] detected an unexplained increase of catalase activity in IDA, and Tekin et al. [36] reported no differences in SOD and catalase

activities between IDA patients and controls. Bay et al. [37] compared antioxidant capacity between IDA and normal subjects and detected no significant differences.

Increased OxS have been reported in patients with IDA [3, 21, 35], which occurs primarily in RBC membrane. ROS membrane surface contributes to deformability alteration [38] and phosphatidylserine exposure, which have been used to explain the reduction of RBCs life in IDA [39]. Also, in BTT an altered oxidative state was reported by some investigators [28, 30]. Therefore, OxS is present in the most common hypochromic microcytic anemia, IDA and BTT, being one of the determining factors of altered catalase activity. Hypochromic microcytic RBCs of BTT and IDA individuals have been studied in the past decades and OxS contribution in reducing the RBCs useful life has been documented. Previous studies on the catalase activity of hypochromic microcytic anemia such as IDA and BTT have reported disagreeing results [20, 21, 25, 26, 34, 35]. In the present work, catalase activity was decreased in IDA and increased in some BTT subjects, with no significant differences between beta-thalassemia mutations. These results will help to clarify how the catalase activity works in these anemia types. The low number of samples is a limitation of this report. Probably, the incorporation of a larger number of participants will allow revealing hidden differences in current work.

Consent

All patients signed an informed consent previously approved by the *Comité de Bioética de la Facultad de Medicina, UNT*.

Conflict of Interests

The authors declare that there is no conflict of interests regarding the publication of this paper.

Acknowledgments

This work was supported by grants from the *Consejo de Investigaciones de la Universidad Nacional de Tucumán*

(CIUNT 26/D520). The authors thank Biochemist Specialist Guillermo Fabián Vechetti and Laboratorio Tucumán for the use of its molecular biology equipment.

References

[1] A. Lolascon, L. De Falco, and C. Beaumont, "Molecular basis of inherited microcytic anemia due to defects in iron acquisitionor heme synthesis," *Haematologica*, vol. 94, no. 3, pp. 395–408, 2009.

[2] A. Coopersmith and M. Ingram, "Red cell volumes and erythropoiesis. II. Age: density: volume relationships of macrocytes," *American Journal of Physiology*, vol. 216, no. 3, pp. 473–482, 1969.

[3] J. L. V. Corrons, A. Miguel-Garcia, M. A. Pujades et al., "Increased susceptibility of microcytic red blood cells to in vitro oxidative stress," *European Journal of Haematology*, vol. 55, no. 5, pp. 327–331, 1995.

[4] WHO Global Database on Anaemia, *Worldwide Prevalence of Anaemia 1993-2005*, 2008, http://whqlibdoc.who.int/publications/2008/9789241596657_eng.pdf.

[5] OMS, "Talasemia y otras hemoglobinopatías. Informe de la Secretaría," mayo de 2006, http://apps.who.int/gb/archive/pdf_files/EB118/B118_5-sp.pdf.

[6] M. S. Abreu and J. A. Peñalver, "S hemoglobinopathies in Argentina," *Medicina (Buenos Aires)*, vol. 52, no. 4, pp. 341–346, 1992.

[7] S. Lazarte, B. Issé, and G. Agüero, "Hemoglobinophaties and thalassemia syndromes in Tucumán: preliminary study," *Biocell*, vol. 25, no. 1, 2001.

[8] A. Larregina, E. Reimer, N. Suldrup, S. Luis, J. Zavatti, and N. N. Polini, "Diagnóstico diferencial de anemias microcíticas," *Acta Bioquimica Clinica Latinoamericana*, vol. 38, no. 4, pp. 465–469, 2004.

[9] S. L. Thein, "The molecular basis of β-thalassemia," *Cold Spring Harbor Perspectives in Medicine*, vol. 3, no. 5, Article ID a011700, 2013.

[10] B. E. Clark and S. L. Thein, "Molecular diagnosis of haemoglobin disorders," *Clinical and Laboratory Haematology*, vol. 26, no. 3, pp. 159–176, 2004.

[11] S. L. Thein, "Pathophysiology of beta thalassemia—a guide to molecular therapies," *Hematology/American Society of Hematology. Education Program*, pp. 31–37, 2005.

[12] M. D. Cappellini, D. Tavazzi, L. Duca et al., "Metabolic indicators of oxidative stress correlate with haemichrome attachment to membrane, band 3 aggregation and erythrophagocytosis in β-thalassaemia intermedia," *British Journal of Haematology*, vol. 104, no. 3, pp. 504–512, 1999.

[13] R. Evstatiev and C. Gasche, "Iron sensing and signalling," *Gut*, vol. 61, no. 6, pp. 933–952, 2012.

[14] C. Kattamis, C. Lazaropoulou, P. Delaporta, F. Apostolakou, A. Kattamis, and I. Papassotiriou, "Disturbances of biomarkers of iron and oxidant-antioxidant homeostasis in patients with beta-thalassemia intermedia," *Pediatric Endocrinology Reviews*, vol. 8, pp. 256–262, 2011.

[15] Q. Shazia, Z. H. Mohammad, T. Rahman, and H. U. Shekhar, "Correlation of oxidative stress with serum trace element levels and antioxidant enzyme status in beta thalassemia major patients: a review of the literature," *Anemia*, vol. 2012, Article ID 270923, 7 pages, 2012.

[16] E. Fibach and E. Rachmilewitz, "The role of oxidative stress in hemolytic anemia," *Current Molecular Medicine*, vol. 8, no. 7, pp. 609–619, 2008.

[17] T. Nagy, E. Paszti, M. Kaplar, H. P. Bhattoa, and L. Goth, "Further acatalasemia mutations in human patients from Hungary with diabetes and microcytic anemia," *Mutation Research—Fundamental and Molecular Mechanisms of Mutagenesis*, vol. 772, pp. 10–14, 2015.

[18] L. G. Macdougall, "Red cell metabolism in iron deficiency anemia III. The relationship between glutathione peroxidase, catalase, serum vitamin E, and susceptibility of iron-deficient red cells to oxidative hemolysis," *The Journal of Pediatrics*, vol. 80, no. 5, pp. 775–782, 1972.

[19] E. Nagababu, S. Gulyani, C. J. Earley, R. G. Cutler, M. P. Mattson, and J. M. Rifkind, "Iron-deficiency anaemia enhances red blood cell oxidative stress," *Free Radical Research*, vol. 42, no. 9, pp. 824–829, 2008.

[20] N. L. Madhikarmi and K. R. S. Murthy, "Antioxidant enzymes and oxidative stress in the erythrocytes of iron deficiency anemic patients supplemented with vitamins," *Iranian Biomedical Journal*, vol. 18, no. 2, pp. 82–87, 2014.

[21] E. Kurtoglu, A. Ugur, A. K. Baltaci, and L. Undar, "Effect of iron supplementation on oxidative stress and antioxidant status in iron-deficiency anemia," *Biological Trace Element Research*, vol. 96, no. 1–3, pp. 117–123, 2003.

[22] L. Góth, "Two cases of acatalasemia in Hungary," *Clinica Chimica Acta*, vol. 207, no. 1-2, pp. 155–158, 1992.

[23] S. S. Lazarte, M. E. Mónaco, A. C. Haro, C. L. Jiménez, M. E. Ledesma Achem, and B. A. Issé, "Molecular characterization and phenotypical study of β-thalassemia in Tucumán, Argentina," *Hemoglobin*, vol. 38, no. 6, pp. 394–401, 2014.

[24] F. Simsek, G. Ozturk, S. Kemahli, D. Erbas, and A. Hasanoglu, "Oxidant and antioxidant status in beta thalassemia major patients," *Ankara Üniversitesi Tıp Fakültesi Mecmuası*, vol. 58, pp. 34–38, 2005.

[25] Z. Kósa, T. Nagy, E. Nagy, F. Fazakas, and L. Góth, "Decreased blood catalase activity is not related to specific beta-thalassemia mutations in Hungary," *International Journal of Laboratory Hematology*, vol. 34, no. 2, pp. 172–178, 2012.

[26] G. C. Gerli, L. Beretta, M. Bianchi, A. Pellegatta, and A. Agostoni, "Erythrocyte superoxide dismutase, catalase and glutathione peroxidase activities in β-thalassemia (major and minor)," *Scandinavian Journal of Haematology*, vol. 25, no. 1, pp. 87–92, 1980.

[27] N. Boudrahem-Addour, M. Izem-Meziane, K. Bouguerra et al., "Oxidative status and plasma lipid profile in β-thalassemia patients," *Hemoglobin*, vol. 39, no. 1, pp. 36–41, 2015.

[28] S. Selek, M. Aslan, M. Horoz, M. Gur, and O. Erel, "Oxidative status and serum PON1 activity in beta-thalassemia minor," *Clinical Biochemistry*, vol. 40, no. 5-6, pp. 287–291, 2007.

[29] L. D. S. Ondei, I. D. F. Estevão, M. I. P. Rocha et al., "Oxidative stress and antioxidant status in beta-thalassemia heterozygotes," *Revista Brasileira de Hematologia e Hemoterapia*, vol. 35, no. 6, pp. 409–413, 2013.

[30] H. A. Labib, R. L. Etewa, O. A. Gaber, M. Atfy, T. M. Mostafa, and I. Barsoum, "Paraoxonase-1 and oxidative status in common Mediterranean β-thalassaemia mutations trait, and their relations to atherosclerosis," *Journal of Clinical Pathology*, vol. 64, no. 5, pp. 437–442, 2011.

[31] M. Vitai and L. Góth, "Reference ranges of normal blood catalase activity and levels in familial hypocatalasemia in Hungary," *Clinica Chimica Acta*, vol. 261, no. 1, pp. 35–42, 1997.

[32] S. Gardenghi, R. W. Grady, and S. Rivella, "Anemia, ineffective erythropoiesis, and hepcidin: interacting factors in abnormal iron metabolism leading to iron overload in β-thalassemia," *Hematology/Oncology Clinics of North America*, vol. 24, no. 6, pp. 1089–1107, 2010.

[33] P. Brissot, M. Ropert, C. Le Lan, and O. Loréal, "Non-transferrin bound iron: a key role in iron overload and iron toxicity," *Biochimica et Biophysica Acta—General Subjects*, vol. 1820, no. 3, pp. 403–410, 2012.

[34] F. Amirkhizi, F. Siassi, S. Minaie, M. Djalali, A. Rahimi, and M. Chamari, "Assessment of lipid peroxidation and activities of erythrocyte cytoprotective enzymes in women with iron deficiency anemia," *Journal of Research in Medical Sciences*, vol. 13, no. 5, pp. 248–254, 2008.

[35] J.-H. Yoo, H.-Y. Maeng, Y.-K. Sun et al., "Oxidative status in iron-deficiency anemia," *Journal of Clinical Laboratory Analysis*, vol. 23, no. 5, pp. 319–323, 2009.

[36] D. Tekin, S. Yavuzer, M. Tekin, N. Akar, and S. Cin, "Possible effects of antioxidant status on increased platelet aggregation in childhood iron-deficiency anemia," *Pediatrics International*, vol. 43, no. 1, pp. 74–77, 2001.

[37] A. Bay, M. Dogan, K. Bulan, S. Kaba, N. Demir, and A. F. Öner, "A study on the effects of pica and iron-deficiency anemia on oxidative stress, antioxidant capacity and trace elements," *Human and Experimental Toxicology*, vol. 32, no. 9, pp. 895–903, 2013.

[38] A. Vayá, M. Simó, M. Santaolaria, J. Todolí, and J. Aznar, "Red blood cell deformability in iron deficiency anaemia," *Clinical Hemorheology and Microcirculation*, vol. 33, no. 1, pp. 75–80, 2005.

[39] D. S. Kempe, P. A. Lang, C. Duranton et al., "Enhanced programmed cell death of iron-deficient erythrocytes," *The FASEB Journal*, vol. 20, no. 2, pp. 368–370, 2006.

11

Impaired Fibrinolysis in Angiographically Documented Coronary Artery Disease

Adriano Basques Fernandes,[1] **Luciana Moreira Lima,**[1]
Marinez Oliveira Sousa,[1] **Vicente de Paulo Coelho Toledo,**[1] **Rashid Saeed Kazmi,**[2]
Bashir Abdulgader Lwaleed,[3] **and Maria das Graças Carvalho**[1]

[1]*Faculty of Pharmacy, Federal University of Minas Gerais, Avenida Antonio Carlos 6627, 31270-901 Belo Horizonte, MG, Brazil*
[2]*Department of Haematology, University Hospital Southampton, Southampton, UK*
[3]*Faculty of Health Sciences, University of Southampton, Southampton, UK*

Correspondence should be addressed to Rashid Saeed Kazmi; rashid.kazmi@uhs.nhs.uk

Academic Editor: Owen McCarty

Impaired fibrinolysis may predispose to coronary artery disease (CAD). Hypofibrinolysis due to high levels of plasminogen activator inhibitor-1 (PAI-1) has been reported in CAD. A novel regulator of fibrinolytic activity, thrombin activatable fibrinolysis inhibitor (TAFI), has attracted attention in recent years. It acts by blocking the formation of a ternary complex of plasminogen, fibrin, and tissue plasminogen activator (t-PA). Previously ambiguous results regarding TAFI levels have been reported in CAD. We measured plasma levels of PAI-1 and TAFI antigen in 123 patients with age ranging from 40 to 65 years who had been submitted to coronary angiography and assessed the association of these markers with the extent of stenosis in three groups: angiographically normal artery (NAn), mild to moderate atheromatosis (MA), and severe atheromatosis (SA). Plasma levels of PAI-1 were increased in patients with severe atheromatosis compared to mild/moderate atheromatosis or to normal patients (66.60, 40.50, and 34.90 ng/mL, resp.; $P < 0.001$). For TAFI no difference was found between different groups. When patients were grouped in only two groups based on clinical cut-off point for intervention (stenosis less than or above 70%) we found increased plasma levels for PAI-1 (37.55 and 66.60 ng/mL, resp.; $P < 0.001$) and decreased plasma levels for TAFI (5.20 and 4.53 μg/mL, resp.; $P = 0.04$) in patients with stenosis above 70%. No difference was found in PAI-1 or TAFI levels comparing the number of affected vessels. *Conclusion*. As evidenced by a raised level of PAI-1 antigen, one can suggest an impaired fibrinolysis in stable CAD, although no correlation with the number of affected vessels was found. Curiously, a decreased plasma level of total TAFI levels was observed in patients with stenosis above 70%. Further studies measuring functional TAFI are required in order to elucidate its association with the extent of degree of atheromatosis.

1. Introduction

The endothelium mediates a variety of vital physiological functions. While in health it maintains vascular integrity by expressing vasoprotective and thromboresistant molecules, on activation endothelial cells (ECs) acquire a phenotype that promotes atherosclerosis [1]. The thrombin catalyzed conversion of plasma fibrinogen into fibrin is the final step of coagulation cascade during haemostasis. The formation of thrombus is followed by the process of fibrinolysis which consists of an enzymatic dissolution of the fibrin clot by plasmin.

It is controlled by endothelial cells through secretion of physiological plasminogen activators like tissue type plasminogen activator (t-PA) and urokinase type plasminogen activator (u-PA). Fibrinolysis is initiated when both plasminogen and t-PA bind to fibrin surface to generate plasmin [2]. However, plasmin is generated on the surface of endothelial cells in the presence or absence of fibrin. In the absence of fibrin plasmin generation is dependent on the constitutively expressed plasminogen and t-PA receptor, annexin 2A. The endothelium also exerts an inhibitory effect on fibrinolysis through the synthesis of an inhibitor, type 1 plasminogen activator inhibitor (PAI-1). High levels of PAI-1 have been shown to be associated with CAD [3, 4]. Yet another fibrinolytic inhibitor is thrombin activatable fibrinolysis inhibitor (TAFI), a plasma zymogen that potently inhibits fibrinolysis when converted to an active enzyme by thrombin, plasmin, trypsin, and, more efficiently, thrombin-thrombomodulin complex [5]. Activated TAFI (TAFIa) inhibits fibrinolysis by removing the carboxyterminal lysine (and arginine) residues on partially degraded fibrin, blocking the formation of a ternary complex of plasminogen, and t-PA. Some studies have shown a trend for increased TAFI levels in CAD patients [6–8]. On the contrary other investigators have found decreased levels of TAFI in CAD patients [9].

The aim of this study was to investigate the association of PAI-1 and TAFI antigen levels with increasing degrees of coronary atheromatosis in patients undergoing angiography.

2. Material and Methods

The population investigated consisted of 123 subjects with age ranging from 40 to 65 years, who had been consecutively submitted to coronary angiography in the Department of Haemodynamics of Socor Hospital, Belo Horizonte, Brazil. This protocol was submitted to the local ethical committees in research of Socor Hospital and Federal University of Minas Gerais. Signed informed consent was required for all subjects enrolled in this study.

This study assessed a population of intermediate to high risk of CAD who had been referred for catheterization due to worsening clinical features on a background of a history of stable angina. Patients with acute coronary syndrome in the preceding 3 months were excluded from the study as were those having concomitant treatment with anticoagulants, lipid lowering drugs, or estrogens, patients with known bleeding or thrombotic disorders, and those with renal, hepatic, autoimmune, or malignant diseases.

Coronary angiography was performed in all 123 subjects by percutaneous transfemoral approach. The images were recorded digitally and all angiograms were analyzed by three experienced cardiologists. The patients were grouped according to the angiographic findings as follows: no stenosis (Group I), stenosis of up to 30% of the luminal diameter in at least one coronary artery (Group II), stenosis of 30 to 70% of the luminal diameter in at least one coronary artery (Group III), and stenosis of more than 70% of the luminal diameter in at least one coronary artery (Group IV).

Blood samples were collected from 12 h fasting patients after coronary angiography (since patients stratification was dependent on this procedure), however, before any other intervention following angiography, into vacuum tubes containing 3.2 w/v sodium citrate as anticoagulant. Blood samples were immediately centrifuged at 2100 g for 20 minutes and plasma samples were separated and stored at −70°C until analysis.

Plasma level of TAFI was performed using a commercially available ELISA Kit (TAFI Antigen Kit, Affinity Biologicals Inc., Canada) according to the manufacturer's instructions.

Quantitative determination of plasma TAFI was performed using citrated set diagnostic Visualize TAFI Antigen Kit (Affinity Biologicals Inc., Canada) whose analytical principle is the enzyme-linked immunosorbent assay (ELISA capture), strictly following the instructions provided by the manufacturer. A microplate reader, BIO-RAD 550-USA, was used for reading the reaction. The reference curve was performed using the standard provided by the manufacturer obtaining the points of 6.8, 3.4, 1.7, 0.850, 0.425, and 0.213 mg/mL and two plasma controls provided by the kit were used to verify the assay performance. The concentration of TAFI in the sample was obtained using the following equation:

$$\log(y) = A + Bx \log(x), \tag{1}$$

with reference value from 5.8 to 10.0 μg/mL.

PAI-1 level was determined using a commercial ELISA Kit (IMUBIND PAI-1 ELISA Kit, American Diagnostica Inc., USA). The intra- and interassay coefficients were 9.0% and 6.6%, respectively (IMUBIND PAI-1 ELISA Kit, American Diagnostica Inc., USA). For both, TAFI and PAI-1, control plasmas were used to verify the assay performance.

Normal distribution of the data was checked by Shapiro-Wilks test. The results were presented as mean and standard deviation (SD) when normally distributed and otherwise as median and interquartile ranges (25th and 75th percentiles). For normally distributed data, ANOVA was used to compare three groups. Mann-Whitney and Kruskal-Wallis tests followed by Dunn's test were used in case of non-normally data for comparison of three groups. Statistical analysis was performed by Sigma Stat version 1.0 software system. A value of $P < 0.05$ was chosen for statistical significance.

3. Results

The baseline characteristics of the study participants are presented in Table 1. The three groups showed homogeneity in relation to age, sex, and body mass index and no statistically significant difference was noted. The incidence for hypertension was high in all three groups. The differences in the incidence of smoking, sedentary lifestyle, and previous history of CAD were statistically significant amongst different degrees of severity of CAD.

Plasma levels of PAI-1 were increased in patients with severe atheromatosis (Group IV) compared to mild/moderate atheromatosis (Groups II/III) ($P < 0.001$) or to angiographically normal (Group I) patients. For TAFI no statistically significant difference was found between groups. Plasma levels of PAI-1 and TAFI are presented in Table 2.

Considering that a clinical intervention must be made in all patients presenting with stenosis above 70%, all of them were rescored in two groups: stenosis of up to 70% of the luminal diameter in at least one coronary artery and stenosis of more than 70% of the luminal diameter in at least one coronary artery. Table 3 shows results for PAI-1 and TAFI in these two groups.

Based on this clinical cut point for intervention, we found *increased* plasma levels for PAI-1 ($P < 0.001$) and decreased

TABLE 1: Baseline patients' characteristics.

	Group I	Groups II/III	Group IV	P
n (M/F)	35 (16/19)	31 (17/14)	57 (31/26)	ns
Men	16 (45.7%)	17 (54.8%)	31 (54.4%)	ns
Age (years)	59.0 ± 7.5	59.5 ± 9.0	60.5 ± 8.8	ns
BMI (Kg/m^2)	25.3 ± 4.1	26.8 ± 4.7	25.8 ± 3.5	ns
Current smoker	6 (17.1%)	8 (25.8%)	23 (40.4%)[a]	P[a] = 0.020
Hypertension	31 (88.6%)	25 (80.6%)	48 (84.2%)	ns
Sedentary lifestyle	33 (94.3%)	23 (74.2%)[A]	43 (75.4%)[a]	P[a] = 0.021 P[A] = 0.023
Family history of CAD	14 (40.0%)	18 (58.1%)	29 (50.8%)	ns
Diabetes mellitus	5 (14.3%)	7 (22.6%)	8 (14.0%)	ns
Previous history of CAD	7 (20.0%)	12 (38.7%)	35 (61.4%)[a]	P[a] < 0.0001

n = sample size; M = male; F = female; BMI = body mass index; ns = not significant; Group I = normal; Groups II/III = mild/moderate atheromatosis, up to 70% in at least one coronary artery; Group IV = severe atheromatosis, >70% in at least one coronary artery; a/A = significant difference to Group I (ANOVA).

TABLE 2: Plasma fibrinolytic markers.

	Group I	Groups II/III	Group IV	P
n	35	31	57	—
PAI-1	34.90 (27.86; 42.43)	40.50 (34.24; 51.83)	66.60[a,b] (44.70; 91.65)	P < 0.001
TAFI	5.71 ± 1.73	5.21 ± 1.42	4.97 ± 1.41	ns

n = sample size; Group I = normal; Groups II/III = mild/moderate atheromatosis, up to 70% in at least one coronary artery; Group IV = severe atheromatosis, >70% in at least one coronary artery; PAI-1 = type 1 plasminogen activator inhibitor; TAFI = thrombin activatable fibrinolysis inhibitor; [a]versus Group I and [b]versus Groups II/III; ns = not significant.
Values for PAI-1 are given in median (25th and 75th percentiles) and expressed in (ng/mL).
Values for TAFI are given in mean ± SD and expressed in (μg/mL).

TABLE 3: Plasma fibrinolysis markers considering stenosis of 70% as clinical cut point for intervention.

	Stenosis < 70%	Stenosis > 70%	P
n	66	57	—
PAI-1	37.55 (30.90; 49.20)	66.60[a] (44.70; 91.65)	P < 0.001
TAFI	5.20 (4.37; 6.31)	4.53[a] (4.04; 5.63)	P = 0.04

n = sample size; PAI-1 = type 1 plasminogen activator inhibitor; TAFI = thrombin activatable fibrinolytic inhibitor; [a]versus stenosis <70%. Values for PAI-1 and TAFI are given in median (25th and 75th percentiles) and expressed in ng/mL and μg/mL, respectively.

TABLE 4: Plasma fibrinolysis markers considering number of affected vessels.

	1v	2v	3v	P
n	16	13	28	—
PAI-1	92.79 ± 60.45	71.83 ± 39.29	62.15 ± 31.97	ns
TAFI	5.31 ± 1.52	4.75 ± 1.16	4.87 ± 1.46	ns

n = sample size; 1v = stenosis in one vessel; 2v = stenosis in two vessels; 3v = stenosis in three or more vessels; PAI-1 = type 1 plasminogen activator inhibitor; TAFI = thrombin activatable fibrinolytic inhibitor; ns = not significant. Values for PAI-1 and TAFI are given in mean ± SD and expressed in ng/mL and μg/mL, respectively.

plasma levels for TAFI (P = 0.04) in patients with stenosis of more than 70%.

We also explored the severity of CAD through the number of affected vessels in patients with stenosis of more than 70% versus plasma levels of PAI-1 and TAFI. No statistically significant difference was found between groups (Table 4).

4. Discussion

Regulation of blood coagulation is an intricate coordination between different pathways. Maintaining a balance between thrombin-stimulated fibrin clot formation and plasmin-induced clot lysis is essential for optimal haemostasis. Any disturbance in these pathways causes a haemorrhagic or a thrombotic tendency depending on the shift of the balance [10]. The data from this study demonstrate that fibrinolysis is impaired in subjects with angiographically documented CAD. PAI-1 levels were increased in patients with severe atheromatosis compared to mild/moderate atheromatosis (P < 0.001) or angiographically normal patients.

Increased levels of PAI-1 have been described in patients with CAD after myocardial infarction (MI) [3] and are considered a risk factor for recurrence [4]. We tried to correlate the severity of disease with the number of affected vessels and PAI-1 levels, but no significant difference between different groups was found (Table 4). Thrombin also plays an important role in fibrinolytic modulation through activation of TAFI [11]. Activated TAFI inhibits plasmin formation and downregulates fibrinolysis [5] contributing to a hypofibrinolytic state in cardiovascular disease [9]. In the present study, we did not find any significant difference in TAFI levels between groups (Table 2). Interestingly, when we rescored groups based on clinical cut point for intervention (stenosis of more than 70%) TAFI plasma levels were decreased in subjects with stenosis of more than 70% (Table 3) compared to those with stenosis of up to 70%, consistent with a previous study [9]. No difference was found between severity of disease through number of affected vessels and TAFI levels (Table 4). Controversial results regarding TAFI levels in CAD patients have been described possibly because of both different characteristics of patients investigated and methods used for its determination [12].

Different clinical studies have investigated the possible relationship between TAFI and cardiovascular events [12]. The results have been inconsistent and studies have reported high, normal, and low plasma levels of TAFI [6–8].

We could speculate that the amount of TAFI generated during coagulation and fibrinolysis varies in different cardiovascular disease stages and, in addition, different results obtained through different assays demonstrate the variable reactivity of antibodies toward different isoforms of TAFI. An important study [13] comparing different TAFI assays has demonstrated that pro-TAFI assay measures high levels of TAFI in CAD, while TAFI antigen assays can detect no alterations in TAFI plasma levels or a slight decrease of TAFI plasma levels in the same samples. We can also speculate that different antibodies react to different isoforms of TAFI, yielding ambiguous results.

The importance of haemostatic alterations in CAD is being increasingly recognised in cardiovascular diseases. Our study has demonstrated that PAI-1 plasma levels are increased in a limited number of CAD patients in Brazilian patients, in line with previous studies [5, 9]. Although decreased TAFI levels are in agreement with other studies [9], its physiological relevance and pathogenic role remain unclear since only the levels of TAFI antigen were evaluated precluding any conclusion on the TAFI function.

The major limitation of the present study was that our observations were based on a small number of patients, which precludes a specific cut-off for PAI-1 and TAFI antigens in severe disease. Another limitation is the fact that in a cohort cross-sectional study we tried to evaluate associations, not predictions or causation. Finally, our findings are related to a group of patients referred for catheterization due to thoracic pain selected by experienced cardiologists. Thus, our subjects with no stenosis may not be representative of the general population. Further work is required to investigate PAI-1 and TAFI antigens roles in CAD in a greater number of patients and functional assays are also required for clarifying the real role of these fibrinolysis inhibitors. Also known modifiers of PAI-1 levels such as smoking, body mass index, and circadian variation should be considered for result interpretation.

In conclusion, this small study confirms an impaired fibrinolysis in stable CAD considering the increased levels of PAI-1, indicating that this marker is actually associated with the atheromatosis extent, although the number of affected vessels seems not to have contributed to increase of PAI-1 levels.

Conflict of Interests

The authors declare that there is no conflict of interests regarding the publication of this paper.

References

[1] K. K. Wu, N. Aleksic, C. M. Ballantyne, C. Ahn, H. Juneja, and E. Boerwinkle, "Interaction between soluble thrombomodulin and intercellular adhesion molecule-1 in predicting risk of coronary heart disease," *Circulation*, vol. 107, no. 13, pp. 1729–1732, 2003.

[2] B. N. Bouma and L. O. Mosnier, "Thrombin Activatable Fibrinolysis Inhibitor (TAFI) at the interface between coagulation and fibrinolysis," *Pathophysiology of Haemostasis and Thrombosis*, vol. 33, no. 5-6, pp. 375–381, 2004.

[3] W. Koenig, D. Rothenbacher, A. Hoffmeister, M. Griesshammer, and H. Brenner, "Plasma fibrin D-dimer levels and risk of stable coronary artery disease: results of a large case-control study," *Arteriosclerosis, Thrombosis, and Vascular Biology*, vol. 21, no. 10, pp. 1701–1705, 2001.

[4] A. M. Thögersen, J.-H. Jansson, K. Boman et al., "High plasminogen activator inhibitor and tissue plasminogen activator levels in plasma precede a first acute myocardial infarction in both men and women: evidence for the fibrinolytic system as an independent primary risk factor," *Circulation*, vol. 98, no. 21, pp. 2241–2247, 1998.

[5] A. Paola Cellai, E. Antonucci, A. Alessandrello Liotta et al., "TAFI activity and antigen plasma levels are not increased in acute coronary artery disease patients admitted to a coronary care unit," *Thrombosis Research*, vol. 118, no. 4, pp. 495–500, 2006.

[6] A. Silveira, K. Schatteman, F. Goossens et al., "Plasma procarboxypeptidase U in men with symptomatic coronary artery disease," *Thrombosis and Haemostasis*, vol. 84, no. 3, pp. 364–368, 2000.

[7] V. Schroeder, T. Chatterjee, H. Mehta et al., "Thrombin activatable fibrinolysis inhibitor (TAFI) levels in patients with coronary artery disease investigated by angiography," *Thrombosis and Haemostasis*, vol. 88, no. 6, pp. 1020–1025, 2002.

[8] A. Santamaría, A. Martínez-Rubio, M. Borrell, J. Mateo, R. Ortín, and J. Fontcuberta, "Risk of acute coronary artery disease associated with functional thrombin activatable fibrinolysis inhibitor plasma level," *Haematologica*, vol. 89, no. 7, pp. 880–881, 2004.

[9] I. Juhan-Vague, P. E. Morange, H. Aubert et al., "Plasma thrombin-activatable fibrinolysis inhibitor antigen concentration and genotype in relation to myocardial infarction in the North and South of Europe," *Arteriosclerosis, Thrombosis, and Vascular Biology*, vol. 22, no. 5, pp. 867–873, 2002.

[10] G. Cesarman-Maus and K. A. Hajjar, "Molecular mechanisms of fibrinolysis," *British Journal of Haematology*, vol. 129, no. 3, pp. 307–321, 2005.

[11] N. H. van Tilburg, F. R. Rosendaal, and R. M. Bertina, "Thrombin activatable fibrinolysis inhibitor and the risk for deep vein thrombosis," *Blood*, vol. 95, no. 9, pp. 2855–2859, 2000.

[12] E. Ceresa, E. Brouwers, M. Peeters, C. Jern, P. J. Declerck, and A. Gils, "Development of ELISAs measuring the extent of TAFI activation," *Arteriosclerosis, Thrombosis, and Vascular Biology*, vol. 26, no. 2, pp. 423–428, 2006.

[13] M. Skeppholm, N. H. Wallén, K. Malmqvist, A. Kallner, and J. P. Antovic, "Comparison of two immunochemical assays for measuring thrombin-activatable fibrinolysis inhibitor concentration with a functional assay in patients with acute coronary syndrome," *Thrombosis Research*, vol. 121, no. 2, pp. 175–181, 2007.

12

Comparable Outcomes for Hematologic Malignancies after HLA-Haploidentical Transplantation with Posttransplantation Cyclophosphamide and HLA-Matched Transplantation

Shannon R. McCurdy and Ephraim J. Fuchs

Sidney Kimmel Comprehensive Cancer Center at Johns Hopkins, Baltimore, MD 21287, USA

Correspondence should be addressed to Shannon R. McCurdy; smccurd2@jhmi.edu

Academic Editor: Suparno Chakrabarti

The implementation of high-dose posttransplantation cyclophosphamide (PTCy) has made HLA-haploidentical (haplo) blood or marrow transplantation (BMT) a cost effective and safe alternative donor transplantation technique, resulting in its increasing utilization over the last decade. We review the available retrospective comparisons of haplo BMT with PTCy and HLA-matched BMT in adults with hematologic malignancies. The examined studies demonstrate no difference between haplo BMT with PTCy and HLA-matched BMT with regard to acute graft-versus-host disease (aGVHD), nonrelapse mortality, and overall survival. Chronic GVHD occurred less frequently after haplo BMT with PTCy compared with HLA-matched BMT utilizing standard GVHD prophylaxis. In addition, patients with a high risk of relapse by the disease risk index had a suggestion of improved progression-free and overall survival after haplo BMT with PTCy when compared with a historical cohort of HLA-matched BMT in one analysis. Furthermore, in Hodgkin lymphoma relapse and progression-free survival were improved in the haplo BMT with PTCy compared with the HLA-matched BMT cohort. These findings support the use of this transplantation platform when HLA-matched related donors (MRDs) are unavailable and suggest that clinical scenarios exist in which haplo BMT may be preferred to HLA-matched BMT, which warrant further investigation.

1. Introduction

HLA-haploidentical (haplo) blood or marrow stem cell transplantation (BMT) has historically been limited by unacceptable rates of graft-versus-host disease (GVHD), graft failure, and nonrelapse mortality (NRM). However, modern transplant techniques, specifically the use of high-dose posttransplantation cyclophosphamide (PTCy) on days +3 and +4, have remarkably reduced GVHD and led to the increasing utilization of haplo donors. The feasibility of haplo BMT has dramatically expanded the donor pool, making allogeneic transplantation available for the vast majority of patients. While clinical trials revealed the safety of the haplo approach with a 1-year NRM of 7% after haplo BMT and a 24% NRM after double umbilical cord blood transplantation (dUCB), the 1-year relapse rates of 45% and 31%, respectively [1], led

to concern that haplo BMT with PTCy was associated with a high risk of relapse. However, the inflated rate may be more apparent than real, as the observed lower incidence of NRM puts a greater pool of patients at risk of relapse. The ease of application, the reduced cost, and the ready availability of haplo donors have led to the widespread adoption of haplo BMT with PTCy as an alternative donor approach. With its expanded use, an increasing number of retrospective studies (Table 1) have been published showing the safety and efficacy of this transplant platform in adults with hematologic malignancies (two of the examined studies contained a small number of adolescent patients) [2, 3]. We review the available publications that compare haplo BMT with PTCy and HLA-matched BMT in an effort to understand the role of haplo BMT and the prioritization of graft type.

TABLE 1: Summary of included studies.

Study	Disease	HLA type and patient number	Conditioning regimens	GVHD prophylaxis	Graft source
McCurdy et al. Blood 2015 [11]	Hematologic malignancies	Haplo $n = 372$	Haplo: Flu 30 mg/m² D-6–2 Cy 14.5 mg/kg D-6–5 TBI 200 cGY D-1	Haplo: PTCy 50 mg/kg D3 and D4, MMF D5–35, Tac D5–90 or 180	BM
		Historical MRD or MUD cohort $n = 614^*$	MRD/MUD: Flu 120 mg/m² Bu 3.2–6.4 IV mg/kg ±ATG	MRD/MUD: CNI + MTX ± sirolimus or CSP with MMF	BM or PBSC
Ciurea et al. Blood 2015 [6]	AML	MUD $n = 1982$	MAC: TBI/Cy TBI/Flu Bu/Cy Mel/Thiotepa/Flu Bu/Flu Bu/Flu/ATG Bu/Thiotepa/Flu NMA: Flu/Cy/TBI	MUD: CNI + MTX or MMF	PBSC > BM
		Haplo $n = 192$		Haplo: PTCy 50 mg/kg D3 and D4, MMF, and CNI	BM > PBSC
Bashey et al. BBMT [7]	Hematologic malignancies	MRD $n = 181$ MUD $n = 178$	MRD or MUD: Bu/Cy Flu/Bu Flu/Bu/Cy Flu/Mel Etop/TBI Flu/Cy Flu/Cy/TBI Cy/TBI Mel/TBI Flu/TBI	MRD or MUD: Tac + MTX ± ATG ± alemtuzumab	PBSC ≫ BM
		Haplo $n = 116$	NMA haplo: Bu/Cy/Etop Flu/Cy/TBI MAC haplo: Flu/Bu/Cy Flu/TBI	Haplo: PTCy 50 mg/kg D3 and D4, MMF, and CNI	NMA haplo: BM ≫ PBSC MAC haplo: PBSC only

TABLE 1: Continued.

Study	Disease	HLA type and patient number	Conditioning regimens	GVHD prophylaxis	Graft source
Raiola et al. BBMT 2014 [3]	Hematologic malignancies	MRD n = 176, MUD n = 43, mmUD n = 43, UCB n = 105, Haplo n = 92	MAC: Thio/Bu/Flu, Bu/Cy, Flu/TBI, Cy/TBI; RIC: Flu/Cy/TBI, Thio/Cy ± Mel	MRD: CSP + mini-MTX; MUD: CSP + mini-MTX + ATG; UCB: CSP + MMF + ATG; Haplo: PTCy 50 mg/kg D3 and D4 + CSP + MMF	BM, PBSC, UCB
		MRD n = 117, MUD n = 101	RIC or MAC	Standard regimens	PBSC or BM
Bashey et al. JCO 2013 [5]	Hematologic malignancies	Haplo n = 53	NMA haplo: Flu 30 mg/m^2 D-6–2, Cy 14.5 mg/kg D-6–5, TBI 200 cGY D-1 or MAC haplo: Flu 25 mg/m^2 D-6–2, Bu 110–130 mg/m^2 IV D-7–4, Cy 14.5 mg/kg D-3–2	Haplo: PTCy 50 mg/kg D3 and D4, MMF D5–35, and Tac D5–180	BM for NMA, PBSC for MAC
Di Stasi et al. BBMT 2014 [4]	AML or MDS	MRD n = 87, MUD n = 108; Haplo n = 32	MRD/MUD: Flu 120–160 mg/m^2 in 4 daily doses Mel 140 mg/m^2 or 100 mg/m^2; Haplo: above + thiotepa 5–10 mg/kg	MRD: Tac + mini-MTX; MUD: Tac + mini-MTX + ATG; Haplo: PTCy 50 mg/kg D3 and D4, MMF D5–100, Tac D5–180	BM or PBSC, BM or PBSC
Kanakry et al. BBMT 2013 [10]	Peripheral T-cell lymphoma	MRD n = 22; Haplo n = 22	Bu/Cy; Cy/TBI, Flu/TBI, Bu/Flu, Flu/Cy/TBI, Fly/Cy/TBI, Bu/Cy, Cy/TBI	MRD: CSP or PTCy 50 mg/kg D3 and D4 ±MMF ±Tac; Haplo: PTCy 50 mg/kg D3 and D4, MMF, Tac, or CSP	BM (1 PBSC)

TABLE 1: Continued.

Study	Disease	HLA type and patient number	Conditioning regimens	GVHD prophylaxis	Graft source
Burroughs et al. BBMT 2008 [2]	Hodgkin lymphoma	MRD $n = 38$ MUD $n = 24$	MRD/MUD: TBI 2 Gy TBI 2 Gy + Flu 30 mg/m^2 days 4–2	MRD/MUD: MMF or CNI	PBSC
		Haplo $n = 28$	Haplo: Flu 30 mg/m^2 D-6–2 Cy 14.5 mg/kg D-6–5 TBI 200 cGY D-1	Haplo: PTCy 50 mg/kg D3 (±D4), MMF D4 or 5–35, Tac D4, or 5–180	BM

HLA: human leukocyte antigen; GVHD: graft-versus-host disease; haplo: HLA-haploidentical; *n*: number; MRD: HLA-matched related donor; MUD: HLA-matched unrelated donor; Flu: fludarabine; D: day; Cy: cyclophosphamide; TBI: total body irradiation; Bu: busulfan; ATG: antithymocyte globulin; PTCy: posttransplantation cyclophosphamide; MMF: mycophenolate mofetil; Tac: tacrolimus; CNI: calcineurin inhibitor; MTX: methotrexate; CSP: cyclosporine; BM: bone marrow; PBSC: peripheral blood stem cells; AML: acute myelogenous leukemia; MAC: myeloablative conditioning; Mel: melphalan; BBMT: biology of blood and marrow transplantation; Etop: etoposide; NMA: nonmyeloablative; mmUD: HLA-mismatched unrelated donor; UCB: umbilical cord blood; JCO: Journal of Clinical Oncology; MDS: myelodysplastic syndrome.
* Armand et al. [12], a disease risk index for patients undergoing allogeneic stem cell transplantation, July 2012; Blood: 120 (4) 905–913.

2. Graft-versus-Host Disease and Immunosuppression Discontinuation

The majority of the reviewed studies showed that the incidence of acute (a) GVHD was either similar [2, 4, 5] or significantly lower after haplo BMT with PTCy ($p < 0.001$) [3, 6] compared with HLA-matched BMT. The cumulative incidence of grades II–IV aGVHD ranged from 24 to 50% after HLA-matched related donor (MRD), 19% to 50% after HLA-matched unrelated donor (MUD), and 14% to 43% after haplo BMT [2–7]. Grades III-IV aGVHD rates were similarly low after MRD, MUD, and haplo BMT, ranging from 4 to 8%, 4 to 13%, and 0 to 11%, respectively [4–6].

The incidence of chronic (c) GVHD was either significantly lower [5, 7] or tended towards being lower [2–4, 6] after haplo compared with HLA-matched donor BMT. Cumulative incidences of moderate or severe cGVHD were 29%, 22%, and 15% ($p = 0.053$) [3], and extensive cGVHD were 54%, 54%, and 38% ($p < 0.05$) [5] for MRD, MUD, and haplo BMT with PTCy, respectively. When transplants only using BM grafts were compared in one analysis, there was no difference in cGHVD rates after MUD and haplo BMT using either myeloablative (MAC) or reduced intensity conditioning (RIC) [6]. However, in another study, when only transplants using peripheral blood stem cell (PBSC) grafts were compared, the 2-year incidence of moderate-severe cGVHD was 45% after MRD, 48% after MUD, and 25% after haplo ($p = 0.01$ for haplo compared with MRD and $p = 0.002$ for haplo versus MUD) [7]. In keeping with the finding of reduced cGVHD, haplo BMT patients were also more likely to discontinue immunosuppression in both univariable analysis at 1 year (81% compared with 55% in the MRD patients ($p < 0.001$)) [3] and multivariable analysis ($p = 0.04$, $p < 0.001$) [2, 7], in the studies that examined this outcome.

3. Immune Reconstitution and Infection

While haplo patients were more likely to have received bone marrow (BM) grafts, which have been associated with engraftment delays [8, 9], neutrophil recovery was similar after haplo BMT with PTCy and HLA-matched BMT. There were low rates of graft failure and time to neutrophil engraftment was similar (18 days in both) [3] or slightly delayed (18 compared with 13 days [4] or 16 compared with 14 [7]) after haplo BMT with PTCy and HLA-matched BMT. In one study, neutrophil recovery was no different after RIC MUD and RIC haplo BMT; however, Day 30 neutrophil recovery was 97% after MAC MUD compared with 90% after MAC haplo BMT, respectively ($p = 0.02$) [6]. Bashey et al. compared neutrophil and platelet engraftment among haplo BMT patients who received either PBSC grafts or BM grafts and found no difference in time to recovery by graft source (16 days to neutrophil engraftment and 26 days to platelet engraftment in both groups) [7]. Immune reconstitution was different at early time points after HLA-matched and haplo BMT, with a decrease in CD3$^+$ and natural killer (NK) cell counts at Day 30 [4] and CD4$^+$ counts at Day 50 [3] in the haplo cohort. However, there were no differences in CD4$^+$,

CD3$^+$, or NK cell counts after these early time points. CD20$^+$ cell counts were similar across transplantation techniques at all time points examined [4].

There was either a trend to an increase [4] or a significant increase [3] in cytomegalovirus (CMV) reactivation after haplo BMT with PTCy compared with MRD and MUD BMT. CMV reactivation rates ranged from 48 to 58%, 54 to 60%, and 71 to 74% after MRD, MUD, and haplo BMT, respectively. Epstein-Barr virus reactivation was either similar with no cases [4] or higher after haplo at 10% compared with 2% after MRD [3]. However, there were no deaths due to post-transplantation lymphoproliferative disease in either cohort of these studies [3, 4].

4. Nonrelapse Mortality

Nonrelapse mortality (NRM) was either not significantly different [3–5, 7, 10] or significantly lower ($p = 0.02$) [2] after haplo compared with MRD BMT. NRM at 1 year ranged from 6% to 24% for MRD, 10% to 35% for MUD, and 4% to 24% for haplo BMT with PTCy (Table 2) [4, 5, 10, 11]. Importantly, NRM was comparable across graft types when conditioning intensity was either similar [3, 5, 6] or more intense [4] for patients undergoing haplo allografting with PTCy. In an analysis that included five graft sources, haplo, MRD, and MUD BMT had equivalent NRM; however, dUCB and HLA-mismatched unrelated donor (mmUD) BMT were both associated with higher NRM [3].

5. Relapse

When examining outcomes for patients with any hematologic malignancy diagnosis who underwent MRD, MUD, or haplo BMT there was no difference in relapse incidence between the graft types [3, 5, 7]. This was notable given the less frequent use of MAC [5, 7] and PBSC grafts [3, 5, 7] and/or the evidence of more advanced disease [3] in the haplo compared with MRD or MUD BMT cohorts in these studies. Raiola et al. also examined outcomes by disease status and showed a tendency towards less relapse in patients with early phase disease (first or second complete remission) after haplo BMT with PTCy at 18% compared with 36% after MRD BMT ($p = 0.09$), with no difference in relapse incidence for patients beyond second complete remission ($p = 0.60$) [3].

Several studies looked at disease specific outcomes. An analysis of acute myelogenous leukemia (AML) and myelodysplastic syndrome (MDS) patients that utilized similar conditioning platforms across graft types found that the relapse rate was not significantly different after MRD, MUD, or haplo BMT at 28%, 23%, and 33% ($p = 0.75$) [4]. In AML, 3-year relapse risks after MAC MUD and MAC haplo were similar, but rates were lower after NMA MUD compared with NMA haplo BMT. The difference in the NMA cohorts may in part be explained by the longer time from diagnosis to transplantation, poorer performance status scores, and higher proportion of patients transplanted beyond first complete remission (despite no difference in disease risk index between the groups) in the haplo BMT compared with the MUD cohort [6]. Patients with peripheral T-cell lymphoma

TABLE 2: Survival outcomes.

Study	NRM		Relapse		PFS or DFS		OS	
	Haplo	Matched (MRD/MUD)	Haplo	Matched (MRD/MUD)	Haplo	Matched (MRD/MUD)	Haplo	Matched (MRD/MUD)
McCurdy et al. Blood 2015 [11]	1 yr: 11%		3 yr: 46% Low: 20% Int: 48% High: 67%		3 yr: 40% Low: 65% Int: 39% High: 25%	66%* 31% 15%	3 yr: 50% Low: 73% Int: 49% High: 37%	70% 47% 25%
Ciurea et al. Blood 2015 [6]	MAC: 1 yr: 12% RIC: 1 yr: 6%	14% 16%	MAC: 3 yr: 44% RIC: 3 yr: 58%	39% 42%			MAC: 3 yr: 45% RIC: 3 yr: 46%	50% 44%
Bashey et al. BBMT 2015 [7]	2 yr: 17%	(14%/16%)	2 yr: 29%	(30%/34%)	2 yr: 54%	(56%/50%)	2 yr: 57%	(72%/59%)
Raiola et al. BBMT 2014 [3]	D1000: 18%	(24%/33%)	35%	(40%/23%)	4 yr: 43%	(32%/36%)	4 yr: 52%	(45%/43%)
Bashey et al. JCO 2013 [5]	1 yr: 4%	(10%/10%)	2 yr: 33%	(34%/34%)	2 yr: 60%	(53%/52%)	2 yr: 64%	(76%/67%)
Di Stasi et al. BBMT 2014 [4]	1 yr: 24%	(20%/35%)	1 yr: 33%	(28%/23%)	3 yr: 30%	(36%/27%)		
Kanakry et al. BBMT 2013 [10]	1 yr: 8%	MRD 6%	1 yr: 34%	MRD 38%				
Burroughs et al. BBMT 2008 [2]	2 yr: 9%	(21%/8%)	2 yr: 40%	(56%/63%)	2 yr: 51%	(23%/29%)	2 yr: 58%	(53%/58%)

NRM: nonrelapse mortality; haplo: human leukocyte antigen- (HLA-) haploidentical; matched: HLA-matched; MRD: HLA-matched related donor; MUD: HLA-matched unrelated donor; PFS: progression-free survival; DFS: disease-free survival; OS: overall survival; yr: year; low: low risk by disease risk index; Int: intermediate risk by disease risk index; high: high or very high risk by disease risk index; BBMT: biology of blood and marrow transplantation; D: day; JCO: Journal of Clinical Oncology.
*Data based on 614 recipients of reduced intensity conditioning and HLA-matched stem cell transplantation from the original disease risk index study cohort [12] whose outcomes were tabulated and received from P. Armand Dana-Farber Cancer Institute, email, July 24, 2014, personal communication.

also had equivalent 1-year cumulative incidence of relapse after MAC MRD at 38% compared with 34% after NMA haplo BMT [10], which is notable given the decreased conditioning intensity in the haplo BMT with PTCy cohort. Notably, in a study of Hodgkin lymphoma, the occurrence of relapse or progressive disease was significantly lower after haplo BMT with PTCy at 40% compared with 56% ($p = 0.01$) and 63% ($p = 0.03$) after MRD and MUD, respectively [2].

6. Progression-Free and Overall Survival

Progression-free survival (PFS) and disease-free survival (DFS) were similar after both haplo and HLA-matched BMT in the studies that included either a variety of hematologic malignancies [3, 5, 7, 11] or AML and MDS [4] ranging from 30 to 40% at 3 years [4, 11]. One analysis looked at PFS by disease risk index (DRI) [12] and found that patients with low-risk and intermediate-risk disease had similar PFS after haplo BMT with PTCy and HLA-matched BMT at 65% and 66%, and 39% and 31%, respectively. There was, however, a suggestion of improved outcomes in patients with high or very high-risk disease after haplo BMT with a 3-year PFS of 25% compared with 15% in the HLA-matched setting [11]. In another report, early phase disease was associated with a tendency towards improved DFS at 60% after haplo compared with 38% for MRD, 25% for MUD, 40% for mmUD, and 38% for UCB BMT ($p = 0.10$) [3]. For advanced phase disease, DFS was no different at 32% for haplo, 22% for MRD, 39% for MUD, 18% for mmUD, and 28% for UCB transplantation ($p = 0.60$).

In Hodgkin lymphoma an improvement in PFS was seen after haplo at 51% compared with 23% and 29% after MRD ($p = 0.0008$) and MUD ($p = 0.03$) BMT, respectively [2]. In peripheral T-cell lymphoma, despite the higher median age in the haplo cohort (59 years compared with 46 years), there was no difference in PFS after MRD BMT and haplo BMT with PTCy [10].

Overall survival (OS) was not significantly different in the majority of the analyses and ranged from 53 to 76% after MRD, 58 to 67% after MUD, and 58 to 64% after haplo BMT at 2 years (Table 2) [2, 5]. Three-year OS by DRI was 70% and 73% for low-risk patients, 47% and 49% for intermediate-risk patients, and 25% and 37% for high or very high-risk patients, after HLA-matched and haplo BMT, respectively. In a comparison of haplo, MRD, MUD, mmUD, and UCB transplantation, there was no difference in 4-year actuarial survival at 53%, 45%, 43%, 40%, and 34% ($p = 0.10$), respectively. However, UCB BMT had inferior survival in multivariable analysis ($p = 0.03$), with haplo and MRD having similar survival ($p = 0.80$) [3]. Finally, 4-year OS in advanced disease by BMT platform was 47%, 30%, 31%, 20%, and 27%, after haplo, MRD, MUD, mmUD, and UCB transplantation, respectively ($p = 0.20$) [3].

7. Discussion

PTCy has decreased the incidence of GVHD, graft failure, and NRM associated with haplo BMT and led to its increasing adoption for patients without an HLA-matched donor. We review the existing retrospective comparisons of HLA-matched BMT and haplo BMT with PTCy in adults with hematologic malignancies. With the use of PTCy based GVHD prophylaxis, rates of aGVHD after haplo BMT appear comparable to that after MRD BMT utilizing standard prophylaxis. While we found similar rates of aGVHD, cGVHD incidence was reduced in the haplo compared with the MRD BMT cohorts. We believe this finding is attributable to PTCy, the use of which was limited to the haplo cohorts in these studies. PTCy, when given early posttransplant, is cytotoxic to alloreactive T-cells that would eventually contribute to cGVHD development. Traditional immunosuppressants, such as calcineurin inhibitors, methotrexate, or mycophenolate mofetil, only inhibit the immune system and flare of GVHD can occur with their cessation. With PTCy, cGVHD prevention is mediated early after transplant and does not require continued use of immunosuppression. Engraftment and immune reconstitution of $CD3^+$, $CD4^+$, and NK cells also appear similar in haplo and MRD BMT after the early posttransplant time period. While the slight delay in neutrophil engraftment and reduction in T-cell counts before Day 50 may be associated with either the haplo graft or the PTCy, it is possible that the use of BM as a stem cell source, which has been associated with engraftment delay [8, 9] and was used preferentially in the haplo cohort, may have contributed. However, the one study that compared neutrophil engraftment after haplo PBSC and haplo BM allografting found no difference in time to neutrophil or platelet recovery [7].

With comparable aGVHD and graft failure rates and a reduced incidence of cGVHD, we would expect a similar NRM. As demonstrated in the early studies of haplo BMT with PTCy, NRM rates were low in these reports, comparable to that seen after MRD BMT. As such, there is now strong evidence for the safety of this transplant platform.

Relapse rates, on the other hand, were a purported weakness associated with haplo BMT with PTCy, owing to the original Phase II study, which found a 45% relapse rate at 1 year [1]. This was an unexpected finding given that the increasing HLA-mismatch could potentially lead to more graft-versus-tumor effects and less relapse after haplo BMT compared with HLA-matched grafts. Critics believed that the PTCy inhibited not only the negative effects of HLA-mismatch, namely, GVHD and graft failure, but the positive graft-versus-tumor effects as well. After reviewing the existing literature comparing HLA-matched and haplo BMT there appears to be no difference in relapse rate in the majority of these retrospective studies. In fact, in certain diseases, relapse may be decreased after haplo BMT. This has been suggested in a study of Hodgkin lymphoma in which relapse and PFS were significantly improved in the haplo cohort compared with the MRD and MUD cohorts, despite the use of BM as a graft source in the haplo cohort and PBSC in the HLA-matched cohort (PBSC have been associated with reduction in relapse in prior analyses [13]). In a single armed study of haplo BMT with PTCy for relapsed Hodgkin lymphoma after prior autologous grafting, Raiola et al. reported a 3-year EFS of 63% [14]. These results support the efficacy of haplo BMT for patients with poor risk Hodgkin lymphoma. Furthermore, MAC has been associated with decreased relapse and increased NRM, equating to no difference in OS when compared with NMA conditioning in prior studies [15]. Despite decreasing conditioning intensity, relapse in peripheral T-cell lymphoma patients was equivocal after with MAC MRD and NMA haplo, suggesting that haplo BMT with PTCy may play an important role in relapse reduction in this disease. However, given the limited and retrospective nature of this data, further study is warranted to better clarify the hierarchy of haplo in transplantation for lymphoma and the effects of haplo BMT with PTCy on relapse.

Outside of lymphoma, stage or risk of disease may also present a scenario in which haplo grafts may be preferred. In the analysis of outcomes by the DRI, there was a suggestion of improved PFS and OS in high and very high-risk disease (risk is determined by disease characteristics and disease stage at transplantation) [11, 12]. This finding reflects the very early clinical data of haplo BMT before the era of PTCy, in which patients with early phase disease did worse after haplo compared with MRD BMT, owing to an increased NRM. However, survival in patients with advanced leukemia after haplo BMT was more similar to those after MRD BMT in that study [16]. The difference in outcomes by disease risk may have been due to a higher risk of death from relapse in high-risk patients. Therefore, the outcomes of high-risk patients depended less on the risk of NRM and more on relapse reduction, which was more effective after haplo BMT. However, Raiola et al. found a trend towards reduction of relapse in early phase disease after haplo BMT with PTCy compared with MRD BMT and similar relapse rates in advanced disease [3]. In the early phases of MAC haplo BMT with PTCy, patients with active leukemia were transplanted and outcomes were poor due to progressive disease early after BMT. As a result, Johns Hopkins adopted a policy to avoid transplantation of patients not in remission. Similarly, with HLA-matched transplant platforms, active disease at the time of transplantation has been associated with poor outcomes, especially in the setting of RIC [17]. Given these contradictory findings, the preferential use of haplo grafts for a given disease stage or risk warrants further investigation.

In all, OS and PFS were not different after haplo and MRD BMT in the studies that compared the two transplant platforms. This suggests that, at a minimum, haplo is an acceptable alternative to HLA-matched transplantation, but further studies are needed to elucidate the clinical scenarios in which haplo BMT with PTCy may be preferred. In the future, other donor factors such as age, sex mismatch, ABO match, CMV compatibility, or NK cell alloreactivity may be more critical than HLA match for donor selection.

Conflict of Interests

The authors declare that there is no conflict of interests regarding the publication of this paper.

References

[1] C. G. Brunstein, E. J. Fuchs, S. L. Carter et al., "Alternative donor transplantation after reduced intensity conditioning: results of parallel phase 2 trials using partially HLA-mismatched related bone marrow or unrelated double umbilical cord blood grafts," *Blood*, vol. 118, no. 2, pp. 282–288, 2011.

[2] L. M. Burroughs, P. V. O'Donnell, B. M. Sandmaier et al., "Comparison of outcomes of HLA-matched related, unrelated, or HLA-haploidentical related hematopoietic cell transplantation following nonmyeloablative conditioning for relapsed or refractory hodgkin lymphoma," *Biology of Blood and Marrow Transplantation*, vol. 14, no. 11, pp. 1279–1287, 2008.

[3] A. M. Raiola, A. Dominietto, C. di Grazia et al., "Unmanipulated haploidentical transplants compared with other alternative donors and matched sibling grafts," *Biology of Blood and Marrow Transplantation*, vol. 20, no. 10, pp. 1573–1579, 2014.

[4] A. Di Stasi, D. R. Milton, L. M. Poon et al., "Similar transplantation outcomes for acute myeloid leukemia and myelodysplastic syndrome patients with haploidentical versus 10/10 human leukocyte antigen-matched unrelated and related donors," *Biology of Blood and Marrow Transplantation*, vol. 20, no. 12, pp. 1975–1981, 2014.

[5] A. Bashey, X. Zhang, C. A. Sizemore et al., "T-cell-replete HLA-haploidentical hematopoietic transplantation for hematologic malignancies using post-transplantation cyclophosphamide results in outcomes equivalent to those of contemporaneous HLA-matched related and unrelated donor transplantation," *Journal of Clinical Oncology*, vol. 31, no. 10, pp. 1310–1316, 2013.

[6] S. O. Ciurea, M. J. Zhang, A. A. Bacigalupo et al., "Haploidentical transplant with posttransplant cyclophosphamide vs matched unrelated donor transplant for acute myeloid leukemia," *Blood*, vol. 126, no. 8, pp. 1033–1040, 2015.

[7] A. Bashey, X. Zhang, K. Jackson et al., "Comparison of outcomes of hematopoietic cell transplants from T-replete haploidentical donors using post-transplantation cyclophosphamide with 10 of 10 HLA-A, -B, -C, -DRB1, and -DQB1 allele-matched unrelated donors and HLA-identical sibling donors: a multivariable analysis including disease risk index," *Biology of Blood and Marrow Transplantation*, 2015.

[8] J. Storek, M. A. Dawson, B. Storer et al., "Immune reconstitution after allogeneic marrow transplantation compared with blood stem cell transplantation," *Blood*, vol. 97, no. 11, pp. 3380–3389, 2001.

[9] G. Gahrton, S. Iacobelli, G. Bandini et al., "Peripheral blood or bone marrow cells in reduced-intensity or myeloablative conditioning allogeneic HLA identical sibling donor transplantation for multiple myeloma," *Haematologica*, vol. 92, no. 11, pp. 1513–1518, 2007.

[10] J. A. Kanakry, Y. L. Kasamon, C. D. Gocke et al., "Outcomes of related donor HLA-identical or HLA-haploidentical allogeneic blood or marrow transplantation for peripheral T cell lymphoma," *Biology of Blood and Marrow Transplantation*, vol. 19, no. 4, pp. 602–606, 2013, Erratum in: *Biology of Blood and Marrow Transplantation*, vol. 19, no. 10, p. 1530, 2013.

[11] S. R. McCurdy, J. A. Kanakry, M. M. Showel et al., "Risk-stratified outcomes of nonmyeloablative HLA-haploidentical BMT with high-dose posttransplantation cyclophosphamide," *Blood*, vol. 125, no. 19, pp. 3024–3031, 2015.

[12] P. Armand, C. J. Gibson, C. Cutler et al., "A disease risk index for patients undergoing allogeneic stem cell transplantation," *Blood*, vol. 120, no. 4, pp. 905–913, 2012.

[13] Stem Cell Trialists' Collaborative Group, "Allogeneic peripheral blood stem-cell compared with bone marrow transplantation in the management of hematologic malignancies: an individual patient data meta-analysis of nine randomized trials," *Journal of Clinical Oncology*, vol. 23, no. 22, pp. 5074–5087, 2005.

[14] A. Raiola, A. Dominietto, R. Varaldo et al., "Unmanipulated haploidentical BMT following non-myeloablative conditioning and post-transplantation CY for advanced Hodgkin's lymphoma," *Bone Marrow Transplantation*, vol. 49, no. 2, pp. 190–194, 2014.

[15] O. Ringdén, M. Labopin, G. Ehninger et al., "Reduced intensity conditioning compared with myeloablative conditioning using unrelated donor transplants in patients with acute myeloid leukemia," *Journal of Clinical Oncology*, vol. 27, no. 27, pp. 4570–4577, 2009.

[16] R. Szydlo, J. M. Goldman, J. P. Klein et al., "Results of allogeneic bone marrow transplants for leukemia using donors other than HLA-identical siblings," *Journal of Clinical Oncology*, vol. 15, no. 5, pp. 1767–1777, 1997.

[17] A. Shimoni, I. Hardan, N. Shem-Tov et al., "Allogeneic hematopoietic stem-cell transplantation in AML and MDS using myeloablative versus reduced-intensity conditioning: the role of dose intensity," *Leukemia*, vol. 20, no. 2, pp. 322–328, 2006.

13

The Iron Status of Sickle Cell Anaemia Patients in Ilorin, North Central Nigeria

Musa A. Sani,[1] James O. Adewuyi,[2] Abiola S. Babatunde,[2]
Hannah O. Olawumi,[2] and Rasaki O. Shittu[3]

[1]Department of Haematology and Blood Transfusion, Kwara State Specialist Hospital, Sobi, 240001 Ilorin, Nigeria
[2]Department of Haematology and Blood Transfusion, University of Ilorin Teaching Hospital, PMB 1459, 240003 Ilorin, Nigeria
[3]Department of Family Medicine, Kwara State Specialist Hospital, Sobi, 240001 Ilorin, Nigeria

Correspondence should be addressed to Abiola S. Babatunde; asbabs2003@yahoo.com

Academic Editor: Thomas Kickler

Objectives. Sickle cell anaemia (SCA) is one of the commonest genetic disorders in the world. It is characterized by anaemia, periodic attacks of thrombotic pain, and chronic systemic organ damage. Recent studies have suggested that individuals with SCA especially from developing countries are more likely to be iron deficient rather than have iron overload. The study aims to determine the iron status of SCA patients in Ilorin, Nigeria. *Methods*. A cross-sectional study of 45 SCA patients in steady state and 45 non-SCA controls was undertaken. FBC, blood film, sFC, sTfR, and sTfR/log sFC index were done on all subjects. *Results*. The mean patients' serum ferritin (589.33 ± 427.61 ng/mL) was significantly higher than the mean serum ferritin of the controls (184.53 ± 119.74 ng/mL). The mean serum transferrin receptor of the patients (4.24 ± 0.17 μg/mL) was higher than that of the controls (3.96 ± 0.17 μg/mL) ($p = 0.290$). The mean serum transferrin receptor (sTfR)/log serum ferritin index of the patients (1.65 ± 0.27 μg/mL) was significantly lower than that of the control (1.82 ± 0.18 μg/mL) ($p = 0.031$). *Conclusion*. Iron deficiency is uncommon in SCA patients and periodic monitoring of the haematological, biochemical, and clinical features for iron status in SCA patients is advised.

1. Introduction

Sickle cell anaemia (SCA) is one of the commonest genetic disorders in the world and a major cause of significant morbidity and mortality in Africa [1]. In Nigeria, the incidence of sickle cell anaemia is about 1-2% of the population [1].

The disease consists of a variety of pathological disorders resulting from the inheritance of sickled haemoglobin (HbS) gene either in the homozygous state (SS) or in double heterozygous state with another abnormal haemoglobin gene, for example, SC, SD, SβThal, SO Arab, and SG [2, 3]. The gene abnormality results in the tendency of sickle haemoglobin (HbS) when deoxygenated, to polymerize intracellularly and deform red blood cells into a characteristic sickled shape, thereby producing the clinical manifestation of a chronic haemolytic anaemia with potential iron overload.

However, some studies have shown that iron overload may be a problem only in SCA patients on hypertransfusion programmes [4–6]. Most SCA patients are not hypertransfused and should not have iron overload. On the other hand, some studies have suggested that individuals with sickle cell disease particularly from developing countries, who have never been transfused, are more likely to be iron deficient rather than have iron overload [4]. There is thus some doubt regarding occurrence of iron overload in sickle cell anaemia patients and iron deficiency may be more common than expected especially in men, according to Koduri [7].

Although absence of bone marrow iron remains the gold standard for the diagnosis of iron deficiency, serum ferritin concentration (sFC) adequately reflects iron stores [8–10] and low serum ferritin is highly specific for the diagnosis of iron deficiency. However, sensitivity of serum ferritin may be low in sickle cell anaemia because of nonspecific elevation due to increased red cell turnover [7], chronic inflammation, and the role of serum ferritin as an acute phase reactant [11, 12]. Soluble transferrin receptors (sTfR) are disulfide-linked transmembrane proteins that facilitate the entry of transferrin-bound iron into the cells. It is a truncated monomer of the tissue receptor, lacking the first 100 amino acids (the transmembrane and cytoplasmic domain of the cellular receptor) [13]. The circulating TFRC mirrors the amount of cellular receptors. Measuring the concentration of serum TfR is an alternative method to assess iron status because the concentration increases during iron deficiency. It is thought that the serum TfR concentration is not increased in individuals during an acute phase response; therefore the measurement of serum TfR may help to distinguish between individuals with iron deficiency anaemia and anaemia of chronic disease. Serum TfR concentration is elevated in iron deficiency, haemolytic anaemia, polycythemia, myelodysplastic syndromes, and use of erythropoietic stimulating agents while aplastic anaemia and chronic renal failure result in decrease. Transferrin receptor is a more recent iron marker that is not affected by inflammation [14] and is thought to be a more reliable index of iron status in SCA than serum ferritin. sTfR/sFC index is the ratio of soluble transferrin receptor to log serum ferritin. The use of the log of serum ferritin in this ratio decreases the influence of the acute phase response on the ferritin component of the ratio. The ratio of sTfR/ferritin can be used to quantify the entire spectrum of iron status from positive iron stores through negative iron balance. sTfR reflect the functional iron compartment while TfR-F index takes advantage of the relationship between sTFR and sFC, that is, an increase in TfR and a decrease in the ferritin concentration. sTfR/sFC ratio has been found to be a better reflector of body iron stores [15].

The present study investigated the iron stores in patients with sickle cell anaemia by quantifying both serum transferrin receptor (sTfR) and serum ferritin from which the sTFR/log serum ferritin ratio was computed.

2. Subjects

This was a cross-sectional study of sickle cell disease patients attending the Sickle Cell Clinic of University of Ilorin Teaching Hospital, Ilorin, Kwara State, Nigeria. Forty-three confirmed sickle cell anaemia patients attending the clinic were recruited into the study. All subjects were aged 15 years or more and were in a steady state. Forty-three apparently healthy age and sex matched controls with Hb phenotype AA only were recruited from students and patients relatives attending the hospital. Patients were excluded from the study if they have had blood transfusion in the previous 12 weeks or any form of sickle cell crises within 2 weeks of the study. Patients on iron containing haematinics or erythropoiesis stimulating agents, vitamin C, and oral contraceptives were also excluded. So also were patients with history of recent overt blood loss, concurrent medical or surgical conditions like peptic ulcer disease, renal failure, liver disease, malignancy, or chronic inflammatory disease. Ethical clearance was obtained from the Ethical Review and Research Committee of the University of Ilorin Teaching Hospital and written consents for inclusion into the study were obtained from all patients and controls.

3. Methods

A structured questionnaire was administered on all subjects recruited for the study and a review of case record folders and routine physical examination were carried out. Venous blood was taken from each subject into a bottle containing K^+ ethylenediaminetetraacetic acid (EDTA) for estimation of full blood count within 2 hours using Sysmex KX 21N automated cell counter (product of Sysmex Corporation, Tokyo, Japan, with serial number B1786). Blood was also taken into plain specimen bottles and allowed to clot at room temperature to obtain serum. Thin blood film was made from the EDTA sample within 2 hours of collection for microscopic study of red cell morphology. Reticulocyte count preparation was made by the method described by Barbara et al. [16] and the reticulocyte count was expressed as a percentage of cells with blue reticular or granular inclusions over the total red cell counted. From the EDTA sample, Hb genotype was determined by electrophoresis using cellulose acetate membrane at alkaline pH 8.0 as described by Barbara et al. [16]. Serum obtained from the clotted blood sample was used for estimation of serum ferritin concentration (sFC) and transferrin receptors (sTfR) and sTfR/log sFC index was calculated. Quantitative measurement of human soluble transferrin receptor was also done using human sTfR ELISA (enzyme linked immune assay) reagent of Biovendor. Control samples provided were run with duplicates of test sample and OD (optical density) was read at 450 nm and 630 nm. The mean of the difference of the two OD was taken as the OD. Quantitative determination of serum ferritin was done using microwell ferritin enzyme immune assay. Control samples provided were also run with duplicates of test sample and the OD read at 450 nm.

The findings were subjected to statistical analysis in which a p value of 0.05 or less was considered as being statistically significant.

4. Sample Size

The sample size was calculated from the formula

$$N = \frac{(Z_1 - X)^2 (P)(1 - P)}{D^2},\qquad(1)$$

where N is minimal sample size at 95% confidence level $Z_1 - X = 1.96$ from statistical table, P is the best estimate of population, prevalence of SCD obtained from literature 2-3%, and D is precision or degree of accuracy which is usually taken as 0.05.

Therefore

$$N = \frac{(1.96)^2 \times (0.025)(0.97)}{(0.05)^2} = 43.\qquad(2)$$

5. Results

The mean age of the patients was 24.63 ± 9.63 years with a range of 16–60 years. The mean age of the controls was 21.56 ± 6.10 with a range of 16–62 years. All forty-three (43) patients had Hb phenotype S (HbSS). The controls had Hb

TABLE 1: Red blood cell indices in patients and controls.

Parameter	Patient (number = 45)		Control (number = 45)		p value	Remarks
	Mean ± SD	Range	Mean ± SD	Range		
PCV (%)	25.19 ± 4.35	18.40–35.80	40.06 ± 4.07	34.70–46.30	0.018	Significant
Hb conc. (g/dL)	7.81 ± 1.84	5.10–12.80	12.53 ± 1.42	10.60–14.70	<0.001	Significant
RBC (×10⁹/L)	3.00 ± 0.74	1.91–4.94	4.74 ± 0.44	4.80–5.45	0.006	Significant
RETIC index (%)	1.48 ± 1.46	0.19–7.23	0.84 ± 0.82	0.21–4.96	<0.001	Significant
MCV (fL)	84.95 ± 11.10	46.90–110.4	84.69 ± 5.51	75.60–99.30	0.321	Not significant
MCH (pg)	27.49 ± 3.65	20.80–34.40	26.48 ± 2.43	21.90–31.10	0.124	Not significant
MCHC (g/dL)	32.09 ± 2.14	24.10–38.20	31.22 ± 1.30	29.00–33.30	0.019	Significant

PCV: packed cell volume, Hb: haemoglobin concentration, RBC: red blood cell, MCV: mean corpuscular volume, MCH: mean corpuscular haemoglobin, MCHC: mean corpuscular haemoglobin concentration, and RETIC: reticulocyte.

phenotype AA only. The mean MCV of the patients was 84.95 ± 11.10 femtolitres and 84.67 ± 5.56 femtolitres for the controls, $p = 0.321$ (Table 1). Twenty-eight (65.1%) patients had normocytosis (MCV = 76–96 fL), 10 patients (23.3%) had microcytosis (MCV < 76 fL), and 5 (11.6%) patients had macrocytosis (MCV > 96 fL). In the controls, thirty-eight (88.4%) had normocytosis, 3 (7.0%) had microcytosis, and 2 (4.6%) had macrocytosis. The mean MCH for the patients was 27.49 ± 3.65 picograms while that of the control was 26.48 ± 2.43 picograms. There was no statistically significant difference between these results (p value = 0.124). The mean MCHC for the patients was 32.09 ± 2.14 g/dL while that of the control was 31.22 ± 1.30 g/dL. This shows statistically significant difference between these results (p value = 0.019). Twenty-three patients (51.1%) had low MCH (MCH < 27 picograms), 16 patients (37.2%) had normal MCH, and 4 (9.3%) had high MCH (MCH > 32 picograms) (Table 2). The mean reticulocyte index in patients was $1.48 \pm 1.46\%$ while the mean reticulocyte count in controls was 0.83 ± 0.82. There was statistically significant difference between the patients' reticulocytes index and controls' reticulocyte index, p value = 0.001 (Table 1). The mean red cell distribution width (RDW) was 74.64 ± 11.84 and 45.43 ± 3.16 for patients and controls, respectively. There was a significant statistical difference between the mean of the patients and the controls, $p < 0.001$.

Thirty-two (74.4%) patients have had blood transfusion in the past whereas 11 (25.6%) have never had blood transfusion in their lifetime. There was previous history of blood transfusion in only five (11.6%) of the control group. The means of serum ferritin among the nontransfused and transfused patients were 436.54 ± 319.62 ng/mL and 828 ± 452.33 ng/mL, respectively.

The patients' mean serum ferritin was 589.33 ± 427.61 ng/mL and the mean serum ferritin for the controls was 184.53 ± 119.74 ng/mL (Table 3). The mean TfR and mean TfR/sFC index of patients and controls were 4.24 ± 0.17 µg/mL, 1.65 ± 0.27 µg/mL, and 3.96 ± 0.17 µg/mL, 1.82 ± 0.18, respectively (Table 3).

6. Discussion

As expected, there were numerical and statistically significant differences in the absolute red cell indices (PCV, Hb, RBC,

TABLE 2: Prevalence of microcytosis, macrocytosis, hypochromia, hyperchromia, and red cell distribution width in patients and controls.

Indices	Prevalence		Percent	
	Patients	Controls	Patients	Controls
Microcytosis				
MCV <76 fL	10	3	22.2	8.8
Normocytosis				
MCV = 76–96 fL	28	38	66.7	86.7
Macrocytosis				
MCV >96 fL	5	2	11.1	4.4
Total	43.0	43.0	100.0	100.0
Hypochromia				
MCH <27 pg	23	14	53.5	32.6
Normochromia				
MCH = 27–32 pg	16	29	37.2	67.4
Hyperchromia				
MCH >32 pg	4	0	9.3	0
Total	43.0	43.0	100.0	100.0
RDW				
<39.0 fL	0	0	0	0
39–46 fL	2	28	4.4	62.2
>46.0 fL	43	17	95.6	37.8
Total	43.0	43.0	100.0	100.0

MCV: mean corpuscular volume, fL: femtolitre.
MCH: mean corpuscular haemoglobin, pg = picogram.
RDW: red cell distribution width. Normal reference range = 42.5 ± 3.5 fL
$p < 0.001$.

and RDW) between patients and controls. However, the calculated indices (MCV and MCH) showed no significant differences with the exception of MCHC which confirmed the well-known higher intracellular density of sickle cells.

The bulk of the patients' diet consisted of mainly carbohydrates and only thirty-three of the patients agreed to take protein-containing diet for more than twice daily.

The mean serum ferritin concentration among transfused patients was higher than among the nontransfused patients (p value = 0.025). This is in agreement with the study of O'Brien who reported a weak positive correlation ($p = 0.026$) between blood transfusion and ferritin levels of the patients

TABLE 3: Biochemical parameters in patients and controls.

Parameter	Patients		Control		p value
	Mean	SD	Mean	SD	
sFC (ng/mL)	589.33	427.61	184.53	119.74	0.025
TfR (μg/mL)	4.24	0.17	3.96	0.17	0.290
TfR/log sFC index	1.65	0.27	1.82	0.18	0.03

sFC: serum ferritin concentration, TfR: transferrin receptor.

[4]. This is also in keeping with report by Porter and Huehns [17] who obtained a good correlation between serum ferritin and number of blood transfusions.

In this study, twenty-two units of blood was the highest transfusion recorded in a 46-year-old patient which is equivalent to 0.5 units of blood per annum. This observation is in agreement with work of Luzzatto who reported approximately 0.5 units in sickle cell patients [18]. Even the largest number of transfusions does not produce iron overload. There was a linear relationship between age and number of blood transfusions ($r = 0.505$, $p \leq 0.001$). This was previously observed by O'Brien who found that the concentrations of serum ferritin correlated directly and significantly with age of the patients [4].

In our study the mean patients' serum ferritin (559.33 $\pm$ 427.61 ng/mL) was higher than the upper limit of reference range (300 ng/mL) and also statistically significantly ($p = 0.025$) higher when compared with the mean serum ferritin of the controls (184.53 $\pm$ 119.74 ng/mL) which was within the reference range. These findings in the patients indicating increase in body iron stores are in keeping with Peterson et al. who reported a high mean serum ferritin in SCD compared to the control [19].

The mean serum transferrin receptor of the patients (4.24 $\pm$ 0.17 μg/mL) was not statistically significantly higher than that of the controls (3.96 $\pm$ 0.17 μg/mL) ($p = 0.290$).

In this study the reference range of 3.61–4.33 μg/mL was obtained by taking two standard deviations below and above the mean serum transferrin receptor of the controls. Fourteen of our patients had serum transferrin receptor above the study reference range. Transferrin receptor levels are increased during haemolysis which is an expected finding in SCD, thus making it difficult to ascertain the significance of the increase. It has been suggested that serum transferrin receptor seems to be more useful in relation to functional iron compartment than iron stores [20, 21]. It has been further suggested that sTfR in the presence of hypochromia and microcytosis and another parameter, the sTfR/log serum ferritin index may all be diagnostic of iron deficiency in SCD [22]. In this study, the mean serum transferrin receptor (sTfR)/log serum ferritin index of the patients (1.65 $\pm$ 0.27 μg/mL) was significantly lower than that of the controls (1.82 $\pm$ 0.18 μg/mL) ($p = 0.031$). This is in agreement with Khatami et al. who observed significant differences in sTfR concentration and sTfR/log ferritin (sTfR-F index) in iron deficient groups, compared to thalassemia groups [23]. Also Punnonen and colleague confirmed sTfR/log serum ferritin index as an outstanding parameter for the identification of patient with depleted iron sores [24].

Although various researchers have used different markers to asses iron status in sickle cell disease patients, there is paucity of data on studies that have used sTfR as a marker of iron store in sickle cell disease patients in this region. Researchers in western Nigeria have also reported cases of iron deficiency anaemia in SCD [14, 22, 25, 26]. Williams and Etuk in Eastern Nigeria reported 53% prevalence of iron deficiency among children with SCA [27]. Peterson et al. [19] in his study of iron metabolism in a group of 39 patients with sickle cell disease found iron deficiency anaemia in as high as 28% cases.

Based on microcytosis, hypochromia, and high sTfR/log serum ferritin index, the prevalence of iron deficiency of 7% obtained in this study is much lower than what was obtained by other authors who reported deficiency in 20% and 17.1% of SCD patients using the combination of microcytosis and hypochromia alone [22]. Mohanty et al. in India using elevated ZPP/H ratios as marker reported iron deficiency anaemia in sixty-seven per cent of subjects with sickle cell anaemia [28].

Other researchers in Nigeria and elsewhere have also reported either normal or increased iron stores in their sickle cell disease patients [4, 29–33].

7. Conclusion and Recommendations

The results of this study corroborate the findings of previous researchers of normal or high iron stores in SCA patients. On the other hand the prevalence of iron deficiency in sickle cell disease patients in this study was found to be only 7%. Iron deficiency may therefore not be as common as was being reported in some previous studies in sickle cell disease patients. The determination of iron status of SCA patients is better based on measurements of sTfR/log serum ferritin index with or without hypochromia or microcytosis rather than on sFC or hypochromia and microcytosis alone.

There is need to carry out further study on a larger scale on sTfR in this region in order to determine the cutoff value for iron deficiency especially in SCA.

Conflict of Interests

The authors declare that there is no conflict of interests regarding the publication of this paper.

References

[1] N. K. D. Halim, A. A. Famodu, and S. N. C. Wemambu, *Textbook of Clinical Haematology and Immunology*, Ambik, 2nd edition, 2001.

[2] G. A. Nnaji, D. A. Ezeagwuna, I. J. F. Nnaji, J. O. Osakwe, A. C. Nwigwe, and O. W. Onwurah, "Prevalence and pattern of sickle cell disease in premarital couples in Southeastern Nigeria," *Nigerian Journal of Clinical Practice*, vol. 16, no. 3, pp. 309–314, 2013.

[3] A. Lai and E. P. Vinchisky, "Sickle cell disease," in *Postgraduate Haematology*, A. V. Hoffbrand, C. Daniel, and E. G. D. Tuddenham, Eds., pp. 104–118, Blackwell, Malden, Mass, USA, 5th edition, 2005.

[4] R. T. O'Brien, "Iron burden in sickle cell anemia," *The Journal of Pediatrics*, vol. 92, no. 4, pp. 579–582, 1978.

[5] A. Cohen and E. Schwartz, "Excretion of iron in response to deferoxamine in sickle cell anemia," *The Journal of Pediatrics*, vol. 92, no. 4, pp. 659–662, 1978.

[6] B. S. Mahony, D. R. Ambruso, and J. H. Githens, "Iron studies in sickle cell anemia," *Journal of Pediatrics*, vol. 93, no. 6, pp. 1070–1074, 1978.

[7] P. R. Koduri, "Iron in sickle cell disease: a review why less is better," *American Journal of Hematology*, vol. 73, no. 1, pp. 59–63, 2003.

[8] A. B. Blumberg, H. R. M. Marti, and C. G. Graber, "Serum ferritin and bone marrow iron in patients undergoing continuous ambulatory peritoneal dialysis," *The Journal of the American Medical Association*, vol. 250, no. 24, pp. 3317–3319, 1983.

[9] L. A. Rocha, D. V. Barreto, F. C. Barreto et al., "Serum ferritin level remains a reliable marker of bone marrow iron stores evaluated by histomorphometry in hemodialysis patients," *Clinical Journal of the American Society of Nephrology*, vol. 4, no. 1, pp. 105–109, 2009.

[10] M. A. M. Ali, A. W. Luxton, and W. H. C. Walker, "Serum ferritin concentration and bone marrow iron stores: a prospective study," *Canadian Medical Association Journal*, vol. 118, no. 8, pp. 945–946, 1978.

[11] R. D. Baynes, "Assessment of iron status," *Clinical Biochemistry*, vol. 29, no. 3, pp. 209–215, 1996.

[12] L. Thomas, "Transferrin saturation," in *Clinical Laboratory Diagnostics*, L. Thomas, Ed., pp. 275–277, TH-Books, Frankfurt, Germany, 1998.

[13] W. Mark and A. V. Hoffbrand, "Iron metabolism, iron deficiency and disorders of haem synthesis," in *Postgraduate Haematology*, A. V. Hoffbrand, D. Catovsky, and E. G. D. Tuddenham, Eds., pp. 26–43, Blackwell, 5th edition, 2005.

[14] C. Beerenhout, O. Bekers, J. P. Kooman, F. M. van der Sande, and K. M. L. Leunissen, "A comparison between the soluble transferrin receptor, transferrin saturation and serum ferritin as markers of iron state in hemodialysis patients," *Nephron*, vol. 92, no. 1, pp. 32–35, 2002.

[15] J. D. Cook, C. H. Flowers, and B. S. Skikne, "The quantitative assessment of body iron," *Blood*, vol. 101, no. 9, pp. 3359–3364, 2003.

[16] J. B. Barbara, L. Mitchell, and B. Imelda, "Basic haematological techniques," in *Dacie and Lewis Practical Haematology*, J. V. Dacie and S. M. Lewis, Eds., pp. 25–57, Churchill Livingstone, London, UK, 10th edition, 2006.

[17] J. B. Porter and E. R. Huehns, "Transfusion and exchange transfusion in sickle cell anaemias, with particular reference to iron metabolism," *Acta Haematologica*, vol. 78, no. 2-3, pp. 198–205, 1987.

[18] L. Luzzatto, "Haemoglobinopathies including thalassaemia. Part 3. Sickle cell anaemia in tropical Africa," *Clinics in Haematology*, vol. 10, no. 3, pp. 757–784, 1981.

[19] C. M. Peterson, J. H. Graziano, A. de Ciutiis et al., "Iron metabolism, sickle cell disease, and response to cyanate," *Blood*, vol. 46, no. 4, pp. 583–590, 1975.

[20] P. Suominen, K. Punnonen, A. Rajamäki, and K. Irjala, "Serum transferrin receptor and transferrin receptor-ferritin index identify healthy subjects with subclinical iron deficits," *Blood*, vol. 92, no. 8, pp. 2934–2939, 1998.

[21] P. Suominen, T. Möttönen, A. Rajamäki, and K. Irjala, "Single values of serum transferrin receptor and transferrin receptor ferritin index can be used to detect true and functional iron deficiency in rheumatoid arthritis patients with anemia," *Arthritis and Rheumatism*, vol. 43, no. 5, pp. 1016–1020, 2000.

[22] P. Lopez-Sall, P. A. Diop, I. Diagne et al., "Transferrine's soluble receptors' contribution to the assessment of iron status in homozygous drepanocytic anemia," *Annales de Biologie Clinique*, vol. 62, no. 4, pp. 415–421, 2004.

[23] S. Khatami, S. R. Dehnabeh, E. Mostafavi et al., "Evaluation and comparison of soluble transferrin receptor in thalassemia carriers and iron deficient patients," *Hemoglobin*, vol. 37, no. 4, pp. 387–395, 2013.

[24] K. Punnonen, K. Irjala, and A. Rajamäki, "Serum transferrin receptor and its ratio to serum ferritin in the diagnosis of iron deficiency," *Blood*, vol. 89, no. 3, pp. 1052–1057, 1997.

[25] S. Davies, J. S. Henthorn, M. Brozovic, and A. A. Win, "Effect of blood transfusion on iron status in sickle cell anaemia," *Clinical and Laboratory Haematology*, vol. 6, no. 1, pp. 17–22, 1984.

[26] O. A. Oluboyede, "Iron studies in pregnant and non-pregnant women with haemoglobin SS or SC disease," *British Journal of Obstetrics and Gynaecology*, vol. 87, no. 11, pp. 989–996, 1980.

[27] I. O. Williams and I. S. Etuk, "Iron status of children with sickle cell anaemia attending clinic at the University of Calabar Teaching Hospital (UCTH), Calabar—Nigeria," *American Journal of Medicine and Medical Sciences*, vol. 3, no. 3, pp. 51–55, 2013.

[28] D. Mohanty, M. B. Mukherjee, R. B. Colah et al., "Iron deficiency anaemia in sickle cell disorders in India," *Indian Journal of Medical Research*, vol. 127, no. 4, pp. 366–369, 2008.

[29] A. A. Akinbami, A. O. Dosunmu, A. A. Adediran et al., "Serum ferritin levels in adults with sickle cell disease in Lagos, Nigeria," *Journal of Blood Medicine*, vol. 4, pp. 59–63, 2013.

[30] Y. A. Aken'Ova, I. Adeyefa, and M. Okunade, "Ferritin and serum iron levels in adult patients with sickle cell anaemia at Ibadan, Nigeria," *African Journal of Medicine and Medical Sciences*, vol. 26, no. 1-2, pp. 39–41, 1997.

[31] M. F. Anderson, "The iron status of pregnant women with hemoglobinopathies," *American Journal of Obstetrics and Gynecology*, vol. 113, no. 7, pp. 895–900, 1972.

[32] A. F. Fleming, "Iron status of anaemic pregnant Nigerians," *The Journal of Obstetrics and Gynaecology of the British Common Wealth*, vol. 76, no. 11, pp. 1013–1017, 1969.

[33] N. Stettler, B. S. Zemel, D. A. Kawchak, K. Ohene-Frempong, and V. A. Stallings, "Iron status of children with sickle cell disease," *Journal of Parenteral and Enteral Nutrition*, vol. 25, no. 1, pp. 36–38, 2001.

14

Crosstalk between Platelets and the Immune System: Old Systems with New Discoveries

Conglei Li,[1, 2] June Li,[1, 2] Yan Li,[2, 3] Sean Lang,[1, 2, 3] Issaka Yougbare,[2] Guangheng Zhu,[2] Pingguo Chen,[2, 3] and Heyu Ni[1, 2, 3, 4]

[1] Department of Laboratory Medicine and Pathobiology, University of Toronto, Toronto, ON, Canada M5S 1A8
[2] Department of Laboratory Medicine, Keenan Research Centre, Li Ka Shing Knowledge Institute, St. Michael's Hospital, and Toronto Platelet Immunobiology Group, University of Toronto, Toronto, ON, Canada M5S 1A8
[3] Canadian Blood Services, Toronto, ON, Canada M5G 2M1
[4] Department of Medicine and Department of Physiology, University of Toronto, Toronto, ON, Canada M5S 1A8

Correspondence should be addressed to Heyu Ni, Nih@smh.ca

Academic Editor: Helen A. Papadaki

Platelets are small anucleate cells circulating in the blood. It has been recognized for more than 100 years that platelet adhesion and aggregation at the site of vascular injury are critical events in hemostasis and thrombosis; however, recent studies demonstrated that, in addition to these classic roles, platelets also have important functions in inflammation and the immune response. Platelets contain many proinflammatory molecules and cytokines (e.g., P-selectin, CD40L, IL-1β, etc.), which support leukocyte trafficking, modulate immunoglobulin class switch, and germinal center formation. Platelets express several functional Toll-like receptors (TLRs), such as TLR-2, TLR-4, and TLR-9, which may potentially link innate immunity with thrombosis. Interestingly, platelets also contain multiple anti-inflammatory molecules and cytokines (e.g., transforming growth factor-β and thrombospondin-1). Emerging evidence also suggests that platelets are involved in lymphatic vessel development by directly interacting with lymphatic endothelial cells through C-type lectin-like receptor 2. Besides the active contributions of platelets to the immune system, platelets are passively targeted in several immune-mediated diseases, such as autoimmune thrombocytopenia, infection-associated thrombocytopenia, and fetal and neonatal alloimmune thrombocytopenia. These data suggest that platelets are important immune cells and may contribute to innate and adaptive immunity under both physiological and pathological conditions.

1. Platelets in Hemostasis and Thrombosis: Classical Role and Nonclassical Mechanisms

Platelets, which were first identified around 130 years ago, are small anucleate cells circulating in the blood with a diameter of 1-2 microns [1–5]. They are the second most abundant cells, after red blood cells, in the blood circulation with a normal concentration of $150–400 \times 10^9$/L in humans. Platelets are produced from their precursor megakaryocytes in the bone marrow [4–8]; immature larger proplatelets are initially released by megakaryocytes into the blood due to local shear stresses in the bone marrow. These proplatelets may further mature in the lung, although the process is largely unknown [8, 9].

The major physiological role of platelets is to accumulate at sites of damaged blood vessel endothelium and initiate the blood clotting process. Platelet adhesion, activation, and subsequent aggregation at sites of vascular injury are critical to the normal arrest of bleeding [10–12]. When the vessel endothelium is injured, collagen and other subendothelial matrix proteins are exposed allowing platelets in the circulation to bind, which results in platelet activation. Activated platelets release certain intracellular soluble mediators, leading to the recruitment and activation of additional platelets at the injury site [10–12]. This platelet response is one key mechanism required to stop bleeding (i.e., the first wave of hemostasis); the other is the coagulation system, which is initiated by tissue factor (extrinsic) pathway or contact factor (intrinsic) pathway to generate thrombin and polymerized fibrin [10, 13–15]. There are many interactions between these two mechanisms which lead to clotting. For example, platelets (particularly activated platelets) accelerate coagulation by providing a negatively charged phosphatidylserine- (PS-) rich membrane surface that enhances the generation of thrombin, which converts fibrinogen (Fg) to fibrin [16, 17]. Conversely, thrombin generated via the coagulation process is a potent platelet activator [18–20] that induces platelet activation and granule release (e.g., P-selectin translocation to the cell surface). Fibrin (especially polymerized fibrin) also stabilizes the platelet plug [21]. Deficiencies in platelet adhesion/aggregation or coagulation are associated with bleeding disorders [14, 22–25]. However, inappropriate platelet plug formation may also result in thrombosis/vessel obstruction. Unstable angina and myocardial infarction typically result from platelet adhesion/aggregation at ruptured atherosclerotic lesions in coronary arteries. Thrombosis in the coronary or cerebral arteries is the major cause of morbidity and mortality worldwide [26, 27]. In addition, it has been demonstrated that thrombus formation in the placenta can lead to fetal loss during pregnancy in several disease conditions, such as antiphospholipid syndrome and estrogen sulfotransferase deficiency [28–31]. Recently, our group also found in murine models that some maternal antifetal platelet antibodies can cause platelet activation and excessive thrombosis in the placenta, which may lead to miscarriage [17]. Thus, the same processes (platelet adhesion and aggregation) play contrasting but critical roles (physiological, i.e., hemostasis versus pathological, i.e., thrombosis).

1.1. Molecular Events of Platelet Adhesion and Aggregation.
It is now clear that platelet receptors, GPIIbIIIa (αIIbβ3 integrin) and the GPIbα complex, which are two abundant glycoproteins expressed on platelets, play the predominant roles in platelet adhesion and aggregation at the site of vascular injury [10–12]. It has been recognized that platelet GPIbα, primarily via binding to immobilized von Willebrand factor (VWF) on collagen, is essential for initiation of platelet-vessel wall interaction, particularly at high shear stress [26, 32, 33]. The GPIb-VWF interaction and/or various platelet agonists (e.g., ADP, thrombin, collagen, and thromboxane A$_2$) can cause platelet activation resulting in a conformational change in αIIbβ3 integrin on the platelet surface [34, 35], which allows for ligand binding (e.g., fibrinogen) [35–37]. When bound to activated αIIbβ3 integrin, fibrinogen is able to cross-link adjacent platelets, leading to platelet aggregation and subsequent formation of a platelet plug [38, 39].

Although it has been well documented since the 1960s that Fg is required for platelet aggregation [40], using an FeCl$_3$ injury intravital microscopy thrombosis model, we demonstrated that occlusive thrombus formation still occurred in both Fg$^{-/-}$ and Fg/VWF double deficient (Fg/VWF$^{-/-}$) mice [41]. We further demonstrated that Fg/VWF-independent platelet aggregation can be induced in vitro under more physiological conditions (i.e., nonanticoagulated blood) [42]. This concept of Fg- and VWF-independent thrombus formation has been confirmed by

several groups in both animal models [43] and human afibrinogenemic patients [44], although the effects of Fg and VWF deficiency on clot formation may be different between mice and humans. In contrast, neither platelet aggregation nor platelet-rich thrombi were observed in β3 integrin-deficient (β3$^{-/-}$) mice (lacking the β subunit of αIIbβ3 and αVβ3 integrins) [41, 45]. These data suggest that nonclassical β3 integrin ligands (i.e., not Fg or VWF) exist, which can support robust platelet aggregation independent from Fg and VWF.

1.2. Role of Plasma Fibronectin in Thrombosis and Hemostasis.
Interestingly, fibronectin, another ligand of β3 integrin, is increased 3–5-fold in platelets from either Fg$^{-/-}$ or Fg/VWF$^{-/-}$ mice, although no obvious change in plasma fibronectin levels was observed [41, 46]. We further observed that platelets from an afibrinogenemic patient had enhanced fibronectin content [23]. Our subsequent studies revealed that the increase in fibronectin content in Fg$^{-/-}$ platelets was due to enhanced plasma fibronectin internalization in the absence of Fg, which competitively binds to β3 integrin for internalization into platelets [21].

To test whether fibronectin is the ligand-mediating platelet aggregation in Fg/VWF$^{-/-}$ mice, Fg/VWF/pFn triple deficient mice were generated. Surprisingly, we found that platelet aggregation was not abolished but was actually enhanced in Fg/VWF/pFn$^{-/-}$ mice compared to Fg/VWF$^{-/-}$ mice [47], indicating that fibronectin is unlikely the ligand of β3 integrin that mediates thrombosis in the absence of both Fg and VWF. Identification and characterization of these novel β3 integrin ligands that mediate Fg/VWF-independent platelet aggregation will provide insights into the mechanisms of hemostasis and thrombosis in both normal and gene-deficient human populations and may lead to new targets for antithrombotic therapies.

In addition to their classic roles in hemostasis and thrombosis, recent studies suggest that platelets are also involved in many other physiological and pathophysiological processes, such as inflammation, angiogenesis, and tumor growth [48–51]. Interestingly, although platelets are anucleate cells, they can still de novo synthesize proteins following stimulation by platelet outside-in signalling [52]. We recently demonstrated that interactions between β3 integrins and their ligands (e.g., plasma Fg [53] and fibronectin (Andrews M and Ni H, unpublished data)) induced platelet P-selectin synthesis, which may affect not only hemostasis and thrombosis but also inflammation and immune responses. In this paper, we will mainly focus on the interaction between platelets and the immune system.

2. The Interaction between Platelets and Immune System

In vertebrates, there are two types of immunity to protect the host from infection: innate and adaptive. The innate immune system is genetically programmed to detect invariant features of invading microbial pathogens, while the adaptive immune system employs antigen-specific receptors that are generated de novo in each species [54]. Phagocytosis was first described by Metchnikoff more than a century ago, but research into innate immunity was largely overshadowed by the discovery of antibodies, CD4$^+$ and CD8$^+$ T cells, and other components of the adaptive immune response [55]. However, the recent discovery of pathogen recognition receptors (PRRs), such as Toll-like receptors (TLRs), Nod-like receptors, and RIG-I-like receptors, which recognize pathogen-associated molecular patterns (PAMPs) that are conserved among microbial pathogens, has greatly advanced our understanding of innate immunity. Platelets express many immunomodulatory molecules (e.g., P-selectin, TLRs, CD40L) and cytokines (e.g., IL-1β, TGF-β) and have the ability to interact with various immune cells. These properties confer platelets the ability to influence both innate and adaptive immune responses [48]. Alternatively, the immune system (e.g., antibodies, cytokines, immune cells) may target platelets and lead to several immune-mediated diseases, such as autoimmune thrombocytopenia, infection-associated thrombocytopenia, and fetal and neonatal alloimmune thrombocytopenia.

2.1. Platelets are Part of the Innate Immune System. Anucleate platelets are found only in mammals. In lower vertebrates, cells involved in hemostasis and blood coagulation are nucleated, termed thrombocytes. In many invertebrates, only one type of cell circulates in the blood, which is responsible for multiple defence mechanisms of the host, including hemostasis and immune functions [56]. Interestingly, mammalian platelets possess many capabilities that are similar to these defensive circulating cells in invertebrates. Platelets contribute to innate immunity in various ways: (1) platelets possess rudimentary antibacterial and phagocytic activity and have been shown to interact with bacteria, viruses, and parasites [57–59]. The interaction of bacteria with platelets induces platelet activation and secretion of antimicrobial peptides [60]; (2) platelets contain many proinflammatory cytokines (e.g., IL-1), which modulate the inflammatory/immune response [48, 49, 61–65]. It has been reported that platelet IL-1α drives cerebrovascular inflammation by inducing brain endothelial cell activation and enhancing their release of the chemokine CXCL1 [66]. Platelet-derived IL-1 also stimulates cytokine production (e.g., IL-6 and IL-8) by vascular smooth muscle cells [67]; (3) platelets express several functional Toll-like receptors (TLRs), such as TLR-2, TLR-4, and TLR-9 [68]. By interacting with TLR-4 on platelets, lipopolysaccharide (LPS) from the gram-negative bacteria activates platelets and induces platelet-neutrophil interactions, leading to neutrophil degranulation and release of extracellular traps that can kill the bacteria [69]. It has been demonstrated that LPS-stimulated platelet secretion potentiates platelet aggregation and thrombus formation via a TLR-4/MyD88 pathway, thus linking innate immunity with thrombosis [70]. However, it remains to be determined whether ligand interaction with other platelet TLRs, such as TLR-2 and TLR-9, also enhances thrombus formation; (4) vessel occlusion by thrombotic events in small vessels may play a role in the containment of invasive microorganisms,

which prevents spreading of this micropathogen-mediated septicaemia and viraemia and contributes to innate immunity. It also remains unclear whether platelets express other kinds of PRRs, such as Nod-like receptors and RIG-I-like receptors; (5) a recent discovery found that, during malaria infection, platelets can adhere to red blood cells infected with *Plasmodium falciparum* (*P. falciparum*) and induce apoptosis of these intracellular malaria parasites by releasing platelet granule components [71]. Mice deficient in C-mpl (Mpl$^{-/-}$), which have one-tenth as many circulating platelets as wild-type controls [72], are more susceptible to death induced by *P. falciparum* infection. The lethal effects of platelets on *P. falciparum* parasites appear to require platelet activation, since aspirin or other inhibitors of platelet function abrogated these effects [71]. Consistent with these observations, recent studies demonstrated that thrombocytopenia in patients with primary chronic autoimmune thrombocytopenia is associated with a significantly higher long-term risk of infection [73]. Thus, platelets are proinflammatory cells and are an important part of innate immunity.

It is very interesting that platelets also contain multiple anti-inflammatory cytokines (e.g., transforming growth factor-β, TGF-β). TGF-β is a potent immune suppressive factor. It has been reported that metastasizing tumor cells induce platelets to secrete TGF-β, which inhibits the antitumor activity of natural killer (NK) cells by downregulating the expression of the activating receptor, natural killer group 2 member D (NKG2D), on NK cells [74]. Neutralization of TGF-β in platelet releasate prevented the downregulation of NKG2D on NK cells and restored their antitumor activity [74]. It remains unknown whether malignant tumor cells can drive platelets to release TGF-β, which inhibits the function of other tumor-infiltrating lymphocytes (besides NK cells) in the tumor microenvironment, allowing the tumor cells to evade the host's immunosurveillance. It has also been demonstrated that platelets may assist tumor cells in evading immune cells via transfer of major histocompatibility complex (MHC) I from platelets to tumor cells [75]. Furthermore, platelets contain a large amount of thrombospondin-1 (TSP-1), which comprises around 25% of the total protein content of platelet α-granules [76]. It has been demonstrated that TSP-1 not only activates the anti-inflammatory cytokine TGF-β1 [77] but also inhibits the phagocytic capacity of macrophages. Murine macrophages deficient in TSP-1 have increased phagocytic function and TSP-1-deficient mice are protected from sepsis-associated mortality [78]. TSP-1 expression is significantly elevated on the surface of platelets in sepsis patients [79], and polymorphisms of TSP-1 have been linked with the development of sepsis-related organ failure [78]. Therefore, platelets are likely not only proinflammatory cells but also modulators that balance inflammation and immune responses.

It is intriguing whether a platelet can decide to support or inhibit inflammation since it contains both pro- and anti-inflammatory cytokines. Platelets also contain both angiogenesis inhibitors (e.g., endostatin, angiostatin, TSP-1, and platelet factor 4) and stimulators (e.g., vascular endothelial growth factor, angiopoietin 1, platelet-derived growth factor and insulin-like growth factor). It has been reported that proangiogenic and antiangiogenic molecules are stored in different α-granules inside platelets and megakaryocytes [50] and that these molecules are selectively released depending on the pathway of platelet activation [80, 81]. Interestingly, angiogenesis may be seen as an inflammatory response, since the newly formed vessels can transport inflammatory cells to sites of inflamed tissues and supply nutrients and oxygen to enhance proliferation of these tissues [82–85]. Since platelets also contain both proinflammatory (e.g., IL-1β) and anti-inflammatory cytokines (TGF-β and TSP-1), it remains to be determined whether they are also stored in different platelet granules and whether these cytokines are selectively released depending on local inflammation status.

Platelets also contain many chemokines. It has been demonstrated in vitro that the platelet-derived chemokine platelet factor 4 prevented monocytes from undergoing spontaneous apoptosis and instead induced the differentiation of monocytes into macrophages [86]. However, it remains to be determined whether platelets are involved in modulating the function of activated macrophages, although it is very likely. Considering the abundance of platelets in the circulation, it is reasonable to assume that platelets may act as sentinel cells and sense the invasion of foreign microorganisms via platelet TLRs, and by releasing chemokines, platelets may recruit more inflammatory cells (e.g., neutrophils) to sites of infection. Further studies are necessary to test these possibilities.

2.2. Platelets Contribute to Adaptive Immunity. It has been reported that P-selectin (CD62P) plays an important role in the development of the Th-1 immune response [87]. Upon platelet activation, P-selectin is translocated from the α-granule to the platelet surface. P-selectin can then interact with peripheral nodes addressin (PNAd) on high endothelial venules (HEV) and P-selectin glycoprotein ligand-1 (PSGL-1) on lymphocytes simultaneously, thus mediating the rolling and recruitment of lymphocytes to HEV of peripheral lymph nodes [88]. Our recent study demonstrated that plasma Fg, which is a key molecule for blood coagulation and platelet aggregation, through interaction with platelet $\beta3$ integrin, can deliver signals to platelets and induce de novo synthesis of P-selectin, which is required for maintenance of the P-selectin content in platelets [53]. This study provided a new link between coagulation/hemostasis and inflammation/immune responses.

In addition to P-selectin, activated platelets also express CD40L on their surface, which plays an important role in supporting immunoglobulin class switch and augmenting CD8$^+$ T-cell function during viral infection [89]. These events can directly affect B-cell differentiation and proliferation, which ultimately affects germinal center formation and antibody production [90]. Thus, platelets are also actively involved in adaptive immunity. Since platelets contain functional TGF-β, which is essential for the development of naturally occurring Foxp3$^+$ regulatory T cells (nTreg) or T helper 17 cells (Th17) depending on the local cytokine environment [91], it remains unknown whether platelets

modulate the balance of immune tolerance and inflammation, contributing to autoimmune diseases.

It has been reported that the effects of platelets on adaptive immunity may play a significant role in the host's defense against bacterial or viral infections. Platelets can actively bind gram-positive bacteria (e.g., *Listeria monocytogenes*) in the circulation and deliver them to splenic CD8α^+ dendritic cells, promoting antibacterial CD8$^+$ T-cell expansion [92]. It has also been reported that platelets contain a large amount of serotonin, which prolongs the activation of CD8$^+$ T cells via an unknown mechanism and aggravates virus-induced liver immunopathology [93].

2.3. Platelets are Involved in Lymphatic Vascular Development. Blood and vessels have shared developmental origins and function together to nourish the developing embryo [94, 95]. Definitive hematopoietic stem cells are derived from a subset of endothelial cells of the dorsal aorta in the aorta-gonad-mesonephros region of the developing embryo [96, 97]. The lymphatic vessels are a specialized vascular system that is parallel but separate from the blood vessels [98]. They form an extensive collecting network that maintains tissue fluid homeostasis, absorbs dietary lipids in the intestine, and facilitates immune cell trafficking and surveillance [99]. These specialized vessels are mainly composed of lymphatic endothelial cells (LECs) that originate in the cardinal vein [98]. During embryonic development, LECs migrate away from the cardinal vein and assemble into vessels to form a de novo collecting vascular system [98, 100]. It has been demonstrated that this blood-lymphatic vessel separation is regulated by a SYK-SLP-76 signalling pathway in blood cells, but the cell type and molecular regulation mechanisms were not well understood [99, 101]. Recently, several independent groups have identified platelets as the cell type in which SLP-76 signalling is essential to regulate lymphatic vessel development [101–103]. It was found that platelet C-type lectin-like receptor 2 (CLEC-2) can bind podoplanin (PDPN) on the surface of lymphatic endothelial cells and activate SLP-76 signalling to mediate blood and lymphatic vessel separation during embryonic development [101]. This interaction is required for blood-lymphatic separation in nonhematopoietic cells. This mechanism is further confirmed by the findings that platelet-specific deletion of SLP-76 is sufficient to induce a phenotype in which blood and lymphatic vessels commingle and that platelet-deficient embryos also exhibit the same phenotype [101, 102]. Considering the versatility of platelets, it would not be surprising if platelets play additional roles in embryonic/fetal development [104], including possible contributions to the development of the immune system.

3. Pathogenesis of Immune-Mediated Thrombocytopenia

Thrombocytopenia is a disorder in which the number of circulating platelets is abnormally low ($<150 \times 10^9$/L). Decreased platelet counts may lead to a severe bleeding diathesis, which, in some cases, may be life-threatening [48].

There are several major categories of thrombocytopenia, grouped according to the cause of the disease: (1) immune-mediated thrombocytopenia, (2) genetic deficiency-associated thrombocytopenia, and (3) malignancy-associated thrombocytopenia, which may occur in diseases such as chronic lymphocytic leukemia and lymphomas, prostate, breast, and ovarian cancers [105–109].

Immune-mediated thrombocytopenia can be further divided into autoimmune and alloimmune thrombocytopenia. Autoimmune thrombocytopenia is due to an abnormal immune response which develops against one's own platelets. The main types of autoimmune thrombocytopenia are primary immune thrombocytopenia (ITP; termed by a group of researchers in ITP) [110], infection-associated thrombocytopenia and drug-induced thrombocytopenia [111]. Alloimmune thrombocytopenia is due to alloantibody-mediated platelet destruction, in which antiplatelet alloantibodies develop following an immune response against transfused platelets from genetically different donors (termed post-transfusion purpura; PTP) or against paternally-derived alloantigens on fetal platelets during pregnancy (termed fetal and neonatal alloimmune thrombocytopenia (FNAIT or FNIT)) [112].

3.1. Platelets in Autoimmune Thrombocytopenia

3.1.1. Autoimmune Thrombocytopenia/Immune Thrombocytopenia (ITP).

Autoimmune thrombocytopenia (ITP) is a bleeding disorder characterized by autoantibody-mediated platelet destruction and impaired platelet production, with an increased bleeding diathesis [113, 114]. The incidence of ITP has been estimated at around 1–2.4 per 10,000 persons [115]. The characteristic of primary ITP is isolated thrombocytopenia (platelet count $< 100 \times 10^9$/L), in the absence of other conditions that may be associated with thrombocytopenia [110].

To date, the exact mechanisms of primary ITP are unclear [116]. Proposed mechanisms include both enhanced platelet destruction and impaired platelet production [117–122]. The GPIIbIIIa and GPIbα complex are the two major antigens targeted by autoantibodies in ITP. In adult ITP patients, approximately 70% of platelet autoantibodies are directed against GPIIbIIIa, and about 20–40% have specificity for the GPIbα complex, or both [123]. The antiplatelet antibodies in ITP may accelerate platelet clearance by Fcγ-receptor (FcγR)-bearing macrophages of the reticuloendothelial system, particularly those in the spleen. The autoantibodies in ITP patients may also affect platelet function, via effects on the binding of ligands (e.g., Fg and VWF) to platelet surface receptors [124, 125], which may further enhance the severity of bleeding in these patients. Furthermore, recent studies demonstrated that antiplatelet antibodies from ITP patients suppress megakaryocyte development and induce megakaryocyte apoptosis, thus inhibiting platelet production [121, 122, 126, 127]. Interestingly, there are some ITP patients who are thrombocytopenic but do not have detectable antiplatelet autoantibodies. It is currently unknown whether some low-affinity antibodies exist in these patients or their antibodies

recognize conformation-dependent epitopes that are lost during current monoclonal platelet antigen capture assays (MAIPA) procedures. It has also been suggested that in this antibody-negative group of ITP patients, cytotoxic CD8$^+$ T cells might be involved in the pathogenesis [128, 129].

To study the pathophysiology of primary ITP, as well as the efficacy and mechanisms of therapies, several laboratory-induced animal models of ITP have been established, such as (NZW × BXSB) F1 mice [130], the antiplatelet antibody passive-transfer model [131, 132], and the splenocyte-engraftment active ITP model [133]. The passive model of ITP was established by the injection of antiplatelet serum or monoclonal antibodies into recipient mice, in which short-term thrombocytopenia subsequently developed [134]. Using this model, it was demonstrated by Nieswandt and his colleagues that rat anti-mouse anti-GPIbα monoclonal antibodies (mAbs), but not anti-GPIIbIIIa mAbs, may cause thrombocytopenia in an Fc-independent manner [132]. We further demonstrated that these anti-GPIbα mAbs were able to cause thrombocytopenia in Fc receptor γ-chain-deficient mice, suggesting that anti-GPIbα-mediated thrombocytopenia may occur via an Fc-independent pathway [135]. Intravenous IgG (IVIG), prepared from pooled plasma from more than 1,000 healthy donors, has been considered a first-line therapy for ITP patients [136]. We found that IVIG effectively ameliorated thrombocytopenia induced by all anti-GPIIbIIIa mAbs, but not anti-GPIbα mAbs (with the exception of the anti-GPIbα antibody p0p4) [135]. Retrospective studies in ITP patients support these data. Go et al. demonstrated that IVIG was an effective therapy in ITP patients without anti-GPIbα antibodies (7/7), whereas most patients with anti-GPIbα antibodies were refractory to this treatment (7/10) [137]. More recently, Peng et al. observed that approximately 82% of ITP patients with anti-GPIIbIIIa antibodies responded to IVIG therapy, while only 49% of the patients with anti-GPIbα antibodies were responsive [138]. Taken together, these data suggest that IVIG is less effective in attenuating ITP mediated by anti-GPIbα antibodies compared to anti-GPIIbIIIa antibodies. Steroid treatment is the most commonly used first-line therapy for ITP patients worldwide. Our recent retrospective study demonstrated that ITP patients with anti-GPIIbIIIa antibodies had a 2-3-fold greater response to steroid treatment than patients with anti-GPIbα antibodies [139]. This is the first study in which a difference in therapeutic responsiveness to steroids was revealed between anti-GPIIbIIIa- and anti-GPIbα-mediated ITP, and the mechanisms underlying this difference are currently under investigation.

The major shortcomings of the passive antiplatelet antibody transfer model of ITP are that this model does not mimic primary chronic (i.e., long-term) ITP, and therefore, it is not feasible to investigate how antiplatelet autoimmunity initiates. To better accommodate these requirements, we have recently established a novel active animal model of ITP [133]. In this model, $\beta3^{-/-}$ mice were transfused with wild-type (WT) platelets, and spleen cells from these immunized $\beta3^{-/-}$ mice were engrafted into irradiated severe combined immunodeficiency (SCID) mice. Platelet counts and bleeding phenotypes were monitored in the SCID recipients. By depleting specific groups of lymphocytes prior to the transfer of splenocytes, CD19+ B-cell- (antibody-) and CD8+ T-cell- (cytotoxic T-cell-) mediated platelet destruction was observed. Both of these types of immune-mediated platelet destruction were dependent on the presence of CD4+ T cells, as CD4+ T-cell depletion completely abrogated the ability of the β3 integrin-reactive splenocytes to induce severe thrombocytopenia or bleeding symptoms, suggesting that CD4+ helper T cells may be responsible for the initiation of immunopathology in ITP [133]. Differences in the responsiveness to IVIG treatment were observed between antibody- and cell-mediated thrombocytopenia, as antibody-mediated thrombocytopenia and associated bleeding were ameliorated by IVIG, while cytotoxic T-cell-mediated severe ITP failed to respond to this therapy [133]. However, the clinical relevance of this study remains to be determined.

3.1.2. Platelets in Infection-Associated Thrombocytopenia.
Chronic infections, such as *Helicobacter pylori* (*H. pylori*) [140], human immunodeficiency virus (HIV) [111, 141, 142], hepatitis virus [143, 144], Epstein-Barr virus [145], cytomegalovirus [146], rubella virus [147], and the recently discovered novel Bunyavirus [148], have been linked with secondary ITP. Thrombocytopenia in these infections has been mainly attributed to antigenic mimicry, whereby antibodies targeting the micropathogens cross-react with platelet glycoproteins resulting in accelerated platelet clearance [111, 149].

The gram-negative bacterium *H. pylori*, which colonizes the stomach, has been associated with many gastrointestinal disorders, such as gastritis and gastric adenocarcinoma [150, 151]. Recent studies demonstrated that *H. pylori* infection is also implicated in the pathogenesis of secondary ITP [140], and that eradication of *H. pylori* infection may lead to disease regression [152, 153]. The prevalence of *H. pylori* infection among ITP patients varies by geographical area, ranging from 22% in North America to 85% in Japan [111, 154, 155]. The pathogenesis of *H. pylori*-associated ITP is not well understood, although antigenic mimicry has been implicated [111].

Human immunodeficiency virus (HIV) was first discovered as the cause of acquired immune deficiency syndrome (AIDS). Thrombocytopenia has been observed in HIV-infected patients with an estimated incidence of 4% to 24% [111, 141, 142] and the rate of thrombocytopenia has been strongly associated with the stage of AIDS progression[156]. Most antiplatelet antibodies isolated from HIV-infected patients react with the β3 integrin (GPIIIa)-(49–66) peptide, suggesting that GPIIIa-(49–66) is a major antigenic determinant for antiplatelet antibodies in these patients [157]. These anti-GPIIIa-(49–66) antibodies, which cross-react with many HIV proteins (e.g., nef, gag, env, and pol) [149], cause platelet destruction via the induction of reactive oxygen species, independent of complement activation [158].

Hepatitis C virus (HCV) infection has also been linked with thrombocytopenia, and the prevalence of HCV in ITP patients varies from 10% to 36% [143, 144]. Mechanistically,

HCV core protein 1 has been shown to induce the generation of antibodies that cross-react with GPIIIa-(49–66), leading to platelet destruction [159]. However, it has been reported that sequestration of platelets in the enlarged spleen (due to portal hypertension and decreased production of thrombopoietin) may also contribute to the pathogenesis of HCV-associated thrombocytopenia [160, 161].

3.2. Platelets in Alloimmune Thrombocytopenia

3.2.1. Fetal and Neonatal Alloimmune Thrombocytopenia.
Fetal and neonatal alloimmune thrombocytopenia (FNAIT or FNIT) is a life-threatening alloimmune disorder, which results from fetal platelet opsonization and destruction by maternal antibodies that develop during pregnancy [162–165]. The maternal immune system targets paternally derived antigens on fetal platelets, due to platelet gene polymorphisms and generates alloantibodies. These maternal alloantibodies can cross the placenta and enter the fetal circulation. The neonatal Fc receptor (FcRn) has been implicated in mediating the maternofetal transfer of IgG [166, 167]. The maternal alloantibodies bind to fetal or neonatal platelets and cause their destruction. The mechanisms of fetal or neonatal platelet destruction in FNAIT are not well understood, although it is thought that these mechanisms may be similar to those in ITP [168].

FNAIT is the most common cause of severe thrombocytopenia in liveborn neonates. The incidence of FNAIT has been estimated at 0.5–1.5 per 1,000 liveborn neonates [169–172]; however, this number does not include miscarriage caused by the disease, since the rate of fetal mortality in affected pregnant women has not been adequately studied, although miscarriage has been reported by several groups [173–177]. Furthermore, the mechanisms of miscarriage and the potential therapies to prevent miscarriage in these women are unknown. The major risk of FNAIT is severe bleeding, especially intracranial hemorrhage (ICH), which may lead to neurological impairment or death in affected fetuses and neonates [162–165]. Contrary to haemolytic disease of the newborn, almost half of FNAIT cases occur during the first pregnancy [174], thus challenging current diagnostic and therapeutic methods. Furthermore, the rate of recurrence among subsequent platelet antigen-positive siblings is close to 100%, with subsequently affected siblings having either a similar or more severe degree of thrombocytopenia [165, 178].

Similar to ITP, the major antigen target in patients with FNAIT is GPIIbIIIa, as most reported FNAIT cases (around 75%) have been characterized by maternal alloantibodies to human platelet antigen-1a (HPA-1a), which is located on fetal β3 integrin [179, 180]. However, there are very few reported cases of FNAIT associated with anti-GPIbα antibodies [181–186], which is in clear contrast to the 20–40% prevalence of anti-GPIbα complex antibodies in patients with ITP [187–189]. The underlying reason for the surprisingly low incidence of FNAIT mediated by anti-GPIbα antibodies has not been explored and the maternal immune responses to fetal platelet antigens remain to be elucidated.

Recent studies suggest that $\beta 3$ integrin is expressed on human placental syncytiotrophoblast cells as early as the first trimester of pregnancy [190, 191]. Thus, the maternal immune system may mount an immune response against "platelet" antigens on placental syncytiotrophoblasts or on fetal platelets that "leak" into the maternal circulation through fetomaternal hemorrhage during pregnancy [112, 190, 191]. Approximately 2–2.5% of the Caucasian population is HPA-1a negative, and maternal alloantibodies to HPA-1a can be formed in homozygous HPA-1bb women carrying a HPA-1a-positive fetus. However, it has been reported that only around 10% of HPA-1a negative pregnant women carrying an HPA-1a-positive fetus will generate anti-HPA-1a antibodies [179]. The human leukocyte antigen- (HLA-) DRB3*0101 allele, which encodes MHC molecule DR52a, has been associated with anti-HPA-1a antibody generation, suggesting that it may be important in presenting the HPA-1a antigen to CD4$^+$ T cells that can provide cytokines to "help" B cells to generate anti-HPA-1a antibodies [179, 192]. It has been further demonstrated that HPA-1a, but not HPA-1b, binds to DR52a and forms stable complexes, which can potentially stimulate the response of CD4$^+$ T cells [193–195]. By culturing peripheral blood mononuclear cells in the presence of the HPA-1a peptide, HPA-1a-specific CD4$^+$ T cells have been isolated from HPA-1a-immunized women that give birth to children with FNAIT, indicating that the T-cell response is involved in the pathogenesis of FNAIT [195, 196].

Our laboratory has recently established animal models of FNAIT using $\beta 3^{-/-}$ mice. $\beta 3^{-/-}$ female mice were transfused with wild-type (WT) platelets before breeding with WT males [197]. The fetuses from this breeding are $\beta 3$ heterozygous (i.e., antigen positive) and are expected to be targeted by the maternal immune response during pregnancy. We first demonstrated that $\beta 3^{-/-}$ mice generated specific antibodies against platelet $\beta 3$ integrin after WT platelet transfusions [197]. The immunized $\beta 3^{-/-}$ females were bred with WT males, and we found that neonatal thrombocytopenia and severe bleeding symptoms (e.g., ICH) were observed in the heterozygous pups from immunized $\beta 3^{-/-}$ mothers, which recapitulated FNAIT in humans [197]. We found that maternal administration of IVIG during pregnancy downregulated the pathogenic anti-$\beta 3$ antibody levels in both the maternal and fetal/neonatal circulation and markedly ameliorated FNAIT symptoms [197]. Our laboratory has demonstrated that anti-$\beta 3$ antibodies generated in our anti-$\beta 3$-mediated FNAIT model may cross-react with $\beta 3$ integrin on fetal endothelial cells and inhibit proliferation and vascular-like tube formation by endothelial cells in vitro [198].

To investigate the potential reasons for the rarity of reported cases of anti-GPIbα-mediated FNAIT in humans, we developed another animal model of FNAIT using GPIb$\alpha^{-/-}$ mice and compared the pathogenesis with our anti-$\beta 3$ integrin-mediated FNAIT model [17, 199]. We found, unexpectedly, that miscarriage occurred in most of the anti-GPIbα-mediated FNAIT, which is far more frequent than that mediated by anti-$\beta 3$ antibodies. Mothers with anti-GPIbα antibodies exhibited extensive fibrin deposition and apoptosis/necrosis in their placentas, which severely

impaired placental function. We further demonstrated, for the first time, that anti-GPIbα (but not anti-$\beta 3$) antisera activated platelets and enhanced fibrin formation in vitro and thrombus formation in vivo [17]. Furthermore, anti-GPIbα antibodies purified from the anti-GPIbα antisera inhibited the binding of α-thrombin to platelet GPIbα, which may lead to increased free circulating thrombin. This thrombin can convert fibrinogen into fibrin and activate platelets via protease-activated receptors 1 and 4, which may further enhance thrombus formation. Thus, the maternal immune response to fetal GPIbα may cause a previously unidentified, nonclassical FNAIT (i.e., spontaneous miscarriage but not neonatal bleeding), which may mask the severity and frequency of anti-GPIbα-mediated FNAIT in humans [17, 199]. We demonstrated that IVIG or anti-FcRn therapy efficiently prevented this life-threatening disease, suggesting potential therapeutic interventions for human FNAIT patients affected by miscarriage [17]. The efficacy of IVIG in anti-GPIbα-mediated FNAIT may be due to IVIG-mediated downregulation of maternal pathogenic antibodies and blockade of these maternal antibodies from crossing the placenta during pregnancy (via occupancy of FcRn). It is currently unknown whether the maternal immune response against fetal GPIbα is indeed a significant cause of miscarriage in humans. Screening the polymorphisms of GPIbα (e.g., HPA-2) in women suffering from miscarriage and habitual abortion and detecting anti-GPIbα antibodies during pregnancy may provide important information to address this critical question. If anti-GPIbα antibodies are indeed a risk factor for miscarriage in humans, identifying these women and treating them during early in pregnancy with IVIG or anti-FcRn therapies may be able to prevent this nonclassical, but devastating, FNAIT.

To further characterize the role of FcRn in the pathogenesis of FNAIT, we developed another murine model of FNAIT using $\beta 3$/FcRn double deficient ($\beta 3^{-/-}$/FcRn$^{-/-}$) mice [200, 201]. In this model, we transfused $\beta 3^{-/-}$/FcRn$^{-/-}$ female mice with $\beta 3^{+/+}$/FcRn$^{-/-}$ platelets and bred them with $\beta 3^{+/+}$/FcRn$^{-/-}$ male mice [200]. We observed that the transfused $\beta 3^{-/-}$/FcRn$^{-/-}$ mice generated specific antibodies against platelet $\beta 3$ integrin and maintained these antibodies at levels that sufficiently induced thrombocytopenia in adult $\beta 3^{+/+}$/FcRn$^{-/-}$ mice. However, no FNAIT developed in these $\beta 3^{-/-}$/FcRn$^{-/-}$ female mice when bred with $\beta 3^{+/+}$/FcRn$^{-/-}$ males, suggesting that FcRn is essential for the induction of FNAIT [200]. Using our newly generated mouse anti-mouse $\beta 3$ integrin antibodies, we further demonstrated that FcRn is required for the transfer of all IgG isotypes from the maternal circulation to the fetus. Although fetal and maternal sides of the placenta both express FcRn, we found that fetal, but not maternal, FcRn was required for transplacental transfer of anti-$\beta 3$ integrin IgG and the induction of FNAIT. This finding may have broad implications for the basic understanding of how maternal antibodies are transported across the placenta and for infectious diseases [200]. We found that anti-FcRn is a more efficient therapy than IVIG, since the dose of anti-FcRn required for therapeutic efficacy in this FNAIT model is much lower than that of IVIG (at least 200-fold less) [200]. In addition, anti-FcRn has the advantage of not being prepared from human plasma (as is IVIG), thus having less chances of transmitting blood-borne micropathogens. Furthermore, our data suggest that anti-FcRn may be useful to prevent the transplacental transport of maternal pathogenic antibodies in other alloimmune diseases, including alloimmune neonatal neutropenia and haemolytic disease of the newborn, or pathogenic antibody transfer from mothers with autoimmune diseases, such as ITP, systemic lupus erythematosus, and autoimmune haemolytic anemia [200].

3.2.2. Posttransfusion Purpura. Posttransfusion purpura (PTP) is a rare but severe alloimmune complication that usually occurs within 7–10 days following a blood transfusion [112, 202]. The true incidence of PTP is unclear, since this disorder is frequently underdiagnosed or misdiagnosed [112]. Patients with PTP are initially sensitized against the offending platelet antigens either during pregnancy or a blood product transfusion. Upon reexposure to the same platelet antigens (typically via a blood transfusion), the antiplatelet alloimmune response is further stimulated and a sudden rise in antiplatelet antibody titers occurs leading to rapid clearance of both transfused platelets and the patient's endogenous platelets. The mechanisms leading to the destruction of the patient's own antigen-negative platelets are unclear [112]. On most occasions, PTP patients present with sudden onset of widespread purpura following a blood transfusion, but life-threatening bleeding symptoms, such as ICH, have been described in some severe cases, sometimes with a fatal outcome [112]. Although it has been reported that some PTP patients recover spontaneously, therapeutic interventions may be required for patients with severe thrombocytopenia and resulting bleeding diathesis. The administration of IVIG, with or without corticosteroids, has been considered as the first-line therapy for PTP [112, 202].

4. Concluding Remarks

It is well known that platelets play critical roles in hemostasis and thrombosis. However, exciting recent studies have revealed many new roles of platelets, such as inflammation/immune responses, tumour growth and metastasis, angiogenesis, and so forth. These new data have revolutionized our understanding of platelet functions. Platelets contain many immunologically functional molecules and contribute to both innate and adaptive immunity, which establishes platelets as immune cells. Considering their abundance in the blood, platelets may act as sentinels to identify invading microorganisms through platelet TLRs. In addition, platelets are also involved in lymphatic vessel development. In addition to the active contributions of platelets to immunity, platelets are also passively targeted in several immune-mediated diseases, although the pathogenesis is not well understood. It remains unknown whether platelets themselves contribute to the initiation or development of these platelet-targeted immune-mediated diseases. Further exploration of the interaction between platelets and the

immune system may provide insights into autoimmune diseases, including the chronic process of atherosclerosis, and lead to the development of new therapies to control diseases such as infection and malignant tumors, as well as bleeding disorders.

Conflict of Interests

The authors declare no competing financial interests.

Acknowledgments

This work was supported in part by the Canadian Institutes of Health Research (MOP 68986 and MOP 119551), Bayer/Canadian Blood Services/Hema-Quebec/Talecris partnership, Equipment Funds from St. Michael's Hospital, Canadian Blood Services, and Canada Foundation for Innovation. Conglei Li is a recipient of the Connaught Scholarship, University of Toronto; Yan Li is a recipient of Canadian Blood Services Postdoctoral Fellowship; Sean Lang is a recipient of the Heart and Stroke Foundation of Canada (Ontario) Master's Studentship Award and Ph.D. Graduate Fellowship from Canadian Blood Services; June Li is a recipient of Laboratory Medicine and Pathobiology Departmental Fellowship, University of Toronto.

References

[1] B. Coller, *A Brief History of Ideas about Platelets in Health and Disease, Platelets*, Edited by A. D. Michelson, Academic Press, Amsterdam, The Netherlands, 2nd edition, 2007.

[2] W. Oler and E. Schaefer, "Ueber einige im Blute vorhandene bakterienbildende Massen," in *Centralblatt Für Die Medicinischen Wissenschaften*, vol. 11, p. 577, 1873.

[3] W. Oler, "An account of certain organisms occurring in the liquor sanguinis," *Proceedings of the Royal Society of London*, vol. 22, pp. 391–398, 1874.

[4] G. Bizzozero, "Su di un nuovo elemento morfologico del sangue dei mammiferi e della sua importanza nella trombosi e nella coagulazione," *L'Osservatore*, vol. 17, pp. 785–787, 1881.

[5] J. Bizzozero, "Ueber einen neuen formbestandtheil des blutes und dessen rolle bei der thrombose und der blutgerinnung—untersuchungen," *Archiv für Pathologische Anatomie und Physiologie und für Klinische Medicin*, vol. 90, no. 2, pp. 261–332, 1882.

[6] J. Wright, "The origin and nature of blood plates," *The Boston Medical and Surgical Journal*, vol. 154, pp. 643–645, 1906.

[7] J. E. Italiano Jr., P. Lecine, R. A. Shivdasani, and J. H. Hartwig, "Blood platelets are assembled principally at the ends of proplatelet processes produced by differentiated megakaryocytes," *Journal of Cell Biology*, vol. 147, no. 6, pp. 1299–1312, 1999.

[8] T. Junt, H. Schulze, Z. Chen et al., "Dynamic visualization of thrombopoiesis within bone marrow," *Science*, vol. 317, no. 5845, pp. 1767–1770, 2007.

[9] R. Fuentes, Y. Wang, J. Hirsch et al., "Infusion of mature megakaryocytes into mice yields functional platelets," *Journal of Clinical Investigation*, vol. 120, no. 11, pp. 3917–3922, 2010.

[10] Z. M. Ruggeri, "Mechanisms initiating platelet thrombus formation," *Thrombosis and Haemostasis*, vol. 78, no. 1, pp. 611–616, 1997.

[11] D. R. Phillips, I. F. Charo, and R. M. Scarborough, "GPIIb-IIIa: the responsive integrin," *Cell*, vol. 65, no. 3, pp. 359–362, 1991.

[12] R. K. Andrews and M. C. Berndt, "Platelet physiology and thrombosis," *Thrombosis Research*, vol. 114, no. 5-6, pp. 447–453, 2004.

[13] K. G. Mann, "Thrombin formation," *Chest*, vol. 124, pp. 4S–10S, 2003.

[14] H. Ni and J. Freedman, "Platelets in hemostasis and thrombosis: role of integrins and their ligands," *Transfusion and Apheresis Science*, vol. 28, no. 3, pp. 257–264, 2003.

[15] M. W. C. Hatton, B. Ross, S. M. R. Southward, M. Timleck-DeReske, and M. Richardson, "Platelet and fibrinogen turnover at the exposed subendothelium measured over 1 year after a balloon catheter de-endothelializing injury to the rabbit aorta: thrombotic eruption at the late re-endothelialization stage," *Atherosclerosis*, vol. 165, no. 1, pp. 57–67, 2002.

[16] G. X. Shen, "Inhibition of thrombin: relevance to anti-thrombosis strategy," *Frontiers in Bioscience*, vol. 11, no. 1, pp. 113–120, 2006.

[17] C. Li, S. Piran, P. Chen et al., "The maternal immune response to fetal platelet GPIbalpha causes frequent miscarriage in mice that can be prevented by intravenous IgG and anti-FcRn therapies," *The Journal of Clinical Investigation*, vol. 121, pp. 4537–4547, 2011.

[18] G. R. Sambrano, E. J. Weiss, Y. W. Zheng, W. Huang, and S. R. Coughlin, "Role of thrombin signalling in platelets in haemostasis and thrombosis," *Nature*, vol. 413, no. 6851, pp. 74–78, 2001.

[19] M. L. Kahn, Y. W. Zheng, W. Huang et al., "A dual thrombin receptor system for platelet activation," *Nature*, vol. 394, no. 6694, pp. 690–694, 1998.

[20] T. K. H. Vu, D. T. Hung, V. I. Wheaton, and S. R. Coughlin, "Molecular cloning of a functional thrombin receptor reveals a novel proteolytic mechanism of receptor activation," *Cell*, vol. 64, no. 6, pp. 1057–1068, 1991.

[21] H. Ni, J. M. Papalia, J. L. Degen, and D. D. Wagner, "Control of thrombus embolization and fibronectin internalization by integrin αIIbβ3 engagement of the fibrinogen γ chain," *Blood*, vol. 102, no. 10, pp. 3609–3614, 2003.

[22] D. Lillicrap, "Genotype/phenotype association in von Willebrand disease: is the glass half full or empty?" *Journal of Thrombosis and Haemostasis*, vol. 7, supplement 1, pp. 65–70, 2009.

[23] Z. Zhai, J. Wu, X. Xu et al., "Fibrinogen controls human platelet fibronectin internalization and cell-surface retention," *Journal of Thrombosis and Haemostasis*, vol. 5, no. 8, pp. 1740–1746, 2007.

[24] T. Gui, A. Reheman, W. K. Funkhouser et al., "In vivo response to vascular injury in the absence of factor IX: examination in factor IX knockout mice," *Thrombosis Research*, vol. 121, no. 2, pp. 225–234, 2007.

[25] T. Gui, A. Reheman, H. Ni et al., "Abnormal hemostasis in a knock-in mouse carrying a variant of factor IX with impaired binding to collagen type IV," *Journal of Thrombosis and Haemostasis*, vol. 7, no. 11, pp. 1843–1851, 2009.

[26] Z. M. Ruggeri, "Platelets in atherothrombosis," *Nature Medicine*, vol. 8, no. 11, pp. 1227–1234, 2002.

[27] S. Falati, P. Gross, G. Merrill-skoloff, B. C. Furie, and B. Furie, "Real time in vivo imaging of platelets, tissue factor and fibrin during arterial thrombus formation in the mouse," *Nature Medicine*, vol. 8, no. 10, pp. 1175–1180, 2002.

[28] A. Lynch, R. Marlar, J. Murphy et al., "Antiphospholipid antibodies in predicting adverse pregnancy outcome: a prospective study," *Annals of Internal Medicine*, vol. 120, no. 6, pp. 470–475, 1994.

[29] G. R. V. Hughes, "Thrombosis, abortion, cerebral disease, and the lupus anticoagulant," *British Medical Journal*, vol. 287, no. 6399, pp. 1088–1089, 1983.

[30] S. M. Bates, "Consultative hematology: the pregnant patient pregnancy loss," *Hematology*, vol. 2010, pp. 166–172, 2010.

[31] M. H. Tong, H. Jiang, P. Liu, J. A. Lawson, L. F. Brass, and W. C. Song, "Spontaneous fetal loss caused by placental thrombosis in estrogen sulfotransferase-deficient mice," *Nature Medicine*, vol. 11, no. 2, pp. 153–159, 2005.

[32] Z. M. Ruggeri, "Von Willebrand factor, platelets and endothelial cell interactions," *Journal of Thrombosis and Haemostasis*, vol. 1, no. 7, pp. 1335–1342, 2003.

[33] W. Bergmeier, C. L. Piffath, T. Goerge et al., "The role of platelet adhesion receptor GPIbα far exceeds that of its main ligand, von Willebrand factor, in arterial thrombosis," *Proceedings of the National Academy of Sciences of the United States of America*, vol. 103, no. 45, pp. 16900–16905, 2006.

[34] M. Moroi, S. M. Jung, K. Shinmyozu, Y. Tomiyama, A. Ordinas, and M. Diaz-Ricart, "Analysis of platelet adhesion to a collagen-coated surface under flow conditions: the involvement of glycoprotein VI in the platelet adhesion," *Blood*, vol. 88, no. 6, pp. 2081–2092, 1996.

[35] T. Xia, J. Takagi, B. S. Coller, J. H. Wang, and T. A. Springer, "Structural basis for allostery in integrins and binding to fibrinogen-mimetic therapeutics," *Nature*, vol. 432, no. 7013, pp. 59–67, 2004.

[36] S. J. Shattil, J. A. Hoxie, M. Cunningham, and L. F. Brass, "Changes in the platelet membrane glycoprotein IIb.IIIa complex during platelet activation," *Journal of Biological Chemistry*, vol. 260, no. 20, pp. 11107–11114, 1985.

[37] J. P. Xiong, T. Stehle, B. Diefenbach et al., "Crystal structure of the extracellular segment of integrin αVβ3," *Science*, vol. 294, no. 5541, pp. 339–345, 2001.

[38] Z. M. Ruggeri, "Old concepts and new developments in the study of platelet aggregation," *Journal of Clinical Investigation*, vol. 105, no. 6, pp. 699–701, 2000.

[39] M. M. Frojmovic, "Platelet aggregation in flow: differential roles for adhesive receptors and ligands," *American Heart Journal*, vol. 135, pp. S119–S131, 1998.

[40] M. J. Cross, "Effect of fibrinogen on the aggregation of platelets by adenosine diphosphate," *Thrombosis et Diathesis Haemorrhagica*, vol. 12, pp. 524–527, 1964.

[41] H. Ni, C. V. Denis, S. Subbarao et al., "Persistence of platelet thrombus formation in arterioles of mice lacking both von Willebrand factor and fibrinogen," *Journal of Clinical Investigation*, vol. 106, no. 3, pp. 385–392, 2000.

[42] H. Yang, A. Reheman, P. Chen et al., "Fibrinogen and von willebrand factor-independent platelet aggregation in vitro and in vivo," *Journal of Thrombosis and Haemostasis*, vol. 4, no. 10, pp. 2230–2237, 2006.

[43] M. Jiroušková, I. Chereshnev, H. Väänänen, J. L. Degen, and B. S. Coller, "Antibody blockade or mutation of the fibrinogen γ-chain C-terminus is more effective in inhibiting murine arterial thrombus formation than complete absence of fibrinogen," *Blood*, vol. 103, no. 6, pp. 1995–2002, 2004.

[44] S. Tsuji, M. Sugimoto, S. Miyata, M. Kuwahara, S. Kinoshita, and A. Yoshioka, "Real-time analysis of mural thrombus formation in various platelet aggregation disorders: distinct

shear-dependent roles of platelet receptors and adhesive proteins under flow," *Blood*, vol. 94, no. 3, pp. 968–975, 1999.

[45] R. O. Hynes and K. M. Hodivala-Dilke, "Insights and questions arising from studies of a mouse model of Glanzmann thrombasthenia," *Thrombosis and Haemostasis*, vol. 82, no. 2, pp. 481–485, 1999.

[46] H. Ni, "Unveiling the new face of fibronectin in thrombosis and hemostasis," *Journal of Thrombosis and Haemostasis*, vol. 4, no. 5, pp. 940–942, 2006.

[47] A. Reheman, H. Yang, G. Zhu et al., "Plasma fibronectin depletion enhances platelet aggregation and thrombus formation in mice lacking fibrinogen and von Willebrand factor," *Blood*, vol. 113, no. 8, pp. 1809–1817, 2009.

[48] J. W. Semple, J. E. Italiano, and J. Freedman, "Platelets and the immune continuum," *Nature Reviews Immunology*, vol. 11, no. 4, pp. 264–274, 2011.

[49] P. Von Hundelshausen and C. Weber, "Platelets as immune cells: bridging inflammation and cardiovascular disease," *Circulation Research*, vol. 100, no. 1, pp. 27–40, 2007.

[50] J. E. Italiano Jr., J. L. Richardson, S. Patel-Hett et al., "Angiogenesis is regulated by a novel mechanism: pro- and antiangiogenic proteins are organized into separate platelet α granules and differentially released," *Blood*, vol. 111, no. 3, pp. 1227–1233, 2008.

[51] B. Ho-Tin-Noé, T. Goerge, S. M. Cifuni, D. Duerschmied, and D. D. Wagner, "Platelet granule secretion continuously prevents intratumor hemorrhage," *Cancer Research*, vol. 68, no. 16, pp. 6851–6858, 2008.

[52] G. A. Zimmerman and A. S. Weyrich, "Signal-dependent protein synthesis by activated platelets: new pathways to altered phenotype and function," *Arteriosclerosis, Thrombosis, and Vascular Biology*, vol. 28, pp. s17–s24, 2008.

[53] H. Yang, S. Lang, Z. Zhai et al., "Fibrinogen is required for maintenance of platelet intracellular and cell-surface P-selectin expression," *Blood*, vol. 114, no. 2, pp. 425–436, 2009.

[54] A. Iwasaki and R. Medzhitov, "Regulation of adaptive immunity by the innate immune system," *Science*, vol. 327, no. 5963, pp. 291–295, 2010.

[55] A. M. Silverstein, "Darwinism and immunology: from Metchnikoff to Burnet," *Nature Immunology*, vol. 4, no. 1, pp. 3–6, 2003.

[56] J. Hose, G. Martin, and A. Gerard, "A decapod hemocyte classification scheme integrating morphology, cytochemistry, and function," *The Biological Bulletin*, vol. 178, pp. 33–45, 1990.

[57] T. Youssefian, A. Drouin, J. M. Massé, J. Guichard, and E. M. Cramer, "Host defense role of platelets: engulfment of HIV and *Staphylococcus aureus* occurs in a specific subcellular compartment and is enhanced by platelet activation," *Blood*, vol. 99, no. 11, pp. 4021–4029, 2002.

[58] M. Joseph, C. Auriault, A. Capron, H. Vorng, and P. Viens, "A new function for platelets: IgE-dependent killing of schistosomes," *Nature*, vol. 303, no. 5920, pp. 810–812, 1983.

[59] B. F. Kraemer, R. A. Campbell, H. Schwertz et al., "Novel anti-bacterial activities of beta-defensin 1 in human platelets: suppression of pathogen growth and signaling of neutrophil extracellular trap formation," *PLoS Pathogens*, vol. 7, Article ID e1002355, 2011.

[60] D. Cox, S. W. Kerrigan, and S. P. Watson, "Platelets and the innate immune system: mechanisms of bacterial-induced platelet activation," *Journal of Thrombosis and Haemostasis*, vol. 9, no. 6, pp. 1097–1107, 2011.

[61] D. D. Wagner and P. C. Burger, "Platelets in inflammation and thrombosis," *Arteriosclerosis, Thrombosis, and Vascular Biology*, vol. 23, pp. 2131–2137, 2003.

[62] P. von Hundelshausen, R. R. Koenen, and C. Weber, "Platelet-mediated enhancement of leukocyte adhesion," *Microcirculation*, vol. 16, no. 1, pp. 84–96, 2009.

[63] V. Henn, J. R. Slupsky, M. Gräfe et al., "CD40 ligand on activated platelets triggers an inflammatory reaction of endothelial cells," *Nature*, vol. 391, no. 6667, pp. 591–594, 1998.

[64] J. W. Semple and J. Freedman, "Platelets and innate immunity," *Cellular and Molecular Life Sciences*, vol. 67, no. 4, pp. 499–511, 2010.

[65] C. M. Hawrylowicz, S. A. Santoro, F. M. Platt, and E. R. Unanue, "Activated platelets express IL-1 activity," *Journal of Immunology*, vol. 143, no. 12, pp. 4015–4018, 1989.

[66] P. Thornton, B. W. McColl, A. Greenhalgh, A. Denes, S. M. Allan, and N. J. Rothwell, "Platelet interleukin-1α drives cerebrovascular inflammation," *Blood*, vol. 115, no. 17, pp. 3632–3639, 2010.

[67] H. Loppnow, R. Bil, S. Hirt et al., "Platelet-derived interleukin-1 induces cytokine production, but not proliferation of human vascular smooth muscle cells," *Blood*, vol. 91, no. 1, pp. 134–141, 1998.

[68] R. Aslam, E. R. Speck, M. Kim et al., "Platelet Toll-like receptor expression modulates lipopolysaccharide-induced thrombocytopenia and tumor necrosis factor-α production in vivo," *Blood*, vol. 107, no. 2, pp. 637–641, 2006.

[69] S. R. Clark, A. C. Ma, S. A. Tavener et al., "Platelet TLR4 activates neutrophil extracellular traps to ensnare bacteria in septic blood," *Nature Medicine*, vol. 13, no. 4, pp. 463–469, 2007.

[70] G. Zhang, J. Han, E. J. Welch et al., "Lipopolysaccharide stimulates platelet secretion and potentiates platelet aggregation via TLR4/MyD88 and the cGMP-dependent protein kinase pathway," *Journal of Immunology*, vol. 182, no. 12, pp. 7997–8004, 2009.

[71] B. J. McMorran, V. M. Marshall, C. De Graaf et al., "Platelets kill intraerythrocytic malarial parasites and mediate survival to infection," *Science*, vol. 323, no. 5915, pp. 797–800, 2009.

[72] W. S. Alexander, A. W. Roberts, N. A. Nicola, R. Li, and D. Metcalf, "Deficiencies in progenitor cells of multiple hematopoietic lineages and defective megakaryocytopoiesis in mice lacking the thrombopoietin receptor c-Mpl," *Blood*, vol. 87, no. 6, pp. 2162–2170, 1996.

[73] M. Nørgaard, A. Ø. Jensen, M. C. Engebjerg et al., "Long-term clinical outcomes of patients with primary chronic immune thrombocytopenia: a Danish population-based cohort study," *Blood*, vol. 117, no. 13, pp. 3514–3520, 2011.

[74] H. G. Kopp, T. Placke, and H. R. Salih, "Platelet-derived transforming growth factor-β down-regulates NKG2D thereby inhibiting natural killer cell antitumor reactivity," *Cancer Research*, vol. 69, no. 19, pp. 7775–7783, 2009.

[75] T. Placke, H. G. Kopp, and H. R. Salih, "The wolf in sheep's clothing: platelet-derived, "pseudo self" impairs cancer cell, "missing self" recognition by NK cells," *Oncoimmunology*, vol. 1, pp. 557–559, 2012.

[76] N. L. Baenziger, G. N. Brodie, and P. W. Majerus, "A thrombin-sensitive protein of human platelet membranes," *Proceedings of the National Academy of Sciences of the United States of America*, vol. 68, no. 1, pp. 240–243, 1971.

[77] S. E. Crawford, V. Stellmach, J. E. Murphy-Ullrich et al., "Thrombospondin-1 is a major activator of TGF-β1 in vivo," *Cell*, vol. 93, no. 7, pp. 1159–1170, 1998.

[78] S. McMaken, M. C. Exline, P. Mehta et al., "Thrombospondin-1 contributes to mortality in murine sepsis through effects on innate immunity," *PLoS ONE*, vol. 6, no. 5, Article ID e19654, 2011.

[79] M. Gawaz, T. Dickfeld, C. Bogner, S. Fateh-Moghadam, and F. J. Neumann, "Platelet function in septic multiple organ dysfunction syndrome," *Intensive Care Medicine*, vol. 23, no. 4, pp. 379–385, 1997.

[80] E. M. Battinelli, B. A. Markens, and J. E. Italiano Jr., "Release of angiogenesis regulatory proteins from platelet alpha granules: modulation of physiologic and pathologic angiogenesis," *Blood*, vol. 118, pp. 1359–1369, 2011.

[81] M. Chatterjee, Z. Huang, W. Zhang et al., "Distinct platelet packaging, release, and surface expression of proangiogenic and antiangiogenic factors on different platelet stimuli," *Blood*, vol. 117, no. 14, pp. 3907–3911, 2011.

[82] A. Marrelli, P. Cipriani, V. Liakouli et al., "Angiogenesis in rheumatoid arthritis: a disease specific process or a common response to chronic inflammation?" *Autoimmunity Reviews*, vol. 10, pp. 595–598, 2011.

[83] K. Grote, H. Schütt, and B. Schieffer, "Toll-like receptors in angiogenesis," *The Scientific World Journal*, vol. 11, pp. 981–991, 2011.

[84] B. A. Imhof and M. Aurrand-Lions, "Angiogenesis and inflammation face off," *Nature Medicine*, vol. 12, no. 2, pp. 171–172, 2006.

[85] U. Fiedler, Y. Reiss, M. Scharpfenecker et al., "Angiopoietin-2 sensitizes endothelial cells to TNF-α and has a crucial role in the induction of inflammation," *Nature Medicine*, vol. 12, no. 2, pp. 235–239, 2006.

[86] B. Scheuerer, M. Ernst, I. Dürrbaum-Landmann et al., "The CXC-chemokine platelet factor 4 promotes monocyte survival and induces monocyte differentiation into macrophages," *Blood*, vol. 95, no. 4, pp. 1158–1166, 2000.

[87] F. Austrup, D. Vestweber, E. Borges et al., "P- and E-selectin mediate recruitment of T-helper-1 but not T-helper-2 cells into inflamed tissues," *Nature*, vol. 385, no. 6611, pp. 81–83, 1997.

[88] T. G. Diacovo, K. D. Puri, R. A. Warnock, T. A. Springer, and U. H. Von Andrian, "Platelet-mediated lymphocyte delivery to high endothelial venules," *Science*, vol. 273, no. 5272, pp. 252–255, 1996.

[89] B. D. Elzey, J. Tian, R. J. Jensen et al., "Platelet-mediated modulation of adaptive immunity: a communication link between innate and adaptive immune compartments," *Immunity*, vol. 19, no. 1, pp. 9–19, 2003.

[90] B. D. Elzey, J. F. Grant, H. W. Sinn, B. Nieswandt, T. J. Waldschmidt, and T. L. Ratliff, "Cooperation between platelet-derived CD154 and CD4⁺ T cells for enhanced germinal center formation," *Journal of Leukocyte Biology*, vol. 78, no. 1, pp. 80–84, 2005.

[91] D. R. Littman and A. Y. Rudensky, "Th17 and regulatory T cells in mediating and restraining inflammation," *Cell*, vol. 140, no. 6, pp. 845–858, 2010.

[92] A. Verschoor, M. Neuenhahn, A. A. Navarini et al., "A platelet-mediated system for shuttling blood-borne bacteria to CD8⁺ dendritic cells depends on glycoprotein GPIb and complement C3," *Nature Immunology*, vol. 12, pp. 1194–1201, 2011.

[93] P. A. Lang, C. Contaldo, P. Georgiev et al., "Aggravation of viral hepatitis by platelet-derived serotonin," *Nature Medicine*, vol. 14, no. 7, pp. 756–761, 2008.

[94] F. Shalaby, J. Rossant, T. P. Yamaguchi et al., "Failure of blood-island formation and vasculogenesis in Flk-1 deficient mice," *Nature*, vol. 376, no. 6535, pp. 62–66, 1995.

[95] D. Y. R. Stainier, B. M. Weinstein, H. W. Detrich III, L. I. Zon, and M. C. Fishman, "cloche, an early acting zebrafish gene, is required by both the endothelial and hematopoietic lineages," *Development*, vol. 121, no. 10, pp. 3141–3150, 1995.

[96] M. F. T. R. De Bruijn, N. A. Speck, M. C. E. Peeters, and E. Dzierzak, "Definitive hematopoietic stem cells first develop within the major arterial regions of the mouse embryo," *EMBO Journal*, vol. 19, no. 11, pp. 2465–2474, 2000.

[97] A. T. Chen and L. I. Zon, "Zebrafish blood stem cells," *Journal of Cellular Biochemistry*, vol. 108, no. 1, pp. 35–42, 2009.

[98] R. S. Srinivasan, M. E. Dillard, O. V. Lagutin et al., "Lineage tracing demonstrates the venous origin of the mammalian lymphatic vasculature," *Genes and Development*, vol. 21, no. 19, pp. 2422–2432, 2007.

[99] C. C. Bertozzi, P. R. Hess, and M. L. Kahn, "Platelets: covert regulators of lymphatic development," *Arteriosclerosis, Thrombosis, and Vascular Biology*, vol. 30, no. 12, pp. 2368–2371, 2010.

[100] Y. Xu, L. Yuan, J. Mak et al., "Neuropilin-2 mediates VEGF-C-induced lymphatic sprouting together with VEGFR3," *Journal of Cell Biology*, vol. 188, no. 1, pp. 115–130, 2010.

[101] C. C. Bertozzi, A. A. Schmaier, P. Mericko et al., "Platelets regulate lymphatic vascular development through CLEC-2-SLP-76 signaling," *Blood*, vol. 116, no. 4, pp. 661–670, 2010.

[102] L. Carramolino, J. Fuentes, C. García-Andrés, V. Azcoitia, D. Riethmacher, and M. Torres, "Platelets play an essential role in separating the blood and lymphatic vasculatures during embryonic angiogenesis," *Circulation Research*, vol. 106, no. 7, pp. 1197–1201, 2010.

[103] K. Suzuki-Inoue, O. Inoue, and Y. Ozaki, "Novel platelet activation receptor CLEC-2: from discovery to prospects," *Journal of Thrombosis and Haemostasis*, vol. 9, supplement 1, pp. 44–55, 2011.

[104] K. Echtler, K. Stark, M. Lorenz et al., "Platelets contribute to postnatal occlusion of the ductus arteriosus," *Nature Medicine*, vol. 16, no. 1, pp. 75–82, 2010.

[105] D. B. Rubinstein and D. L. Longo, "Peripheral destruction of platelets in chronic lymphocytic leukemia: recognition, prognosis and therapeutic implications," *American Journal of Medicine*, vol. 71, no. 4, pp. 729–732, 1981.

[106] A. W. Berkman, T. Kickler, and H. Braine, "Platelet-associated IgG in patients with lymphoma," *Blood*, vol. 63, no. 4, pp. 944–948, 1984.

[107] C. Nieder, E. Haukland, A. Pawinski, and A. Dalhaug, "Anaemia and thrombocytopenia in patients with prostate cancer and bone metastases," *BMC Cancer*, vol. 10, article 284, 2010.

[108] J. Ballot, D. McDonnell, and J. Crown, "Successful treatment of thrombocytopenia due to marrow metastases of breast cancer with weekly docetaxel," *Journal of the National Cancer Institute*, vol. 95, no. 11, pp. 831–832, 2003.

[109] A. Chehal, A. Taher, M. Seoud, and A. Shamseddine, "Idiopathic thrombocytopenic purpura and ovarian cancer," *European Journal of Gynaecological Oncology*, vol. 24, no. 6, pp. 539–540, 2003.

[110] F. Rodeghiero, R. Stasi, T. Gernsheimer et al., "Standardization of terminology, definitions and outcome criteria in immune thrombocytopenic purpura of adults and children: report from an international working group," *Blood*, vol. 113, no. 11, pp. 2386–2393, 2009.

[111] H. Liebman, "Other immune thrombocytopenias," *Seminars in Hematology*, vol. 44, pp. S24–S34, 2007.

[112] C. Kaplan, H. Ni, and J. Freedman, "Alloimmune thrombocytopenia," in *Platelets*, A. D. Michelson, Ed., chapter 46, 3rd edition, 2011.

[113] B. Godeau, D. Provan, and J. Bussel, "Immune thrombocytopenic purpura in adults," *Current Opinion in Hematology*, vol. 14, no. 5, pp. 535–556, 2007.

[114] B. Psaila and J. B. Bussel, "Refractory immune thrombocytopenic purpura: current strategies for investigation and management," *British Journal of Haematology*, vol. 143, no. 1, pp. 16–26, 2008.

[115] P. E. Abrahamson, S. A. Hall, M. Feudjo-Tepie, F. S. Mitrani-Gold, and J. Logie, "The incidence of idiopathic thrombocytopenic purpura among adults: a population-based study and literature review," *European Journal of Haematology*, vol. 83, no. 2, pp. 83–89, 2009.

[116] N. Cooper and J. Bussel, "The pathogenesis of immune thrombocytopaenic purpura," *British Journal of Haematology*, vol. 133, no. 4, pp. 364–374, 2006.

[117] D. B. Cines, J. B. Bussel, H. A. Liebman, and E. T. Luning Prak, "The ITP syndrome: pathogenic and clinical diversity," *Blood*, vol. 113, no. 26, pp. 6511–6521, 2009.

[118] D. Stoll, D. B. Cines, R. H. Aster, and S. Murphy, "Platelet kinetics in patients with idiopathic thrombocytopenic purpura and moderate thrombocytopenia," *Blood*, vol. 65, no. 3, pp. 584–588, 1985.

[119] P. J. Ballem, G. M. Segal, J. R. Stratton, T. Gernsheimer, J. W. Adamson, and S. J. Slichter, "Mechanisms of thrombocytopenia in chronic autoimmune thrombocytopenic purpura. Evidence of both impaired platelet production and increased platelet clearance," *Journal of Clinical Investigation*, vol. 80, no. 1, pp. 33–40, 1987.

[120] T. Gernsheimer, J. Stratton, P. J. Ballem, and S. J. Slichter, "Mechanisms of response to treatment in autoimmune thrombocytopenic purpura," *New England Journal of Medicine*, vol. 320, no. 15, pp. 974–980, 1989.

[121] M. Chang, P. A. Nakagawa, S. A. Williams et al., "Immune thrombocytopenic purpura (ITP) plasma and purified ITP monoclonal autoantibodies inhibit megakaryocytopoiesis in vitro," *Blood*, vol. 102, no. 3, pp. 887–895, 2003.

[122] E. J. Houwerzijl, N. R. Blom, J. J. L. Van Der Want et al., "Ultrastructural study shows morphologic features of apoptosis and para-apoptosis in megakaryocytes from patients with idiopathic thrombocytopenic purpura," *Blood*, vol. 103, no. 2, pp. 500–506, 2004.

[123] D. S. Beardsley and M. Ertem, "Platelet autoantibodies in immune thrombocytopenic purpura," *Transfusion and Apheresis Science*, vol. 19, no. 3, pp. 237–244, 1998.

[124] A. Olsson, P. O. Andersson, L. Tengborn, and H. Wadenvik, "Serum from patients with chronic idiopathic thrombocytopenic purpura frequently affect the platelet function," *Thrombosis Research*, vol. 107, no. 3-4, pp. 135–139, 2002.

[125] M. Yanagu, M. Suzuki, T. Soga et al., "Influences of antiplatelet autoantibodies on platelet function in immune thrombocytopenic purpura," *European Journal of Haematology*, vol. 46, no. 2, pp. 101–106, 1991.

[126] R. McMillan, L. Wang, A. Tomer, J. Nichol, and J. Pistillo, "Suppression of in vitro megakaryocyte production by antiplatelet autoantibodies from adult patients with chronic ITP," *Blood*, vol. 103, no. 4, pp. 1364–1369, 2004.

[127] L. Yang, L. Wang, C. H. Zhao et al., "Contributions of TRAIL-mediated megakaryocyte apoptosis to impaired megakaryocyte and platelet production in immune thrombocytopenia," *Blood*, vol. 116, no. 20, pp. 4307–4316, 2010.

[128] B. Olsson, P. O. Andersson, M. Jernås et al., "T-cell-mediated cytotoxicity toward platelets in chronic idiopathic thrombocytopenic purpura," *Nature Medicine*, vol. 9, no. 9, pp. 1123–1124, 2003.

[129] E. Sayeh, K. Sterling, E. Speck, J. Freedman, and J. W. Semple, "IgG antiplatelet immunity is dependent on an early innate natural killer cell-derived interferon-γ response that is regulated by CD8+ T cells," *Blood*, vol. 103, no. 7, pp. 2705–2709, 2004.

[130] N. Oyaizu, R. Yasumizu, M. Miyama-Inaba et al., "(NZW x BXSB)F1 mouse. A new animal model of idiopathic thrombocytopenic purpura," *Journal of Experimental Medicine*, vol. 167, no. 6, pp. 2017–2022, 1988.

[131] A. R. Crow, S. Song, J. W. Semple, J. Freedman, and A. H. Lazarus, "IVIg inhibits reticuloendothelial system function and ameliorates murine passive-immune thrombocytopenia independent of anti-idiotype reactivity," *British Journal of Haematology*, vol. 115, no. 3, pp. 679–686, 2001.

[132] B. Nieswandt, W. Bergmeier, K. Rackebrandt, J. Engelbert Gessner, and H. Zirngibl, "Identification of critical antigen-specific mechanisms in the development of immune thrombocytopenic purpura in mice," *Blood*, vol. 96, no. 7, pp. 2520–2527, 2000.

[133] L. Chow, R. Aslam, E. R. Speck et al., "A murine model of severe immune thrombocytopenia is induced by antibody- and CD8+ T cell-mediated responses that are differentially sensitive to therapy," *Blood*, vol. 115, no. 6, pp. 1247–1253, 2010.

[134] J. W. Semple, "Animal models of immune thrombocytopenia (ITP)," *Annals of Hematology*, vol. 89, pp. S37–S44, 2010.

[135] M. L. Webster, E. Sayeh, M. Crow et al., "Relative efficacy of intravenous immunoglobulin G in ameliorating thrombocytopenia induced by antiplatelet GPIIbIIIa versus GPIbα antibodies," *Blood*, vol. 108, no. 3, pp. 943–946, 2006.

[136] A. Cuker and D. B. Cines, "Immune thrombocytopenia," *Hematology*, vol. 2010, pp. 377–384, 2010.

[137] R. S. Go, K. L. Johnston, and K. C. Bruden, "The association between platelet autoantibody specificity and response to intravenous immunoglobulin G in the treatment of patients with immune thrombocytopenia," *Haematologica*, vol. 92, no. 2, pp. 283–284, 2007.

[138] J. Peng, S. Ma, X. Liu et al., "Autoantibody to platelet GPIb/IX is a predictive factor for poor response to intrevenous immunoglobulin in adults with severe immune thrombocytopenia," *Journal of Thrombosis and Haemostasis*, 2011, XXIII Congress of the International Society on Thrombosis and Haemostasis.

[139] Q. Zeng, L. Zhu, L. Tao et al., "Relative efficacy of steroid therapy in immune thrombocytopenia mediated by anti-platelet GPIIbIIIa versus GPIbalpha antibodies," *American Journal of Hematology*, vol. 87, no. 2, pp. 206–208, 2012.

[140] B. François, F. Trimoreau, P. Vignon, P. Fixe, V. Praloran, and H. Gastinne, "Thrombocytopenia in the sepsis syndrome: role of hemophagocytosis and macrophage colony-stimulating factor," *American Journal of Medicine*, vol. 103, no. 2, pp. 114–120, 1997.

[141] J. Y. Peltier, P. Lambin, C. Doinel, A. M. Courouce, P. Rouger, and J. J. Lefrere, "Frequency and prognostic importance of thrombocytopenia in symptom-free HIV-infected individuals: a 5-year prospective study," *AIDS*, vol. 5, no. 4, pp. 381–384, 1991.

[142] E. M. Sloand, H. G. Klein, S. M. Banks, B. Vareldzis, S. Merritt, and P. Pierce, "Epidemiology of thrombocytopenia in HIV infection," *European Journal of Haematology*, vol. 48, no. 3, pp. 168–172, 1992.

[143] J. M. Pawlotsky, M. Bouvier, P. Fromont et al., "Hepatitis C virus infection and autoimmune thrombocytopenic purpura," *Journal of Hepatology*, vol. 23, no. 6, pp. 635–639, 1995.

[144] S. Pivetti, A. Novarino, F. Merico et al., "High prevalence of autoimmune phenomena in hepatitis C virus antibody positive patients with lymphoproliferative and connective tissue disorders," *British Journal of Haematology*, vol. 95, no. 1, pp. 204–211, 1996.

[145] T. A. Steeper, C. A. Horwitz, S. B. Moore et al., "Severe thrombocytopenia in Epstein-Barr virus-induced mononucleosis," *Western Journal of Medicine*, vol. 150, no. 2, pp. 170–173, 1989.

[146] J. G. Wright, "Severe thrombocytopenia secondary to asymptomatic cytomegalovirus infection in an immunocompetent host," *Journal of Clinical Pathology*, vol. 45, no. 11, pp. 1037–1038, 1992.

[147] H. P. Staub, "Postrubella thrombocytopenic purpura. A report of eight cases with discussion of hemorrhagic manifestations of rubella," *Clinical Pediatrics*, vol. 7, no. 6, pp. 350–356, 1968.

[148] X. J. Yu, M. F. Liang, S. Y. Zhang et al., "Fever with thrombocytopenia associated with a novel bunyavirus in China," *New England Journal of Medicine*, vol. 364, no. 16, pp. 1523–1532, 2011.

[149] Z. Li, M. A. Nardi, and S. Karpatkin, "Role of molecular mimicry to HIV-1 peptides in HIV-1-related immunologic thrombocytopenia," *Blood*, vol. 106, no. 2, pp. 572–576, 2005.

[150] S. Suerbaum and P. Michetti, "Helicobacter pylori infection," *New England Journal of Medicine*, vol. 347, no. 15, pp. 1175–1186, 2002.

[151] R. P. H. Logan and M. M. Walker, "ABC of the upper gastrointestinal tract: epidemiology and diagnosis of Helicobacter pylori infection," *British Medical Journal*, vol. 323, no. 7318, pp. 920–922, 2001.

[152] A. Gasbarrini, F. Franceschi, R. Tartaglione, R. Landolfi, P. Pola, and G. Gasbarrini, "Regression of autoimmune thrombocytopenia after eradication of Helicobacter pylori," *The Lancet*, vol. 352, no. 9131, p. 878, 1998.

[153] T. Inaba, M. Mizuno, S. Take et al., "Eradication of Helicobacter pylori increases platelet count in patients with idiopathic thrombocytopenic purpura in Japan," *European Journal of Clinical Investigation*, vol. 35, no. 3, pp. 214–219, 2005.

[154] M. Michel, N. Cooper, C. Jean, C. Frissora, and J. B. Bussel, "Does Helicobater pylori initiate or perpetuate immune thrombocytopenic purpura?" *Blood*, vol. 103, no. 3, pp. 890–896, 2004.

[155] T. Ando, T. Tsuzuki, T. Mizuno et al., "Characteristics of Helicobacter pylori-induced gastritis and the effect of H. pylori eradication in patients with chronic idiopathic thrombocytopenic purpura," *Helicobacter*, vol. 9, no. 5, pp. 443–452, 2004.

[156] P. S. Sullivan, D. L. Hanson, S. Y. Chu, J. L. Jones, and C. A. Ciesielski, "Surveillance for thrombocytopenia in persons infected with HIV: results from the multistate adult and adolescent spectrum of disease project," *Journal of Acquired Immune Deficiency Syndromes and Human Retrovirology*, vol. 14, no. 4, pp. 374–379, 1997.

[157] M. A. Nardi, L. X. Liu, and S. Karpatkin, "GPIIIa-(49–66) is a major pathophysiologically relevant antigenic determinant for anti-platelet GPIIIA of HIV-1-related immunologic thrombocytopenia," *Proceedings of the National Academy of Sciences of the United States of America*, vol. 94, no. 14, pp. 7589–7594, 1997.

[158] M. Nardi, S. Tomlinson, M. A. Greco, and S. Karpatkin, "Complement-independent, peroxide-induced antibody lysis of platelets in HIV-1-related immune thrombocytopenia," *Cell*, vol. 106, no. 5, pp. 551–561, 2001.

[159] W. Zhang, M. A. Nardi, W. Borkowsky, Z. Li, and S. Karpatkin, "Role of molecular mimicry of hepatitis C virus protein with platelet GPIIIa in hepatitis C-related immunologic thrombocytopenia," *Blood*, vol. 113, no. 17, pp. 4086–4093, 2009.

[160] K. Yabu, K. Kiyosawa, S. Ako et al., "Type C chronic hepatitis associated with thrombocytopenia in two patients," *Journal of Gastroenterology and Hepatology*, vol. 9, no. 1, pp. 99–104, 1994.

[161] L. E. Adinolfi, M. G. Giordano, A. Andreana et al., "Hepatic fibrosis plays a central role in the pathogenesis of thrombocytopenia in patients with chronic viral hepatitis," *British Journal of Haematology*, vol. 113, no. 3, pp. 590–595, 2001.

[162] J. H. Herman, M. I. Jumbelic, R. J. Ancona, and T. S. Kickler, "In utero cerebral hemorrhage in alloimmune thrombocytopenia," *American Journal of Pediatric Hematology/Oncology*, vol. 8, no. 4, pp. 312–317, 1986.

[163] E. Weiner, N. Zosmer, R. Bajoria et al., "Direct fetal administration of immunoglobulins: another disappointing therapy in alloimmune thrombocytopenia," *Fetal Diagnosis and Therapy*, vol. 9, no. 3, pp. 159–164, 1994.

[164] S. Gaddipati, R. L. Berkowitz, A. A. Lembet, R. Lapinski, J. G. McFarland, and J. B. Bussel, "Initial fetal platelet counts predict the response to intravenous gammaglobulin therapy in fetuses that are affected by PLA1 incompatibility," *American Journal of Obstetrics and Gynecology*, vol. 185, no. 4, pp. 976–980, 2001.

[165] J. B. Bussel, M. R. Zabusky, R. L. Berkowitz, and J. G. McFarland, "Fetal alloimmune thrombocytopenia," *New England Journal of Medicine*, vol. 337, no. 1, pp. 22–26, 1997.

[166] V. Ghetie and E. S. Ward, "Multiple roles for the major histocompatibility complex class I-related receptor FcRn," *Annual Review of Immunology*, vol. 18, pp. 739–766, 2000.

[167] D. C. Roopenian and S. Akilesh, "FcRn: the neonatal Fc receptor comes of age," *Nature Reviews Immunology*, vol. 7, no. 9, pp. 715–725, 2007.

[168] R. McMillan, R. L. Longmire, M. Tavassoli, S. Armstrong, and R. Yelenosky, "In vitro platelet phagocytosis by splenic leukocytes in idiopathic thrombocytopenic purpura," *New England Journal of Medicine*, vol. 290, no. 5, pp. 249–251, 1974.

[169] J. B. Bussel and A. Primiani, "Fetal and neonatal alloimmune thrombocytopenia: progress and ongoing debates," *Blood Reviews*, vol. 22, no. 1, pp. 33–52, 2008.

[170] C. Kaplan, "Foetal and neonatal alloimmune thrombocytopaenia," *Orphanet Journal of Rare Diseases*, vol. 1, no. 1, article 39, 2006.

[171] V. S. Blanchette, L. Chen, Z. Salomon De Friedberg, V. A. Hogan, E. Trudel, and F. Decary, "Alloimmunization to the Pl(A1) platelet antigen: results of a prospective study," *British Journal of Haematology*, vol. 74, no. 2, pp. 209–215, 1990.

[172] M. Dreyfus, C. Kaplan, E. Verdy, N. Schlegel, I. Durand-Zaleski, and G. Tchernia, "Frequency of immune thrombocytopenia in newborns: a prospective study," *Blood*, vol. 89, no. 12, pp. 4402–4406, 1997.

[173] G. Bertrand, M. Drame, C. Martageix, and C. Kaplan, "Prediction of the fetal status in noninvasive management of alloimmune thrombocytopenia," *Blood*, vol. 117, no. 11, pp. 3209–3213, 2011.

[174] C. Mueller-Eckhardt, A. Grubert, M. Weisheit et al., "348 cases of suspected neonatal alloimmune thrombocytopenia," *The Lancet*, vol. 1, no. 8634, pp. 363–366, 1989.

[175] M. F. Murphy, H. Hambley, K. Nicolaides, and A. H. Waters, "Severe fetomaternal alloimmune thrombocytopenia presenting with fetal hydrocephalus," *Prenatal Diagnosis*, vol. 16, pp. 1152–1155, 1996.

[176] C. Ghevaert, K. Campbell, J. Walton et al., "Management and outcome of 200 cases of fetomaternal alloimmune thrombocytopenia," *Transfusion*, vol. 47, no. 5, pp. 901–910, 2007.

[177] J. Kjeldsen-Kragh, M. K. Killie, G. Tomter et al., "A screening and intervention program aimed to reduce mortality and serious morbidity associated with severe neonatal alloimmune thrombocytopenia," *Blood*, vol. 110, no. 3, pp. 833–839, 2007.

[178] C. Kaplan, F. Daffos, F. Forestier et al., "Management of alloimmune thrombocytopenia: antenatal diagnosis and in utero transfusion of maternal platelets," *Blood*, vol. 72, no. 1, pp. 340–343, 1988.

[179] L. M. Williamson, G. Hackett, J. Rennie et al., "The natural history of fetomaternal alloimmunization to the platelet-specific antigen HPA-1a (Pl^{A1}, Zw^a) as determined by antenatal screening," *Blood*, vol. 92, no. 7, pp. 2280–2287, 1998.

[180] H. Kroll, V. Kiefel, and S. Santoso, "Clinical aspects and typing of platelet alloantigens," *Vox Sanguinis*, vol. 74, supplement 2, pp. 345–354, 1998.

[181] N. Bizzaro and G. Dianese, "Neonatal alloimmune amegakaryocytosis. Case report," *Vox Sanguinis*, vol. 54, no. 2, pp. 112–114, 1988.

[182] M. Goldman, E. Trudel, L. Richard, S. Khalife, and G. M. Spurll, "Neonatal alloimmune thrombocytopenia due to anti-HPA-2b (anti-Koa)," *Immunohematology*, vol. 19, no. 2, pp. 43–46, 2003.

[183] H. Kroll, V. Kiefel, W. Muntean, and C. Mueller-Eckhardt, "Anti-KO^a as the cause of neonatal alloimmune thrombocytopenia," *Vox Sang*, vol. 12, pp. 52–67, 1994.

[184] I. H. A. Al-Sheikh, M. Khalifa, A. Rahi, M. I. Qadri, and K. Al Abad, "A rare case of neonatal alloimmune thrombocytopenia due to anti-HPA-2b," *Annals of Saudi Medicine*, vol. 18, no. 6, pp. 547–549, 1998.

[185] P. Grenet, J. Dausset, M. Dugas, D. Petit, J. Badoual, and Y. Tangun, "Neonatal thrombopenic purpura with anti-Ko-a feto-maternal isoimmunization," *Archives Francaises de Pediatrie*, vol. 22, no. 10, pp. 1165–1174, 1965.

[186] A. Davoren, B. R. Curtis, R. H. Aster, and J. G. McFarland, "Human platelet antigen-specific alloantibodies implicated in 1162 cases of neonatal alloimmune thrombocytopenia," *Transfusion*, vol. 44, no. 8, pp. 1220–1225, 2004.

[187] D. B. Cines and V. S. Blanchette, "Medical progress: immune thrombocytopenic purpura," *New England Journal of Medicine*, vol. 346, no. 13, pp. 995–1008, 2002.

[188] R. McMillan, "Antiplatelet antibodies in chronic immune thrombocytopenia and their role in platelet destruction and defective platelet production," *Hematology/Oncology Clinics of North America*, vol. 23, no. 6, pp. 1163–1175, 2009.

[189] R. He, D. M. Reid, C. E. Jones, and N. R. Shulman, "Spectrum of Ig classes, specificities, and titers of serum antiglycoproteins in chronic idiopathic thrombocytopenic purpura," *Blood*, vol. 83, no. 4, pp. 1024–1032, 1994.

[190] B. Kumpel, M. J. King, S. Sooranna et al., "Phenotype and mRNA expression of syncytiotrophoblast microparticles isolated from human placenta," *Annals of the New York Academy of Sciences*, vol. 1137, pp. 144–147, 2008.

[191] B. M. Kumpel, K. Sibley, D. J. Jackson, G. White, and P. W. Soothill, "Ultrastructural localization of glycoprotein IIIa (GPIIIa, β3 integrin) on placental syncytiotrophoblast microvilli: implications for platelet alloimmunization during pregnancy," *Transfusion*, vol. 48, no. 10, pp. 2077–2086, 2008.

[192] F. Décary, D. L'Abbé, L. Tremblay, and P. Chartrand, "The immune response to the HPA-1a antigen: association with HLA-DRw52a," *Transfusion Medicine*, vol. 1, no. 1, pp. 55–62, 1991.

[193] S. Wu, K. Maslanka, and J. Gorski, "An integrin polymorphism that defines reactivity with alloantibodies generates an anchor for MHC class II peptide binding: a model for unidirectional alloimmune responses," *Journal of Immunology*, vol. 158, no. 7, pp. 3221–3226, 1997.

[194] C. S. Parry, J. Gorski, and L. J. Stern, "Crystallographic structure of the human leukocyte antigen DRA, DRB33*0101: models of a directional alloimmune response and autoimmunity," *Journal of Molecular Biology*, vol. 371, no. 2, pp. 435–446, 2007.

[195] T. B. Stuge, B. Skogen, M. T. Ahlen, A. Husebekk, S. J. Urbaniak, and H. Bessos, "The cellular immunobiology associated with fetal and neonatal alloimmune thrombocytopenia," *Transfusion and Apheresis Science*, vol. 45, pp. 53–59, 2011.

[196] M. T. Ahlen, A. Husebekk, M. K. Killie, B. Skogen, and T. B. Stuge, "T-cell responses associated with neonatal alloimmune thrombocytopenia: Isolation of HPA-1a-specific, HLA-DRB3*0101-restricted CD4$^+$ T cells," *Blood*, vol. 113, no. 16, pp. 3838–3844, 2009.

[197] H. Ni, P. Chen, C. M. Spring et al., "A novel murine model of fetal and neonatal alloimmune thrombocytopenia: response to intravenous IgG therapy," *Blood*, vol. 107, no. 7, pp. 2976–2983, 2006.

[198] S. Lang, H. Yang, S. Boyd et al., "Impaired angiogenesis contributes to pathogenesis of fetal and neonatal immune thrombocytopenia," *Journal of Thrombosis and Haemostasis*, 2011, XXIII Congress of the International Society on Thrombosis and Haemostasis.

[199] A. H. Schmaier, "Are maternal antiplatelet antibodies a prothrombotic condition leading to miscarriage?" *The Journal of Clinical Investigation*, vol. 121, pp. 4241–4243, 2011.

[200] P. Chen, C. Li, S. Lang et al., "Animal model of fetal and neonatal immune thrombocytopenia: role of neonatal Fc receptor in the pathogenesis and therapy," *Blood*, vol. 116, no. 18, pp. 3660–3668, 2010.

[201] C. Kaplan, "FNAIT: the fetus pleads guilty!," *Blood*, vol. 116, pp. 3384–3386, 2010.

[202] C. E. Gonzalez and Y. M. Pengetze, "Post-transfusion purpura," *Current Hematology Reports*, vol. 4, no. 2, pp. 154–159, 2005.

15

Sucrose-Formulated Recombinant Factor VIII Dosing Flexibility in Prophylaxis Regimens: Experience from Postmarketing Surveillance Studies

Thomas J. Humphries,[1] Stephan Rauchensteiner,[2] Claudia Tückmantel,[3] Alexander Pieper,[4] Monika Maas Enriquez,[5] and Prasad Mathew[1]

[1]*Bayer HealthCare, 100 Bayer Boulevard, P.O. Box 915, Whippany, NJ 08981-0915, USA*
[2]*Bayer Pharma AG, Global Medical Affairs Therapeutic Areas (GMA), Muellerstrasse 178, 13353 Berlin, Germany*
[3]*Bayer Pharma AG, Aprather Weg 18a, Building 470, 42096 Wuppertal, Germany*
[4]*M.A.R.C.O. GmbH & Co. KG, Moskauer Strasse 25, 40227 Düsseldorf, Germany*
[5]*Bayer Pharma AG, Global Clinical Development Therapeutic Area NOHI, Aprather Weg, 42096 Wuppertal, Germany*

Correspondence should be addressed to Thomas J. Humphries; thomas.humphries@bayer.com

Academic Editor: David Varon

Objectives. Prophylaxis regimens for severe hemophilia A allowing more flexible dosing while maintaining efficacy may improve adherence and decrease the cost of prophylaxis. Here, we compared the clinical effectiveness of once- or twice-weekly versus ≥3-times-weekly prophylaxis with sucrose-formulated recombinant factor VIII (rFVIII-FS) in a "real-world" practice setting. *Methods.* Data from 3 postmarketing studies were pooled. Patients with severe hemophilia A receiving ≥1 prophylaxis infusion/wk of rFVIII-FS for ≥80% of a prophylaxis observation period (≥5 months) were included. Patients were categorized based on physician-assigned treatment regimens of 1-2 prophylaxis injections/wk ($n = 63$) or ≥3 prophylaxis injections/wk ($n = 76$). Descriptive statistics were determined for annualized bleeding rates (ABRs). *Results.* Median (quartile 1; quartile 3) ABR for all bleeds was 2.0 (0; 4.0) in the 1-2 prophylaxis injections/wk group and 3.9 (1.5; 9.3) in the ≥3 prophylaxis injections/wk group. Median ABRs for joint, spontaneous, and trauma-related bleeds were numerically lower with 1-2 prophylaxis injections/wk. As an estimate of prophylaxis success, 63% (≥3 prophylaxis injections/wk) to 84% of patients (1-2 prophylaxis injections/wk) had ≤4 annualized joint bleeds. *Conclusions.* Dosing flexibility and successful prophylaxis with rFVIII-FS were demonstrated. Very good bleeding control was achieved with both once-twice-weekly and ≥3-times-weekly prophylaxis dosing regimens.

1. Introduction

Prophylaxis with factor VIII (FVIII) replacement products is the standard of care for patients with severe hemophilia in developed countries. Compared with on-demand treatment, prophylaxis confers several clinical benefits and is therefore recommended by World Federation of Hemophilia and National Hemophilia Foundation guidelines [1, 2]. However, standard prophylaxis generally requires injections ≥3 times per week [2], which can be a barrier to treatment adherence and may not be needed for all patients. Frequent infusions may be particularly challenging for young patients in whom venous access can be difficult [3]. Prophylaxis regimens that allow less frequent and more flexible dosing while maintaining efficacy may improve adherence and decrease the cost of prophylaxis.

A number of studies have demonstrated the efficacy of sucrose-formulated recombinant FVIII (rFVIII-FS) using a ≥3-times-weekly dosing regimen [4–8]. Although only 2 prospective clinical studies have investigated the efficacy of rFVIII-FS using a once- or twice-weekly dosing regimen [9, 10], postmarketing studies of rFVIII-FS have collected data from patients using various prophylaxis regimens [11, 12]. Using pooled data from 3 postmarketing studies, the objective of this analysis was to compare the clinical effectiveness of once- or twice-weekly versus ≥3-times-weekly prophylaxis dosing with rFVIII-FS in patients with severe hemophilia A in the routine, or "real-world," clinical setting.

2. Patients and Methods

Patients with hemophilia A included in this analysis receiving treatment with rFVIII-FS were enrolled in 1 of 3 postmarketing surveillance studies conducted in Austria, Denmark, France, Greece, Italy, Netherlands, Spain, Sweden [11], Taiwan [12], and Germany (KG0301-DE. Data on File, Berlin, Germany: Bayer Pharma AG, 2005). The studies included patients with hemophilia A who used rFVIII-FS for routine treatment for up to 24 months. For the current pooled analysis, patients with severe hemophilia with FVIII:C <1% who had a total prophylaxis observation period of ≥5 months and received ≥1 prophylaxis infusion per week for ≥80% of the prophylaxis observation period and who were considered valid for the efficacy analysis in the respective postmarketing surveillance study were selected. Patients with documented inhibitors or who were receiving rFVIII-FS for immune tolerance induction were excluded from the analysis. Data were collected in paper-based patient diaries during the postmarketing studies.

2.1. Dosing Regimens. The dosing regimen for each patient was determined by the treating physician. Patients who met the criteria for the pooled analysis were categorized into either the 1-2 prophylaxis injections/wk group, defined as 1 or 2 documented prophylaxis injections per week in ≥70% of the weeks during the prophylaxis observation period, or the ≥3 prophylaxis injections/wk group. In the real-world settings for these studies, presumably the treating physicians evaluated the global status of their patients before assigning dosing frequency.

2.2. Data Collection and Analysis. Descriptive summary statistics were determined for demographic characteristics, the number of days in the prophylaxis observation period, number of prophylaxis injections per week, time between injections, prophylaxis dose per week, and the annualized bleeding rate (ABR) for total, joint, trauma-related, and spontaneous bleeding events. The results were analyzed overall and by the age subgroups of patients <18 versus ≥18 years.

Periods of prophylaxis treatment interruption (defined as no prophylaxis injection for >28 days) were excluded from the main analysis. Descriptive summary statistics were determined for the number of days excluded from the analysis based on this definition. In a sensitivity analysis, the number of exposure days and the ABR were analyzed for the total observation period from the first prophylaxis injection onward (i.e., including prophylaxis treatment interruptions) to assess the impact of excluded injections and bleeds that occurred during prophylaxis treatment interruption.

3. Results

3.1. Patients. Among 322 patients from the 3 postmarketing studies [11, 12] [KG0301-DE. Data on File, Berlin, Germany:

Bayer Pharma AG; 2005], 139 were eligible for analysis based on the selection criteria for this analysis; 45% ($n = 63$) were grouped into the 1-2 prophylaxis injections/wk group and 55% ($n = 76$) were in the ≥3 prophylaxis injections/wk group. Of the 322 original patients, 183 (56%) were excluded from the pooled analysis for not fulfilling the criteria for prophylaxis treatment ($n = 114$), for having FVIII:C ≥1% ($n = 57$) or a history of inhibitors ($n = 8$), or for the fact that their rFVIII-FS use was for immune tolerance induction ($n = 4$). Demographic and prophylaxis dosing information by dosing group is shown in Table 1; overall, half of the patients were <18 years of age and most patients were white. The median (range) age was higher in the 1-2 prophylaxis injections/wk dosing group compared with the ≥3 prophylaxis injections/wk group (20 [0–63] years and 15 [1–71] years, resp.). Also, a higher percentage of patients aged <18 years were assigned to the ≥3 prophylaxis injections/wk group compared with the 1-2 prophylaxis injections/wk group (57% versus 44%). Fewer patients in the 1-2 prophylaxis injections/wk dosing group compared with the ≥3 prophylaxis injections/wk group had a target joint present at the time of enrollment into the respective studies (27% and 43%, resp., Table 1). This difference may be a result of physician evaluations prior to the assignment of dosing frequency.

3.2. Treatment. The median total prophylaxis observation time per patient was approximately 2 years (range, 140–839 days), and the majority of patients had no relevant prophylaxis treatment interruptions (nonprophylaxis periods, Table 1). The prophylaxis dose per week was lower in the 1-2 prophylaxis injections/wk group compared with the ≥3 prophylaxis injections/wk group. Patients in the 1-2 prophylaxis injections/wk group received an actual mean of 1.6 prophylaxis injections/week compared with 2.8 actual prophylaxis injections/wk for patients in the ≥3 prophylaxis injections/wk group. The mean annual dose for prophylaxis injections was 2300.1 IU/kg/y in the 1-2 prophylaxis injections/wk group and 3834.3 IU/kg/y in the ≥3 prophylaxis injections/wk group (Table 1).

3.3. Prophylaxis Efficacy. The median (quartile 1; quartile 3 [Q1; Q3]) ABR for all bleeds was 2.0 (0; 4.0) in the 1-2 prophylaxis injections/wk group and 3.9 (1.5; 9.3) in the ≥3 prophylaxis injections/wk group (Figure 1); mean ± SD ABR was 4.1 ± 6.4 and 7.0 ± 10.7, respectively. Similarly, the median ABRs for joint bleeds, spontaneous bleeds, and trauma-related bleeds were numerically lower in the 1-2 prophylaxis injections/wk group compared with the ≥3 prophylaxis injections/wk group (Table 2).

When analyzed by age subgroup, the trend toward lower ABRs for all bleeds in the 1-2 prophylaxis injections/wk group was observed for both the <18 and ≥18 year subgroups (Table 3). However, the ABRs were higher in patients ≥18 years compared with patients <18 years. The lowest median ABR (Q1; Q3) for all bleeds was observed in patients <18 years receiving 1-2 prophylaxis injections/wk (1.9 [0; 3.0]), and the highest was observed in patients ≥18 years receiving ≥3 prophylaxis injections/wk (4.7 [1.9; 11.2]). The ABRs for joint and spontaneous bleeds were also higher in patients ≥18

TABLE 1: Demographic and dosing characteristics.

	Prophylaxis 1-2x/wk (n = 63)	Prophylaxis ≥3x/wk (n = 76)	Total (N = 139)
Age, y			
Mean	23	21	22
Median (range)	20 (0–63)	15 (1–71)	17 (0–71)
<18 y, n (%)	28 (44)	43 (57)	71 (51)
Race, n (%)			
White	52 (83)	61 (80)	113 (81)
Asian	5 (8)	4 (5)	9 (7)
Others	2 (3)	3 (4)	5 (4)
Missing	4 (6)	8 (11)	12 (9)
Target joint present, n (%)	17 (27)	33 (43)	50 (36)
Prophylaxis observation period, d			
Mean ± SD	573 ± 220	609 ± 207	593 ± 213
Median (range)	695 (151–826)	731 (140–839)	726 (140–839)
Number of excluded nonprophylaxis days/patient*			
Mean ± SD	41 ± 108	34 ± 96	37 ± 101
Median (range)	0 (0–516)	0 (0–506)	0 (0–516)
Number of all injections/wk/patient			
Mean ± SD	1.8 ± 0.5	3.1 ± 0.5	2.5 ± 0.8
Median (range)	1.9 (1.0–3.2)	3.0 (2.0–4.8)	2.6 (1.0–4.8)
Number of prophylaxis injections/wk/patient			
Mean ± SD	1.6 ± 0.4	2.8 ± 0.4	2.3 ± 0.7
Median (range)	1.6 (0.9–2.2)	2.8 (1.5–3.8)	2.3 (0.9–3.8)
Time between prophylaxis injections,† d			
Mean ± SD	4.4 ± 1.4	2.2 ± 0.4	3.2 ± 1.5
Median (range)	4.0 (3.0–7.0)	2.0 (2.0–3.0)	3.0 (2.0–7.0)
Prophylaxis dose/wk, IU/kg			
Mean ± SD	44.1 ± 26.8	73.5 ± 33.9	60.2 ± 34.1
Median (range)	33.5 (11.4–101.9)	71.5 (17.1–166.5)	56.2 (11.4–166.5)
Prophylaxis dose/injection, IU/kg			
Mean ± SD	27.0 ± 13.5	26.2 ± 11.2	26.6 ± 12.2
Median (range)	26.6 (6.3–56.4)	27.0 (6.5–54.2)	26.9 (6.3–56.4)
Prophylaxis dose/y, IU/kg			
Mean ± SD	2300.1 ± 1396.5	3834.3 ± 1768.9	3139.0 ± 1778.8
Median (range)	1750.3 (594.8–5318.1)	3732.8 (890.7–8687.3)	2930.6 (594.8–8687.3)

*Interruptions in prophylaxis treatment, defined as periods of ≥28 days without any prophylaxis injection, were excluded from the main analysis.
†Median time per patient between 2 prophylaxis infusions was analyzed.

years compared with patients <18 years in each dosing group, whereas the ABR for trauma-related bleeds was lower in patients ≥18 years compared with patients <18 years (Table 3).

A greater percentage of patients in the 1-2 prophylaxis injections/wk group had 0 annualized bleeds and 0 annualized joint bleeds compared with patients in the ≥3 prophylaxis injections/wk group (30% and 40% versus 7% and 17%, resp., Table 4). In the 1-2 prophylaxis injections/wk group, 81% had ≤8 annualized bleeds compared with 68% of patients in the ≥3 prophylaxis injections/wk group. For joint bleeds, 84%

of patients in the 1-2 prophylaxis injections/wk group had ≤4 annualized joint bleeds compared with 63% of patients in the ≥3 prophylaxis injections/wk group. Patients in the 1-2 prophylaxis injections/wk group were still more likely to have 0 annualized bleeds, regardless of age subgroup (data not shown). However, the lower percentage of patients in the total population receiving 1-2 prophylaxis injections/wk with >8 annualized bleeds compared with patients in the ≥3 prophylaxis injections/wk group was only observed in patients <18 years. For joint bleeds, the frequency pattern

TABLE 2: Annualized bleeding rates by dosing group.

Annualized bleeding rates	Prophylaxis 1-2x/wk ($n = 63$)	Prophylaxis ≥3x/wk ($n = 76$)
All bleeds		
Mean ± SD	4.1 ± 6.4	7.0 ± 10.7
Median (Q1; Q3)	2.0 (0; 4.0)	3.9 (1.5; 9.3)
Joint bleeds		
Mean ± SD	2.8 ± 5.2	4.5 ± 7.0
Median (Q1; Q3)	0.9 (0; 2.6)	2.4 (0.6; 5.5)
Spontaneous bleeds		
Mean ± SD	2.4 ± 5.0	3.1 ± 6.2
Median (Q1; Q3)	0 (0; 1.9)	0.9 (0; 3.7)
Trauma-related bleeds		
Mean ± SD	1.6 ± 3.7	3.4 ± 5.4
Median (Q1; Q3)	0.6 (0; 2.0)	1.5 (0.5; 4.6)

Q1 = quartile 1; Q3 = quartile 3.

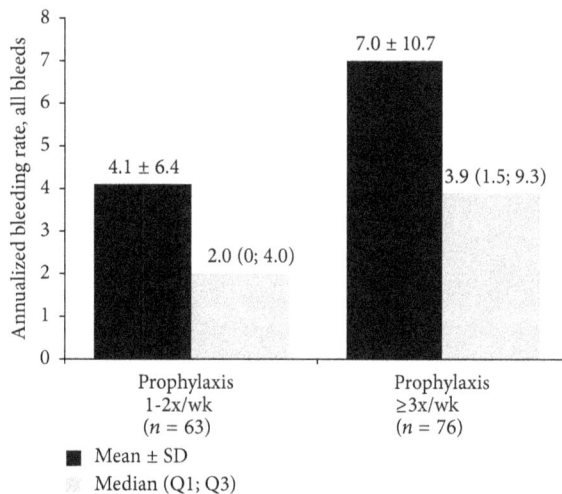

FIGURE 1: Annualized bleeding rate for all bleeds by dosing group. Q1 = quartile 1; Q3 = quartile 3.

was generally similar to the overall population, but there were more patients <18 years of age with 0 annualized joint bleeds compared with patients ≥18 years of age in both dosing groups.

Analyses using different prophylaxis regimen definitions (receiving 1-2 or ≥3 prophylaxis injections/wk in 50% of the weeks during the observation period versus 70%) resulted in similar results as the primary analysis. A sensitivity analysis included the total observation time from the first prophylaxis injection until the end of the observation time irrespective of any interruption of prophylaxis treatment. The reason for this sensitivity analysis was to make sure that bleeding treatment periods were not wrongly interpreted as interruptions of prophylaxis treatment. Results from this analysis showed that there were no major changes in bleeding results and, especially, that the approach of the primary analysis did not

introduce bias in favor of the 1-2 prophylaxis injections/wk group.

4. Discussion

In this pooled analysis of data from 3 postmarketing studies, 1-2 weekly infusions of rFVIII-FS were at least as effective as ≥3-times-weekly dosing in preventing bleeding episodes in patients with severe hemophilia A, demonstrating effective prophylaxis dosing flexibility with rFVIII-FS for some patients under real-life conditions. Almost half of the patients (45%) treated with prophylaxis were using a regimen of 1-2 prophylaxis injections/wk; adult patients and patients without target joints were more likely to be prescribed this regimen. The median ABR for all, joint, trauma-related, and spontaneous bleeds was numerically lower for patients receiving 1-2 prophylaxis injections/wk compared with those receiving ≥3 prophylaxis injections/wk. Furthermore, the percentage of patients with 0 bleeding episodes was higher in the 1-2 prophylaxis injections/wk group compared with the ≥3 prophylaxis injections/wk group.

In these postmarketing studies, dosing frequency was assigned by the treating physician. Patients following a 1-2 prophylaxis injections/wk regimen may have had a milder bleeding phenotype, had fewer target joints, or had other factors that influenced FVIII half-life; therefore, patients in this group may have been less prone to bleeds in general or experienced a longer duration of protection from bleeding, resulting in numerically better outcomes compared with patients treated ≥3 times/wk. Bleeding history information, such as the number of bleeding episodes in the previous year, was not available to investigate this hypothesis. However, since physicians base their treatment assignment in clinical practice on specifics of patient medical history and characteristics, it can be assumed that the assignment to a lower frequency of prophylaxis occurred for those patients with a milder bleeding phenotype in the past. The effect of different types of prophylaxis regimens on joint outcomes was not the subject of this analysis. The fact that the percentage of patients with target joints was lower in the 1-2 prophylaxis injections/wk group compared with the ≥3 prophylaxis injections/wk group suggests that the lower frequency regimen was most likely assigned to patients with a milder bleeding phenotype. Indeed, results from a randomized, double-blind study indicated that, while receiving 3-times-weekly prophylaxis with rFVIII-FS, significantly more bleeds were reported in patients with target joints versus without target joints [4].

Analysis by age subgroup revealed that the trend toward lower ABRs observed in the 1-2 prophylaxis injections/wk group compared with the ≥3 prophylaxis injections/wk group was not age dependent. However, there was a trend toward higher joint bleeding rates in patients ≥18 years of age compared with patients <18 years of age and more trauma-related bleeds in the lower age group. An analysis of bleeding patterns in patients with severe hemophilia A receiving prophylaxis during prospective clinical trials found lower bleeding rates in adults compared with children [13]. However, this same analysis also reported a trend toward increasing frequency of joint bleeds with increasing age and higher trauma-related

TABLE 3: Annualized bleeding rates by dosing and age subgroups.

Annualized bleeding rates	Prophylaxis 1-2x/wk ($n = 63$)		Prophylaxis ≥3x/wk ($n = 76$)	
	Age <18 y $n = 28$	Age ≥18 y $n = 35$	Age <18 y $n = 43$	Age ≥18 y $n = 33$
All bleeds				
Mean ± SD	3.0 ± 5.6	5.0 ± 6.9	5.8 ± 5.9	8.7 ± 14.7
Median (Q1; Q3)	1.9 (0; 3.0)	2.4 (0; 8.4)	3.5 (1.1; 8.5)	4.7 (1.9; 11.2)
Joint bleeds				
Mean ± SD	1.5 ± 3.4	3.9 ± 6.1	2.9 ± 3.2	6.6 ± 9.6
Median (Q1; Q3)	0.5 (0; 1.5)	1.7 (0; 3.5)	1.8 (0.5; 4.2)	3.8 (1.5; 8.5)
Spontaneous bleeds				
Mean ± SD	0.5 ± 1.0	3.9 ± 6.3	1.1 ± 2.2	5.8 ± 8.5
Median (Q1; Q3)	0 (0; 0.5)	1.1 (0; 6.8)	0.5 (0; 1.0)	3.0 (0; 8.8)
Trauma-related bleeds				
Mean ± SD	2.4 ± 5.1	1.1 ± 1.9	4.3 ± 4.5	2.4 ± 6.2
Median (Q1; Q3)	1.0 (0; 2.4)	0 (0; 1.1)	2.5 (0.9; 7.0)	0.7 (0; 1.9)

Q1 = quartile 1; Q3 = quartile 3.

TABLE 4: Annualized bleeding frequency.

	Number (%) of patients		
	Prophylaxis 1-2x/wk ($n = 63$)	Prophylaxis ≥3x/wk ($n = 76$)	Total ($N = 139$)
Total bleeds			
0	19 (30.2)	5 (6.6)	24 (17.3)
>0 to ≤2	12 (19.0)	19 (25.0)	31 (22.3)
>2 to ≤8	20 (31.7)	28 (36.8)	48 (34.5)
>8	12 (19.0)	24 (31.6)	36 (25.9)
Joint bleeds			
0	25 (39.7)	13 (17.1)	38 (27.3)
>0 to ≤2	18 (28.6)	23 (30.3)	41 (29.5)
>2 to ≤4	10 (15.9)	12 (15.8)	22 (15.8)
>4	10 (15.9)	28 (36.8)	38 (27.3)

bleeding rates in children [13], which is in agreement with the results of this pooled analysis.

The data from this pooled analysis support the hypothesis that not all patients need the standard 3-times-weekly dosing regimen to achieve bleeding control [14]. This hypothesis is further supported by data from the Canadian Hemophilia Primary Prophylaxis (CHPS) study, a prospective, long-term study that investigated the efficacy of tailored prophylaxis for severe hemophilia A [10]. Of the 56 boys in the study at study year 13, 36 (64%) had escalated from once-weekly prophylaxis to twice-weekly prophylaxis to control bleeding; 17 of these 36 patients escalated from twice-weekly prophylaxis to alternate-day prophylaxis [15, 16].

A limitation of this analysis is that the data are pooled from observational, noninvestigational "real-world" studies. The results must be considered without pharmacokinetic data or data on time to fall below a certain FVIII trough level. In addition, historical bleeding data are not available to investigate possible reasons for the differences in bleeding rates observed between the 2 dosing groups nor is information available on the treating physicians' rationale for selecting a specific dosing frequency. Also, unlike the CHPS study, joint outcomes were not assessed in the current study, and only annualized bleeding rates were evaluated. Another potential limitation of the analysis was that periods without documentation of injections or bleeds could have biased results or assignment of patients to analysis groups. To avoid this bias, periods of prophylaxis treatment interruption ≥28 days were excluded from the analysis. A cut-off threshold of 28 days is theoretically a long enough time period to be representative of a true prophylaxis treatment interruption without excluding data from bleeding treatment periods; however, it was possible that some bleeds may have required treatment for >28 days. A sensitivity analysis that included all data during the prophylaxis treatment interruptions showed no major differences compared with the primary analysis.

A definition of successful prophylaxis in the clinical practice setting has not yet been determined. In these post-marketing data, 81% of the once-twice-weekly dosing group had ≤8 total annualized bleeds compared with 68% of those in the ≥3-times-weekly dosing group. The results for annualized joint bleeds, perhaps a better gauge of prophylaxis success, were 84% and 63% for ≤4 joint bleeds for the 2 groups, respectively. In the absence of data on patient adherence, these results might be considered successful prophylaxis in a practice setting. Nevertheless, one-third of the patients treated with a standard prophylaxis regimen of 3x/week did not demonstrate an acceptable outcome of joint bleed control with the dosages used for prophylaxis injection. A possible explanation is the difference in incidence of target joints at baseline between the dosing groups. In patients <12 years of age, target joints at baseline were present in 5.9% in the once-twice-weekly group versus 22.6% in the ≥3-times-weekly group. The corresponding figures for those ≥12 years of age were 34.8% versus 57.8%. It can only be speculated that higher dosages may provide better outcomes in terms of prevention of joint bleeds in these patients.

5. Conclusions

Dosing flexibility with rFVIII-FS was demonstrated in this pooled analysis from 3 postmarketing studies. Very good bleeding control as shown by ABR for all bleeds and joint bleeds was achieved by both a standard ≥3-times-weekly dosing regimen and by a less frequent once-twice-weekly regimen. The prophylaxis success achieved was reasonable in the absence of an agreed definition of success in the clinical setting. The selection of dosing regimen was made by the treating physician. The patients prescribed the less frequent regimen were likely to be older and to be without target joints.

Conflict of Interests

T. J. Humphries, S. Rauchensteiner, C. Tückmantel, M. Maas Enriquez, and P. Mathew are employees of Bayer. A. Pieper is an employee of M.A.R.C.O. GmbH & Co. KG and was fully funded by Bayer HealthCare AG (Leverkusen, Germany).

Acknowledgments

This study was funded by Bayer HealthCare AG (Leverkusen, Germany). Medical writing assistance was provided by Erin P. Scott for Complete Healthcare Communications, Inc. (Chadds Ford, PA), and was fully funded by Bayer HealthCare Pharmaceuticals.

References

[1] National Hemophilia Foundation, *Medical and Scientific Advisory Council (MASAC) Recommendations Concerning Prophylaxis (Regular Administration of Clotting Factor Concentrate to Prevent Bleeding)*, Document #179, National Hemophilia Foundation, 2014, http://www.hemophilia.org/sites/default/files/document/files/masac179.pdf.

[2] A. Srivastava, A. K. Brewer, E. P. Mauser-Bunschoten et al., "Guidelines for the management of hemophilia," *Haemophilia*, vol. 19, no. 1, pp. e1–e7, 2013.

[3] P. Petrini, "Identifying and overcoming barriers to prophylaxis in the management of haemophilia," *Haemophilia*, vol. 13, supplement 2, pp. 16–22, 2007.

[4] S. Lalezari, A. Coppola, J. Lin et al., "Patient characteristics that influence efficacy of prophylaxis with rFVIII-FS three times per week: a subgroup analysis of the LIPLONG study," *Haemophilia*, vol. 20, no. 3, pp. 354–361, 2014.

[5] P. Collins, A. Faradji, M. Morfini, M. M. Enriquez, and L. Schwartz, "Efficacy and safety of secondary prophylactic vs. on-demand sucrose-formulated recombinant factor VIII treatment in adults with severe hemophilia A: results from a 13-month crossover study," *Journal of Thrombosis and Haemostasis*, vol. 8, no. 1, pp. 83–89, 2010.

[6] T. C. Abshire, H. H. Brackmann, I. Scharrer et al., "Sucrose formulated recombinant human antihemophilic factor VIII is safe and efficacious for treatment of hemophilia A in home therapy—international Kogenate-FS study group," *Thrombosis and Haemostasis*, vol. 83, no. 6, pp. 811–816, 2000.

[7] M. J. Manco-Johnson, T. C. Abshire, A. D. Shapiro et al., "Prophylaxis versus episodic treatment to prevent joint disease in boys with severe hemophilia," *The New England Journal of Medicine*, vol. 357, no. 6, pp. 535–544, 2007.

[8] M. J. Manco-Johnson, C. L. Kempton, M. T. Reding et al., "Randomized, controlled, parallel-group trial of routine prophylaxis vs. on-demand treatment with sucrose-formulated recombinant factor VIII in adults with severe hemophilia A (SPINART)," *Journal of Thrombosis and Haemostasis*, vol. 11, no. 6, pp. 1119–1127, 2014.

[9] V. V. Vdouin, T. A. Andreeva, T. A. Chernoua et al., "Prophylaxis with once, twice or three-times weekly dosing of rFVIII-FS Prevents joint bleeds in a previously treated pediatric population with moderate/severe hemophilia A," *Journal of Coagulation Disorders*, vol. 3, no. 1, pp. 1–8, 2011.

[10] B. M. Feldman, M. Pai, G. E. Rivard et al., "Tailored prophylaxis in severe hemophilia A: interim results from the first 5 years of the Canadian hemophilia primary prophylaxis study," *Journal of Thrombosis and Haemostasis*, vol. 4, no. 6, pp. 1228–1236, 2006.

[11] R. Musso, E. Santagostino, A. Faradji et al., "Safety and efficacy of sucrose-formulated full-length recombinant factor VIII: experience in the standard clinical setting," *Thrombosis and Haemostasis*, vol. 99, no. 1, pp. 52–58, 2008.

[12] J.-H. Young, H.-C. Liu, E.-J. Hsueh et al., "Efficacy and safety evaluation of sucrose-formulated recombinant factor VIII for Taiwanese patients with haemophilia A," *Haemophilia*, vol. 15, no. 4, pp. 968–970, 2009.

[13] K. Fischer, P. Collins, S. Björkman et al., "Trends in bleeding patterns during prophylaxis for severe haemophilia: observations from a series of prospective clinical trials," *Haemophilia*, vol. 17, no. 3, pp. 433–438, 2011.

[14] M. Carcao, H. Chambost, and R. Ljung, "Devising a best practice approach to prophylaxis in boys with severe haemophilia: evaluation of current treatment strategies," *Haemophilia*, vol. 16, supplement 2, pp. 4–9, 2010.

[15] P. Hilliard, N. Zourikian, V. Blanchette et al., "Musculoskeletal health of subjects with hemophilia A treated with tailored prophylaxis: Canadian Hemophilia Primary Prophylaxis (CHPS) study," *Journal of Thrombosis and Haemostasis*, vol. 11, no. 3, pp. 460–466, 2013.

[16] M. X. Hang, V. S. Blanchette, E. Pullenayegum, M. Mclimont, and B. M. Feldman, "Age at first joint bleed and bleeding severity in boys with severe hemophilia A: Canadian Hemophilia Primary Prophylaxis study," *Journal of Thrombosis and Haemostasis*, vol. 9, no. 5, pp. 1067–1069, 2011.

16

Frequency and Prognostic Relevance of *FLT3* Mutations in Saudi Acute Myeloid Leukemia Patients

Ghaleb Elyamany,[1,2] **Mohammad Awad,**[2] **Kamal Fadalla,**[3] **Mohamed Albalawi,**[3]
Mohammad Al Shahrani,[4] **and Abdulaziz Al Abdulaaly**[3]

[1] *Department of Hematology and Blood Bank, Theodor Bilharz Research Institute, Giza 12411, Egypt, Egypt*
[2] *Department of Central Military Laboratory, Prince Sultan Military Medical City, P.O. Box 7897, Riyadh 11159, Saudi Arabia*
[3] *Department of Adult Clinical Hematology and Stem Cell Therapy, Prince Sultan Military Medical City, Riyadh, Saudi Arabia*
[4] *Department of Pediatric Hematology/Oncology, Prince Sultan Military Medical City, P.O. Box 7897, Riyadh 11159, Saudi Arabia*

Correspondence should be addressed to Ghaleb Elyamany; ghalebelyamany@yahoo.com

Academic Editor: Andreas Neubauer

The Fms-like tyrosine kinase-3 (*FLT3*) is a receptor tyrosine kinase that plays a key role in cell survival, proliferation, and differentiation of hematopoietic stem cells. Mutations of *FLT3* were first described in 1997 and account for the most frequent molecular mutations in acute myeloid leukemia (AML). AML patients with *FLT3* internal tandem duplication (ITD) mutations have poor cure rates the prognostic significance of point mutations; tyrosine kinase domain (TKD) is still unclear. We analyzed the frequency of *FLT3* mutations (ITD and D835) in patients with AML at diagnosis; no sufficient data currently exist regarding *FLT3* mutations in Saudi AML patients. This study was aimed at evaluating the frequency of *FLT3* mutations in patients with AML and its significance for prognosis. The frequency of *FLT3* mutations in our study (18.56%) was lower than many of the reported studies, *FLT3*-ITD mutations were observed in 14.4%, and *FLT3*-TKD in 4.1%, of 97 newly diagnosed AML patients (82 adult and 15 pediatric). Our data show significant increase of *FLT3* mutations in male more than female (13 male, 5 female). Our results support the view that *FLT3*-ITD mutation has strong prognostic factor in AML patients and is associated with high rate of relapse, and high leucocytes and blast count at diagnosis and relapse.

1. Introduction

FLT3 (Fms-like tyrosine kinase-3), also known as FLK2 (fetal liver kinase-2) and STK1 (human stem cell kinase-1), was originally isolated as a hematopoietic progenitor cell-specific kinase and belongs to Class-III receptor tyrosine kinase (RTK) family to which c-Fms, c-Kit, and the PDGFR (platelet derived growth factor receptor) also belong [1]. Normal expression of *FLT3* is restricted to hematopoietic progenitor cells in the bone marrow (BM), thymus, and lymph nodes but is also found in other tissues such as placenta, brain, cerebellum, and gonads [2].

FLT3 plays a key role in cell survival, proliferation, and differentiation of hematopoietic stem cells [3]. The human *FLT3* gene is located on chromosome 13q12 and encompasses 24 exons. It encodes a membrane-bound glycosylated protein

of 993 amino acids with a molecular weight of 158–160 kDa, as well as a nonglycosylated isoform of 130–143 kDa that is not associated with the plasma membrane [4]. The structure of *FLT3* is shown in Figure 1. *FLT3* is frequently overexpressed in acute leukemia. *FLT3* mutations occur in approximately 30% of acute myeloid leukemia (AML) patients and confer a poor prognosis [5].

The two major types of mutation that occur are internal tandem duplication (ITD) mutations of the juxtamembrane region and point mutations in tyrosine kinase domain (TKD), which frequently involve aspartic acid 835 of the kinase domain (D835). Both mutations result in constitutive activation of the receptor's tyrosine kinase activity in the absence of ligand [6].

Many studies have shown that AML patients with *FLT3*-ITD mutations have poor cure rates due to relapse. This

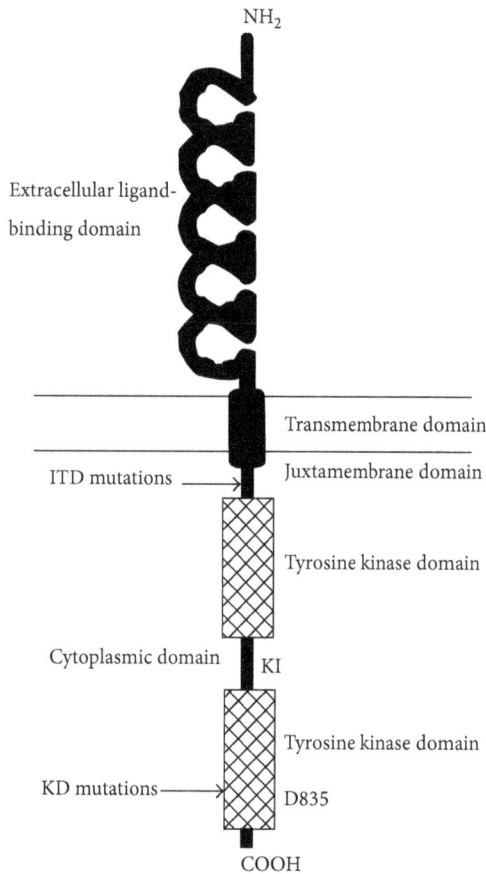

FIGURE 1: Diagram of *FLT3* structure. Shown in schematic fashion are the 5 immunoglobulin-like folds that make up the ligand-binding extracellular domain, single transmembrane domain, and cytoplasmic domain made up of a kinase domain interrupted by a kinase insert. The juxtamembrane domain where internal tandem duplications (ITDs) occur and aspartic acid 835 where most kinase domain mutations occur are indicated by arrows (Small D. *FLT3* Mutations: Biology and Treatment. Hematology Am Soc Hematol Educ Program. 2006).

has led to the development of a number of small molecule tyrosine kinase inhibitors (TKI) with activity against *FLT3* [7]. Adult patients usually have a higher prevalence of *FLT3*-ITD (24%) than pediatric AML patients. This observation may partially explain why adult AML has a poorer clinical outcome than pediatric AML [8]. Moreover, the clinical significance of *FLT3*-TKD mutation which is found in approximately 5–10% of AML patients is not clear yet, but several studies indicate that it is also an adverse prognostic indicator [8]. Clinically AML patients with *FLT3*-ITD tend to have higher WBC counts and an increased percentage of leukemic blasts [9]. *FLT3* mutations have also been seen in myelodysplastic syndrome (MDS) in about 3–5% of newly diagnosed patients and in MDS patients without *FLT3* mutations, they sometimes appear when these patients progress to AML [10].

This study which is considered the first study done in Saudi Arabia focuses on frequency and prognosis of the

presence of *FLT3* mutations in adult and pediatric acute myeloid leukemia patients; only one study was done for detection of *FLT3* oncogene mutations in adult acute myeloid leukemia using conformation sensitive gel electrophoresis [11].

2. Materials and Methods

2.1. Patients. Bone marrow samples or blood samples from 97 patients with AML at diagnosis (66 BM and 31 blood samples) were screened for *FLT3* mutations. The range of age was one year old to 82 years (median 36 years, mean 37.8 years). Of the 97 patients, 94 (96.9%) had de novo AML, 1 (1%) had secondary AML after myelodysplastic syndrome (MDS) (s-AML), and 2 (2.1%) had AML after transformation from CML. The study was approved by the ethics and research committee of the institution.

Samples were evaluated by cytomorphology, multiparameter flow cytometry, cytogenetics, fluorescence in situ hybridization (FISH), and molecular genetics in parallel.

2.2. Methods. DNA was extracted using QIAamp DNA Kit (Qiagen) according to the manufacturer's instruction.

2.2.1. Analysis of the ITD of the FLT3 Gene. PCR reaction was composed of 200 ng of DNA, 50 mM KCL, 10 mM Tris-HCL, pH 8.3, 1.5 mM $MgCL_2$, 0.001% (wt/vol) gelatin, 200 μM dNTPs, 0.4 μM of each published primer [29], and 1 U of gold *Taq* polymerase, in a volume of 50 μL.

The PCR consisted of an initial incubation step at 95°C for 10 minutes followed by 35 cycles at 94°C for 30 seconds, 57°C for 60 seconds, and 72°C for 90 seconds and final extension step at 72°C for 10 minutes on a GeneAmp PCR system 9700 (Applied Biosystems). PCR products were analyzed on standard 3% agarose gels, and samples showing additional longer PCR products were considered *FLT3*/ITD+.

2.2.2. Analysis of the D835 Mutation of the FLT3 Gene. PCR reaction was set up as above using published primers [28]. PCR product was digested with EcoRV (Promega), at 37°C for 2 h. The digestion products were separated on a 3% agarose gel, and incomplete digestion indicated the presence of a mutant.

3. Statistical Analysis

The Kaplan-Meier technique was used to analyze the probability of overall survival (OS) and event-free survival (EFS). OS was calculated from time of diagnosis to death and EFS from time of diagnosis to death, evidence of persistent leukemia, or relapse. Continuous variables, such as white blood cell count and hemoglobin, were compared by using the Kruskal-Wallis test. Differences between means were considered as significant at $P < 0.05$.

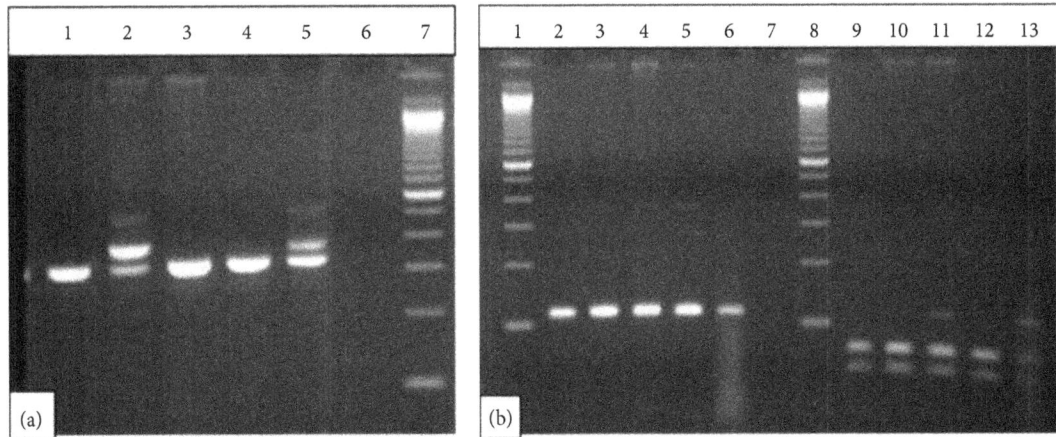

FIGURE 2: PCR analysis of *FLT3*-ITD and D835 mutations. (a) This gel shows patients positive for ITD lanes 2 and 5, patients negative for ITD lanes 1, 3, and 4, water control lane 6, and marker lane 7. (b) This gel shows undigested sample for D835 lanes 2–6, water control lane 7, marker lanes 1 and 8, digested sample lanes 9–13, positive patients lanes 11 and 13, and negative patients lanes 9, 10, and 12.

4. Results

Table 1 summarizes the characteristics of the patients included in the study. Of the 97 AML patients studied, 47 were males (48.5%) and 50 were females (51.5%); 18 cases (13 males, 5 females) were positive for *FLT3* mutations with overall frequency of 18.55%. In these 18 *FLT3*-positive cases, 14/97 (14.43%) had *FLT3*-ITD and 4/97 (4.12%) were found to contain the D835 mutations (Figures 2(a) and 2(b)). None of the 3 secondary AML (MDS and CML) patients examined showed *FLT3*-ITD or D835 mutations. None of the patients had combination of *FLT3*-ITD and D835 mutation in the *FLT3* gene.

In *FLT3*-mutated patients median WBC was 65×10^9/L compared to 12.5×10^9/L in the rest of the patients. Peripheral blood blasts were elevated in *FLT3*-mutated group compared to *FLT3*-wild type (WT) patients (40% versus 8%, resp.).

Among *FLT3*-mutated patients, 8 cases died, 5 during induction chemotherapy and 3 during consolidation chemotherapy (1/8 D835+ and 7/8 ITD+), 7 cases relapsed within 4–20 months (1/7 D835 and 6/7 ITD+), and 3 cases (2/3 D835+ and 1/3 ITD+) achieved complete remission (CR).

As cytogenetic study was available only in a limited number of cases, correlation for cytogenetic analysis was not possible. In mutated group, cytogenetic and molecular studies revealed that 4 cases (22.2%) are associated with AML specific abnormalities, namely, PML-RARA/t (15; 17)(q22; q21), AML-ETO t(8; 21)(q22; q22), CBFB/inv(16)(p13; q22), and MLL (DC,BAR)/11q23. By conventional karyotype, it was not available for 5 cases because of a low number of analyzed metaphases; 3 cases were trisomy (2 cases with trisomy 8 and one case with trisomy 5) and 6 cases were with normal karyotype. Median overall survival was 10.0 months for *FLT3*-mutated patients and 20.0 months for WT patients ($P = 0.031$), and *FLT3*-positive patients had also a significantly shorter 2-year event-free survival (EFS) than *FLT3*/WT patients ($P = 0.040$) because of a higher relapse rate.

5. Discussion

FLT3 mutations are one of the most frequent gene defects so far reported in AML, occurring in approximately 25–35% of patients [3, 28, 30–32]. *FLT3*-ITD represents one of the most frequent genetic alterations in AML. They show a frequency of 20% to 27% in AML in adults [22, 28] and of 10% to 16% in childhood cases [33, 34].

The overall frequency of *FLT3* mutations in our study (18.55%) is lower than most of the reported studies [3, 28, 30–32]; however, some reports agree with our report [21]. Also, the only study which was conducted in Saudi Arabia for *FLT3* mutations in AML patients showed frequency of 20.15% (26/129), close to our results [11]. The explanations of lower frequency of *FLT3* mutations in our study from other several studies may be explained by differences in the sizes of examined groups or might be due to population genetics, environmental factors, selected patient population studies, or because of differences of age as the median age of patients in this study was 36 years in comparison to comparative studies or a combination of the all.

Adult patients usually have a higher prevalence of *FLT-3*-ITD mutation than pediatric AML patients; this observation may partially explain why adult AML has a poorer clinical outcome than pediatric AML [8]. In our study, the frequency of *FLT3*-ITD mutation in adult AML was 14.43% which is lower than reported in other published studies [8, 19, 20, 22, 28, 35], but still in the variation range of frequency of ITD mutations (13–27%) reported by some study group [12, 21] (Table 2). In contrast to published studies the rate of *FLT3*-ITD mutation in pediatric AML (20%) is more than the adult and higher than most of the reported studies [33, 34, 36]. This difference in the rate most likely is attributed to small size of samples of pediatric AML (15 cases).

Similarly, the rate of *FLT3*-TKD mutation (D835) in our study is 4.12% (4/97) which is less frequent than *FLT3*-ITD mutation (14/97), these results are in accordance with the published studies on the frequency of *FLT3*-TKD in AML

TABLE 1: Summary of the characteristics of the patients included in the study.

Parameter	*FLT3*-mutated patients ($n = 18$)	*FLT3* WT patients ($n = 79$)
Male : female	13 : 5	34 : 45
Median age (years)	38	35
Median WBCs count	65×10^9/L	12.5×10^9/L
Median platelets count	53×10^9/L	71×10^9/L
Median hemoglobin	9.1 g/dL	10 g/dL
Median PB blasts	40%	8%
History of AML		
De novo AML	18/94	76/94
Secondary s-AML	0/3	3/3
FLT3 mutation rate and OS		
FLT3-ITD	14/97 (14.43%)	NA
FLT3-D835	4/97 (4.12%)	NA
Total	**18/97 (18.55%)**	NA
Median OS (months)	10	20
Cytogeneticanalysis		
Available for FISH	18	56
Available for karyotype	13	40
t (8; 21)	1	6
t (15; 17)	1	3
inv 16/t (16; 16)	1	3
11q23/MLL	1	2
Non recurrent translocations	0	5
+8	2	5
+5	1	1
+13	0	2
+21	0	1
−8	0	1
5q−/−5	0	2
7q−/−7	0	2
Complex karyotype	0	2
Hyperdiploid	0	2
Other aberrations	0	4

WT: wild type; OS: overall survival; FISH: fluorescence in situ hybridization.

performed by many study groups [20, 22, 27, 28]; the rate of *FLT3*-TKD mutation (D835) in our study is almost very close to the largest study done by Bacher et al. [23] in which *FLT3*-TKD mutations were detected in 147 of 3082 (4.8%) patients. However, our results are slightly lower than many studies on the frequency of *FLT3*-TKD in AML (Table 3) which were performed by Abu-Duhier et al. [27], Yamamoto et al. [28], Thiede et al. [22], Moreno et al. [26], and Fröhling et al. [8]; according to these studies, *FLT3*-TKD mutation shows an incidence of 5.8% to 7.7% in AML. However, some of the reported studies show incidence higher than these studies ranged from 8 to 12% [22].

Our data are in accordance with those published by other groups [8, 13, 14, 17, 22, 29, 37–41] and showed that *FLT3*-ITD mutation has a strong prognostic factor in AML patients and associated disease progression with high rate of relapse and shorter overall survival; median overall survival was 10.0 months for *FLT3*-mutated patients and 20.0 months for WT

patients ($P = 0.031$), and event-free survival (EFS) was also worse for *FLT3*-positive patients than *FLT3*-WT patients ($P = 0.040$) because of a higher relapse rate. Also high leucocytes count, high blast cells count in peripheral blood, resistant to therapy and confers a poor prognosis, Table 1. This has led to the development of a number of small molecule tyrosine kinase inhibitors (TKI) with activity against *FLT3* [7, 42]. Moreover, patients with low or absent levels of WT *FLT3*, consistent with homozygosity for the *FLT3*-ITD allele, appear to have a particularly dismal outcome [22].

Because of the low frequency, the prognostic significance of *FLT3*-TKD mutations is still unclear [23]. Many recent studies [21, 23, 43] showed that *FLT3*-TKD has little or no prognostic significance in AML patients. In this study, according to our data unlike the *FLT3*-ITD mutation, which are associated with inferior survival, prognosis was not influenced by mutation of *FLT3*-TKD. Moreover, Bacher et al. [23] found an additional favorable impact of *FLT3*-TKD on

Table 2: Frequency of *FLT3*/ITD mutations in the current study and in previous studies.

Reference (year)	Total, n	FLT-ITD+ %
Our study (2013)	97	14.4
Ishfaq et al. [12] (2012)	30	13.3
Xu et al. [13] (2012)	216	20.8
Ding et al. [14] (2012)	656	27.1
Zaker et al. [15] (2010)	212	18.0
Wang et al. [16] (2010)	76	19.7
Al-Tonbary et al. [17] (2009)	30	20.0
Gari et al. [11] (2008)	129	11.6
Suzuki et al. [18] (2007)	60	20.0
Wang et al. [19] (2005)	143	25.9
Auewarakul et al. [20] (2005)	256	27.3
Sheikhha et al. [21] (2003)	80	10.0
Fröhling et al. [8] (2002)	224	32.0
Thiede et al. [22] (2002)	979	20.4

Table 3: Frequency of *FLT3*/TKD mutations in the current study and in previous studies.

Reference (year)	Total, n	FLT-TKD %
Our Study (2013)	97	4.1
Ding et al. [14] (2012)	656	7.0
Zaker et al. [15] (2010)	212	6.0
Gari et al. [11] (2008)	129	8.5
Bacher et al. [23] (2008)	3082	4.8
Mead et al. [24] (2007)	1107	11.5
Auewarakul et al. [20] (2005)	256	5.9
Wang et al. [19] (2005)	143	6.3
Andersson et al. [25] (2004)	109 (<60 y)	10.1
Moreno et al. [26] (2003)	208	9.6
Sheikhha et al. [21] (2003)	80	7.5
Thiede et al. [22] (2002)	979	7.7
Fröhling et al. [8] (2002)	224	14.0
Abu-Duhier et al. [27] (2001)	97	7.2
Yamamoto et al. [28] (2001)	429	7.0

EFS in prognostically favorable AML with NPM1 or CEBPA mutations. However, Yamamoto et al. [28] revealed that, in contrast to our study, D835 mutations were not significantly related to the leukocytosis but tended to worsen disease-free survival.

As a surprising finding in our study, the rate of *FLT3* mutations in male (13/18; 72.2%) is higher than in female (5/18; 27.8%); this finding may be the first one reported in English literature showing the significant difference between male and female ($P = 0.025$). One small study was done on 30 AML patients with frequency of *FLT3*/ITD mutation in AML which was 4/30 (13.3%); three were males and one female [12]. However, these results should be treated with reservation, due to the relatively small sample sizes. These differences in male/female ratio in our study from several reported studies may be due to population genetics, environmental factors,

relative small sample sizes, or a combination of all and further research and investigation are required.

As one interesting rare finding, one adult AML patient in our cohort study who did not have *FLT3* mutations at diagnosis has been found to acquire *FLT3*/ITD at the time of relapse; this finding was reported by another study group [10] and raises the importance of assessing *FLT3* gene on all relapses. This finding also suggests that *FLT3* mutations are unstable and that there is potential clinical value in continuously monitoring *FLT3* mutation status [44].

6. Conclusion

Currently no sufficient data exist regarding *FLT3* mutations in Saudi patients. This study was aimed at evaluating the prevalence of *FLT3* mutations in patients with AML and its significance for prognosis. The frequency of *FLT3* mutations in our study was lower than (18.56%) other reported studies; however, some reports agree with our report or are very close. Our data as other several reports support the view that *FLT3*/ITD has strong prognostic factor in AML patients and is associated with high rate of relapse, is resistant to therapy, and confers a poor prognosis. Our data show increase of *FLT3* mutations in male more than female which need more research studies using large size samples. This study also raises the importance of assessing *FLT3* gene on all relapses as one case which did not have *FLT3* mutations at diagnosis has been found to acquire *FLT3*/ITD at the time of relapse. Early detection of *FLT3* mutations and an intensification of induction therapy might thus be useful for this group of patients to overcome the poor prognosis.

Abbreviations

FLT3: Fms-like tyrosine kinase-3
FLK2: Fetal liver kinase-2
STK1: Human stem cell kinase-1
BM: Bone marrow
AML: Acute myeloid leukemia
ITD: Internal tandem duplication
TKD: Tyrosine kinase domain
RTK: Receptor tyrosine kinase
PDGFR: Platelet derived growth factor receptor
MDS: Myelodysplastic syndrome
WT: Wild type
OS: Overall survival
FISH: Fluorescence in situ hybridization
EFS: Event-free survival
TKI: Tyrosine kinase inhibitors.

Conflict of Interests

The authors declare that they have no competing interests.

Acknowledgments

The authors thank Dr. Omar Alsuhaibani, Head Division of Hematology and Blood Bank, for general support. They also thank all the Hematology, Cytogenetic and Molecular Laboratories staffs and data managers, especially Mr. Mohamed Asiri and Dalal Alkhammash from Hematology Laboratory for data collection and management and Ms. Nadia Halawani from Molecular Laboratory for great help in molecular work of this study. Finally, they thank Ms. Khowla Al-Fayez and Inesse Abdullah from Cytogenetic Laboratory for excellent help and data collection in cytogenetic aspect of this study.

References

[1] D. Small, M. Levenstein, E. Kim et al., "STK-1, the human homolog of Flk-2/Flt-3, is selectively expressed in CD34+ human bone marrow cells and is involved in the proliferation of early progenitor/stem cells," *Proceedings of the National Academy of Sciences of the United States of America*, vol. 91, no. 2, pp. 459–463, 1994.

[2] O. Rosnet, H.-J. Bühring, S. Marchetto et al., "Human FLT3/FLK2 receptor tyrosine kinase is expressed at the surface of normal and malignant hematopoietic cells," *Leukemia*, vol. 10, no. 2, pp. 238–248, 1996.

[3] D. Gary Gilliland and J. D. Griffin, "The roles of FLT3 in hematopoiesis and leukemia," *Blood*, vol. 100, no. 5, pp. 1532–1542, 2002.

[4] A. Markovic, K. L. MacKenzie, and R. B. Lock, "FLT-3: a new focus in the understanding of acute leukemia," *International Journal of Biochemistry and Cell Biology*, vol. 37, no. 6, pp. 1168–1172, 2005.

[5] F. Kuchenbauer, W. Kern, C. Schoch et al., "Detailed analysis of FLT3 expression levels in acute myeloid leukemia," *Haematologica*, vol. 90, no. 12, pp. 1617–1625, 2005.

[6] M. Nakao, S. Yokota, T. Iwai et al., "Internal tandem duplication of the flt3 gene found in acute myeloid leukemia," *Leukemia*, vol. 10, no. 12, pp. 1911–1918, 1996.

[7] D. Small, "FLT3 mutations: biology and treatment," *Hematology/the Education Program of the American Society of Hematology*, pp. 178–184, 2006.

[8] S. Fröhling, R. F. Schlenk, J. Breitruck et al., "Prognostic significance of activating FLT3 mutations in younger adults (16 to 60 years) with acute myeloid leukemia and normal cytogenetics: a study of the AML study group Ulm," *Blood*, vol. 100, no. 13, pp. 4372–4380, 2002.

[9] H. Kiyoi and T. Naoe, "FLT3 mutations in acute myeloid leukemia," *Methods in Molecular Medicine*, vol. 125, pp. 189–197, 2006.

[10] L.-Y. Shih, C.-F. Huang, P.-N. Wang et al., "Acquisition of FLT3 or N-ras mutations is frequently associated with progression of myelodysplastic syndrome to acute myeloid leukemia," *Leukemia*, vol. 18, no. 3, pp. 466–475, 2004.

[11] M. Gari, A. Abuzenadah, A. Chaudhary et al., "Detection of FLT3 oncogene mutations in acute myeloid leukemia using conformation sensitive gel electrophoresis," *International Journal of Molecular Sciences*, vol. 9, no. 11, pp. 2194–2204, 2008.

[12] M. Ishfaq, A. Malik, M. Faiz et al., "Molecular characterization of FLT3 mutations in acute leukemia patients in Pakistan," *Asian Pacific Journal of Cancer Prevention*, vol. 13, no. 9, pp. 4581–4585, 2012.

[13] Y. Y. Xu, L. Gao, Y. Ding et al., "Detection and clinical significance of FLT3-ITD gene mutation in patients with acute myeloid leukemia," *Zhongguo Shi Yan Xue Ye Za Zhi*, vol. 20, no. 6, pp. 1312–1315, 2012.

[14] Z. X. Ding, H. J. Shen, J. C. Miao et al., "NPM1 and FLT3 gene mutation patterns and their prognostic significance in 656 Chinese patients with acute myeloid leukemia," *Zhonghua Xue Ye Xue Za Zhi*, vol. 33, no. 10, pp. 829–834, 2012.

[15] F. Zaker, M. Mohammadzadeh, and M. Mohammadi, "Detection of KIT and FLT3 mutations in acute myeloid leukemia with different subtypes," *Archives of Iranian Medicine*, vol. 13, no. 1, pp. 21–25, 2010.

[16] Y. Wang, Z. Li, C. He et al., "MicroRNAs expression signatures are associated with lineage and survival in acute leukemias," *Blood Cells, Molecules, and Diseases*, vol. 44, no. 3, pp. 191–197, 2010.

[17] Y. Al-Tonbary, A. K. Mansour, H. Ghazy, D. M. Elghannam, and H. A. Abd-Elghaffar, "Prognostic significance of foetal-like tyrosine kinase 3 mutation in Egyptian children with acute leukaemia," *International Journal of Laboratory Hematology*, vol. 31, no. 3, pp. 320–326, 2009.

[18] R. Suzuki, M. Onizuka, M. Kojima et al., "Prognostic significance of FLT3 internal tandem duplication and NPM1 mutations in acute myeloid leukemia in an unselected patient population," *International Journal of Hematology*, vol. 86, no. 5, pp. 422–428, 2007.

[19] L. Wang, D. Lin, X. Zhang, S. Chen, M. Wang, and J. Wang, "Analysis of FLT3 internal tandem duplication and D835 mutations in Chinese acute leukemia patients," *Leukemia Research*, vol. 29, no. 12, pp. 1393–1398, 2005.

[20] C. U. Auewarakul, N. Sritana, C. Limwongse, W. Thongnoppakhun, and P.-T. Yenchitsomanus, "Mutations of the FLT3 gene in adult acute myeloid leukemia: determination of incidence and identification of a novel mutation in a Thai population," *Cancer Genetics and Cytogenetics*, vol. 162, no. 2, pp. 127–134, 2005.

[21] M. H. Sheikhha, A. Awan, K. Tobal, and J. A. Liu Yin, "Prognostic significance of FLT3 ITD and D835 mutations in AML patients," *Hematology Journal*, vol. 4, no. 1, pp. 41–46, 2003.

[22] C. Thiede, C. Steudel, B. Mohr et al., "Analysis of FLT3-activating mutations in 979 patients with acute myelogenous leukemia: association with FAB subtypes and identification of subgroups with poor prognosis," *Blood*, vol. 99, no. 12, pp. 4326–4335, 2002.

[23] U. Bacher, C. Haferlach, W. Kern, T. Haferlach, and S. Schnittger, "Prognostic relevance of FLT3-TKD mutations in AML: the combination matters an analysis of 3082 patients," *Blood*, vol. 111, no. 5, pp. 2527–2537, 2008.

[24] A. J. Mead, D. C. Linch, R. K. Hills, K. Wheatley, A. K. Burnett, and R. E. Gale, "FLT3 tyrosine kinase domain mutations are biologically distinct from and have a significantly more favorable prognosis than FLT3 internal tandem duplications in patients with acute myeloid leukemia," *Blood*, vol. 110, no. 4, pp. 1262–1270, 2007.

[25] A. Andersson, B. Johansson, C. Lassen, F. Mitelman, R. Billström, and T. Fioretos, "Clinical impact of internal tandem duplications and activating point mutations in FLT3 in acute myeloid leukemia in elderly patients," *European Journal of Haematology*, vol. 72, no. 5, pp. 307–313, 2004.

[26] I. Moreno, G. Martin, P. Bolufer et al., "Incidence and prognostic value of FLT3 internal tandem duplication and D835 mutations in acute myeloid leukemia," *Haematologica*, vol. 88, no. 1, pp. 19–24, 2003.

[27] F. M. Abu-Duhier, A. C. Goodeve, G. A. Wilson, R. S. Care, I. R. Peake, and J. T. Reilly, "Identification of novel FLT-3 Asp835

mutations in adult acute myeloid leukaemia," *British Journal of Haematology*, vol. 113, no. 4, pp. 983–988, 2001.

[28] Y. Yamamoto, H. Kiyoi, Y. Nakano et al., "Activating mutation of D835 within the activation loop of *FLT3* in human hematologic malignancies," *Blood*, vol. 97, no. 8, pp. 2434–2439, 2001.

[29] H. Kiyoi, T. Naoe, Y. Nakano et al., "Prognostic implication of *FLT3* and N-RAS gene mutations in acute myeloid leukemia," *Blood*, vol. 93, no. 9, pp. 3074–3080, 1999.

[30] H. Kiyoi, M. Towatari, S. Yokota et al., "Internal tandem duplication of the *FLT3* gene is a novel modality of elongation mutation which causes constitutive activation of the product," *Leukemia*, vol. 12, no. 9, pp. 1333–1337, 1998.

[31] M. Levis and D. Small, "*FLT3*: ITDoes matter in leukemia," *Leukemia*, vol. 17, no. 9, pp. 1738–1752, 2003.

[32] D. L. Stirewalt and J. P. Radich, "The role of *FLT3* in haematopoietic malignancies," *Nature Reviews Cancer*, vol. 3, no. 9, pp. 650–665, 2003.

[33] S. Meshinchi, W. G. Woods, D. L. Stirewalt et al., "Prevalence and prognostic significance of *FLT3* internal tandem duplication in pediatric acute myeloid leukemia," *Blood*, vol. 97, no. 1, pp. 89–94, 2001.

[34] D. C. Liang, L.-Y. Shih, I.-J. Hung et al., "Clinical relevance of internal tandem duplication of the *FLT3* gene in childhood acute myeloid leukemia," *Cancer*, vol. 94, no. 12, pp. 3292–3298, 2002.

[35] S. Yokota, H. Kiyoi, M. Nakao et al., "Internal tandem duplication of the *FLT3* gene is preferentially seen in acute myeloid leukemia and myelodysplastic syndrome among various hematological malignancies. A study on a large series of patients and cell lines," *Leukemia*, vol. 11, no. 10, pp. 1605–1609, 1997.

[36] P. Chang, M. Kang, A. Xiao et al., "*FLT3* mutation incidence and timing of origin in a population case series of pediatric leukemia," *BMC Cancer*, vol. 10, article 513, 2010.

[37] S. Horiike, S. Yokota, M. Nakao et al., "Tandem duplications of the *FLT3* receptor gene are associated with leukemic transformation of myelodysplasia," *Leukemia*, vol. 11, no. 9, pp. 1442–1446, 1997.

[38] E. Ishii, M. Zaitsu, K. Ihara, T. Hara, and S. Miyazaki, "High expression but no internal tandem duplication of *FLT3* in normal hematopoietic cells," *Pediatric Hematology and Oncology*, vol. 16, no. 5, pp. 437–441, 1999.

[39] P. D. Kottaridis, R. E. Gale, M. E. Frew et al., "The presence of a *FLT3* internal tandem duplication in patients with acute myeloid leukemia (AML) adds important prognostic information to cytogenetic risk group and response to the first cycle of chemotherapy: analysis of 854 patients from the United Kingdom Medical Research Council AML 10 and 12 trials," *Blood*, vol. 98, no. 6, pp. 1752–1759, 2001.

[40] S. Schnittger, C. Schoch, M. Dugas et al., "Analysis of *FLT3* length mutations in 1003 patients with acute myeloid leukemia: correlation to cytogenetics, FAB subtype, and prognosis in the AMLCG study and usefulness as a marker for the detection of minimal residual disease," *Blood*, vol. 100, no. 1, pp. 59–66, 2002.

[41] S. P. Whitman, K. J. Archer, L. Feng et al., "Absence of the wild-type allele predicts poor prognosis in adult de novo acute myeloid leukemia with normal cytogenetics and the internal tandem duplication of *FLT3*: a cancer and leukemia group B study," *Cancer Research*, vol. 61, no. 19, pp. 7233–7239, 2001.

[42] A. Y. H. Leung, C.-H. Man, and Y.-L. Kwong, "*FLT3* inhibition: a moving and evolving target in acute myeloid," *Leukemia*, vol. 27, pp. 260–268, 2013.

[43] W. Li, L. Zhang, L. Huang, Y. Mi, and J. Wang, "Meta-analysis for the potential application of *FLT3*-TKD mutations as prognostic indicator in non-promyelocytic AML," *Leukemia Research*, vol. 36, no. 2, pp. 186–191, 2012.

[44] M. Warren, R. Luthra, C. C. Yin et al., "Clinical impact of change of *FLT3* mutation status in acute myeloid leukemia patients," *Modern Pathology*, vol. 25, no. 10, pp. 1405–1412, 2012.

17

Plasma and Red Cell Reference Intervals of 5-Methyltetrahydrofolate of Healthy Adults in Whom Biochemical Functional Deficiencies of Folate and Vitamin B_{12} Had Been Excluded

Agata Sobczyńska-Malefora, Dominic J. Harrington, Kieran Voong, and Martin J. Shearer

The Nutristasis Unit, The Centre for Haemostasis and Thrombosis, GSTS Pathology (Part of King's Healthcare Partners), St. Thomas' Hospital, London SE1 7EH, UK

Correspondence should be addressed to Agata Sobczyńska-Malefora; agata.malefora@gsts.com

Academic Editor: David Varon

5-Methyltetrahydrofolate (5-MTHF) is the predominant form of folate and a strong determinant of homocysteine concentrations. There is evidence that suboptimal 5-MTHF availability is a risk factor for cardiovascular disease independent of homocysteine. The analysis of folates remains challenging and is almost exclusively limited to the reporting of "total" folate rather than individual molecular forms. The purpose of this study was to establish the reference intervals of 5-MTHF in plasma and red cells of healthy adults who had been prescreened to exclude biochemical evidence of functional deficiency of folate and/or vitamin B_{12}. Functional folate and vitamin B_{12} status was assessed by respective plasma measurements of homocysteine and methylmalonic acid in 144 healthy volunteers, aged 19–64 years. After the exclusion of 10 individuals, values for 134 subjects were used to establish the upper reference limits for homocysteine (13 μmol/L females and 15 μmol/L males) and methylmalonic acid (430 nmol/L). Subjects with values below these cutoffs were designated as folate and vitamin B_{12} replete and their plasma and red cell 5-MTHF reference intervals determined, N = 126: 6.6–39.9 nmol/L and 223–1041 nmol/L, respectively. The application of these intervals will assist in the evaluation of folate status and facilitate studies to evaluate the relationship of 5-MTHF to disease.

1. Introduction

5-MTHF, the predominant form of folate (vitamin B_9) in plasma and red cells, is a substrate for the methionine synthase and vitamin B_{12} (methylcobalamin form—methyl-Cbl) mediated conversion of homocysteine (tHcy) to methionine (Figure 1). Suboptimal 5-MTHF availability leads to an increase in circulating homocysteine (hyperhomocysteinaemia) which has been associated with many diseases and health complications including cardiovascular disease [1, 2]. There is also evidence to suggest that 5-MTHF deficiency may be a cardiovascular risk factor independent of homocysteine [3, 4].

In the plasma of healthy humans, 5-MTHF typically constitutes 80–90% of total folate [5, 6]. Circulatory concentrations of 5-MTHF are partly dependant on methylenetetrahydrofolate reductase (MTHFR) genotype [7, 8]. Conversely, the 5-MTHF content of red cells has been reported to vary greatly [9, 10].

Tissue folate status is typically assessed by measurement of "total" folate concentration in blood because commonly available assays are unable to differentiate between the various circulatory forms. Analysis of folate in red cells is considered to be a strong indicator of folate adequacy because it reflects intracellular status and is not influenced by recent or transient changes in dietary folate intake. Traditionally a value of 317 nmol/L (140 μg/L) for red cell folate (RCF) has been considered as the cutoff concentration for folate adequacy [11]. Serum levels <7.9 nmol/L (<3 μg/L) usually indicate folate insufficiency. However, there is little consensus for the reference intervals for plasma and red cell folate [12].

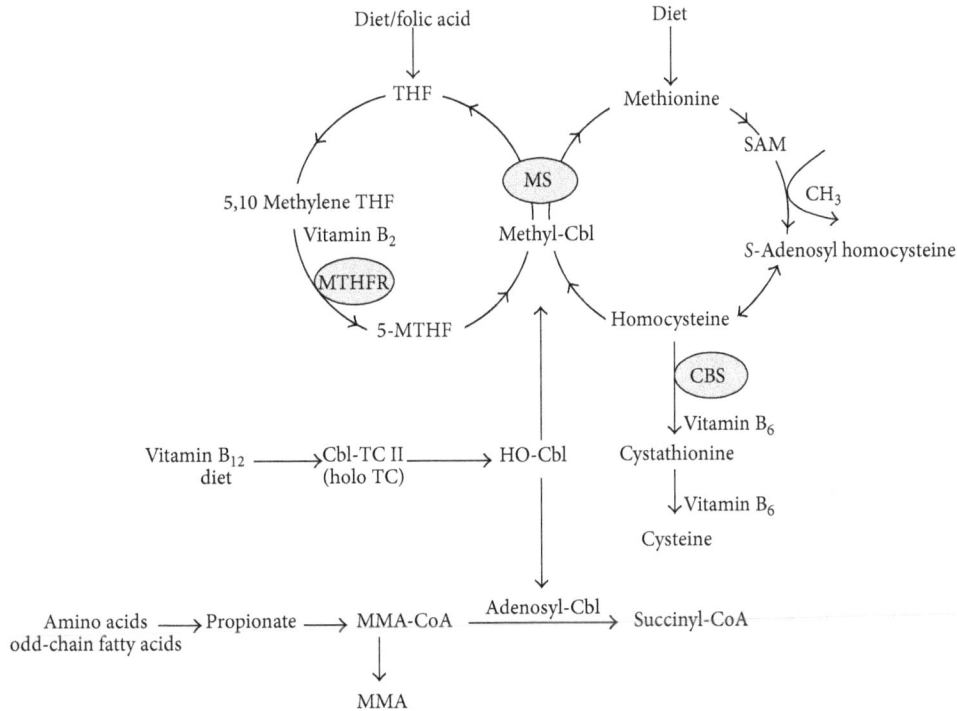

FIGURE 1: Homocysteine, folate, and vitamin B_{12} metabolism. THF (tetrahydrofolate), 5-MTHF (5-methyltetrahydrofolate), MTHFR (methylene tetrahydrofolate reductase), MS (methionine synthase), CBS (cystathionine beta-synthase), SAM (S-adenosyl methionine), Cbl (cobalamin), TC II (transcobalamin), holo TC (holotrascobalamin), OH-Cbl (hydroxocobalamin), MMA-CoA (methylmalonyl-CoA), and MMA (methylmalonic acid).

Furthermore, methodology bias is very common in folate assays and particularly pronounced for RCF values, as a consequence of variation in approach to the preparation and storage of red cell lysates [12]. This lack of harmonisation of folate methods prevents the interlaboratory adoption of reference intervals.

The purpose of this study was to establish reference intervals for plasma and red cell 5-MTHF in adults, using a fully validated HPLC assay, after excluding subjects in whom functional folate and/or vitamin B_{12} deficiency was biochemically indicated by elevated concentrations of tHcy and/or MMA, respectively. The basis of an elevated MMA concentration as a sensitive functional indicator of vitamin B_{12} deficiency is that 5-deoxyadenosylcobalamin is an essential cofactor for the conversion of methylmalonyl-CoA to succinyl-CoA. In vitamin B_{12} insufficiency/deficiency (5-deoxyadenosylcobalamin form) the excess of methylmalonyl-CoA is hydrolysed to MMA causing the circulatory concentration of MMA to increase (Figure 1) [13].

2. Materials and Methods

2.1. Study Participants and Study Design. One hundred and forty-four volunteers, aged 19–64 years, were recruited from members of staff from St. Thomas' Hospital by advertisement. Subjects were excluded from participation if they were pregnant or taking vitamin supplements or drugs (e.g., phenytoin) known to interfere with folate or homocysteine

metabolism. Recruited subjects were then screened to assess their functional folate and vitamin B_{12} status. This led to the exclusion of ten subjects who had either outlying values of tHcy and/or MMA or who admitted to previously undeclared use of relevant dietary supplements and/or drugs. Of the remaining 134 subjects, those with tHcy and MMA values above their respective 97.5th percentiles were deemed to be potentially folate or vitamin B_{12} deficient and were excluded from our reported reference intervals for 5-MTHF. The study was approved by St. Thomas' Hospital Local Research Ethics Committee and written consent was obtained from all participants.

2.2. Blood Collection and Analytical Methods. Nonfasting, venous blood samples were collected into EDTA-containing tubes and immediately placed on ice and protected from light. Following hematocrit determinations, lysates were prepared by the addition of $100\,\mu$L whole blood to $900\,\mu$L of $5\,$g/L ascorbic acid solution. Plasma was prepared by centrifugation. All samples were stored at $-70°$C until analysis.

Plasma tHcy was measured by automated fluorescence polarization immunoassay (IMx, Abbott Laboratories). The intra- and inter-CVs for this assay were 2.0% and 2.7%, respectively. Plasma MMA was analysed using HPLC [14]. The differences of duplicate analysis of 16 samples ranged from 0.0 to 10.9%, while the interassay CVs for five samples (concentration range: 177–1114 nmol/L) were between 6 and 12%.

Plasma and red blood cell 5-MTHF were measured by HPLC as previously described [15]. In brief, 4-aminoacetophenone was used as an internal standard [16] and Bond Elut C_{18} (100 mg, 1 mL reservoir) cartridges (Varian Inc.) were utilised for SPE with an elution strategy based on that of Pfeiffer et al. [6] with some in-house modifications. Sample components were separated using a ACE C_{18}, 3 μm column (125 × 4.6 mm) supplied by Hichrom, UK, with a mobile phase composition of 0.033 mol/L potassium phosphate buffer (pH 2.3) : acetonitrile : methanol (89 : 6.6 : 4.4, by volume) at a flow rate of 0.34 mL/min. The fluorescence detector wavelength settings were: excitation 290 nm and emission 365 nm.

A primary stock solution of 5-MTHF was prepared by dissolving ~5 mg of 5-MTHF powder in 10 mL of 20 mM potassium phosphate buffer pH 7.2 with 1 g/L cysteine. An aliquot (1 mL) of this stock solution was removed to determine the concentration by UV spectrophotometry and 90 mg of ascorbic acid powder was immediately added to the remaining stock solution. The absorbance of 5-MTHF was measured at 290 nm using the molar absorptivity value of $32000\,\mathrm{L\,mol^{-1}\,cm^{-1}}$ after 1 in 40 and 1 in 33.3 dilution with 20 mmol/L potassium phosphate buffer pH 7.2 containing 1 g/L cysteine.

The primary stock solution (1018.70 μmol/L) was diluted 1 in 5 in 10 g/L ascorbic acid and this stock solution was aliquoted and stored at −70°C (secondary stock: 203.74 μmol/L). One aliquot of the secondary stock solution was diluted further with 1 g/L ascorbic acid to the concentration of 20.37 μmol/L (tertiary stock). This stock was used on the day of analysis to prepare a calibration curve of a minimum of four points.

The accuracy of our 5-MTHF calibration standard was checked against the Standard Reference Material (SRM) 1955 (National Institute of Standards & Technology, USA) which included three reference samples with certified 5-MTHF concentrations (uncertainties) of 4.26 ± 0.25, 9.73 ± 0.24, and 37.1 ± 1.4 nmol/L [17]. These reference samples were used to construct a calibration curve to verify the 5-MTHF concentration of our secondary stock solution with the theoretical concentration (by UV spectroscopy) of 203.74 μmol/L. The calculated concentration of our secondary stock using the SRM 1955 generated standard curve was 196.13 μmol/L (3.6% difference). In another analytical run the standard curve was prepared by serial dilutions of the 20.37 μmol/L 5-MTHF tertiary stock (as in the typical HPLC run) and SRM 1955 samples were analysed. The CVs for the means derived from the values assigned by the manufacturer of SRM 1955 and obtained in these analyses ranged from 2.1 to 5.9% for samples with the concentration of 4.26 and 37.1 nmol/L, respectively.

The 5-MTHF red cell folate concentration was calculated according to the formula

5-MTHF in red cells

= {whole blood 5-MTHF

− [plasma 5-MTHF (1 − hematocrit)]}

× hematocrit^{-1} (1)

[4, 18].

2.3. Statistical Analysis. Normality of data was checked by the Kolmogorov-Smirnov test. Where the variables were not normally distributed; nonparametric tests or $\log_{10}$ transformed values were used. Subjects with outlying tHcy, MMA, and 5-MTHF values were excluded using the Tukey test [19, 20]. For the lower (where appropriate) and upper reference limits the 2.5th and 97.5th percentiles were used. The z-test was used to establish whether to partition reference values by sex [19, 21]. The independent samples Student's t-test was applied to compare the values between sexes. Confidence intervals for the lower and upper reference limits were obtained using the rank numbers [19, 22]. Pearson's or Spearman's correlations were carried out to examine relationships between two continuous variables. Results were considered statistically significant if the observed, two-sided P value was <0.05. Statistical analyses were carried out using SPSS for Windows (SPSS Inc., USA).

3. Results

3.1. Screening for Subjects with Outlying tHcy and MMA Results and the 97.5th Percentiles for tHcy and MMA. Of the 144 subjects initially recruited, 72 (50%) were represented by laboratory staff, 36 (25%) held administrative positions, 24 (16%) were from supporting services, and 12 (8%) held clinical posts. The majority of participants were Caucasian $N = 107$ (74%), with 20 (14%) of Asian and 17 (12%) of Afro-Caribbean origins. Ten of these subjects were excluded before the determination of the upper cutoff values for plasma tHcy and MMA. Three of these 10 subjects were taking vitamin supplements and one subject was taking opiates which are known to affect folate metabolism [23, 24]. Two subjects with tHcy >15 μmol/L, on further investigation, were found to be taking medication that interfered with tHcy metabolism [23, 25]. The remaining four subjects were identified as outliers (Tukey method). Two of these four subjects had an MMA >1000 nmol/L (suggestive of vitamin B_{12} deficiency); one had a family history of pernicious anaemia whilst the other individual was on medications and consumed a vegetarian diet. One of these four subjects had a plasma tHcy of 25.7 μmol/L with low MMA (121 nmol/L) suggesting folate deficiency and in another both markers were elevated. To the best of our knowledge no other volunteers participating in the study were taking vitamins or any drugs/medications interfering with folate/homocysteine metabolism. The remaining 134 subjects were used to establish the upper cutoff values for tHcy.

Plasma tHcy was normally distributed ($P = 0.348$), whilst plasma MMA was positively skewed ($P = 0.007$). There was a gender difference in tHcy concentrations ($P = 0.01$) with males having higher values. Plasma MMA concentration did not differ between genders ($P = 0.440$). After the exclusion of the upper 2.5th percentile, upper reference limits for

TABLE 1: Summary of results of $N = 126$ subjects used to derive 5-MTHF reference intervals.

	Females $N = 69$ mean (SD); median	Males $N = 57$ mean (SD); median	Student's t-test P value	All $N = 126$ mean (SD); median
Age (range)	38 (10); 38 (23–60)	38 (12); 36 (19–64)	0.730	38 (11); 37
tHcy (μmol/L)	8.4 (1.8); 7.9	9.7 (2.1); 9.7	<0.001	8.9 (2.1); 8.9
MMA (nmol/L)	116 (93); 101	112 (76); 100	0.794	114 (85); 100
Plasma 5-MTHF (nmol/L)	19.4 (8.5); 19.1	18.7 (8.2); 17.8	0.624	19.1 (8.3); 18.2
Redcell 5-MTHF (nmol/L)*	583 (222); 572	585 (164); 557	0.975	586 (197); 560
Whole blood 5-MTHF (nmol/L)	618 (229); 592	611 (172); 582	0.838	615 (205); 584

*Result adjusted for plasma 5-MTHF content.

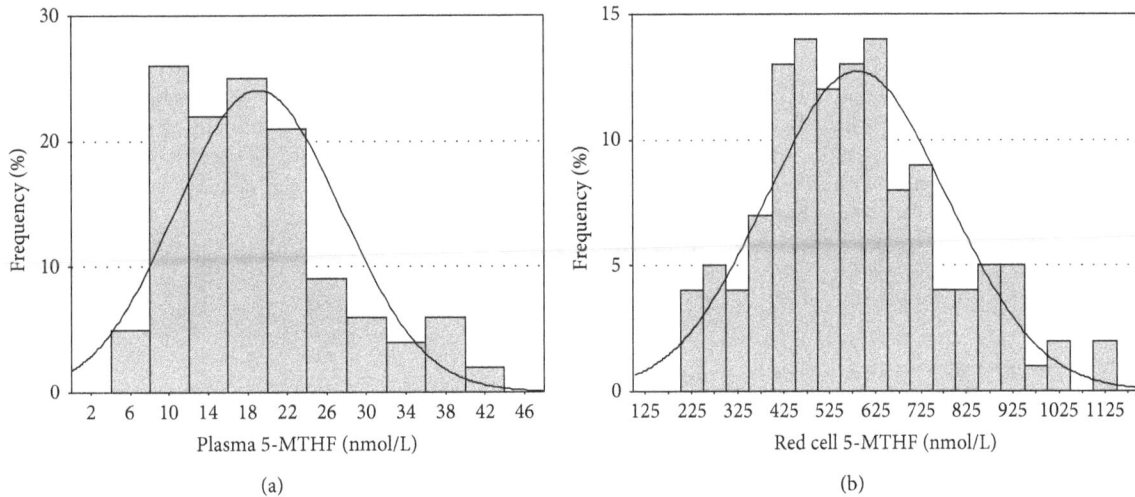

FIGURE 2: Distribution of the 5-MTHF concentrations in plasma and red cells.

tHcy were established as 13 μmol/L (females, $N = 72$) and 15 μmol/L (males, $N = 62$) and for MMA as 430 nmol/L (all 134 subjects).

3.2. Establishing Reference Intervals for 5-MTHF.

Five subjects with functional deficiencies of folate and/or vitamin B_{12} as defined by elevated tHcy (>13 μmol/L for females and >15 μmol/L for males) and MMA (>430 nmol/L for both genders) were excluded from further analysis. In addition, three subjects had highly elevated red cells 5-MTHF of >1143 nmol/L (identified by the Tukey test as outlying values) and these subjects were also excluded. There were no outlying plasma 5-MTHF values. Hence, 126 subjects were eligible for the construction of the reference intervals for 5-MTHF. The ethnic distribution of these 126 subjects was 93 Caucasian (73%), 17 Afro-Caribbean (14%), and 16 Asian (13%). The proportion of women within these ethnic groups was 41% Caucasian, 65% Afro-Caribbean, and 44% Asian. The age and summary of all results for females and males used to derive 5-MTHF reference intervals is given in Table 1. Age and all the parameters measured followed a normal distribution. The values remained normally distributed after partition by sex. Reference intervals together with 90% confidence intervals for the lower and upper 95% reference limits are displayed in Table 2. The distribution of 5-MTHF concentrations in plasma and red blood cells is shown in Figure 2. Plasma 5-MTHF correlated with whole blood 5-MTHF ($r = 0.565$,

TABLE 2: Reference intervals for 5-MTHF with 90% confidence intervals for lower and upper 95% reference limits.

Analyte	Reference intervals	Lower reference limit	Upper reference limit
Plasma 5-MTHF (nmol/L)	6.6–39.9	5.3–8.9	36.9–41.7
Redcell 5-MTHF (nmol/L)	223–1040	206–291	930–1110
Whole blood 5-MTHF (nmol/L)	245–1102	224–311	969–1184

$P < 0.001$), red cell 5-MTHF ($r = 0.523$, $P < 0.001$) but did not correlate with age ($r = 0.087$, $P = 0.332$), tHcy ($r = -0.122$, $P = 0.172$), or MMA ($r = -0.103$, $P = 0.256$). Red cell 5-MTHF correlated with whole blood 5-MTHF ($r = 0.998$, $P < 0.001$) and age ($r = 0.204$, $P = 0.022$) but did not correlate with tHcy ($r = -0.172$, $P = 0.054$) and MMA ($r = -0.047$, $P = 0.605$). Whole blood 5-MTHF, in addition to its correlations with age, plasma, and red cell 5-MTHF, correlated with tHcy ($r = -0.181$, $P = 0.043$).

4. Discussion

Reference intervals of 5-MTHF were determined for plasma (6.6–39.9 nmol/L) and red cells (223–1040 nmol/L) for healthy adults aged 19–64 years. Separate reference intervals are also shown for the whole blood 5-MTHF which can be utilised if plasma 5-MTHF is not available to correct for red cell 5-MTHF contents. Many laboratories performing the standard RCF assay do not adjust their results for folate contents in plasma. Although this approach reduces assay costs, it may provide misleading RCF status, especially when plasma folate concentrations are >45 nmol/L [26].

Subjects with likely functional folate and/or vitamin B_{12} deficiency/insufficiency were excluded from the construction of 5-MTHF reference intervals after the determination of cohort specific upper limits for plasma tHcy and MMA. The upper limits for plasma tHcy and MMA were established prior to removal of six subjects who on subsequent review were discovered to be taking previously nondeclared medications or supplements and four subjects with outlying tHcy and/or MMA values. This process is in agreement with expert recommendations [27]. The value for the upper reference limit for tHcy of 13 μmol/L for females and 15 μmol/L for males established in our current study is similar to the upper limits of 12.8 and 14.7 μmol/L observed for females and males, respectively (nonsmokers aged 40–42 years with high folate intakes and low-moderate coffee consumption), resident in western Norway [28]. The difference of 2 μmol/L between the upper tHcy reference limit for females and males is consistent with a study reported by Jacques et al. [29]. Although it has been well documented that tHcy is influenced by gender and age [29], laboratories often still choose to adopt a single cutoff value to distinguish normal from elevated tHcy concentrations.

The measurement of plasma MMA is accepted as a sensitive functional marker of cobalamin deficiency/insufficiency and avoids the ambiguities associated with commonly used serum cobalamin assays [13]. As with tHcy, the upper limit above which an MMA concentration is considered to be elevated differs between laboratories [30] and a variety of approaches to determine reference intervals have been used. For example, Rasmussen et al. [31] reported an inner 95% reference intervals for MMA of 80–280 nmol/L established in 235 subjects prior to exclusion of those with a high probability of cobalamin deficiency (based on MMA decrease post cobalamin supplementation), outliers and those with high tHcy. In another study, an MMA concentration >470 nmol/L (inner 95%) was used as the upper limit in healthy adults with no clinical laboratory evidence of cobalamin deficiency [32].

Population-based reference intervals for 5-MTHF have not previously been reported. We are therefore unable to compare our findings with those of others. However the values for 5-MTHF concentrations obtained are in good agreement with data from other studies [6, 33]. In comparison with the median of 427 nmol/L (range: 92–1086) for red cell 5-MTHF from 109 healthy subjects, aged 18–65 years, reported by Smulders et al. [8], the values in our study were higher: median 560 nmol/L (range: 206–1110). This might be attributed to differences in methodologies and the fact that individuals with mild to moderate B-vitamin deficiencies were not excluded in that study [8].

A positive correlation between red cell 5-MTHF concentrations and age observed in this study is consistent with previous observations [34, 35]. Conversely, higher red cell

5-MTHF values in older participants are not reflected by a corresponding decrease in tHcy levels, suggesting that age is a folate-independent determinant of tHcy. It is not clear why folate concentrations are higher in the elderly. It has been suggested that this could represent an oversupply of the vitamin (diet) or it could reflect the tendency, as opposed to the younger group, to retain folate both in plasma and red blood cells [35]. Surprisingly, plasma 5-MTHF did not correlate with tHcy in our selected cohort used to establish 5-MTHF reference intervals. However, the whole blood 5-MTHF correlated weakly with tHcy (P = 0.043) and correlations of red cell 5-MTHF with tHcy were approaching statistical significance (P = 0.054). These weak or lack of correlations may be attributed to the relatively small sample size and the fact that all subjects with outlying tHcy and above our reference cutoffs were removed. To support this, Spearman's correlations (data not shown) on all subjects initially recruited N = 144 demonstrated stronger and expected significant correlations of plasma or red cell (whole blood) 5-MTHF with tHcy.

One caveat to our study is that the 5-MTHF reference intervals are unlikely to apply to children. Opladen et al. reported that serum 5-MTHF levels are the highest in the first year of life, followed by a continuous decrease until the age of 16 years [36].

5. Conclusions

In conclusion, the plasma and red cell 5-MTHF reference intervals for an adult population were determined from 126 subjects without evidence of functional folate and/or vitamin B_{12} deficiency as assessed by tHcy and MMA analyses. The application of these intervals will assist in the evaluation of folate status and facilitate the evaluation of 5-MTHF as an independent risk factor for disease states.

Ethical Approval

The study was approved by St. Thomas' Hospital Local Research Ethics Committee and written consent was obtained from all participants, no. 07/H0804/148.

Conflict of Interests

The authors declare that there is no conflict of interests regarding the publication of this paper.

Acknowledgments

The authors would like to thank Mrs. Renata Gorska (Centre for Haemostasis and Thrombosis) for preparation of the figures.

References

[1] H. McNulty, K. Pentieva, L. Hoey, and M. Ward, "Homocysteine, B-vitamins and CVD," *Proceedings of the Nutrition Society*, vol. 67, no. 2, pp. 232–237, 2008.

[2] K. S. McCully, "Homocysteine, vitamins, and vascular disease prevention," *The American Journal of Clinical Nutrition*, vol. 86, no. 5, pp. 1563S–1568S, 2007.

[3] C. Antoniades, C. Shirodaria, N. Warrick et al., "5-methyltetrahydrofolate rapidly improves endothelial function and decreases superoxide production in human vessels: effects on vascular tetrahydrobiopterin availability and endothelial nitric oxide synthase coupling," *Circulation*, vol. 114, no. 11, pp. 1193–1201, 2006.

[4] I. Quéré, T. V. Perneger, J. Zittoun et al., "Red blood cell methylfolate and plasma homocysteine as risk factors for venous thromboembolism: a matched case-control study," *The Lancet*, vol. 359, no. 9308, pp. 747–752, 2002.

[5] R. J. Leeming, A. Pollock, L. J. Melville, and C. G. B. Hamon, "Measurement of 5-methyltetrahydrofolic acid in man by high-performance liquid chromatography," *Metabolism*, vol. 39, no. 9, pp. 902–904, 1990.

[6] C. M. Pfeiffer, Z. Fazili, L. McCoy, M. Zhang, and E. W. Gunter, "Determination of folate vitamers in human serum by stable-isotope-dilution tandem mass spectrometry and comparison with radioassay and microbiologic assay," *Clinical Chemistry*, vol. 50, no. 2, pp. 423–432, 2004.

[7] Z. Fazili and C. M. Pfeiffer, "Measurement of folates in serum and conventionally prepared whole blood lysates: application of an automated 96-well plate isotope-dilution tandem mass spectrometry method," *Clinical Chemistry*, vol. 50, no. 12, pp. 2378–2381, 2004.

[8] Y. M. Smulders, D. E. C. Smith, R. M. Kok et al., "Red blood cell folate vitamer distribution in healthy subjects is determined by the methylenetetrahydrofolate reductase C677T polymorphism and by the total folate status," *The Journal of Nutritional Biochemistry*, vol. 18, no. 10, pp. 693–699, 2007.

[9] F. M. T. Loehrer, C. P. Angst, W. E. Haefeli, P. P. Jordan, R. Ritz, and B. Fowler, "Low whole-blood S-adenosylmethionine and correlation between 5-methyltetrahydrofolate and homocysteine in coronary artery disease," *Arteriosclerosis, Thrombosis, and Vascular Biology*, vol. 16, no. 6, pp. 727–733, 1996.

[10] M. Lucock and Z. Yates, "Measurement of red blood cell methylfolate," *The Lancet*, vol. 360, no. 9338, pp. 1021–1022, 2002.

[11] Food and Nutrition Board IoM, *Dietary Reference Intakes for Thiamin, Riboflavin, Niacin, Vitamin B_6, Folate, Vitamin B_{12}, Pantothenic Acid, Biotin and Choline*, National Academy Press, Washington, DC, USA, 1998.

[12] UK NEQAS Haematinics, "Report on reference range data collected from haematinics scheme participants in July 2007," Tech. Rep., Good Hope Hospital, Haematology Department, Heart of England Foundation Trust, 2008.

[13] G. Hølleland, J. Schneede, P. M. Ueland, P. K. Lund, H. Refsum, and S. Sandberg, "Cobalamin deficiency in general practice. Assessment of the diagnostic utility and cost-benefit analysis of methylmalonic acid determination in relation to current diagnostic strategies," *Clinical Chemistry*, vol. 45, no. 2, pp. 189–198, 1999.

[14] P. J. Babidge and W. J. Babidge, "Determination of methylmalonic acid by high-performance liquid chromatography," *Analytical Biochemistry*, vol. 216, no. 2, pp. 424–426, 1994.

[15] A. Sobczynska-Malefora, D. J. Harrington, M. C. E. Lomer et al., "Erythrocyte folate and 5-methyltetrahydrofolate levels decline during 6 months of oral anticoagulation with warfarin," *Blood Coagulation and Fibrinolysis*, vol. 20, no. 4, pp. 297–302, 2009.

[16] J. Chladek, L. Sispera, and J. Martinkova, "High-performance liquid chromatographic assay for the determination of 5-methyltetrahydrofolate in human plasma," *Journal of Chromatography B*, vol. 744, pp. 307–313, 2000.

[17] H. Ihara, T. Watanabe, N. Hashizume et al., "Commutability of National Institute of Standards and Technology standard reference material 1955 homocysteine and folate in frozen human serum for total folate with automated assays," *Annals of Clinical Biochemistry*, vol. 47, no. 6, pp. 541–548, 2010.

[18] A. V. Hoffbrand, F. A. Newcombe, and D. L. Mollin, "Method of assay of red cell folate activity and the value of the assay as a test for folate deficiency," *Journal of Clinical Pathology*, vol. 19, no. 1, pp. 17–28, 1966.

[19] CLSI, *Defining, Establishing, and Verifying Reference Intervals in the Clinical Laboratory, Approved Guideline*, CLSI document C28-A3, Clinical and Laboratory Standards Institute, Wayne, Pa, USA, 3rd edition, 2008.

[20] J. W. Tukey, *Exploratory Data Analysis*, Addison-Wesley, Reading, Mass, USA, 1977.

[21] E. K. Harris and J. C. Boyd, "On dividing reference data into subgroups to produce separate reference ranges," *Clinical Chemistry*, vol. 36, no. 2, pp. 265–270, 1990.

[22] H. E. Solberg, "International Federation of Clinical Chemistry (IFCC). Scientific Committee, Clinical Section. Expert Panel on Theory of Reference Values, and International Committee for Standardization in Haematology (ICSH). Standing Committee on Reference Values. Approved Recommendation (1986) on the theory of reference values. Part 1. The concept of reference values," *Journal of Clinical Chemistry and Clinical Biochemistry*, vol. 25, no. 5, pp. 337–342, 1987.

[23] E. H. Reynolds, R. J. Wrighton, A. L. Johnson, J. Preece, and I. Chanarin, "Inter-relations of folic acid and vitamin B_{12} in drug-treated epileptic patients," *Epilepsia*, vol. 12, no. 2, pp. 165–171, 1971.

[24] W.-Y. Au, S.-K. Tsang, B. K. L. Cheung, T.-S. Siu, E. S. K. Ma, and S. Tam, "Cough mixture abuse as a novel cause of folate deficiency: a prospective, community-based, controlled study," *Haematologica*, vol. 92, no. 4, pp. 562–563, 2007.

[25] U. Sener, Y. Zorlu, O. Karaguzel, O. Ozdamar, I. Coker, and M. Topbas, "Effects of common anti-epileptic drug monotherapy on serum levels of homocysteine, vitamin B_{12}, folic acid and vitamin B6," *Seizure*, vol. 15, no. 2, pp. 79–85, 2006.

[26] N. Philpott, B. P. Kelleher, O. P. Smith, and S. D. O'Broin, "High serum folates and the simplification of red cell folate analysis," *Clinical and Laboratory Haematology*, vol. 23, no. 1, pp. 15–20, 2001.

[27] H. Refsum, A. D. Smith, P. M. Ueland et al., "Facts and recommendations about total homocysteine determinations: an expert opinion," *Clinical Chemistry*, vol. 50, no. 1, pp. 3–32, 2004.

[28] O. Nygård, H. Refsum, P. M. Ueland, and S. E. Vollset, "Major lifestyle determinants of plasma total homocysteine distribution: the hordaland homocysteine study," *The American Journal of Clinical Nutrition*, vol. 67, no. 2, pp. 263–270, 1998.

[29] P. F. Jacques, I. H. Rosenberg, G. Rogers et al., "Serum total homocysteine concentrations in adolescent and adult Americans: results from the third National Health and Nutrition Examination Survey," *The American Journal of Clinical Nutrition*, vol. 69, no. 3, pp. 482–489, 1999.

[30] E. Nexo and E. Hoffmann-Lücke, "Holotranscobalamin, a marker of vitamin B-12 status: analytical aspects and clinical utility," *The American Journal of Clinical Nutrition*, vol. 94, no. 1, pp. 359S–365S, 2011.

[31] K. Rasmussen, J. Moller, M. Lyngbak, A. M. Pedersen, and L. Dybkjaer, "Age- and gender-specific reference intervals for total homocysteine and methylmalonic acid in plasma before and after vitamin supplementation," *Clinical Chemistry*, vol. 42, pp. 630–636, 1996.

[32] A. Goringe, R. Ellis, I. McDowell et al., "The limited value of methylmalonic acid, homocysteine and holotranscobalamin in the diagnosis of early B_{12} deficiency," *Haematologica*, vol. 91, no. 2, pp. 231–234, 2006.

[33] Z. Fazili, C. M. Pfeiffer, and M. Zhang, "Comparison of serum folate species analyzed by LC-MS/MS with total folate measured by microbiologic assay and Bio-Rad radioassay," *Clinical Chemistry*, vol. 53, no. 4, pp. 781–784, 2007.

[34] J. D. Wright, K. Bialostosky, E. W. Gunter et al., "Blood folate and vitamin B_{12}: United States, 1988–94," *Vital and Health Statistics*, no. 243, pp. 1–78, 1998.

[35] J. Selhub, P. F. Jacques, G. Dallal, S. Choumenkovitch, and G. Rogers, "The use of blood concentrations of vitamins and their respective functional indicators to define folate and vitamin B_{12} status," *Food and Nutrition Bulletin*, vol. 29, no. 2, pp. S67–S73, 2008.

[36] T. Opladen, V. T. Ramaekers, G. Heimann, and N. Blau, "Analysis of 5-methyltetrahydrofolate in serum of healthy children," *Molecular Genetics and Metabolism*, vol. 87, no. 1, pp. 61–65, 2006.

18

The Observation Report of Red Blood Cell Morphology in Thailand Teenager by Using Data Mining Technique

Sarawut Saichanma, Sucha Chulsomlee, Nonthaya Thangrua, Pornsuri Pongsuchart, and Duangmanee Sanmun

Division of Clinical Microscopy, Faculty of Medical Technology, Huachiew Chalermprakiet University, Samut Prakan 10540, Thailand

Correspondence should be addressed to Sarawut Saichanma; sarawut@hcu.ac.th

Academic Editor: Elvira Grandone

It is undeniable that laboratory information is important in healthcare in many ways such as management, planning, and quality improvement. Laboratory diagnosis and laboratory results from each patient are organized from every treatment. These data are useful for retrospective study exploring a relationship between laboratory results and diseases. By doing so, it increases efficiency in diagnosis and quality in laboratory report. Our study will utilize J48 algorithm, a data mining technique to predict abnormality in peripheral blood smear from 1,362 students by using 13 data set of hematological parameters gathered from automated blood cell counter. We found that the decision tree which is created from the algorithm can be used as a practical guideline for RBC morphology prediction by using 4 hematological parameters (MCV, MCH, Hct, and RBC). The average prediction of RBC morphology has true positive, false positive, precision, recall, and accuracy of 0.940, 0.050, 0.945, 0.940, and 0.943, respectively. A newly found paradigm in managing medical laboratory information will be helpful in organizing, researching, and assisting correlation in multiple disciplinary other than medical science which will eventually lead to an improvement in quality of test results and more accurate diagnosis.

1. Introduction

Data mining technique is a process of discovering pattern of data. The patterns discovered must be meaningful in that they lead to some advantage. The overall goal of the data mining process is to extract information from a data set and transform it into an understandable data in order to aid user decision making. It utilizes methods such as statistics and mathematics to explore a relationship of data set or suitable conditions of those data, which leads to the extract of needed information or knowledge of relations. The decision tree is a supported modeling that represents the classification process of input data as a tree-like graph. It is based on Divide and Conquer concept, which is formed by many rules that branched out from the tree until the decision is made. There are many methods of decision tree algorithm such as AD-Tree, C4.5 decision (J48), or Random-Tree.

The J48 algorithm is an open source JAVA implementing C4.5 in WEKA (Waikato Environment for Knowledge Analysis) software. The tree is constructed from gain ratio, the element with a highest gain ratio assigned as the root and uses gain ratio as the splitting branch of the tree [1].

The data mining has been used widely in many fields such as marketing, public relations, prediction of economy, and weather forecast. In hematology laboratory, it has become a powerful tool in managing uncountable laboratory information in order to seek knowledge that is underlying or within any given information. Many applications of data mining in hematology were proposed such as evaluated risk factors and relationship with life-threatening infection in children with febrile neutrophilia [2], created diagnosis approached to polycythemia vera [3], and proposed an original method to identify the immunophenotypic signature of chronic lymphocytic leukemia [4].

TABLE 1: The data set in this study.

Number	Code	Description	Domain
1	Sex	Sex	Male, female
2	WBC	White blood cell count (cell/uL)	Integer
3	RBC	Red blood cell count	Integer
4	Hb	Hemoglobin (g/dL)	Integer
5	Hct	Hematocrit (%)	Integer
6	MCV	Mean corpuscular volume (fL)	Integer
7	MCH	Mean corpuscular hemoglobin (pg)	Integer
8	MCHC	Mean corpuscular hemoglobin concentration (g/dL)	Integer
9	PLT	Platelet count (cell/uL)	Integer
10	NEU	Neutrophil count (%)	Integer
11	LYMP	Lymphocyte count (%)	Integer
12	MONO	Monocyte count (%)	Integer
13	EO	Eosinophil count (%)	Integer
14	BASO	Basophil count (%)	Integer
15	RBC morphology	Red blood cell morphology	Normal, abnormal

The authors applied data mining technique to dismiss bias from individual skill which makes the report very subjective. The relationships between red blood cell morphology reporting and hematological parameters (WBC, RBC, Hb, Hct, MCV, MCH, MCHC, PLT, NEU, LYMP, MONO, EO, and BASO) from blood cell analyzer were investigated. This study shows that by applying data mining, using hematological parameters from automated blood cell analyzer can help predicting the abnormality of RBC morphology as good as the RBC morphology which reported by individual skill. In the future, this guideline can be used as tools for laboratory improvement.

2. Material and Method

2.1. Sample and Data Set. The retrospective study used 1362 results from teenagers (17–19 years old) first-year undergraduate student checkup at Huachiew Chalermprakiet University in 2011. The data set included sex, hematological parameters, and RBC morphology. The hematological parameters from automated blood cell analyzer are composed of WBC, RBC, Hb, Hct, MCV, MCH, MCHC, PLT, NEU, LYMP, MONO, EO, and BASO (SysMex XT1800i, Sysmex corporation, Kobe, Japan). The peripheral blood smear was prepared and stained by ICSH standard protocol [5]; RBC morphology was manually evaluated by medical technologist who has a license certification from the medical technology council of Thailand. Collected data are assigned to two groups: normal RBC morphology and abnormal RBC morphology. The peripheral blood smears that are reported as normochromic and normocytic are categorized as normal RBC morphology while others fall into abnormal RBC morphology category (more details about data set are shown in Table 1).

2.2. Data Analysis by Data Mining Technique. The data mining analysis was analyzed by using WEKA version 3.6.9 which the collection of machine learning algorithms for data mining

tasks [1]. The J48 which ones of decision tree of data mining technique was approached to this study. The evaluation of all the classifiers accuracy used a ten-fold cross-validation. The performance evaluation was averaged from all of ten separated evaluations. True positive (TP) was the number of abnormal RBC morphology predicted to be abnormal RBC morphology. False negative (FN) was the number of abnormal RBC morphologies predicted to be normal RBC morphology. True negative (TN) was the number of normal RBC morphologies predicted to be normal RBC morphology. False positive (FP) was the number of normal RBC morphologies predicted to be abnormal morphology. The validation measurements were investigated by accuracy, sensitivity, and specificity of result when compared with RBC morphology report. We focus on the following validation measures:

$$\text{Precision} = \text{TP}/(\text{TP} + \text{FN}),$$

$$\text{Specificity} = \text{TN}/(\text{TN} + \text{FP}),$$

$$\text{Recall} = \text{TP} / (\text{TP} + \text{TN}),$$

$$\text{Accuracy} = (\text{TP} + \text{TN})/(\text{TP} + \text{TN} + \text{FN} + \text{FP}),$$

$$F\text{-measure} = 2 * \text{Precision} * \text{Specificity}/(\text{Precision} + \text{Specificity}).$$

2.3. Statistics. All data were presented as the mean ± standard deviation (SD). The significant evaluation between different categories was performed with the independent t-test. The P value less than 0.05 was considered as statistically significant.

3. Results

The hematological parameters from blood cell analyzer and RBC morphology report of 1362 cases were evaluated. There are 260 male cases (19.1%) and 1102 female cases (80.9%). The 1362 cases of RBC morphology were evaluated. Abnormal RBC morphology was found in 354 cases (25.99%) which

TABLE 2: The hematological parameters which were categorized by RBC morphology and sex.

Hematological parameters	Female			Male		
	Abnormal blood smear (mean ± SD)	Normal blood smear (mean ± SD)	Significant (P < 0.05)	Abnormal blood smear (mean ± SD)	Normal blood smear (mean ± SD)	Significant (P < 0.05)
WBC ($\times 10^3$ cell/μL)	7.87 ± 1.85	7.62 ± 1734.89	S	8.27 ± 2.07	7.31 ± 1.66	S**
RBC (cell/μL)	5.28 ± 0.56	4.73 ± 0.36	S	6.41 ± 0.58	5.45 ± 0.38	S
Hb (mg/dL)	11.64 ± 1.22	13.02 ± 0.83	S	13.86 ± 1.11	15.34 ± 0.86	S
Hct (%)	36.18 ± 3.33	40.03 ± 2.41	S	42.66 ± 2.89	46.17 ± 2.35	S
MCV (fL)	69.09 ± 7.45	84.9 ± 4.93	S	66.98 ± 6.55	84.88 ± 4.53	S
MCH (pg)	22.22 ± 2.56	27.62 ± 1.78	S	21.76 ± 2.41	28.21 ± 1.64	S
MCHC (g/dL)	32.16 ± 1.36	32.53 ± 0.76	S	32.48 ± 1.32	33.23 ± 0.72	S
PLT ($\times 10^3$ cell/μL)	313.85 ± 69.64	273.12 ± 54.92	S	282.08 ± 61.59	253.15 ± 47.35	S
NEU (%)	57.09 ± 8.23	57.22 ± 8.06	NS	59.67 ± 9.16	57.54 ± 7.85	NS*
LYMP (%)	37.57 ± 7.58	37.45 ± 7.41	NS	34.89 ± 8.26	36.83 ± 6.98	NS
MONO (%)	2.96 ± 1.03	2.99 ± 1.05	NS	2.67 ± 0.93	2.88 ± 1.06	NS
EO (%)	2.18 ± 1.95	2.12 ± 1.93	NS	2.51 ± 1.9	2.49 ± 2.45	NS
BASO (%)	0.2 ± 0.4	0.22 ± 0.41	NS	0.27 ± 0.45	0.26 ± 0.44	NS
Total	318	784		36	224	

*NS: no statistically significant; **S: statistically significant.

classified as male 36 cases (2.64%) and female 318 cases (23.35%). The WBC, RBC, Hb, Hct, MCV, MCH, MCHC, and PLT of abnormal RBC morphology cases were significant from the normal RBC morphology cases in both male and female ($P < 0.05$). In the contrast to NEU, LYMP, MONO, EOS, and BASO were not significant RBC morphology (more details are shown in Table 2).

The data were analyzed by using J48 algorithm. The performance of J48 algorithm was evaluated by TP, FP, precision, recall, F-measure, and accuracy. The average RBC morphology prediction has TP, FP, precision, recall F-measure, and accuracy of 0.940, 0.050, 0.945, 0.940, 0.941, and 0.943, respectively. Interestingly, when all 13 data sets were analyzed by the algorithm, the program dismissed all but 4 data sets (MCV, MCH, Hct, and RBC) which were useful in predicting RBC morphology. According to the decision tree, if the MCV is less than or equal to 78.3 fL, it was labeled as abnormal RBC morphology. On the other hand, the MCV of greater than 78.3 fL, the interrelationship of MCH, Hct, and RBC are considered. In addition, this decision trees of both male and female show similarity which means that the decision tree was sex independent (more details were shown in Tables 3 and 4 and in Figure 1).

4. Discussion

The RBC morphology report is common, basic, and fundamental in hematology testing. Thus, it is needed in screening red blood cell abnormality before investigation into more specific diseases. RBC morphology reports in hematology laboratory are done manually. Undoubtedly, this report takes time, and at the end, it is very subjective and varies from one technologist to another due to individual laboratory skill and decision making skill.

TABLE 3: The confusion matrix of predicted RBC morphology by J48 algorithm.

Actual class from manual RBC morphology report	Predicted class from J48 model	
	Abnormal	Normal
Abnormal	TP (338)	FN (16)
Normal	FP (66)	TN (942)

The authors studied the mean and SD of parameters and found that no parameter can clearly classify RBC morphology whether normal or abnormal. Some data are still overlapped but those data are not applicable to use mean and SD to differentiate. Though, there are some parameters such as WBC, Hb, Hct, RBC, MCV, MCH, MCHC, and PLT that are significantly different. According to what we found, Hb, Hct, RBC, MCV, MCH, and MCHC are all indication of overall red blood cell, so the variations in those parameters are related to the variation of changes in red blood cell morphology. MCV, MCH, Hct, and RBC are related to changes found in RBC morphology on blood smear more than those found in RBC and MCHC. Hence, when analyzed with J48 algorithm, we found these parameters on decision tree arranged in order of degree of changes in RBC morphology on blood smear (MCV, MCH, Hct, and RBC, resp.). Whichever a parameter that has minimal or no effect is not specific to RBC morphology as seen in MCHC. Though MCHC is the parameter that reflects mean corpuscular hemoglobin concentration of individual red blood cell, report from previous studies has shown that MCHC showed the least change but the use of MCHC is limited to only in quality control purpose more than in diagnostic purpose [6]. WBC and PLT are differently found in normal and abnormal RBC morphology which is expected

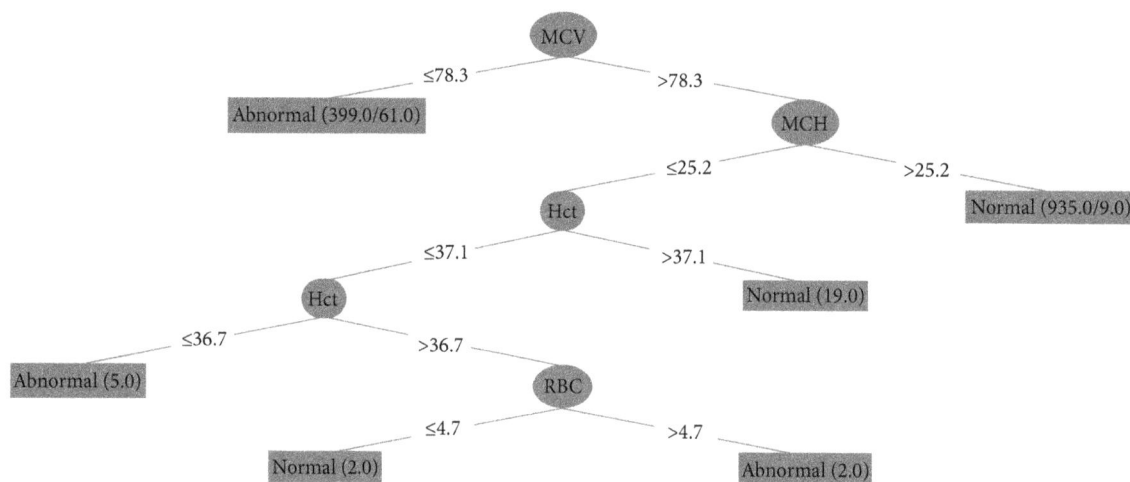

FIGURE 1: The decision tree from J48 algorithm in predicting RBC morphology. If MCV is less than or equal to 78.3 fL, RBC is labeled as abnormal RBC morphology but if MCV is more than 78.3 fL and MCH is more than 25.2 pg, RBC is still labeled as normal. And if MCH is less than or equal to 25.2 pg but Hct is greater than 37.1%, RBC is normal. On the other hand, if Hct is less than or equal to 36.7%, RBC is abnormal. But if Hct is between 36.7 and 37.1% and RBC is less than or equal to 4.7×10^{12} cell/L, it will most likely be normal RBC morphology. However, if RBC is more than 4.7×10^{12} cell/L, it is abnormal RBC morphology.

TABLE 4: The performance evaluation of predicted normal and abnormal RBC morphology.

Class	Abnormal	Normal	Average
TP	0.955	0.935	0.940
FP	0.065	0.045	0.050
Precision	0.837	0.983	0.945
Recall	0.955	0.935	0.940
F-Measure	0.892	0.958	0.941
Accuracy	0.943	0.943	0.943

to see in other parameters. This occurrence is unsupported by any previous studies, so it is only an occasional agreement.

This study has shown the benefit of applying data mining technique by creating a practical guideline in blood smear examination from decision tree (as seen in Figure 1). An advantage of a decision tree is to assist in decision making. That is the number appears in decision tree is an exactly value which is easier to make a decision than using a normal range in laboratory, thus it will reduce uncertainty in decision making. Moreover, it can be used as a practical guideline for RBC morphology from hematological parameter. However, what we have shown is only a practical guideline, however scanning a peripheral blood smear is encouraged. In addition, due to the limitation of samples, we have only normal and microcytic red blood cell in thalassemia and hemoglobinopathies which a common anemia in Thailand [7]. The study did not cover macrocytic anemia, because of it low percentage and only found in older Thai. In the future, data collection should include macrocytic anemia in order to make the complete practical guideline for clinical laboratory improvement.

5. Conclusion

Data mining by using J48 algorithm shows a distinctive point of data mining in analyzing a relationship of a complex data that exceeds capability of a common statistics. The J48 is a mathematic calculation cooperates with simulation model and a simple decision tree in order to create a practical guideline in predicting RBC morphology from hematological parameters of 4 data sets (MCV, MCH, Hct, and RBC) from 13 datasets which can be used for RBC morphology from hematological parameters such as teenager for baseline data.

Conflict of Interests

This research has no financial supports to disclose.

References

[1] M. Hall, E. Frank, G. Holmes, B. Pfahringer, P. Reutemann, and I. H. Witten, *The WEKA Data Mining Software: An Update: SIGKDD Explorations*, 2009.

[2] Z. Badiei, M. Khalesi, M. H. Alami et al., "Risk factors associated with life-threatening infections in children with febrile neutropenia: a data mining approach," *Journal of Pediatric Hematology/Oncology*, vol. 33, no. 1, pp. e9–e12, 2011.

[3] M. Kantardzic, B. Djulbegovic, and H. Hamdan, "A data-mining approach to improving Polycythemia Vera diagnosis," *Computers and Industrial Engineering*, vol. 43, no. 4, pp. 765–773, 2002.

[4] A. Zucchetto, I. Cattarossi, P. Nanni et al., "Cluster analysis of immunophenotypic data: the example of chronic lymphocytic leukemia," *Immunology Letters*, vol. 134, no. 2, pp. 137–144, 2011.

[5] B. Houwen, "Blood film preparation and staining procedures," *Clinics in Laboratory Medicine*, vol. 22, no. 1, pp. 1–14, 2002.

[6] B. S. Bull, R. Aller, and B. Houwen, "MCHC—red cell index or quality control parameter?" in *Proceedings of the 16th World Congress of the International Society of Haematology*, pp. 25–29, Singapore, August 1996.

[7] K. Sanchaisuriya, S. Fucharoen, T. Ratanasiri et al., "Thalassemia and hemoglobinopathies rather than iron deficiency are major causes of pregnancy-related anemia in northeast Thailand," *Blood Cells, Molecules, and Diseases*, vol. 37, no. 1, pp. 8–11, 2006.

19

Association of ABO Blood Group Phenotype and Allele Frequency with Chikungunya Fever

Pairaya Rujirojindakul,[1] Virasakdi Chongsuvivatwong,[2] and Pornprot Limprasert[1]

[1]*Department of Pathology, Faculty of Medicine, Prince of Songkla University, Hat Yai, Songkhla 90110, Thailand*
[2]*Epidemiology Unit, Faculty of Medicine, Prince of Songkla University, Hat Yai, Songkhla 90110, Thailand*

Correspondence should be addressed to Pairaya Rujirojindakul; rupairay@medicine.psu.ac.th

Academic Editor: Bashir A. Lwaleed

Background. The objective of this study was to investigate the association of the ABO blood group phenotype and allele frequency with CHIK fever. *Methods.* A rural community survey in Southern Thailand was conducted in August and September 2010. A total of 506 villagers were enrolled. Cases were defined as individuals having anti-CHIK IgG by hemagglutination $\geq 1:10$. *Results.* There were 314 cases (62.1%) with CHIK seropositivity. Females were less likely to have positive anti-CHIK IgG with odds ratio (OR) (95% CI) of 0.63 (0.43, 0.93). All samples tested were Rh positive. Distribution of CHIK seropositivity versus seronegativity (P value) in A, B, AB, and O blood groups was 80 versus 46 (0.003), 80 versus 48 (0.005), 24 versus 20 (0.55), and 130 versus 78 (<0.001), respectively. However, chi-square test between ABO and CHIK infection showed no statistical significance ($P = 0.76$). Comparison of the ABO blood group allele frequency between CHIK seropositivity and seronegativity was not statistically significant. *Conclusion.* This finding demonstrated no association of the ABO blood group phenotypes and allele frequencies with CHIK infection.

1. Introduction

Chikungunya (CHIK) is a disease caused by arthropod-borne viruses transmitted by *Aedes* mosquitoes. Classically, acute infection manifests as the sudden onset of high-grade fever, rash, and severe joint pain [1]. The outbreak in Thailand during 2008–2010 showed that the highest attack rate, 1130.67 per 100,000 of population, was in Southern Thailand [2]. Compared with other arboviral diseases such as dengue disease, relatively few studies have been conducted in the host factors for CHIK infection.

ABO and Rhesus (Rh) blood groups are the most clinically important in transfusion practice and have been widely researched in population genetics, anthropological studies, and disease susceptibility studies [3–5]. Associations between the ABO blood group and various viral infections have been demonstrated, including dengue [6] and hepatitis C [7]. Currently, results from genome-wide association studies (GWAS) suggest an association of the ABO blood group antigen with systemic inflammation [8, 9].

Although the ABO blood group has been shown to play an important role in resistance or susceptibility to infections [10, 11], well-designed studies aimed at defining the relationship of the ABO blood group phenotype or allele frequency and susceptibility to CHIK infection are limited. Therefore, this study was undertaken to investigate the association of the ABO and Rh blood group phenotype, as well as allele frequency, with anti-CHIK IgG seropositivity in a community setting.

2. Material and Methods

We conducted this study in three villages in Phatthalung province in Southern Thailand because they had the highest reported CHIK infection rate, 45.89 per 100,000 of population, in 2010. Thai villagers aged ≥18 years, living in the study area during the CHIK outbreak, were enrolled. Exclusion criteria were as follows: having laboratory confirmation of other infections, congenital or acquired immune deficiencies, or a history of chronic small joint diseases. During August

TABLE 1: Univariate analysis for CHIK seropositivity.

Variables	Anti-CHIK IgG		P value	OR (95% CI)
	Positive (%) N = 314	Negative (%) N = 192		
Age (years)			0.13	
<40	97 (30.9)	76 (39.6)		Reference
40–60	148 (47.1)	80 (41.7)		1.45 (0.97, 2.17)
>60	69 (22)	36 (18.8)		1.5 (0.91, 2.48)
Gender			**0.03**	
Male	110 (35)	49 (25.5)		Reference
Female	204 (65)	143 (74.5)		0.64 (0.43, 0.95)
ABO blood group			0.76	
O	130 (41.4)	78 (40.6)	<0.001	Reference
A	80 (25.5)	46 (24)	0.003	1.04 (0.66, 1.65)
B	80 (25.5)	48 (25)	0.005	1 (0.63, 1.58)
AB	24 (7.6)	20 (10.4)	0.55	0.72 (0.37, 1.39)

and September 2010, 506 subjects were enrolled. This study was approved by the Ethics Committee of Prince of Songkla University (EC 53-317-05-1-3), and written informed consent was obtained from all the participants.

2.1. ABO, Rh, and Anti-CHIK Serological Testing. We collected EDTA blood and tested blood groups at the Blood Bank, Songklanagarind Hospital. Within six hours after collection, both the ABO and Rh blood groups were determined with cell grouping using anti-A, anti-B, and anti-D antibodies (National Blood Centre, Thai Red Cross Society, Bangkok, Thailand). For the ABO blood group, we also performed serum grouping using A-cell and B-cell (National Blood Centre, Thai Red Cross Society, Bangkok, Thailand). Plasma was kept at $-70°C$ before sending samples to the Armed Forces Research Institute of Medical Science (AFRIMS), Bangkok, for Anti-CHIK IgG hemagglutination inhibition (HI) test. We defined cases of CHIK infection as participants who had HI titre ≥1 : 10 [12, 13].

2.2. Statistical Analysis. Analyses were performed using R software with Epicalc packages. The blood group frequency was tested with chi-square or Fisher's exact tests, and odds ratios (ORs) with 95% confidence intervals (CI) were calculated. Symptomatic infection was defined as individuals with anti-CHIK IgG ≥ 1 : 10 who reported having acute fever with pain at the small joints during the CHIK outbreak. For symptomatic variables with three-category outcomes, including noninfected, symptomatic, and asymptomatic groups, we used polytomous logistic regression to calculate ORs and 95% CI.

To estimate the allele frequencies of the ABO blood group, we applied the Bernstein method as previously described [14, 15]. Briefly, the allelic frequencies of alleles A, B, and O were assigned as p, q, and r, respectively. Then, p = 1 − square root of [frequency (B) + frequency (O)], q = 1 − square root of [frequency (A) + frequency (O)], and r = 1 − square root of frequency (O). If $p + q + r$ was not

equal to 1, a deviation $(D) = 1 - (p + q + r)$ was used to adjust the allelic frequencies as follows: $p' = p(1 + D/2)$, $q' = q(1 + D/2)$, and $r' = (r + D/2)(1 + D/2)$. The Hardy-Weinberg equilibrium (HWE) was tested using the goodness-of-fit chi-square test. The calculation for allelic frequencies and HWE was done using S2 ABOestimator software version 1.1.0.2 (Pedro J.N., Silva, Lisbon, Portugal). All P values less than 0.05 were considered significant.

3. Results

From a sample size of 506, we found 314 laboratory-confirmed CHIK cases (62.1%). Of the 314 cases, 166 had symptomatic infection. Median ages (IQR) of cases and controls were 47 (39, 58) and 45 (35.5, 58.5) years, respectively ($P = 0.20$).

All tested samples were Rh positive. No ABO discrepancy between cell and serum grouping was found. Distribution of positive and negative anti-CHIK IgG was significantly different in blood group O, A, and B (Table 1). The 95% CI of OR for blood groups A, B, and AB compared with O included unity, as shown in Table 1. The chi-square test between the ABO blood group and CHIK seropositivity showed no statistical significance (P value = 0.76).

For symptomatic manifestation with noninfection as a reference, the odds of being asymptomatic increased by 1.8-fold in age group of 40–60 years and decreased by 0.6 times in females (Table 2).

Allelic frequencies of the ABO blood group in each group, including CHIK seronegativity, seropositivity, and asymptomatic and symptomatic infection, are displayed in Table 3. There was no significant difference between the ABO allele frequencies and each outcome compared with CHIK seronegativity.

4. Discussion

This study demonstrated a very high rate of CHIK seropositivity confirmed by anti-CHIK IgG in a community-based

TABLE 2: Univariate analysis for symptomatic manifestations.

Variables	Asymptomatic		Symptomatic	
	RRR	95% CI	RRR	95% CI
Age (years)				
<40	Reference		Reference	
40–60	**1.8**	**1.09, 2.97**	1.34	0.84, 2.13
>60	1.79	1, 3.21	0.82	0.45, 1.49
Gender				
Male	Reference		Reference	
Female	**0.6**	**0.38, 0.95**	0.66	0.42, 1.05
ABO blood group				
O	Reference		Reference	
A	1.05	0.65, 1.8	1.07	0.63, 1.82
B	1.13	0.67, 1.92	0.91	0.53, 1.55
AB	0.56	0.24, 1.31	0.86	0.41, 1.78

RRR: relative risk ratio.

TABLE 3: Allelic frequencies of ABO blood group in each group.

Group	Allelic frequency			HWE test P value
	p(A)	q(B)	r(O)	
CHIK seronegativity	0.19	0.19	0.62	0.06
CHIK seropositivity	0.18	0.18	0.64	0.38
(i) Asymptomatic infection	0.17	0.19	0.64	0.71
(ii) Symptomatic infection	0.19	0.17	0.63	0.12

HWE: the Hardy-Weinberg equilibrium.

study after an outbreak in Thailand. We also provided serological and allelic frequencies of the ABO blood group in Thais. However, the results did not show any significant association of ABO phenotype or allele frequencies with CHIK seropositivity and asymptomatic or symptomatic infection using CHIK seronegativity as a reference.

The ABO blood group distribution in this study was similar to other studies carried out in blood donors in Thailand [16, 17]. During an Indian outbreak in 2005–2009, two studies were conducted to investigate the relationship between ABO/Rh blood groups and CHIK infection based on self-declared symptoms. The results showed an increased susceptibility to CHIK infection in the Rh positive individuals [18]. The differences of the ABO blood group system between infected and noninfected groups were observed when combined with Rh status [19]. Generally, complex diseases especially host susceptibility to infection are influenced by more than one genetic or environmental factor. Therefore, extensive genetic studies are required to answer this question.

The limitation of the present study is that there was no anti-CHIK IgM or convalescent samples of IgG tested for confirming acute CHIK infection because we conducted this study one year after the outbreak. However, Panning et al. [20] reported no evidence of CHIK antibodies before an outbreak in Sri Lanka, where the last severe CHIK epidemic occurred during the same period in Thailand in 1960s [21].

In conclusion, our study demonstrated no association of the ABO blood group phenotype and allele frequencies with CHIK seropositivity. Further research should be undertaken

in order to extensively explore the host and environmental factors associated with susceptibility and resistance to CHIK infection. This knowledge will help to identify susceptible individuals for monitoring and may be applied to other serious infections as well.

Conflict of Interests

The authors declare that there is no conflict of interests regarding the publication of this paper.

Acknowledgments

This work was fully supported by a Grant from Prince of Songkla University (Grant no. MED540025S). The authors are grateful to Ms. Patchani Nakkara and the health volunteers in Tungnaree subdistrict for providing all necessary support during this study. We also would like to thank all the villagers for their participation, Ms. Wanwimon Yindee for her technical support, and the Armed Forces Research Institute of Medical Science (AFRIMS) for CHIK serological testing.

References

[1] G. Borgherini, P. Poubeau, F. Staikowsky et al., "Outbreak of chikungunya on Reunion Island: early clinical and laboratory features in 157 adult patients," *Clinical Infectious Diseases*, vol. 44, no. 11, pp. 1401–1407, 2007.

[2] Bureau of Epidemiology, *Situation of Chikungunya Fever in Thailand*, Bureau of Epidemiology, Department of Disease Control, Ministry of Public Health, Nonthaburi, Thailand, 2010.

[3] L. Ségurel, Z. Gao, and M. Przeworski, "Ancestry runs deeper than blood: the evolutionary history of ABO points to cryptic variation of functional importance," *BioEssays*, vol. 35, no. 10, pp. 862–867, 2013.

[4] B. K. Lee, Z. Zhang, A. Wikman, P. G. Lindqvist, and M. Reilly, "ABO and RhD blood groups and gestational hypertensive disorders: a population-based cohort study," *British Journal of Obstetrics and Gynaecology*, vol. 119, no. 10, pp. 1232–1237, 2012.

[5] U. Pelzer, F. Klein, M. Bahra et al., "Blood group determinates incidence for pancreatic cancer in Germany," *Frontiers in Physiology*, vol. 4, article 118, pp. 1–4, 2013.

[6] S. Kalayanarooj, R. V. Gibbons, D. Vaughn et al., "Blood group AB is associated with increased risk for severe dengue disease in secondary infections," *The Journal of Infectious Diseases*, vol. 195, no. 7, pp. 1014–1017, 2007.

[7] R. Behal, R. Jain, K. K. Behal, and T. N. Dhole, "Variation in the host ABO blood group may be associated with susceptibility to hepatitis C virus infection," *Epidemiology and Infection*, vol. 138, no. 8, pp. 1096–1099, 2010.

[8] G. Paré, D. I. Chasman, M. Kellogg et al., "Novel association of ABO histo-blood group antigen with soluble ICAM-1: results of a genome-wide association study of 6,578 women," *PLoS Genetics*, vol. 4, no. 7, Article ID e1000118, 2008.

[9] D. Melzer, J. R. B. Perry, D. Hernandez et al., "A genome-wide association study identifies protein quantitative trait loci (pQTLs)," *PLoS Genetics*, vol. 4, no. 5, Article ID e1000072, 2008.

[10] P. Greenwell, "Blood group antigens: molecules seeking a function?" *Glycoconjugate Journal*, vol. 14, no. 2, pp. 159–173, 1997.

[11] D. J. Anstee, "The relationship between blood groups and disease," *Blood*, vol. 115, no. 23, pp. 4635–4643, 2010.

[12] W. M. Hammon and G. E. Sather, "Virological findings in the 1960 hemorrhagic fever epidemic (dengue) in Thailand," *The American Journal of Tropical Medicine and Hygiene*, vol. 13, pp. 629–641, 1964.

[13] A. Theamboonlers, P. Rianthavorn, K. Praianantathavorn, N. Wuttirattanakowit, and Y. Poovorawan, "Clinical and molecular characterization of Chikungunya virus in south Thailand," *Japanese Journal of Infectious Diseases*, vol. 62, no. 4, pp. 303–305, 2009.

[14] J. M. Nam and J. J. Gart, "Bernstein's and gene-counting methods in generalized ABO-like systems," *Annals of Human Genetics*, vol. 39, no. 3, pp. 361–373, 1976.

[15] S. T. Ndoula, J. J. N. Noubiap, J. R. N. Nansseu, and A. Wonkam, "Phenotypic and allelic distribution of the ABO and Rhesus (D) blood groups in the Cameroonian population," *International Journal of Immunogenetics*, vol. 41, no. 3, pp. 206–210, 2014.

[16] O. Nathalang, S. Kuvanont, P. Punyaprasiddhi, C. Tasaniyanonda, and T. Sriphaisal, "A preliminary study of the distribution of blood group systems in Thai blood donors determined by the gel test," *The Southeast Asian Journal of Tropical Medicine and Public Health*, vol. 32, no. 1, pp. 204–207, 2001.

[17] D. Chandanayingyong, T. T. Sasaki, and T. J. Greenwalt, "Blood groups of the Thais," *Transfusion*, vol. 7, no. 4, pp. 269–276, 1967.

[18] N. C. Kumar, M. Nadimpalli, V. R. Vardhan, and S. D. Gopal, "Association of ABO blood groups with Chikungunya virus," *Virology Journal*, vol. 7, article 140, 2010.

[19] S. Lokireddy, V. Sarojamma, and V. Ramakrishna, "Genetic predisposition to chikungunya—a blood group study in chikungunya affected families," *Virology Journal*, vol. 6, article 77, 2009.

[20] M. Panning, D. Wichmann, K. Grywna et al., "No evidence of chikungunya virus and antibodies shortly before the outbreak on Sri Lanka," *Medical Microbiology and Immunology*, vol. 198, no. 2, pp. 103–106, 2009.

[21] U. Thavara, A. Tawatsin, T. Pengsakul et al., "Outbreak of chikungunya fever in Thailand and virus detection in field population of vector mosquitoes, *Aedes aegypti* (L.) and *Aedes albopictus* Skuse (Diptera: Culicidae)," *The Southeast Asian Journal of Tropical Medicine and Public Health*, vol. 40, no. 5, pp. 951–962, 2009.

20

Effect of Gender on Coagulation Functions: A Study in Metastatic Colorectal Cancer Patients Treated with Bevacizumab, Irinotecan, 5-Fluorouracil, and Leucovorin

Cemil Bilir, Hüseyin Engin, and Yasemin Bakkal Temi

Bülent Ecevit University School of Medicine, Department of Internal Medicine, Division of Medical Oncology, 67100 Zonguldak, Turkey

Correspondence should be addressed to Cemil Bilir; cebilir@yahoo.com

Academic Editor: Aldo Roccaro

Introduction. We designed this study to evaluate how coagulation parameters are changed in metastatic colorectal cancer (mCRC) patients treated with bevacizumab, irinotecan, 5-fluorouracil, and leucovorin (FOLFIRI). *Methods.* A total of 48 mCRC patients who initially received bevacizumab with FOLFIRI were eligible for this study. Thirty-four patients were analyzed at baseline and on the 4th, 8th, and 12th cycles of chemotherapy. *Results.* There were 19 male and 15 female patients. Baseline characteristics of the groups were similar, but women had better overall survival than men (14 months versus 12 months, $P = 0.044$). D-dimer levels decreased significantly after the 12th cycle compared with baseline in men but not in women. Men and women had increased levels of serum fibrinogen at the early cycles, but these increased fibrinogen levels continued after the 4th cycle of chemotherapy only in women. In addition, serum fibrinogen levels did not significantly change, but aPTT levels decreased in men. *Discussion.* The major finding of this study is that bevacizumab-FOLFIRI chemotherapy does not promote changes in the coagulation system. If chemotherapy treatment and the possible side effects of FOLFIRI-bevacizumab treatment are well managed, then alterations of the coagulation cascade will not have an impact on overall survival and mortality.

1. Introduction

Bevacizumab is typically used in combination with fluoropyrimidine-based chemotherapy for the treatment of patients with metastatic colorectal cancer (mCRC) [1]. In a pivotal phase III trial of first-line mCRC, bevacizumab in combination with standard irinotecan/fluorouracil (FOLFIRI) chemotherapy increased tumor response rate by 10% and significantly lengthened the overall survival [1, 2]. In the bevacizumab arm, the patients had an increased incidence of thrombotic events compared with the control arm (19.4% versus 16.2%, resp.), but this result was not significant [1]. In a meta-analysis, a total of 7956 patients diagnosed with many types of solid tumors from 15 randomized trials were identified. The authors revealed that patients treated with bevacizumab had a statistically significant increased risk of venous thromboembolic events (VTEs), with an RR of 1.33 (95% CI, 1.13–1.56, $P < 0.001$) compared with the controls [3]. Hurwitz et al. reported a meta-analysis of 6,055 patients in 10 randomized studies [4]. This study concluded that the addition of bevacizumab to chemotherapy did not significantly increase the risk of VTEs versus chemotherapy alone. The risk for VTEs was attributed to tumor and host factors [4]. Epistaxis, hemoptysis, hematemesis, gastrointestinal bleeding, vaginal bleeding, and brain hemorrhage have been reported as hemorrhagic toxicities associated with bevacizumab [5]. These controversial findings open the possibility that factors other than bevacizumab, such as drugs, cancer, age, gender, or comorbidities, can cause VTEs. Therefore, we designed this study to evaluate how coagulation parameters, such as the international normalized ratio (INR), activated partial thromboplastin time (aPTT), and fibrinogen and D-dimer levels, can be altered in mCRC patients treated with FOLFIRI-bevacizumab chemotherapy.

2. Materials and Methods

A total of 48 metastatic colorectal cancer patients who had initially received bevacizumab combined with the FOLFIRI regimen were eligible for the study. The study was conducted in the Medical Oncology Clinic of the Bulent Ecevit University School of Medicine between the period of May 2010 and May 2013. Patients with a previous history of hematological disease, those who have been taking anticoagulant therapy, and those with chronic disease, such as liver cirrhosis or renal failure, were excluded from the study. During the bevacizumab treatment period, all patients who had Grade 3-4 bleeding were excluded from the study. Written and verbal consents were obtained from all the patients for chemotherapy and study enrollment. Treatment responses were measured between every 2 and 3 months. If a patient progressed or discontinued bevacizumab for any reason (e.g., bleeding, intestinal perforation, and metastasectomy), he or she was excluded from the study. At the end of the study, a total of 34 patients were included and analyzed.

2.1. Drug Administration. All patients received the following treatment regimen: bevacizumab 5 mg/kg IV combined with irinotecan 180 mg/m^2 IV (Day 1), leucovorin 400 mg/m^2 IV (Day 1), and 5-fluorouracil (400 mg/m^2 IV bolus and then 2400 mg/m^2 continuous infusion 46 h) IV, once every 2 weeks for 12 cycles. All measurements were repeated at baseline and on the 4th, 8th, and 12th cycles of chemotherapy. Chemotherapy was continued beyond the 12th cycle for patients who had a partial response or stable disease.

2.2. Sample Collection. Blood samples were collected before drug administration at baseline and on Day 1 of chemotherapy of the 4th, 8th, and 12th cycles using a 19-gauge needle under minimum stasis. Platelet counts were analyzed using a Beckman Coulter Gen-S (SM, USA) automated blood counting device.

The conventional coagulation parameters, such as the international normalized ratio (INR), activated partial thromboplastin time (aPTT), fibrinogen, and D-dimer, were measured using a fully automated STA compact device from Diagnostica Stago.

2.3. Statistical Analysis. Treatment outcomes were estimated as response rate (RR), disease control rate, OS, and progression-free survival (PFS). OS was defined as the time between the date of metastatic disease diagnosis and the date of death from any cause. PFS was defined as the time from the date of metastatic disease diagnosis to the date of disease progression or death from any cause.

Overall survival was calculated using the Kaplan-Meier method and the log-rank test. $P < 0.05$ was considered to be significant. The appropriateness of data to normal ranges was controlled using the Shapiro-Wilk test. Data were analyzed using the two-way ANOVA and nonparametric tests. Data in the tables are presented as the mean and standard error (SE) or median and interquartile range (IR) of data. A probability value of less than 0.05 was considered to be statistically significant.

3. Results

In this study, there were 19 male and 15 female patients diagnosed with mCRC. The mean age of women was 60.1 ($\pm$7) and that of men was 61.5 ($\pm$9.9); there was no significant difference between the groups ($P = 0.59$). Baseline characteristics of the groups are shown in Table 1. All parameters, except OS, had no statistical significance. Women had greater OS than men. Men had more liver and lung metastases compared with women, but the difference was not significant (15 versus 9, $P = 0.7$).

Results of laboratory parameters at baseline and on Day 1 of the 4th, 8th, and 12th cycles are presented in Figure 1. Delta values were defined as the differences between the baseline and each of the following cycles: 4th, 8th, and 12th. D-dimer levels decreased significantly after the 12th cycle compared with the baseline in men but not in women. Both men and women have increased levels of serum fibrinogen at the early cycles, but increased fibrinogen levels continued after the 4th cycle of chemotherapy only in women. Conversely, fibrinogen levels and serum aPTT levels decreased in men but not in women. Serum INR levels did not change significantly in the first eight cycles of chemotherapy in both men and women. However, after the 12th cycle, INR levels increased significantly in women. This increase was statistically significant but without clinical meaning. Women have a higher risk of anemia than men in the early stages of treatment because their Hb levels decreased from 12.7 to 12.1, whereas there was no decrease detected in men. Cox regression analysis did not find any correlation of laboratory parameters with OS and PFS.

Some coagulation parameters have differences according to metastatic sites. In women, baseline fibrinogen levels were higher in liver metastasis compared with other metastatic sites, such as bone, peritoneum, and lung (381 mg/dL versus 348 mg/dL, $P = 0.007$). Additionally, serum baseline PLT levels were lower in liver metastasis compared with the other sites (170,000/mm^3 versus 262,000/mm^3, $P = 0.007$). With regard to changes in the parameters because of chemotherapy, Hb levels were different in the groups according to the metastatic site. There was a significant decrease in the Hb levels in the early period of chemotherapy especially in women. Dropping Hb levels were more prominent in peritoneal and bone metastases compared with liver metastasis (0.66 gr/dL versus 0.35 gr/dL, $P = 0.04$). There was no correlation between the laboratory parameters and metastatic sites in men. After the study termination, 1 man and 1 woman (6% of the study population) had deep vein thrombosis without pulmonary embolism, and there also was no Grade 3-4 bleeding.

4. Discussion

In this study, we found that FOLFIRI-bevacizumab chemotherapy has some changes on coagulation parameters such as

TABLE 1: Baseline characteristics of the groups.

	Women (minimum–maximum) $n = 15$	Men (minimum–maximum) $n = 19$	P value
Age, years	60	61.5	0.85
Colon cancer	12	14	—
Rectal cancer	3	5	—
Adenocarcinoma	15	19	
Grades 1-2	5	4	
Grade 3	10	15	0.4
Metastases site			
Liver	8	12	
Lung	1	3	
Bone	3	4	0.8
Diabetes	3	4	
Hypertension	2	5	1
D-dimer (mg/dL)	883 (106–2233)	794 (206–2760)	0.88
Fibrinogen (mg/dL)	382 (330–415)	348 (250–630)	0.73
aPTT (sec)	24 (19–29)	26 (19–29)	0.26
INR	0.93 (0.8–1.06)	1.0 (0.8–1.1)	0.44
Platelet count (×1000 mm^3)	185 (160–274)	274 (165–468)	0.057
Hemoglobin, gr/dL	12.7 (11.9–13.3)	12.7 (10.7–16)	0.98
Creatinine, mg/dL	0.9 (0.7–1.1)	0.8 (0.5–1.1)	0.17
White blood cell, mm^3	5600 (4400–13500)	6600 (3900–11000)	0.46
PFS, months	8 (6–11)	9 (4–14)	0.7
OS, months	14 (10–33)	12 (6–28)	0.044

aPTT: activated partial thromboplastin time, INR: international normalized ratio, PFS: progression-free survival, and OS: overall survival.

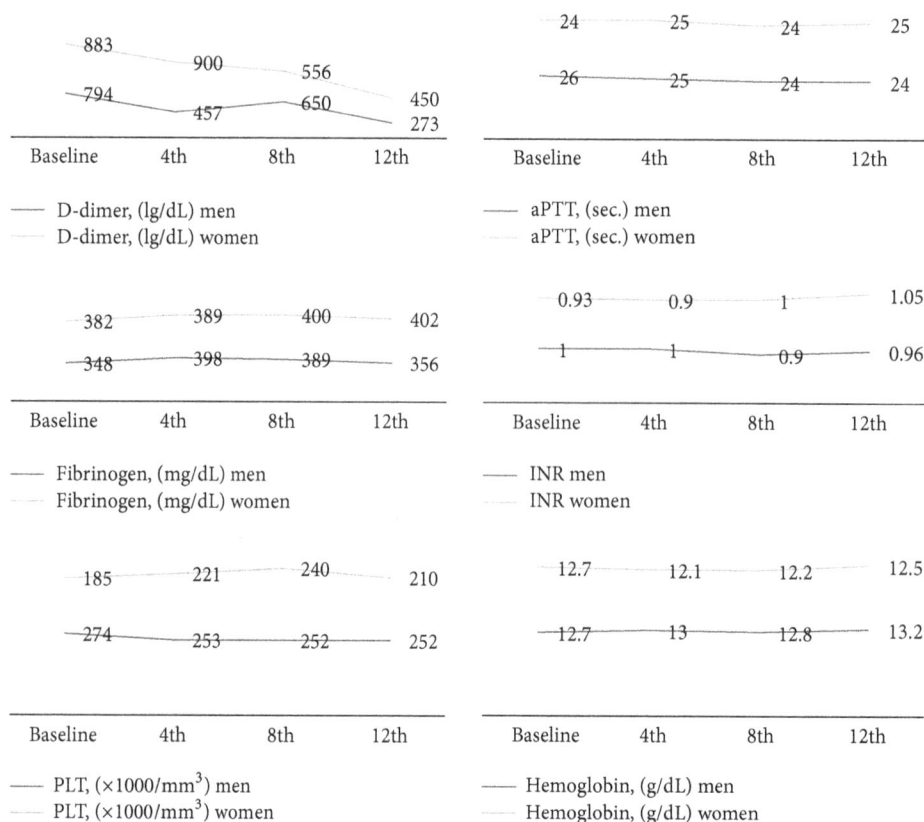

FIGURE 1: Results of laboratory parameters at baseline and on Day 1 of cycles 4, 8, and 12.

decreased D-dimer levels in men, increased fibrinogen levels in both men and women in the early stage of treatment, and increased INR in women. Despite these changes, none of these variables had an effect on OS and/or PFS.

A few small studies have reported changes in coagulation system markers in response to breast cancer chemotherapy, and these reports supported the development of a chemotherapy-induced hypercoagulable state [6]. Kirwan et al. also reported a well-designed prospective study on the markers of hemostasis (thrombin-antithrombin (TAT), fibrinogen, D-dimer, and platelet count) and functional clotting assays (prothrombin time (PT) and aPTT and procoagulants tissue factor (TF), cancer procoagulant (CP), and plasma vascular endothelial growth factor (pVEGF)), which were measured before chemotherapy and at 24 h, 4 days, 8 days, and 3 months after chemotherapy in patients with breast cancer. The authors revealed that the coagulation markers and procoagulants were increased before chemotherapy in patients who subsequently developed VTE [7]. Additionally, the authors revealed that aPTT showed a marked decrease within 24 h of chemotherapy; however, it was more pronounced in patients who subsequently developed VTE. The reduction in aPTT was maintained for up to 3 months [7], whereas a marked prolongation of PT was detected at 8 days and occurred only in patients who subsequently developed VTE [7]. In a lung cancer study, patients receiving chemotherapy revealed an early reduction of aPTT (at Days 2, 5, and 7 after treatment) and a slightly later decrease of PT (at Days 5, 7, and 14 after treatment) [8]. According to these findings, we speculate that there have been some alterations in the coagulation systems in patients who received chemotherapy. In colorectal cancer, there is only one small study published by Ustuner et al. They examined changes in coagulation parameters in 18 metastatic colorectal cancer patients and did not find any significant changes in platelet count, PT, and aPTT at baseline and in the subsequent chemotherapy cycles [5]; however, their study population was small and had no gender differentiation [5]. In our study, we found a shortened aPTT after the 8th cycle in men but not in women. However, this decrease remains within normal limits, and there was no clinical finding, such as VTE, in any patients for the duration of our study. Additionally, similar to previous breast cancer studies, we found minimal INR prolonged from the 0th cycle of the chemotherapy to the 12th cycle in women; only two women had Grade 1-2 bleeding during the study, and INR prolongation was detected after the 12th cycle. We may have been able to show more INR prolongation if we followed the patients beyond the 12th cycle, but we did not have prolonged follow-up results.

In this study, women had greater OS compared with men, and this finding may be a reason for men to have more liver and lung metastases compared with women, so men had a higher metastatic tumor burden.

In patients with cancer, the major causes are direct myelotoxicity from chemotherapeutic drugs and cytokine-mediated inhibition of erythropoiesis [9]. We showed a drop in Hb after the 4th cycle of FOLFIRI-bevacizumab chemotherapy in women but not in men. After the 4th cycle, we did not find any significant change in both men and women, but we must consider that, during the course of treatment, especially after the 4th to 6th cycles, some patients received blood transfusions.

Ustuner et al. did not find any significant changes in D-dimer and fibrinogen levels after the FOLFIRI-bevacizumab treatment [5], but we found a nonsignificant reduction in D-dimer levels in women and a significant decrease after the 12th cycle in men. This result is interesting because it reveals that D-dimer has a prognostic value in patients with colorectal and lung cancers [10]. In addition, Altiay et al. reported a significant correlation between response to chemotherapy and D-dimer levels in patients with both local and advanced lung cancer [11]. In our study, we showed a significant decrease in D-dimer levels in men; this reason may be the cause of higher metastatic tumor burden in men, and thus, after cancer chemotherapy, tumor burden and D-dimer can decrease; however, there was no significant correlation with overall survival. We also found a significant increase in fibrinogen levels in women, but there was no significant correlation with overall survival.

The major limitation of our study was having limited number of patients. We have only 34 patients with colorectal cancer, and we could not show the long-term outcomes such as VTE and/or bleeding complications. Only two patients had deep vein thrombosis after the chemotherapy; thus, a limited number of these patients avoid the statistical analyses. To our knowledge, there are some reports similar to our study that revealed the changes of coagulation parameters with cancer chemotherapy, but our study initially reported that these changes did not have any negative impact on OS in patients with colorectal cancer.

In conclusion, FOLFIRI-bevacizumab chemotherapy altered the coagulation functions according to gender. Although FOLFIRI-bevacizumab chemotherapy has some effects, these changes do not have any negative impact on overall survival and progression-free survival. If chemotherapy treatment and the possible side effects of FOLFIRI-bevacizumab are well managed, then alterations of the coagulation cascade will not have any impact on overall survival and mortality.

Conflict of Interests

All authors have no conflict of interests, and they did not receive any financial support for this study.

References

[1] H. Hurwitz, L. Fehrenbacher, W. Novotny et al., "Bevacizumab plus irinotecan, fluorouracil, and leucovorin for metastatic colorectal cancer," The New England Journal of Medicine, vol. 350, no. 23, pp. 2335–2342, 2004.

[2] P. Ferroni, V. Formica, M. Roselli, and F. Guadagni, "Thromboembolic events in patients treated with anti-angiogenic drugs," Current Vascular Pharmacology, vol. 8, no. 1, pp. 102–113, 2010.

[3] S. R. Nalluri, D. Chu, R. Keresztes, X. Zhu, and S. Wu, "Risk of venous thromboembolism with the angiogenesis inhibitor

bevacizumab in cancer patients: a meta-analysis," *JAMA—Journal of the American Medical Association*, vol. 300, no. 19, pp. 2277–2285, 2008.

[4] H. I. Hurwitz, L. B. Saltz, E. van Cutsem et al., "Venous thromboembolic events with chemotherapy plus bevacizumab: a pooled analysis of patients in randomized phase II and III studies," *Journal of Clinical Oncology*, vol. 29, no. 13, pp. 1757–1764, 2011.

[5] Z. Ustuner, O. M. Akay, M. Keskin, E. Kuş, C. Bal, and Z. Gulbas, "Evaluating coagulation disorders in the use of bevacizumab for metastatic colorectal cancer by thrombelastography," *Medical Oncology*, vol. 29, no. 5, pp. 3125–3128, 2012.

[6] D. Pectasides, D. Tsavdaridis, C. Aggouridaki et al., "Effects on blood coagulation of adjuvant CNF (cyclophosphamide, novantrone, 5-fluorouracil) chemotherapy in stage II breast cancer patients," *Anticancer Research*, vol. 19, no. 4, pp. 3521–3526, 1999.

[7] C. C. Kirwan, G. McDowell, C. N. McCollum, S. Kumar, and G. J. Byrne, "Early changes in the haemostatic and procoagulant systems after chemotherapy for breast cancer," *British Journal of Cancer*, vol. 99, no. 7, pp. 1000–1006, 2008.

[8] E. C. Gabazza, O. Taguchi, T. Yamakami et al., "Coagulation-fibrinolysis system and markers of collagen metabolism in lung cancer," *Cancer*, vol. 70, pp. 2631–2636, 1992.

[9] J. L. Spivak, "The anaemia of cancer: death by a thousand cuts," *Nature Reviews Cancer*, vol. 5, no. 7, pp. 543–555, 2005.

[10] B. Komurcuoglu, S. Ulusoy, M. Gayaf, A. Guler, and E. Ozden, "Prognostic value of plasma D-dimer levels in lung carcinoma," *Tumori*, vol. 97, no. 6, pp. 743–748, 2011.

[11] G. Altiay, A. Ciftci, M. Demir et al., "High plasma d-dimer level is associated with decreased survival in patients with lung cancer," *Clinical Oncology*, vol. 19, no. 7, pp. 494–498, 2007.

21

Practical Approaches to the Use of Lenalidomide in Multiple Myeloma: A Canadian Consensus

Donna Reece,[1] C. Tom Kouroukis,[2] Richard LeBlanc,[3] Michael Sebag,[4] Kevin Song,[5] and John Ashkenas[6]

[1] *Princess Margaret Hospital, University Health Network, 610 University Avenue, Toronto, ON, Canada M5G 2M9*
[2] *Department of Oncology, Juravinski Cancer Centre, 699 Concession Street, Hamilton, ON, Canada L8V 5C2*
[3] *Hôpital Maisonneuve-Rosemont, University of Montreal, Montreal, QC, Canada H1T 2M4*
[4] *McGill University Health Centre, McGill University, Montreal, QC, Canada H3A 1A1*
[5] *Leukemia/BMT Program of British Columbia, Vancouver General Hospital, Vancouver, BC, Canada V5Z 1M9*
[6] *SCRIPT, Toronto, ON, Canada M4S 1Z9*

Correspondence should be addressed to Donna Reece, donna.reece@uhn.on.ca

Academic Editor: Antonio Palumbo

In Canada, lenalidomide combined with dexamethasone (Len/Dex) is approved for use in relapsed or refractory multiple myeloma (RRMM). Our expert panel sought to provide an up-to-date practical guide on the use of lenalidomide in the managing RRMM within the Canadian clinical setting, including management of common adverse events (AEs). The panel concluded that safe, effective administration of Len/Dex treatment involves the following steps: (1) lenalidomide dose adjustment based on creatinine clearance and the extent of neutropenia or thrombocytopenia, (2) dexamethasone administered at 20–40 mg/week, and (3) continuation of treatment until disease progression or until toxicity persists despite dose reduction. Based on available evidence, the following precautions should reduce the risk of common Len/Dex AEs: (1) all patients treated with Len/Dex should receive thromboprophylaxis, (2) erythropoiesis-stimulating agents (ESAs) should be used cautiously, and (3) females of child-bearing potential and males in contact with such females must use multiple contraception methods. Finally, while Len/Dex can be administered irrespective of prior therapy and in all prognostic subsets, patients with chromosomal deletion 17(p13) have less favorable outcomes with all treatments, including Len/Dex. New directions for the use of lenalidomide in RRMM are also considered.

1. Introduction

Multiple myeloma (MM), the second most common hematological malignancy in adults, is associated with various clinical manifestations including anemia, lytic bone lesions, and renal and immune impairments. According to Canadian Cancer statistics, an estimated 2300 Canadians will be diagnosed with MM and 1350 will die from this disease in 2011 [1]. While no cure for MM is available, five-year survival rates have risen substantially in Canada and elsewhere over the last decade, partly due to novel therapies such as thalidomide, bortezomib, and lenalidomide [2, 3]. Nonetheless, regardless of initial treatment, most patients will eventually relapse and require salvage therapy, often consisting of novel agents, alone or in combination.

Lenalidomide is an immunomodulatory drug with direct effects on myeloma cells as well as their microenvironment. Early clinical trials with lenalidomide as a single agent in relapsed or refractory MM (RRMM) patients demonstrated its antimyeloma activity [4]. In preclinical studies, the agent has been shown to kill myeloma cells by upregulating certain cyclin-dependent kinase inhibitors and other early response factors [5]. Lenalidomide can also induce apoptosis by the activation of the intrinsic caspase-8 pathway [6], and it is thought to be more potent than thalidomide at inhibiting MM cell line growth and inhibiting TNF-α secretion from peripheral blood cells following LPS stimulation [7, 8].

Lenalidomide also has antiangiogenic properties, manifested *in vitro* by its ability to inhibit endothelial cell migration [9]. In addition, lenalidomide has properties not shared by thalidomide, such as inhibition of T regulatory cells and enhancement of tumor immunity [10, 11].

As reported in two landmark phase III trials that are the basis of Canadian approval of lenalidomide in RRMM, the efficacy of this agent is greatest when used in combination with dexamethasone [12, 13]. This combination is supported by data showing that lenalidomide can activate caspases 3, 8, and 9 with variable efficiency in different MM cell lines and that the addition of dexamethasone is synergistic and leads to a greater induction of apoptosis [5].

Additional studies, subgroup analyses of available phase III trials, and Canadian postmarketing experiences have all informed current practice regarding the use of lenalidomide in the RRMM patient population. In this paper we aim to provide an up-to-date practical guide on the use of this novel agent in the setting of RRMM, as well as a guide to managing commonly seen adverse events. To the best of our knowledge, the current report provides the first Canadian guidance for using lenalidomide in RRMM.

2. Methods

The expert panel convened in Paris, France, on May 2, 2011, in conjunction with the 13th International Myeloma Workshop. The group met to discuss the use of lenalidomide in the management of RRMM in the Canadian environment. The Chair (DR) invited panelists to research and write individual sections of the paper.

The various sections were collected, compiled, and distributed to the group, which discussed the paper via web conference. Panelists subsequently generated a revised draft in which all sections included specific clinical guidance (i.e., practice considerations). The revised paper was discussed at a final web conference, where all practice recommendations were considered, revised as appropriate, and ultimately adopted by the full panel; any areas of disagreement are noted.

Celgene Canada provided the impetus for the panel to pursue this project freely and independently. Celgene Canada supported the process throughout, including support for the participation of a medical writer (JA) in preparing this paper. The opinions represented here are solely those of the physician-panelists.

3. Indication, Timing, Dose, and Treatment Duration

In October 2008, the combination of lenalidomide and dexamethasone (Len/Dex) was approved in Canada for the treatment of RRMM in patients who had received at least one prior therapy. This approval was based on evidence from two phase III trials, namely, MM009 [12] and MM010 [13], which showed significant benefits in response rate (RR), time to progression (TTP), and overall survival (OS) following Len/Dex therapy, compared with dexamethasone

monotherapy. The benefits of Len/Dex over dexamethasone alone were seen in all age groups and were independent of previous therapy type. Based on the currently approved indication for this agent in Canada and the results of available studies, the initiation of lenalidomide therapy is not limited by the number or type of previous lines of therapy, although OS and progression-free survival are greater among patients with only one prior therapy versus those with two or more prior therapies [35].

In the MM009 and MM010 trials, lenalidomide was given at a dose of 25 mg per day on days 1 to 21 of a 28-day cycle, along with 40 mg of dexamethasone per day on days 1–4, 9–12, and 17–20. After the fourth cycle, 40 mg of dexamethasone was given daily on days 1–4 of every cycle. Cycles were continued until disease progression or until toxicity persisted, despite dose reduction. Noting the lack of prospective randomized trials specifically addressing different approaches to drug administration in the relapsed/refractory setting, the panel agreed that the recommended dose and schedule of Len/Dex therapy need not directly follow those outlined in published clinical trials.

We agreed that the starting dose of lenalidomide should remain at the current standard (25 mg daily on days 1–21) in the absence of baseline renal insufficiency and/or significant cytopenias. Specifically, the dose of lenalidomide must be adjusted based on the creatinine clearance, using standard dose adjustments (Table 1). Either the Cockcroft-Gault or the MDRD (modification of diet in renal disease) formula may be used to calculate creatinine clearance. Caution is urged in calculating the renal function based solely on serum creatinine level in older patients with MM [36].

Lenalidomide treatment should be used with caution in patients with thrombocytopenia (i.e., platelet counts $<50 \times 10^9$/L or $<30 \times 10^9$/L in those with heavy marrow infiltration with myeloma) and absolute neutrophil counts $<1.0 \times 10^9$/L; if lenalidomide is used in this setting, measures for aggressive growth factor supplementation and/or platelet transfusion support must be in place.

Although the pivotal phase III trials in RRMM used the standard high-dose (HD) pulsed dexamethasone (12 doses of 40 mg per month, on days 1–4, 9–12, and 17–20 of a 28-day schedule), it has become common practice in Canada to administer dexamethasone on a weekly schedule (four doses of 20–40 mg per month, on days 1, 8, 15, and 22 of a 28-day schedule). Although dexamethasone dose should be selected on the basis of individual clinical circumstances, the panel notes that such low-dose (LD) dexamethasone administration is particularly suitable for elderly patients, as well as those with uncontrolled diabetes, unmanageable glucocorticoid side effects, or relatively indolent relapses.

Weekly LD dexamethasone now represents the standard of care in newly diagnosed individuals. The panel's preference for LD dexamethasone administration is based in part on the results of a trial on Len/Dex in initial therapy for MM (see New Directions, below) [30]. Here, despite a somewhat lower RR compared to the HD dexamethasone group, patients receiving LD dexamethasone plus lenalidomide experienced improved OS and fewer grade ≥ 3 toxicities. A second line of evidence supporting the use of dexamethasone

TABLE 1: Dose adjustments at the start of therapy according to renal function [14].

Renal function	Dose*
Mild renal impairment ($60 \leq CrCl < 90$ mL/min)	25 mg (normal dose) every 24 hours
Moderate renal impairment ($30 \leq CrCl < 60$ mL/min)	10 mg[†] every 24 hours
Severe renal impairment (CrCl < 30 mL/min, not requiring dialysis)	15 mg every 48 hours
End-stage renal disease (CrCl < 30 mL/min, requiring dialysis)	5 mg once daily. On dialysis days, the dose should be administered following dialysis

* While maintaining a treatment cycle of 21 out of 28 days.
† Dose may be escalated to 15 mg once daily after two cycles if patient does not respond to and is tolerating treatment.
CrCl: creatinine clearance.

TABLE 2: Lenalidomide dose reduction levels with adequate renal function.

Dose level	Lenalidomide dose (mg)
Initial dose	25
First reduction level	15
Second reduction level	10
Third reduction level	5
Fourth reduction level	Discontinuation

at doses lower than employed in MM009 and MM010 comes from a post hoc analysis of stepwise dose reduction in these trials [37]. In this analysis, which did not directly test a weekly dexamethasone regimen, patients who reduced the dose of dexamethasone experienced significantly better RR, TTP, and OS. A final reason for the use of weekly LD dexamethasone is more hypothetical: one purported important mechanism of action of lenalidomide is via its immunomodulatory properties, and laboratory and clinical studies have demonstrated that dexamethasone can antagonize the potentially beneficial immunostimulatory effects of this drug [5, 38]. Therefore, LD dexamethasone may allow better immunomodulatory effects, while preserving the ability of corticosteroids to enhance the antiproliferative activities of lenalidomide.

Finally, with regard to treatment duration, lenalidomide therapy should be maintained continuously in most patients. This is in contrast to regimens in which combination therapy is given to maximal response and then discontinued to allow a treatment hiatus. One study has reported that the duration of lenalidomide therapy is directly related to a longer survival [39]. However, the optimal dose of lenalidomide when administered on a long-term basis is less certain. For example, another post hoc analysis of the MM009/MM010 study examined patients who were still on therapy 12 months after entering the trial and found that those who had dose reductions after 12 months had a significantly longer PFS than those who had reductions less than 12 months earlier, or no dose reduction [40].

The panel makes no specific recommendation on routine dose reduction after a specific period of time. However, we recommend that doses of lenalidomide and/or dexamethasone should be reduced to allow treatment to continue until disease progression occurs. Dose interruptions should occur only in situations of significant toxicities, with a plan to reinstitute therapy as soon as toxicity decreases with appropriate dose modifications. If required, dose reduction to ameliorate toxicity should follow the recommendations outlined in Tables 1, 2, 3, and 4.

Practice considerations are as follows.

(i) Len/Dex is approved for the treatment of RRMM in patients who have received ≥ 1 prior therapy and is appropriate irrespective of the number or type of therapies previously given.

(ii) Lenalidomide dose must be adjusted based on creatinine clearance.

(iii) Dosing should take into account pre-existing and developing cytopenias.

(iv) Dexamethasone is usually administered at doses of 20–40 mg once per week. However, this LD regimen has not been formally studied in the setting of relapsed myeloma, and the results may not be the same as those reported in the pivotal MM009/MM010 trials.

(v) Len/Dex treatment should be maintained as in the pivotal trials, that is, continued until disease progression or until significant toxicity persists despite dose reduction.

4. Treatment of Special Populations

4.1. High-Risk Multiple Myeloma. The definition of high-risk myeloma has evolved considerably over the past decade from one that predominantly relied on clinical and biochemical parameters (Durie-Salmon and ISS (International Staging System) stage, serum LDH (lactate dehydrogenase), CRP (C-reactive protein), proliferating index, etc.) to one that accounts for disease-specific cytogenetic and genomic factors. Several recurrent chromosomal aberrations—including chromosomal deletions (del(13q14), del(17p13)), translocations (t(4; 14), t(14; 16), t(14; 20)), and amplifications (1q21), as well as numerical chromosomal abnormalities (hypodiploid versus hyperdiploid karyotype)—correlate with poor disease outcomes. Similarly, genomewide gene expression profiling (GEP) studies have identified myeloma molecular subgroups with unique gene signatures that correlate with disease outcomes. In particular, a 70-gene signature was validated as a predictor of response to therapy

TABLE 3: Lenalidomide dose adjustment for neutropenia.

Neutrophil count	Recommendations
$<1 \times 10^9$/L on day 1 of a cycle	Delay start of the cycle for a week, until neutrophil count $\geq 1 \times 10^9$/L
$<1 \times 10^9$/L during a cycle	Interruption of lenalidomide until next cycle (dexamethasone should be continued)
Returning to $\geq 1 \times 10^9$/L on next cycle	Continue lenalidomide at same dose $\pm$ addition of G-CSF, if no other significant toxicities needing dose reduction Reduce lenalidomide to the first reduction level if other significant toxicities observed
For each subsequent drop $<1 \times 10^9$/L	Interrupt lenalidomide treatment
Returning to $\geq 1 \times 10^9$/L on next cycle	Resume lenalidomide at next dose reduction level

G-CSF: granulocyte-colony stimulating factor.

TABLE 4: Lenalidomide dose adjustment for thrombocytopenia.

Platelet count	Recommendations
$<30 \times 10^9$/L on day 1 of a cycle	Delay start of the cycle for a week, until platelet count $\geq 30 \times 10^9$/L
$<30 \times 10^9$/L during a cycle	Interruption of lenalidomide until next cycle (dexamethasone should be continued)
Returning to $\geq 30 \times 10^9$/L on next cycle	Reduce lenalidomide to the first reduction level
For each subsequent drop $<30 \times 10^9$/L	Interrupt lenalidomide treatment
Returning to $\geq 30 \times 10^9$/L on next cycle	Resume lenalidomide at next dose reduction level

and disease survival independently of clinical parameters and structural or numerical chromosomal abnormalities. Although most Canadian centers perform FISH cytogenetics for detection of del(13q14), del(17p13), and t(4; 14), genomic analyses are not routinely obtained.

To date, four retrospective studies have assessed the impact of cytogenetic abnormalities on outcomes of Len/Dex treatment among RRMM patients [15–18], as summarized in Table 5. The most consistent finding among these studies is that patients with del(17p13) experience less favorable outcomes when treated with Len/Dex [15, 16] or Len/Dex with bortezomib than those individuals lacking this adverse prognostic factor [18]. However, the presence of del(17p13) has repeatedly been shown to predict a shorter progression-free survival (PFS) and OS among RRMM patients, regardless of therapy [15, 16, 18]. Although patients with del(17p13) derive less benefit, the panel agreed that they may be treated with Len/Dex but should preferentially be considered for clinical trials designed for high-risk patients, if such an option is available. Innovative strategies, not yet defined, are needed for patients with a 17p13 deletion.

Although the trials of Reece et al. [15] and Klein et al. [16] suggest that Len/Dex treatment can overcome the poorer prognosis ordinarily associated with del(13q14) and t(4; 14), these conclusions are in contrast to those of Avet-Loiseau et al. [17]. In this last study, del(13q14) and t(4; 14) were associated with significantly lower RR, PFS, and OS in univariate analysis. In particular, patients with t(4; 14), compared to patients without t(4; 14), experienced significantly lower response and survival rates. However, multivariate regression analysis identified a prior history of progression while on thalidomide as the main adverse prognostic factor, and t(4; 14) per se was not retained in the model. Moreover, the patients in the Avet-Loiseau trial were more heavily pretreated. Evidence to date is also equivocal

regarding the impact on Len/Dex treatment efficacy of chromosome 1q21 amplifications [16, 18].

With regard to high-risk myeloma, as defined by the 70-gene GEP signature, there are currently no studies assessing the impact of lenalidomide-based therapy on the survival of these patients when used in the relapsed setting. However, results of studies incorporating lenalidomide in the frontline treatment regimen (e.g., Total Therapy 3, incorporating multidrug induction therapy, tandem autologous stem cell transplantation, and maintenance with the combination of lenalidomide, bortezomib, and dexamethasone) suggest that the 70-gene GEP signature remains a predictor of poor survival outcomes [41].

Currently, it remains difficult to provide definite recommendations for the use of lenalidomide in relapsed patients with high-risk cytogenetics. Prospective studies in this area are clearly warranted.

Practice considerations are as follows.

(i) Based on the results of a Canadian analysis of the Expanded Access Program of Len/Dex in relapsed/refractory myeloma patients, Len/Dex may be effective in patients with t(4; 14) or del(13q14) identified by FISH (fluorescence in situ hybridization) cytogenetics.

(ii) Patients with del17(p13) have poorer outcomes with all treatments, including Len/Dex treatment, and are high-priority candidates for innovative regimens directed to high-risk patients. However, Len/Dex may be used in the absence of such alternatives.

4.2. Previous Thalidomide Treatment. Although lenalidomide has been shown to be more potent than thalidomide in preclinical studies, the two agents are structurally similar

TABLE 5: Adverse prognostic factors identified by multivariate analysis in patients with relapsed/refractory myeloma treated with lenalidomide and dexamethasone.

Reference	Study population	PFS/TTP	Overall survival
Reece et al., 2009 [15]	130 RRMM patients treated with Len/Dex	Del(17p13) Elevated creatinine Prior bortezomib Prior thalidomide	Del(17p13) Elevated creatinine Prior bortezomib Prior thalidomide Age >65 yrs
Klein et al., 2011 [16]	92 RRMM patients treated with Len/Dex	Del(13q) if associated with other abnormalities	Del(17p13) Amp(1q21)
Avet-Loiseau et al., 2010 [17]	207 "heavily pretreated" RRMM patients treated with Len/Dex	Progression during thalidomide Hemoglobin <100 Del 13q	Progression during thalidomide
Dimopoulos et al., 2010 [18]	99 RRMM patients treated with Len/Dex ($n = 50$) or Len/Dex + bortezomib	t(4;14) Del(17p13) Thalidomide resistance Elevated LDH Extramedullary disease	Del(13q) Amp(1q21) Del(17p13) Thalidomide resistance ISS Bortezomib resistance Elevated LDH Extramedullary disease

PFS: progression-free survival; TTP: time to progression; RRMM: relapsed or refractory multiple myeloma; Len/Dex: lenalidomide combined with dexamethasone; LDH: lactate dehydrogenase; ISS: international staging system.

TABLE 6: The effect of Len/Dex treatment according to prior response to thalidomide. Adapted from Wang et al. [19].

	Thalidomide sensitive[1]			Thalidomide relapsed[2]			Thalidomide resistant[3]		
	Len/Dex	Placebo/Dex	P	Len/Dex	Placebo/Dex	P	Len/Dex	Placebo/Dex	P
Overall response rates (PR or better) %	64.8	17.1	<0.001	41.9	5.9	<0.01	50	20.8	0.042
Response duration, mo (95% CI)	13.4 (7.0 to NE)	3.2 (2.3 to NE)	0.009	8.8 (5.3 to NE)	NE (8.6 to NE)	0.77	NE (6.0 to NE)	NE (6.0 to NE)	0.22
Median PFS, mo (95% CI)	9.3 (5.6 to 18.0)	4.6 (3.9 to 4.7)	<0.001	7.8 (5.2 to 11.1)	3.7 (2.8 to 6.5)	0.002	7.0 (4.9 to 16.9)	3.7 (2.1 to 8.4)	0.013

[1]Sensitive: patients with stable disease or better who did not progress while on thalidomide.
[2]Relapsed: patients with stable disease or better who progressed while on thalidomide.
[3]Resistant: patients who progressed on thalidomide but never responded to thalidomide.
Len/Dex: lenalidomide combined with dexamethasone; PR: partial response; PFS: progression-free survival; NE: not estimable.

and likely exert their antimyeloma effects through similar mechanisms. Retrospective investigations suggest that prior thalidomide exposure [15], progression during thalidomide [17], and thalidomide resistance [18] independently predict reduced PFS and OS.

The MM-009 and MM-010 phase III studies included 154 (44%) and 120 (34%) patients, respectively, who had been previously exposed to thalidomide [12, 13]. A post hoc analysis of these two studies demonstrated that, while the overall RR of lenalidomide treatment was lower in patients previously treated with thalidomide (65% versus 54%), the response duration was not statistically different [19]. Further subgroup analyses of patients with prior thalidomide exposure revealed that those who had responded to thalidomide and did not progress while on therapy had the best overall RR, median duration of response, and PFS when subsequently treated with lenalidomide

(Table 6). RR and PFS among patients who failed to respond to thalidomide were better with Len/Dex than with dexamethasone alone, although duration of response to the assigned agent did not differ. Finally, PFS was superior with Len/Dex over dexamethasone monotherapy, regardless of prior thalidomide response. Another nonrandomized, prospective study of 106 previously thalidomide-treated patients suggested that the overall RR, PFS, and OS were not significantly different between patients who were thalidomide-sensitive versus thalidomide-resistant (56%, 10 months, 17 months, resp.) [42]. A third study, retrospective in nature, looked at retreatment with immunomodulatory agents in patients given this class of drugs as initial therapy for myeloma. For the subset of patients who received Len/Dex after initial thalidomide, the overall RR was 48% and the median TTP was 9 months [43].

Practice considerations are as follows.

(i) Although treatment efficacy may be somewhat reduced, Len/Dex is an appropriate treatment choice among patients previously treated with thalidomide, irrespective of their earlier response.

4.3. Elderly Patients. Up to 37% of newly diagnosed MM patients are older than 75 years [44]. Elderly patients are more likely to have significant comorbidities, tend to be frail, and have lower performance status and poorer tolerance to medications. Nevertheless, elderly patients have often been included in clinical studies of novel agents, and available evidence suggests that, with appropriate management, they can also benefit from these agents. However, a 40 mg dose of dexamethasone can be challenging to deliver to some elderly patients, and this agent may be given at a lower weekly dose of 20 mg.

Practice considerations are as follows.

(i) Among elderly patients, dexamethasone should be started at a dose of 40 mg per week, unless there are significant and/or severe comorbidities.

(ii) Dexamethasone should be started at a dose of 20 mg per week in less fit patients; an initial dose of 16 mg may be considered for very frail patients, as guided by clinical judgment. As noted above, these doses are lower than those used in the MM009/MM010 studies and the results may not be the same as when 4-day pulses are administered.

5. Toxicities and Management of Adverse Events

The safety and toxicity of lenalidomide have been evaluated in published clinical trials [12, 13], as well as in an expanded-access program for Canadian and international patients [45]. Although lenalidomide is well tolerated by most patients, some adverse effects are common during treatment. However, some of the more significant side effects associated with thalidomide are not seen with lenalidomide. Indeed, in the MM-009 and MM-010 studies, the incidences of grade 3-4 constipation, somnolence, and peripheral neuropathies were similar for the Len/Dex-treated group compared to the dexamethasone monotherapy group [12, 13]. Importantly, side effects associated with Len/Dex are not affected by the number of prior therapies [35].

5.1. Hematologic Toxicities. The most common grade 3-4 adverse events in the two phase III pivotal trials of lenalidomide were hematologic, including neutropenia; thrombocytopenia; to a lesser extent, anemia. The risk of grade 3 or 4 febrile neutropenia was slightly increased with the addition of lenalidomide (3.4% in the Len/Dex group versus 0% in the dexamethasone group). Dose reductions typically occur most frequently during the initial cycles. It is not clear whether the risks of neutropenia and thrombocytopenia per se decrease with time or whether the pattern observed

is secondary to dose modifications [46, 47]. At any rate, clinicians should be particularly vigilant during the first few months after initiation of lenalidomide. Given that a standard lenalidomide dose of 25 mg among patients with renal failure is associated with more cytopenias, especially neutropenia and thrombocytopenia [48], reducing the initial dose may ameliorate these risks. Specific recommendations for laboratory monitoring are summarized below.

5.1.1. Neutropenia and Thrombocytopenia. Myelosuppression associated with lenalidomide is dose-dependent and is usually predictable and manageable [47]. To decrease risks of infection and bleeding, lenalidomide should not be started in patients with an absolute neutrophil count (ANC) below 1.0×10^9/L or a platelet count below 50×10^9/L except in exceptional circumstances and with supportive measures in place, as discussed above. Lenalidomide administration should be interrupted whenever neutrophil and platelet counts reach these cutoffs. At the next cycle, if neutropenia is the only dose-limiting toxicity, treatment may resume at the same dose, with the addition of growth factor support such as filgrastim 300 or 480 mcg administered subcutaneously once or twice weekly, in patients with ANC $>1.0 \times 10^9$/L. In the presence of other dose-limiting toxicities, dose reduction is recommended (Table 2). Treatment may also be reintroduced, albeit at a reduced level, when platelet count is over 30×10^9/L. For each subsequent grade 3-4 neutropenia and platelet count less than 30×10^9/L, lenalidomide administration should be withheld and restarted at a lower dose at the next cycle. Dose adjustments for neutropenia and thrombocytopenia associated with lenalidomide are presented in Tables 3 and 4. In some circumstances, especially during the first few cycles, significant neutropenia or thrombocytopenia can result from heavy myeloma bone marrow infiltration rather than pure myelosuppression. In these cases, lenalidomide should probably be continued with the addition of G-CSF (granulocyte-colony stimulating factor) in case of neutropenia and platelet transfusions given to manage thrombocytopenia.

5.1.2. Anemia. Anemia is rarely a significant problem in patients undergoing Len/Dex combination therapy. Thus, clinicians should follow the standard practice established by their institution for transfusions. Some concerns have been raised regarding the potential risk of venous thromboembolic events associated with concomitant use of erythropoietin. Although the MM-010 study [13] suggested that these events are unrelated, the MM-009 [12] study identified a trend toward more venous thromboembolic events with erythropoietin. Accordingly, we recommend that erythropoiesis-stimulating agents (ESAs) be used with caution in patients receiving lenalidomide; if an ESA is given, the hemoglobin level should be maintained at <120 g/L as per the Health Canada label.

5.1.3. Others. Recently, lenalidomide exposure has been associated with failure to mobilize a sufficient number of stem cells using growth factors alone [49–51]. This negative effect on stem cell mobilization can be overcome with the addition of cyclophosphamide [52] or plerixafor [53]. Since use of lenalidomide most commonly follows relapse after autologous stem cell transplant (ASCT) and successful stem cell mobilization in eligible patients, this consideration is rarely problematic in Canada.

Practice considerations are as follows.

(i) MM patients experiencing neutropenia or thrombo-cytopenia should interrupt lenalidomide treatment until their ANC reaches 1.0×10^9/L and/or their platelet count reaches 30×10^9/L. Lenalidomide may then be restarted at a lower dose, as indicated in Table 2.

(ii) The timing of interrupting and restarting lenalido-mide in response to neutropenia and thrombocy-topenia should follow the guidance in Tables 3 and 4, respectively.

(iii) To avoid a potential increase in the risk of venous thromboembolism, ESAs should be utilized cau-tiously with Len/Dex, and the hemoglobin level should be maintained at <120 g/L.

5.2. Nonhematological Toxicities. Many nonhematological adverse effects reported with the combination of Len/Dex are associated with dexamethasone alone, including insomnia, peripheral edema, tremor, muscle weakness, blurred vision, dyspepsia, psychological changes, and hyperglycemia. These adverse events should be managed in the usual manner; if sig-nificant and persistent, they may necessitate dexamethasone dose reduction. Additionally, lenalidomide is potentially associated with gastrointestinal symptoms such as diarrhea, constipation, and nausea, as well as with muscle cramps, fatigue, and muscle weakness. As a general rule, for grade 3-4 nonhematological treatment-related toxicities, lenalidomide treatment should be withheld and restarted at the next lower dose level when toxicity has resolved to grade 2 or lower.

5.2.1. Infections. Despite the immunomodulatory effect of lenalidomide, the infection rate was increased with the addition of lenalidomide in both the MM-009 and MM-010 trials [12, 13]. Most infections were low-grade, with grade 3-4 infections seen in 10–20% of patients. Per study protocol, no antibiotic prophylaxis was provided in either of the two phase III trials. Due to this risk of infection, antibiotic prophylaxis may be considered for patients treated with Len/Dex, especially if HD dexamethasone is used. Unfortunately, there currently exists no recommendation for a single antibiotic class for this purpose, but our own prefer-ence is levofloxacin. Given that use of LD dexamethasone is associated with less frequent infections in newly diagnosed patients [30], it is not clear whether routine antibiotic prophylaxis is necessary.

In the MM-009 and MM-010 studies, reports of grade 3-4 viral or fungal infections were rare [54].

Practice Considerations are as follows.

(i) LD dexamethasone is associated with a lower risk of infection than HD dexamethasone among new MM patients.

(ii) Given the modest elevation in the risk of infection with Len/Dex treatment, antibiotic prophylaxis may be considered. Acceptable agents include trimetho-prim/sulfamethoxazole or levaquin.

5.2.2. Thromboembolic Events. Although the risk of throm-boembolic events is low when lenalidomide is adminis-tered as a single agent [4], this risk increases when it is used in combination with dexamethasone. The incidences of thromboembolic events in the MM-009 and MM-010 studies were 8.8–14.7% with Len/Dex versus 3.4–4.7% with dexamethasone alone. However, thromboprophylaxis was not required in either of these studies.

The risk of venous thromboembolism is higher within the first few months after initiation of therapy with Len/Dex, decreasing dramatically thereafter [46]. This observation might be explained in part by the administration of higher doses of dexamethasone during the first 4 cycles of therapy, followed by a significant decrease. Indeed, an Eastern Cooperative Oncology Group (ECOG) trial has shown that the incidence of thromboembolism is directly related to dexamethasone dose [30]. The risk of venous throm-boembolism among MM patients treated with Len/Dex is comparable to that of other high-risk populations for whom thromboprophylaxis is commonly recommended. A number of prophylactic approaches have been suggested when immunomodulatory agents are administered, includ-ing those based on the number of potential risk factors for venous thromboembolism [55, 56]. However, a recently published phase III trial reported similar rates of throm-bosis when either enoxaparin or ASA was used as throm-boprophylaxis in transplant-eligible patients with newly diagnosed MM treated with lenalidomide-based regimens [57].

In the absence of randomized phase III trials compar-ing the thromboprophylaxis agents with a control/placebo group in an RRMM setting, it is difficult to draw con-clusions concerning the real efficacy of these regimens. Nevertheless, the panel endorsed an approach in which daily ASA was suggested as thromboprophylaxis in patients not known to be at heightened risk of thrombotic events or to be allergic or intolerant to ASA. For those in whom ASA is contraindicated, prophylactic low molecular-weight heparin (LMWH)—such as enoxaparin 40 mg per day—should be used. For patients with a recent his-tory of a thromboembolic event, full anticoagulation with LMWH is recommended, although warfarin could even-tually be considered in patients with robust and stable platelet counts while on lenalidomide. Due to the low risk of venous thromboembolism associated with lenalido-mide monotherapy (see New Directions, to be mentioned later), thromboprophylaxis in this scenario is not indi-cated.

Practice considerations are as follows.

(i) For lenalidomide monotherapy, the decision for thromboprophylaxis should be based on medical considerations. Some panel members felt strongly that thromboprophylaxis should be employed routinely in this setting.

(ii) In the absence of contraindications, all patients on Len/Dex therapy should receive thromboprophylaxis. For patients without a history of thromboembolism or other known thrombotic conditions, ASA 81 or 325 mg per day is recommended. Prophylactic doses of LMWH (e.g., enoxaparin 40 mg sc daily) represent an alternative for such low-risk patients.

(iii) Therapeutic anticoagulation with LMWH is recommended as thromboprophylaxis in patients with a recent history of thromboembolism or other known thrombotic disorder. Warfarin may be considered in patients with stable and reliable platelet counts over 100×10^9/L.

(iv) Thromboprophylaxis should be held if the platelet count drops below 50×10^9/L and restarted when patients recover over that threshold.

5.2.3. Rashes. Rashes occur in up to 29% of patients on the Len/Dex regimen [58]. These rashes occur most frequently during the first few weeks of treatment, are usually self-limited, and are severe in only a minority of patients. Nevertheless, Stevens-Johnson syndrome and toxic epidermal necrolysis have been reported and can be fatal. For localized rashes, antihistamines and topical steroids are usually sufficient. For mild but more extensive rashes, short-duration systemic low-dose steroids are usually needed. When rashes are more severe, dose interruption, reduction, or permanent discontinuation may be required, depending on clinical judgment. Importantly, patients with a past history of a severe rash associated with thalidomide should not receive lenalidomide. Of interest, one case of skin hypersensitivity reaction to lenalidomide with successful desensitization has been reported [59]. A similar case has been described for thalidomide [60], further supporting this intervention for those experiencing type I hypersensitivity to lenalidomide. Recommended management of rashes is summarized in Table 7.

Practice considerations are as follows.

(i) If a rash becomes severe, lenalidomide dose may be reduced, interrupted, or discontinued; otherwise, antihistamines and steroids are usually sufficient.

5.2.4. Teratogenicity. Since lenalidomide could potentially be teratogenic in humans, precautions in females with child-bearing potential and males are important to avoid birth defects. In order to reduce these risks, the RevAid program provides a safe access to lenalidomide by stipulating a number of conditions for potential patients. For females of child-bearing potential, birth control using complete abstinence or two contraception methods is mandatory, beginning four weeks before initiation of lenalidomide and up to four weeks after. For males, complete abstinence or use of latex condoms during sexual contact with females of child-bearing potential is mandatory. While it is unknown whether lenalidomide is excreted in breast milk, breastfeeding is generally not recommended.

Practice considerations are as follows.

(i) Females of child-bearing potential and males in sexual contact with such females who are on Len/Dex treatment must use multiple contraception methods.

5.2.5. Other. General symptoms such as fatigue and asthenia are reported at a similar frequency with Len/Dex as with dexamethasone monotherapy. However, these symptoms can become a reason for lenalidomide dose modification or discontinuation, especially in the elderly. Diarrhea and constipation have both been described, each occurring in approximately 20% of patients [45]. Although these symptoms can be routinely managed, our experience indicates that diarrhea may be particularly problematic in certain patients and that ongoing treatment with loperamide or similar agents may allow continuation of full doses of lenalidomide. The fact that lenalidomide capsules contain lactose might contribute to the gastrointestinal side effects noted in some patients.

For unexplained reasons, Len/Dex combination has been associated with a higher incidence of grade 3-4 atrial fibrillation compared to dexamethasone alone (4% versus 1.1%, resp.) [14]. Other side effects, such as loss of appetite and muscle cramps, may be bothersome to patients receiving treatment on a long-term basis. We have found that the use of quinine sulphate 200–300 mg per day is often effective in reducing the incidence and frequency of muscle cramps in significantly affected patients [61]. Anecdotally, patients with severe muscle cramps not completely controlled with quinine have derived relief from daily low doses of benzodiazepines such as clonazepam.

Tumor lysis syndrome has been described with lenalidomide, but it is more often a concern in chronic lymphocytic leukemia patients treated with this agent. Its occurrence in MM has not been well evaluated but appears to be uncommon. Nevertheless, tumor lysis syndrome can occur in any patient with a hematologic malignancy and a high tumor burden or with renal impairment. Thus, proper hydration and monitoring of electrolytes, creatinine, and uric acid is advisable in patients with a high tumor load and/or rapidly proliferating disease.

In contrast to that of thalidomide, the incidence of peripheral neuropathy with lenalidomide is very low [14]. Some cases of neurologic deterioration have been described with lenalidomide, but they might be due to the evolution of prior neuropathy. A recent observational study on the clinical course of peripheral neuropathy during lenalidomide treatment concluded that this therapy does not worsen peripheral neuropathy [62].

TABLE 7: Management of rashes due to lenalidomide.

Signs/symptoms	Treatment
Localized maculopapular rash	Topical steroids; antihistamines
Widespread maculopapular rash	Hold lenalidomide; topical or oral steroids depending on severity; antihistamines; after resolution, restart lenalidomide at lower dose
Generalize erythroderma or desquamation	Hold lenalidomide; oral steroids; Dermatology consultation; do not restart lenalidomide
Urticaria	Hold lenalidomide; symptomatic management with antihistamines ± oral steroids; after resolution, may attempt desensitization if reinitiation of lenalidomide is planned

Practice considerations are as follows.

(i) Patients with significant diarrhea may require agents such as loperamide on a regular basis.

(ii) Quinine sulphate 200–300 mg per day can reduce muscle cramps in affected patients.

(iii) Although tumor lysis syndrome is considerably more common in patients treated with lenalidomide for chronic lymphocytic leukemia, myeloma patients with a high tumor load and/or rapidly proliferating disease may be at risk for this complication, especially if renal insufficiency is present. Proper hydration and laboratory monitoring is advisable in such patients when lenalidomide is initiated [63, 64].

5.3. *Second Primary Malignancies.* Emerging data from maintenance therapy studies using lenalidomide (IFM 05-02, CALGB 100104, and MM-015) suggest that long-term use of this agent might be associated with the development of second primary malignancies (SPM). However, in RRMM, after a median followup of 48 months for surviving patients, MM-009 and MM-010 have shown a low incidence of SPM. Furthermore, SPM rates were similar for patients on Len/Dex versus those on dexamethasone alone [40].

After an exhaustive review of clinical trials and post-marketing data, the European Medicines Agency issued a statement on September 23, 2011 to the effect that "the benefit-risk balance for lenalidomide remains positive within its approved patient population but advises doctors of the risk of new cancers as a result of treatment with the medicine." This analysis found that there were 3.98 cases of new cancer for every 100 patient-years in patients receiving lenalidomide compared with 1.38 cases in those not receiving lenalidomide in the approved population (Press Release 23 Sept 2011, European Medicines Agency, http://www.ema.europa.eu/). These included skin cancers as well as hematologic malignancies and some invasive solid tumors. Health Canada issued a similar statement in May 2012, recommending careful evaluation of patients "before and during treatment in order to screen for the occurrence of new malignancies" (http://hc-sc.gc.ca/dhp-mps/medeff/advisories-avis/prof/_2012/revlimid_hpc-cps-eng.php, accessed July 2012).

The panel therefore reiterates that patients on lenalidomide should be watched for signs or symptoms of a new cancer. Routine cancer screening should be followed, per Canadian or local guidelines [65, 66].

Practice consideration are as follows.

(i) The efficacy of lenalidomide in RRMM outweighs the small risk of developing a secondary malignancy.

(ii) Physicians and patients should be aware of this small risk; routine Canadian cancer screening measures should be performed, and any signs or symptoms of a possible second cancer should be evaluated and reported, if appropriate, to the RevAid program.

5.4. *Monitoring of Adverse Events.* Proper monitoring is required to note emerging side effects and to prevent potential treatment complications. A complete blood count with differential should be obtained every two weeks during the first 3 cycles and subsequently every month before a new cycle. Serum creatinine should be obtained before each cycle in order to adjust the lenalidomide dose according to impaired renal function. Because of possible liver toxicity [67] or thyroid dysfunction [68] associated with lenalidomide therapy, liver function tests including aspartate aminotransferase (AST), alanine aminotransferase (ALT), and bilirubin, as well as thyroid function tests should be done periodically throughout the treatment. Because atrial fibrillation remains a relatively rare event, serial electrocardiograms (ECGs) are not routinely required. For females of child-bearing potential, two pregnancy tests must be negative before starting lenalidomide: at 7–14 days and at 24 hours before administration of the drug. During the treatment, pregnancy tests should be conducted weekly for the first four weeks, then monthly (or every two weeks if menstrual cycles are irregular) until four weeks after treatment cessation.

5.5. *New Directions.* Given the established efficacy and favorable toxicity profile of lenalidomide in RRMM, this agent has now been evaluated at different time points in the disease course, as well as in combination with drugs other than dexamethasone alone (combination therapy) [20–29, 31–34, 68–75]. Combination of lenalidomide with alkylators, anthracyclines, and/or bortezomib yields very high remission rates (Table 8). So far, no randomized trials have established the superiority of a 3- or 4-drug combination over Len/Dex in terms of PFS or OS. Results of

TABLE 8: Summary of emerging lenalidomide combination therapies in the first- and second-line treatment of multiple myeloma.

Combination	First line		≥Second line	
	Efficacy	Major toxicities	Efficacy	Major toxicities
MPR Palumbo et al., 2007 [20]	81% ≥ PR	Hematological toxicity		
MPR-R Palumbo et al., 2010 [21]			75% ≥ PR	Hematological toxicity, infections
RMPT Palumbo et al., 2010 [22]				
RVD Richardson et al., 2009, 2010 [23, 24]	100% ≥ PR	Hematological toxicity, sensory neuropathy	61% ≥ MR	Hematological toxicity
CPR Reece et al., 2010 [25]			94% ≥ MR	Hematological toxicity
CRD Schey et al., 2010 [26]			81% ≥ PR	Hematological toxicity
RVDC Kumar et al., 2010 [27]	96% ≥ PR	Hematological toxicity, sensory neuropathy		
CRd Kumar et al., 2011 [28]	85% ≥ PR	Hematological toxicity		
RVDD Jakubowiak et al., 2011 [29]	95% ≥ PR	Fatigue, constipation, sensory neuropathy, infection		

MPR: melphalan, prednisone, lenalidomide; PR: partial response; MPR-R: MPR + lenalidomide maintenance until progression; RMPT: lenalidomide, melphalan, prednisone, thalidomide; RVD: lenalidomide, bortezomib, dexamethasone; MR: minimal response; CPR: cyclophosphamide, prednisone, lenalidomide; CRD: cyclophosphamide, lenalidomide, dexamethasone; RVDC: lenalidomide, bortezomib, dexamethasone, cyclophosphamide; CRd: cyclophosphamide, lenalidomide, dexamethasone; RVDD: lenalidomide, bortezomib, pegylated liposomal doxorubicin, dexamethasone.

an induction trial, comparing Len/dex with MPT (MM020), are anticipated later this year.

In addition, even though lenalidomide—given with dexamethasone—is currently approved only for use after one prior therapy, there is considerable interest in employing this drug as part of initial therapy in newly diagnosed patients. Options in this setting include its administration in induction regimens in patients both eligible and ineligible for ASCT, in addition to its use as maintenance therapy after ASCT.

Phase III trials have now been initiated in these settings, and the available results are summarized in Table 9. Two recent randomized trials indicate that posttransplant maintenance therapy with single agent lenalidomide started 60–100 days after ASCT significantly improves PFS, and one of these trials has noted a survival advantage in the lenalidomide arm [27]. Adoption of lenalidomide maintenance as a standard of care will depend on the identification of the subgroups most likely to benefit, the risk of late complications such as SPM, and the cost implications of such a strategy. On balance, it is likely that the results of recent/ongoing randomized studies will lead to expanded applications of lenalidomide in the treatment of patients with MM.

6. Conclusions

Based on available evidence, Len/Dex appears to be an effective and safe treatment strategy for RRMM patients, regardless of the type and number of prior therapies. In order to ensure optimal balance between efficacy and tolerability, lenalidomide dose and schedule should be adjusted based on creatinine clearance and presence of neutropenia and thrombocytopenia; dexamethasone should typically be administered at weekly doses of 20–40 mg, and treatment should be continued until disease progression or toxicity, even in patients requiring dose reduction.

Although certain adverse events can occur with Len/Dex, the following precautions can significantly reduce their impact: (1) Lenalidomide interruption and dose modification should follow established guidelines, with judicious use of G-CSF and transfusions if needed to avoid potential hematological toxicities; (2) all patients should receive thromboprophylaxis unless contraindicated. In most patients without a history of thrombosis, 81 mg of ASA is sufficient; alternatively, prophylactic doses of LMWH may be administered. Patients with a recent history of thromboembolism or known thrombotic disorder require full anticoagulation while on Len/Dex, usually consisting of LMWH; patients with stable platelet counts over $100 \times 10^9/L$ can be considered for coumadin; (3) ESAs should be used cautiously, and if this treatment is used, the hemoglobin target should be <120 g/L; (4) females of child-bearing potential and males in sexual contact with such females must use multiple contraception methods.

Future studies are needed to elucidate the role of lenalidomide as part of initial MM therapy, as well as maintenance therapy after ASCT. Also, while various three- and four-drug combinations including lenalidomide as the

TABLE 9: Summary of phase III trials evaluating new indications for lenalidomide in the treatment of multiple myeloma.

New indications	Trials	Regimens	Response rate	PFS	OS
Induction therapy	ECOG E4A03 Rajkumar et al., 2010 [30]	Len + HD dex	79%	19.1 mos	75% (2-yr)
		Len + LD dex	68%	25.3 mos	87% (2-yr)
	MM-015 Palumbo et al. 2012 [31] $N = 348$ (Age 65–75)	MP	47%	12 mos	65% (3 yrs)
		MPR		15 mos	~70% (3 yrs)
		MPR-R	79%	31 mos	73% (3 yrs)
	MM-020	MPT Len + LD dex until progression Len + LD dex for 18 mos	In progress	In progress	In progress
	Palumbo et al., 2011 [32] $N = 402$	Len + LD dex × 4 cycles → MPR	20%	54% (2 yrs)	87% (2 yrs)
		Len + LD dex × 4 cycles → ASCT × 2	25%	73% (2 yrs)	90% (2 yrs)
Maintenance therapy after ASCT	IFM2005-02 Attal et al, 2010 [33] $N = 614$	Len	—	42 mos	81% (3 yrs)
		Placebo	—	24 mos	81% (3 yrs)
	CALGB 100104 McCarthy et al. 2010 [34] $N = 568$	Len	—	43.6 mos	~80% (3 yrs)
		Placebo	—	21.5 mos	~80% (3 yrs)
Induction and maintenance ± ASCT in newly diagnosed patients	IFM/Dana Farber trial	VRD × 8 → Len maintenance × 1 yr (ASCT at progression) VRD × 3 → ASCT → Len maintenance × 1 yr	In progress	In progress	In progress

CR: compete response; PFS: progression-free survival; OS: overall survival; Len: lenalidomide; HD dex: high-dose dexamethasone; LD dex: low-dose dexamethasone; MP: melphalan, prednisone; MPR: melphalan, prednisone, lenalidomide; MPR-R: MPR + lenalidomide maintenance until progression; MPT: melphalan, prednisone, thalidomide; ASCT: autologous stem cell transplantation; VRD: bortezomib, lenalidomide, dexamethasone.

backbone appear promising, not enough information is available to recommend combination treatment outside of a clinical trial.

Following submission of this manuscript, Chen et al., sponsored by Cancer Care Ontario. Published a guideline on Lenalidomide in Multiple Myeloma [76].

Disclosure

D. Reece research funding from Celgene, Janssen, Millennium Pharmaceuticals, Novartis, Merck, Bristol-Meyers-Squibb and honoraria from Celgene, Janssen, Novartis and Amgen. C. Tom Kouroukis received honoraria and had advisory boards from Celgene and Novartis and Honoraria from Janssen, Amgen. R. LeBlanc received research funding from Janssen, Celgene, The Binding Site and Myeloma Canada and honoraria and advisory board from Celgene, Janssen and Novartis. M. Sebag received research funding from Janssen and honoraria and advisory boards from Celgene, Janssen and Novartis. K. Song received research support from Celgene and honoraria and advisory boards from Celgene, Janssen and Novartis. The participation of J. Ashkenas was supported by Myeloma Canada. J. Ashkenas declares no other areas of possible conflicts, financial or otherwise.

Acknowledgments

The authors thank Myeloma Canada and Celgene Canada for their support of this project through an unrestricted educational grant. They also thank Peter Janiszewski, Ph.D. SCRIPT, Toronto, Ontario, Canada, for assistance in preparing this paper.

References

[1] Canadian Cancer Society's Steering Committee on Cancer Statistics, *Canadian Cancer Statistics*, Canadian Cancer Society, Toronto, ON, 2011.

[2] S. K. Kumar, S. V. Rajkumar, A. Dispenzieri et al., "Improved survival in multiple myeloma and the impact of novel therapies," *Blood*, vol. 111, no. 5, pp. 2516–2520, 2008.

[3] C. P. Venner, J. M. Connors, H. J. Sutherland et al., "Novel agents improve survival of transplant patients with multiple myeloma including those with high-risk disease defined by

early relapse (<12 months)," *Leukemia and Lymphoma*, vol. 52, no. 1, pp. 34–41, 2011.

[4] P. Richardson, S. Jagannath, M. Hussein et al., "Safety and efficacy of single-agent lenalidomide in patients with relapsed and refractory multiple myeloma," *Blood*, vol. 114, no. 4, pp. 772–778, 2009.

[5] A. K. Gandhi, J. Kang, L. Capone et al., "Dexamethasone synergizes with lenalidomide to inhibit multiple myeloma tumor growth, but reduces lenalidomide-induced immunomodulation of T and NK cell function," *Current Cancer Drug Targets*, vol. 10, no. 2, pp. 155–167, 2010.

[6] N. Mitsiades, C. S. Mitsiades, V. Poulaki et al., "Apoptotic signaling induced by immunomodulatory thalidomide analogs in human multiple myeloma cells: therapeutic implications," *Blood*, vol. 99, no. 12, pp. 4525–4530, 2002.

[7] T. Hideshima, D. Chauhan, Y. Shima et al., "Thalidomide and its analogs overcome drug resistance of human multiple myeloma cells to conventional therapy," *Blood*, vol. 96, no. 9, pp. 2943–2950, 2000.

[8] D. Verhelle, L. G. Corral, K. Wong et al., "Lenalidomide and CC-4047 inhibit the proliferation of malignant B cells while expanding normal CD34+ progenitor cells," *Cancer Research*, vol. 67, no. 2, pp. 746–755, 2007.

[9] A. De Luisi, A. Ferrucci, A. M. L. Coluccia et al., "Lenalidomide restrains motility and overangiogenic potential of bone marrow endothelial cells in patients with active multiple myeloma," *Clinical Cancer Research*, vol. 17, no. 7, pp. 1935–1946, 2011.

[10] V. Kotla, S. Goel, S. Nischal et al., "Mechanism of action of lenalidomide in hematological malignancies," *Journal of Hematology and Oncology*, vol. 2, p. 36, 2009.

[11] F. Davies and R. Baz, "Lenalidomide mode of action: Linking bench and clinical findings," *Blood Reviews*, vol. 24, supplement 1, pp. S13–S19, 2010.

[12] D. M. Weber, C. Chen, R. Niesvizky et al., "Lenalidomide plus dexamethasone for relapsed multiple myeloma in North America," *The New England Journal of Medicine*, vol. 357, no. 21, pp. 2133–2142, 2007.

[13] M. Dimopoulos, A. Spencer, M. Attal et al., "Lenalidomide plus dexamethasone for relapsed or refractory multiple myeloma," *The New England Journal of Medicine*, vol. 357, no. 21, pp. 2123–2132, 2007.

[14] Revlimid Product Monograph. Celgene Inc. July 30, 2011.

[15] D. Reece, K. W. Song, T. Fu et al., "Influence of cytogenetics in patients with relapsed or refractory multiple myeloma treated with lenalidomide plus dexamethasone: adverse effect of deletion 17p13," *Blood*, vol. 114, no. 3, pp. 522–525, 2009.

[16] U. Klein, A. Jauch, T. Hielscher et al., "Chromosomal aberrations +1q21 and del(17p13) predict survival in patients with recurrent multiple myeloma treated with lenalidomide and dexamethasone," *Cancer*, vol. 117, no. 10, pp. 2136–2144, 2011.

[17] H. Avet-Loiseau, J. Soulier, J. P. Fermand et al., "Impact of high-risk cytogenetics and prior therapy on outcomes in patients with advanced relapsed or refractory multiple myeloma treated with lenalidomide plus dexaméthasone," *Leukemia*, vol. 24, no. 3, pp. 623–628, 2010.

[18] M. A. Dimopoulos, E. Kastritis, D. Christoulas et al., "Treatment of patients with relapsed/refractory multiple myeloma with lenalidomide and dexamethasone with or without bortezomib: prospective evaluation of the impact of cytogenetic abnormalities and of previous therapies," *Leukemia*, vol. 24, no. 10, pp. 1769–1778, 2010.

[19] M. Wang, M. A. Dimopoulos, C. Chen et al., "Lenalidomide plus dexamethasone is more effective than dexamethasone alone in patients with relapsed or refractory multiple myeloma regardless of prior thalidomide exposure," *Blood*, vol. 112, no. 12, pp. 4445–4451, 2008.

[20] A. Palumbo, P. Falco, P. Corradini et al., "Melphalan, prednisone, and lenalidomide treatment for newly diagnosed myeloma: a report from the GIMEMA—Italian Multiple Myeloma Network," *Journal of Clinical Oncology*, vol. 25, no. 28, pp. 4459–4465, 2007.

[21] A. Palumbo, M. Delforge, J. Catalano et al., "A phase 3 study evaluating the efficacy and safety of lenalidomide combined with melphalan and prednisone in patients >= 65 years with newly diagnosed multiple myeloma (ndmm): continuous use of lenalidomide vs fixed-duration regimens," *Blood*, vol. 116, abstract no. 622, 2010.

[22] A. Palumbo, A. Larocca, P. Falco et al., "Lenalidomide, melphalan, prednisone and thalidomide (RMPT) for relapsed/refractory multiple myeloma," *Leukemia*, vol. 24, no. 5, pp. 1037–1042, 2010.

[23] P. G. Richardson, E. Weller, S. Jagannath et al., "Multicenter, phase I, dose-escalation trial of lenalidomide plus bortezomib for relapsed and relapsed/refractory multiple myeloma," *Journal of Clinical Oncology*, vol. 27, no. 34, pp. 5713–5719, 2009.

[24] P. G. Richardson, E. Weller, S. Lonial et al., "Lenalidomide, bortezomib, and dexamethasone combination therapy in patients with newly diagnosed multiple myeloma," *Blood*, vol. 116, no. 5, pp. 679–686, 2010.

[25] D. E. Reece, E. Masih-Khan, A. Khan et al., "Phase I-II trial of oral cyclophosphamide, prednisone and lenalidomide (Revlimid) for the treatment of patients with relapsed and refractory multiple myeloma," *Blood*, vol. 116, abstract no. 3055, 2010.

[26] S. A. Schey, G. J. Morgan, K. Ramasamy et al., "The addition of cyclophosphamide to lenalidomide and dexamethasone in multiply relapsed/refractory myeloma patients; a phase I/II study," *British Journal of Haematology*, vol. 150, no. 3, pp. 326–333, 2010.

[27] S. K. Kumar, I. Flinn, S. J. Noga et al., "Bortezomib, dexamethasone, cyclophosphamide and lenalidomide combination for newly diagnosed multiple myeloma: phase 1 results from the multicenter EVOLUTION study," *Leukemia*, vol. 24, no. 7, pp. 1350–1356, 2010.

[28] S. K. Kumar, M. Q. Lacy, S. R. Hayman et al., "Lenalidomide, cyclophosphamide and dexamethasone (CRd) for newly diagnosed multiple myeloma: results from a phase 2 trial," *American Journal of Hematology*, vol. 86, no. 8, pp. 640–645, 2011.

[29] A. J. Jakubowiak, K. A. Griffith, D. E. Reece et al., "Lenalidomide, bortezomib, pegylated liposomal doxorubicin, and dexamethasone in newly diagnosed multiple myeloma: a phase 1/2 multiple myeloma research consortium trial," *Blood*, vol. 118, no. 3, pp. 535–543, 2011.

[30] S. V. Rajkumar, S. Jacobus, N. S. Callander et al., "Lenalidomide plus high-dose dexamethasone versus lenalidomide plus low-dose dexamethasone as initial therapy for newly diagnosed multiple myeloma: an open-label randomised controlled trial," *The Lancet Oncology*, vol. 11, no. 1, pp. 29–37, 2010.

[31] A. Palumbo, R. Hajek, M. Delforge et al., "Continuous lenalidomide treatment for newly diagnosed multiple myeloma," *Blood*, vol. 366, pp. 1759–1769, 2012.

[32] A. Palumbo, F. Cavallo, i. Hardan et al., "Melphalan/ Prednisone/Lenalidomide (MPR) Versus High-Dose Melphalan

and Autologous Transplantation (MEL200) in Newly Diagnosed Multiple Myeloma (MM) Patients <65 Years: results of a randomized phase III study," *Blood*, vol. 118, abstract no. 3069, 2011.

[33] M. Attal, V. Cances-Lauwers, G. Marit et al., "Lenalidomide maintenance treatment after stem-cell transplantation for multiple myeloma," *The New England Journal of Medicine*, vol. 366, pp. 1782–1791, 2010.

[34] P. McCarthy, K. Owzar, and K. Anderson, "Phase III Intergroup study of lenalidomide versus placebo maintenance therapy following single autologous hematopoietic stem cell transplantation (AHSC T) for multiple myeloma: CALGB, 100104," *Blood*, vol. 116, abstract no. 37, 2010.

[35] E. A. Stadtmauer, D. M. Weber, R. Niesvizky et al., "Lenalidomide in combination with dexamethasone at first relapse in comparison with its use as later salvage therapy in relapsed or refractory multiple myeloma," *European Journal of Haematology*, vol. 82, no. 6, pp. 426–432, 2009.

[36] M. Kleber, G. Ihorst, B. Deschler et al., "Detection of renal impairment as one specific comorbidity factor in multiple myeloma: multicenter study in 198 consecutive patients," *European Journal of Haematology*, vol. 83, no. 6, pp. 519–527, 2009.

[37] J. F. San Miguel, M. Dimopoulos, D. Weber et al., "Dexamethasone dose adjustments seem to result in better efficacy and improved tolerability in patients with relapsed/refractory multiple myeloma who are treated with lenalidomide/dexamethasone (MM-009/010 sub-analysis)," *Blood*, vol. 110, abstract no. 2712, 2007.

[38] A. K. Hsu, H. Quach, T. Tai et al., "The immunostimulatory effect of lenalidomide on NK-cell function is profoundly inhibited by concurrent dexamethasone therapy," *Blood*, vol. 117, no. 5, pp. 1605–1613, 2011.

[39] J. F. San-Miguel, M. A. Dimopoulos, E. A. Stadtmauer et al., "Effects of lenalidomide and dexamethasone treatment duration on survival in patients with relapsed or refractory multiple myeloma treated with lenalidomide and dexamethasone," *Clinical Lymphoma, Myeloma and Leukemia*, vol. 11, no. 1, pp. 38–43, 2011.

[40] M. Dimopoulos and N. R. Orlowski, "Lenalidomide and dexamethasone (LEN plus DEX) treatment in relapsed/refractory multiple myeloma (RRMM) patients (pts) and risk of second primary malignancies (SPM): analysis of MM-009/010.," *Journal of Clinical Oncology*, vol. 29, abstract no. 8009, 2011.

[41] B. Nair, F. Van Rhee, J. D. Shaughnessy et al., "Superior results of total therapy 3 (2003-33) in gene expression profiling-defined low-risk multiple myeloma confirmed in subsequent trial 2006-66 with VRD maintenance," *Blood*, vol. 115, no. 21, pp. 4168–4173, 2010.

[42] T. Guglielmelli, S. Bringhen, S. Rrodhe et al., "Previous thalidomide therapy may not affect lenalidomide response and outcome in relapse or refractory multiple myeloma patients," *European Journal of Cancer*, vol. 47, no. 6, pp. 814–818, 2011.

[43] S. Madan, M. Q. Lacy, A. Dispenzieri et al., "Efficacy of retreatment with immunomodulatory drugs (IMiDs) in patients receiving IMiDs for initial therapy of newly diagnosed multiple myeloma," *Blood*, vol. 118, pp. 1763–1765, 2011.

[44] K. C. Altekruse SF, M. Krapcho, N. Neyman et al., Eds., *SEER Cancer Statistics Review, 1975–2007*, National Cancer Institute, Bethesda, MD, USA, 2010.

[45] C. Chen, D. E. Reece, D. Siegel et al., "Expanded safety experience with lenalidomide plus dexamethasone in relapsed or refractory multiple myeloma," *British Journal of Haematology*, vol. 146, no. 2, pp. 164–170, 2009.

[46] J. D. Ishak, M. A. Weber, D. Knight et al., "Declining rates of adverse events and dose modifications with lenalidomide in combination with dexamethasone," *Blood*, vol. 112, abstract no. 3708, 2008.

[47] S. B. Lonial, R. Swern, A. S. . Weber et al., "Neutropenia is a predictable and early event in affected patients with relapsed/refractory multiple myeloma treated with lenalidomide in combination with dexamethasone," *Blood*, vol. 114, abstract no. 2879, 2009.

[48] R. Niesvizky, T. Naib, P. J. Christos et al., "Lenalidomide-induced myelosuppression is associated with renal dysfunction: adverse events evaluation of treatment-naïve patients undergoing front-line lenalidomide and dexamethasone therapy," *British Journal of Haematology*, vol. 138, no. 5, pp. 640–643, 2007.

[49] S. Kumar, A. Dispenzieri, M. Q. Lacy et al., "Impact of lenalidomide therapy on stem cell mobilization and engraftment post-peripheral blood stem cell transplantation in patients with newly diagnosed myeloma," *Leukemia*, vol. 21, no. 9, pp. 2035–2042, 2007.

[50] U. Popat, R. Saliba, R. Thandi et al., "Impairment of filgrastim-induced stem cell mobilization after prior lenalidomide in patients with multiple myeloma," *Biology of Blood and Marrow Transplantation*, vol. 15, no. 6, pp. 718–723, 2009.

[51] A. Nazha, R. Cook, D. T. Vogl et al., "Stem cell collection in patients with multiple myeloma: impact of induction therapy and mobilization regimen," *Bone Marrow Transplantation*, vol. 46, no. 1, pp. 59–63, 2011.

[52] T. Mark, J. Stern, J. R. Furst et al., "Stem cell mobilization with cyclophosphamide overcomes the suppressive effect of lenalidomide therapy on stem cell collection in multiple myeloma," *Biology of Blood and Marrow Transplantation*, vol. 14, no. 7, pp. 795–798, 2008.

[53] I. N. M. Micallef, A. D. Ho, L. M. Klein, S. Marulkar, P. J. Gandhi, and P. A. McSweeney, "Plerixafor (Mozobil) for stem cell mobilization in patients with multiple myeloma previously treated with lenalidomide," *Bone Marrow Transplantation*, vol. 46, no. 3, pp. 350–355, 2011.

[54] R. L. Baz, S. Hussein, M. Swern et al., "Lenalidomide (LEN) therapy in combination with dexamethasone (DEX) is associated with a low incidence of viral infections," *Blood*, vol. 116, abstract no. 1950, 2010.

[55] M. Carrier, G. Le Gal, J. Tay, C. Wu, and A. Y. Lee, "Rates of venous thromboembolism in multiple myeloma patients undergoing immunomodulatory therapy with thalidomide or lenalidomide: a systematic review and meta-analysis," *Journal of Thrombosis and Haemostasis*, vol. 9, no. 4, pp. 653–663, 2011.

[56] A. Palumbo, M. Cavo, S. Bringhen et al., "Aspirin, warfarin, or enoxaparin thromboprophylaxis in patients with multiple myeloma treated with thalidomide: a phase III, open-label, randomized trial," *Journal of Clinical Oncology*, vol. 29, no. 8, pp. 986–993, 2011.

[57] A. Larocca, F. Cavallo, S. Bringhen et al., "Aspirin or enoxaparin thromboprophylaxis for newly-diagnosed multiple 11 myeloma patients treated with lenalidomide," *Blood*, vol. 119, no. 4, pp. 933–939, 2012.

[58] H. P. Sviggum, M. D. P. Davis, S. V. Rajkumar, and A. Dispenzieri, "Dermatologic adverse effects of lenalidomide therapy for amyloidosis and multiple myeloma," *Archives of Dermatology*, vol. 142, no. 10, pp. 1298–1302, 2006.

[59] J. Phillips, J. Kujawa, M. Davis-Lorton, and A. Hindenburg, "Successful desensitization in a patient with lenalidomide

hypersensitivity," *American Journal of Hematology*, vol. 82, no. 11, p. 1030, 2007.

[60] E. Nucera, D. Schiavino, S. Hohaus et al., "Desensitization to thalidomide in a patient with multiple myeloma," *Clinical Lymphoma and Myeloma*, vol. 8, no. 3, pp. 176–178, 2008.

[61] S. El-Tawil, T. Al Musa, H. Valli, M. P. Lunn, T. El-Tawil, and M. Weber, "Quinine for muscle cramps," *Cochrane database of systematic reviews*, vol. 12, Article ID CD005044, 2010.

[62] R. Zambello, T. Berno, L. Candiotto et al., "Peripherial neuropathy clinical course during lenalidomide therapy for relapsed/refractory multiple myeloma: a single-centre prospective non interventional study," *Haematologica*, vol. 96, abstract no. P-399, 2011.

[63] C.-M. Wendtner, P. Hillmen, D. Mahadevan et al., "Final results of a multicenter phase 1 study of lenalidomide in patients with relapsed or refractory chronic lymphocytic leukemia," *Leukemia and Lymphoma*, vol. 53, no. 3, pp. 417–423, 2012.

[64] C. S. Chim, "Rapid complete remission in multiple myeloma with bortezomib/thalidomide/ dexamethasone combination therapy following development of tumor lysis syndrome," *Cancer Chemotherapy and Pharmacology*, vol. 62, no. 1, pp. 181–182, 2008.

[65] D. J. Leddin, R. Enns, R. Hilsden et al., "Canadian Association of Gastroenterology position statement on screening individuals at average risk for developing colorectal cancer: 2010," *Canadian Journal of Gastroenterology*, vol. 24, no. 12, pp. 705–714, 2010.

[66] J. Izawa, K. L. D. Siemens et al., "Prostate cancer screening: Canadian guidelines 2011," *Canadian Urological Association Journal*, vol. 5, pp. 235–240, 2010.

[67] S. Hussain, R. Browne, J. Chen, and S. Parekh, "Lenalidomide-induced severe hepatotoxicity," *Blood*, vol. 110, no. 10, p. 3814, 2007.

[68] M. K. Figaro, W. Clayton, C. Usoh et al., "Thyroid abnormalities in patients treated with lenalidomide for hematological malignancies: results of a retrospective case review," *American Journal of Hematology*, vol. 86, no. 6, pp. 467–470, 2011.

[69] F. Gay, S. S. Vincent Rajkumar, P. Falco et al., "Lenalidomide plus dexamethasone vs. lenalidomide plus melphalan and prednisone: a retrospective study in newly diagnosed elderly myeloma," *European Journal of Haematology*, vol. 85, no. 3, pp. 200–208, 2010.

[70] A. J. Jakubowiak, D. Dytfeld, S. Jagannath et al., "Carfilzomib, lenalidomide, and dexamethasone in newly diagnosed multiple myeloma: initial results of phase I/II MMRC trial," *Blood*, vol. 116, abstract no. 862, 2010.

[71] S. Lentzsch, A. O. 'Sullivan, R. Kennedy et al., "Combination of bendamustine, lenalidomide, and dexamethasone in patients with refractory or relapsed multiple myeloma is safe and highly effective: results of a phase i clinical trial," *Blood*, vol. 116, abstract no. 989, 2010.

[72] S. Lonial, R. Vij, J. L. Harousseau et al., "Elotuzumab in combination with lenalidomide and low-dose dexamethasone in patients with relapsed/refractory multiple myeloma: interim results of a phase 1 study," *Blood*, vol. 116, abstract no. 1936, 2010.

[73] A. Palumbo, P. Falco, A. Falcone et al., "Melphalan, prednisone, and lenalidomide for newly diagnosed myeloma: kinetics of neutropenia and thrombocytopenia and time-to-event results," *Clinical Lymphoma and Myeloma*, vol. 9, no. 2, pp. 145–150, 2009.

[74] D. J. White, N. J. Bahlis, D. C. Marcellus et al., "Phase II testing of lenalidomide plus melphalan for previously untreated older patients with multiple myeloma: the NCIC CTG MY. 11 trial," *Blood*, vol. 112, abstract no. 2767, 2008.

[75] W. Bensinger, M. Wang, R. Z. Orlowski et al., "Dose-escalation study of carfilzomib (CFZ) plus lenalidomide (LEN) plus low-dose dexamethasone (Dex) (CRd) in relapsed/refractory multiple myeloma (R/R MM)," *Journal of Clinical Oncology*, vol. 28, abstract no. 8029, 2010.

[76] C. Chen, F. Baldassarre, S. Kanjeekal et al., *Lenalidomide in Multiple Myeloma*, Program in Evidence-Based Care Evidence-Based Series no. 6-5, Cancer Care Ontario, Toronto, Canada, 2012.

22

Frequency of Red Cell Alloimmunization and Autoimmunization in Thalassemia Patients: A Report from Eastern India

Suvro Sankha Datta,[1] **Somnath Mukherjee,**[2] **Biplabendu Talukder,**[3]
Prasun Bhattacharya,[3] **and Krishnendu Mukherjee**[3]

[1]*Department of Transfusion Medicine, The Mission Hospital, Durgapur, West Bengal 713212, India*
[2]*Department of Transfusion Medicine, AIIMS, Bhubaneswar 751019, India*
[3]*Department of Immunohematology & Blood Transfusion, MCH, Kolkata 700073, India*

Correspondence should be addressed to Suvro Sankha Datta; suvro.datta@gmail.com

Academic Editor: Thomas Kickler

Introduction. Red blood cell (RBC) alloimmunization and autoimmunization remain a major problem in transfusion dependent thalassemic patients. There is a paucity of data on the incidence of RBC alloimmunization and autoimmunization in thalassemic patients from eastern part of India, as pretransfusion antibody screening is not routinely performed. *Aims*. To assess the incidence of RBC alloimmunization and autoimmunization in transfusion dependent thalassemic patients in eastern India. *Materials and Methods*. Total 500 thalassemia cases were evaluated. The antibody screening and identification were performed with commercially available panel cells (Diapanel, Bio-rad, Switzerland) by column agglutination method. To detect autoantibodies, autocontrol and direct antiglobulin tests were carried out using polyspecific coombs (IgG + C3d) gel cards in all patients. *Results*. A total of 28 patients developed RBC alloimmunization (5.6%) and 5 patients had autoantibodies (1%). Alloantibody against c had the highest incidence (28.57%) followed by E (21.42%). Five out of 28 (17.85%) patients had developed antibodies against both c and E. *Conclusion*. Data from this study demonstrate that the RBC alloantibody and autoantibody development rates are significant in our region. Thus, pretransfusion antibody screening needs to be initiated in eastern India in order to ensure safe transfusion practice.

1. Introduction

Thalassemia is a congenital hemolytic disorder, caused by a partial or complete defect in α or β globin chain synthesis. In India, it is estimated that around 8000–10000 new thalassemics (homozygous) are born every year and beta thalassemia gene is found more commonly in Punjabis, Sindhis, Bengalis, and Gujaratis [1]. In the absence of stem cell transplantation, the disease is treated by life-long red blood cell (RBC) transfusion [2] to keep the hemoglobin (Hb) level between 9 and 11.5 g/dL. Blood transfusion, despite being lifesaving process, is associated with inherent risks of alloimmunization against red cells antigens. Red blood cell (RBC) alloimmunization occurs due to genetic disparity between donor and recipient red cells antigens [3]. The development

of alloantibodies and autoantibodies against RBC antigens causes laboratory difficulties during RBC crossmatching, shortens in vivo survival of transfused red cells, delays provision of safe transfusions, and may accelerate iron overloading [4, 5]. Alloimmunization rates were reported from 4% to 50% in thalassemic patients and were lower in more homogenous populations [2, 6–8]. Red cells autoantibodies are not very common but they can result in clinical hemolysis and can cause difficulty during crossmatching. Patients with autoantibodies may have a higher transfusion rate and often require immunosuppressive drugs or splenectomy [9, 10]. The term "clinically significant" in relation to alloantibodies may refer to an antibody that causes an obvious, clinical hemolytic transfusion reaction (fever, chills, hemoglobinuria, etc.) or an antibody that does not cause any overt clinical symptoms but is associated with laboratory signs of hemolysis (increased bilirubin, decreased haptoglobin, etc.) or an antibody that is not associated with any clinical or laboratory signs of hemolysis, but RBCs incompatible with it survive less than normal lifespan [11]. In eastern part of India 5.6% of population have beta thalassemia trait and 5% of population have HbE carrier state [12]. But there is a paucity of data on the incidence of RBC alloimmunization and autoimmunization in thalassemic patients from this region, as pretransfusion antibody screening is not routinely performed. Thus this study was conducted to find out the frequency of alloimmunization, autoimmunization, and most common alloantibodies involved to red cell antigens in thalassemic patients. This study helped the authors to formulate transfusion strategies for all multitransfused thalassemic patients in eastern part of India.

2. Materials and Methods

The prospective and observational study was carried out in the Department of Immunohematology & Blood Transfusion, Medical College Hospital Kolkata, for the period of two and half years (January 2012 to June 2014). The study population were all transfusion dependent thalassemic patients of Medical College Hospital Kolkata. Informed consent was obtained from patients or their parents. The study was approved by hospital ethics committee.

2.1. Patients. Total 500 thalassemic patients were evaluated in the age ranging from 2 to 40 years. The inclusion criteria were patients who were dependent on transfusion and had a history of blood transfusion at least once in every month. The exclusion criteria were female patients who were transfusion dependent but had a history of Rh isoimmunization or fetomaternal haemorrhage. Clinical and transfusion records were analyzed in all patients for presence of alloimmunization/autoimmunization with antibody specificity among different age groups and different types of thalassemic (beta thalassemia major and E-beta thalassemia) patients.

2.2. Transfusion Policy. All thalassemia patients were transfused according to institutional transfusion policy to keep target Hb level 9–11.5 g/dL with a transfusion interval of 2–4 weeks (median interval of 3 weeks). As per transfusion strategy of our institute, all thalassemia patients were given ABO and Rh(D) matched packed red cells after compatibility testing by gel card technique in the AHG phase (type and crossmatch policy). In case patients were detected to have alloantibodies, those patients received ABO & Rh(D) matched particular antigen negative (against which they had alloantibody) compatible units for transfusion. Patients who had developed autoantibodies received transfusion with "best matched" units.

2.3. Immunohematological Tests. A volume of 2 mL blood was drawn into an ethylene diamine tetraacetate (EDTA) containing tube, centrifuged at 3000 ×g for 3 minutes to obtain plasma (for crossmatch and antibody screening) and red cells (for detection of autoantibodies) on gel card system. Prior to every transfusion, plasma was tested for the presence of alloantibodies by using commercial three-cell panel (Diacell, Bio-Rad, Switzerland). All alloantibody screening positive samples were evaluated to identify the antibody specificity. Antibody specificity detection was performed using a commercial 11-cell identification panel (Diapanel, Bio-Rad, Switzerland). Autocontrol was performed in each case to identify autoantibodies. It was done by incubating patient's cell with patient's plasma at 37°C for 15 minutes and then centrifuging for 10 minutes on gel card containing polyspecific antihuman globulin (anti-IgG + C3d). A polyspecific direct antiglobulin test was also performed each time using 1% cell suspension of the patient's RBC with antihuman globulin. All the tests were performed using the gel card method by Diamed ID (Switzerland), as per manufacturer's guidelines. Elution and adsorption methods were employed in patients with suspected autoantibodies.

2.4. Statistical Analysis. Statistical analysis was performed through SPSS software (version 17.0; SPSS Inc., Chicago, IL, USA) by making the frequency distribution tables and identifying frequency of alloimmunization and autoimmunization as well as the specificity of the particular alloantibodies. Discrete categorical data were presented as n (%). Comparisons for categorical data were made by Chi-square test. All reported p values are two-sided, with a significance level of 0.05.

3. Results

3.1. Patient Characteristics. During the study period, a total of 500 thalassemia patients were reviewed. Three hundred thirty-three patients (66.6%) had beta thalassemia major and one hundred sixty-seven (33.4%) had E-beta thalassemia or thalassemia intermedia. There were 215 males and 285 females. Male to female ratio in this study was 1 : 1.33. According to blood group of the patients among Rh(D) positive patients, 120 of them were A, 184 of them were B, 106 of them were O, and 52 of them were AB. On the other side among Rh(D) negative patients, 12 of them were A, 11 of them were B, 9 of them were O, and 6 of them were AB (Figure 1).

3.2. Alloimmunization Rate in Different Groups according to Age, Sex, and Thalassemia Subtypes. According to age of distribution patients were divided into 4 age groups. In between 2 and 10 years of age total patients were 216 and among them 3 cases of alloimmunization were detected (1.38%). In 11–20 years of age total 6 patients had alloantibodies among 173 patients (3.47%). In 21–30 years of age total patients were 81 and among them 15 had alloantibodies (18.52%). In 31–40 years of age among 30 patients 4 had alloimmunization (13.33%). So it was found that the rate of alloimmunization increases with the age of the patients' population and approximately 67.86% (19/28) of total cases of alloimmunization were detected in the age group of 21–40 years (Figure 2).

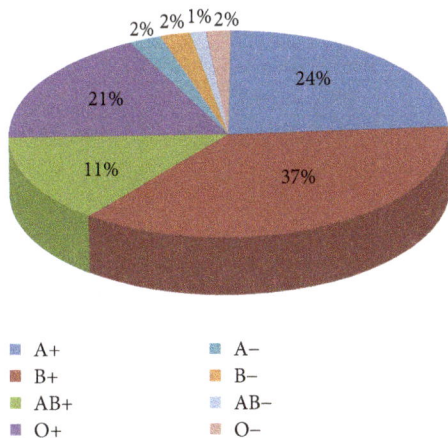

FIGURE 1: Blood groups of patients.

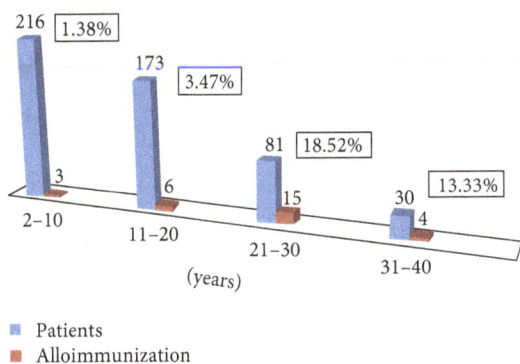

FIGURE 2: Alloimmunization in different age groups.

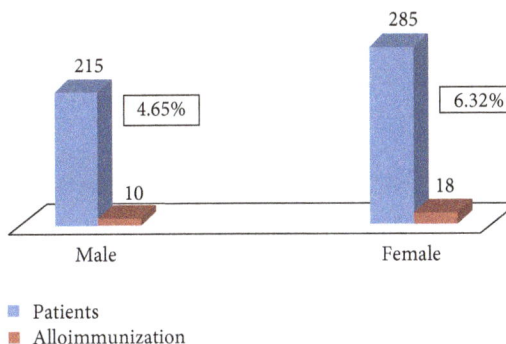

FIGURE 3: Alloimmunization in male and female patients.

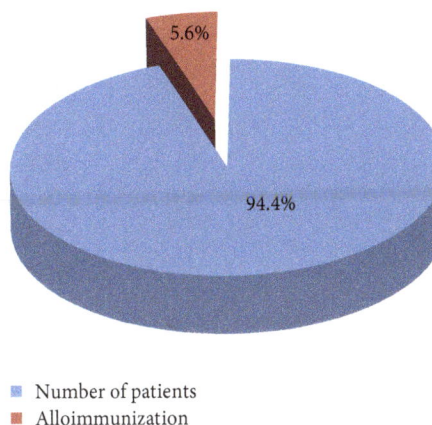

FIGURE 4: Alloimmunization rate.

The rates of alloimmunization among male and female patients population were 10 cases of alloimmunization among 215 of male patients and 18 cases of alloimmunization in 285 of female patients. The rates of alloimmunization among male and female populations were 4.65% (10/215) and 6.32% (18/285), respectively (Figure 3). As the p value was more than 0.05, there were no significant differences observed in rate of alloimmunization between male and female patients population.

The rate of alloimmunization was 5.71% (19/333) in beta thalassemia major patients and 5.39% (9/167) in E-beta thalassemic. As the p value was more than 0.05, therefore no significant differences were observed between beta thalassemia major and E-beta thalassemic patients (Table 1).

3.3. Alloantibody Specificity. A total of 28 patients developed RBC alloimmunization among 500 (5.6%) (Figure 4). Alloantibody against c had the highest incidence (28.57%) followed by E (21.42%), Jk^b (7.14%), Jk^a (3.57%), C (3.57%), D (3.57%), and s (3.57%), respectively. Five out of 28 (17.85%) patients had developed antibodies against c and E and three out of 28 patients had alloimmunization against C and D (3.57%), E and Jk^b (3.57%), and E and Fy^b (3.57%), respectively (Table 2).

3.4. Autoimmunization. Among 500 patients, 5 had (1%) developed autoantibodies as determined by positive autocontrol on gel card (IgG + C3d) as well as positive direct antiglobulin tests.

4. Discussion

There is no study on the frequency of alloimmunization and autoimmunization in transfusion dependent thalassemia patients from eastern part of India till now. In the present study we examined and defined the alloimmunization rate along with rate of autoantibody formation. We also reported the frequency of different alloantibodies in these patients' population that have not been previously described.

The factors for alloimmunization are complex and involve predominantly three contributing elements: the RBC antigenic difference between the blood donor and the recipient; the recipient's immune status; and the immunomodulatory effect of the allogeneic blood transfusions on the recipient's immune system. A low rate of alloimmunization may be expected when there is homogeneity of RBC antigens between the blood providers and recipients. Previous data on presumed homogenous populations in Greece and Italy showed an overall low rate (5% to 10%) of alloimmunization [6, 13, 14]. But data from Asia and Africa varies significantly in different countries. The rate of alloimmunization was reported as high as 23% in few countries [15, 16] to 7.7% in

TABLE 1: Alloimmunization in different types of thalassemic patients.

Alloimmunization	Beta thalassemia major	E-beta thalassemia	p value
Rate	(19/333) = 5.71%	(9/167) = 5.39%	$p > 0.05$

TABLE 2: Alloantibody specificity.

Alloantibody type	Number of cases (n)	Frequency of alloantibody
Anti-c	8	(8/28) = 28.57%
Anti-E	6	(6/28) = 21.42%
Anti-(c + E)	5	(5/28) = 17.85%
Anti-Jk^b	2	(2/28) = 7.14%
Anti-Jk^a	1	(1/28) = 3.57%
Anti-(E + Fy^b)	1	(1/28) = 3.57%
Anti-(E + Jk^b)	1	(1/28) = 3.57%
Anti-C	1	(1/28) = 3.57%
Anti-D	1	(1/28) = 3.57%
Anti-(D + C)	1	(1/28) = 3.57%
Anti-s	1	(1/28) = 3.57%
Total (n)	28	

some other nations [17, 18] depending on demography and homogeneity of population. Different studies were reported from different parts of India showing the alloimmunization rate in between 3.4% and 8.6% [19–22]. In this study the rate of alloimmunization was 5.6% which was consistent with the rate of alloimmunization observed in other parts of India. At our center, most of the patients and blood donors are from West Bengal and adjoining areas. This homogeneity between the patient and blood donors population may be the reason for low rate of alloimmunization in this study.

When we compared the alloimmunization rate in different age groups, we found that most cases of alloimmunization (67.86%) were detected in the age group of 21–40 years as those patients were dependent on blood transfusion for several years. Thus it was assumed that the patients who required blood transfusion for several years with multiple units had more chance to form alloantibody in course of their life. This was consistent with a study which showed that frequency of alloantibody was higher among transfusion recipients of more than one unit of red cell transfusion and approximately 2–9% of those patients had new alloantibodies [23]. As we could not identify the actual starting time of blood transfusion in the study population, the low rate of alloimmunization in paediatric age group might be due to immune tolerance to form alloantibody on exposure to foreign red cell antigens [24, 25].

We did not find any association of gender (male/female) with rate of alloimmunization. In literature, few studies showed that gender was not a significant factor in the development of alloimmunization [26, 27]. However, some reported a significant association between alloimmunization

and gender [28, 29]. Alloimmunization rate was not significantly affected depending on the diagnosis of thalassemia. It was almost same in beta thalassemia major and E-beta thalassemic patients.

In this study it was observed that around 78.5% of alloantibodies detected were against the antigens of Rh system. Similar result was also reported from a center in north India [19]. In this study alloantibody against c antigen was the most common alloantibody against a single red cell antigen (28.57%) followed by alloantibody against E (21.42%). Among the alloantibodies against multiple red cell antigens alloantibody against c and E was the most common (17.85%). This was consistent with the results of other studies [19, 21]. On obtaining a detailed transfusion history from the alloimmunized patients, it was found that the two Rh(D) negative patients who developed anti-D had received transfusions in rural hospitals on two and three occasions. We have no information about whether weak D testing of donor units was done at those hospitals. This could account for the development of anti-D in two of our thalassemic patients. It was reported that, in alloimmunized patients, the probability of additional antibody formation increases approximately threefold [30, 31]. This report alerts us that the transfusion dependent patients with single alloantibody are at risk of developing multiple alloantibodies in further course of time.

In the present study, 5 (1%) patients developed autoantibodies. Previously studies reported 1.7% to 11% rate of autoimmunization in thalassemia patients [32, 33]. No autoantibody was associated with alloimmunization in this study. In all cases elution was performed and elutes were tested with the panel cells on gel card. In all cases IgG autoantibodies were detected with a panagglutinin reaction with the panel cells. The clinical importance of autoantibodies in multitransfused patients is debatable. Although some reports found the existence of warm autoantibodies to be associated with clinically significant hemolysis [34], others did not find any significant association with hemolysis [35].

5. Conclusion

Although the overall incidence of RBC alloimmunization in this study was 5.6%, almost all of the alloimmunized patients had the antibodies which were clinically significant. Thus, pretransfusion antibody screening on patients' sample prior to crossmatching needs to be initiated in eastern India to ensure safe transfusion practice. We also recommended a practical, cost-effective, and feasible approach that the RBC antigen typing should be performed before first transfusion in thalassemic patients and issue of antigen matched blood (at least for Rh and Kell antigen) should be started to reduce the risk of alloimmunization.

Conflict of Interests

The authors declare that there is no conflict of interests regarding the publication of this paper.

References

[1] D. Shah, P. Chowdhary, and A. P. Dubey, "Current trends in management of beta thalassemia," *Indian Journal of Pediatrics*, vol. 36, pp. 1229–1242, 1999.

[2] L.-Y. Wang, D.-C. Liang, H.-C. Liu et al., "Alloimmunization among patients with transfusion-dependent thalassemia in Taiwan," *Transfusion Medicine*, vol. 16, no. 3, pp. 200–203, 2006.

[3] K. S. Trudell, "Detection and identification of antibodies," in *Modern Blood Banking and Transfusion Practices*, D. M. Harmening, Ed., pp. 242–263, FA Davis, Philadelphia, Pa, USA, 5th edition, 2005.

[4] S. Charache, "Problems in transfusion therapy," *The New England Journal of Medicine*, vol. 322, no. 23, pp. 1666–1668, 1990.

[5] J. M. Higgins and S. R. Sloan, "Stochastic modeling of human RBC alloimmunization: evidence for a distinct population of immunologic responders," *Blood*, vol. 112, no. 6, pp. 2546–2553, 2008.

[6] G. Sirchia, A. Zanella, A. Parravicini, F. Morelati, P. Rebulla, and G. Masera, "Red cell alloantibodies in thalassemia major: results of an Italian cooperative study," *Transfusion*, vol. 25, no. 2, pp. 110–112, 1985.

[7] S. T. Singer, V. Wu, R. Mignacca, F. A. Kuypers, P. Morel, and E. P. Vichinsky, "Alloimmunization and erythrocyte autoimmunization in transfusion-dependent thalassemia patients of predominantly Asian descent," *Blood*, vol. 96, no. 10, pp. 3369–3373, 2000.

[8] S. Pahuja, M. Pujani, S. K. Gupta, J. Chandra, and M. Jain, "Alloimmunization and red cell autoimmunization in multitransfused thalassemics of Indian origin," *Hematology*, vol. 15, no. 3, pp. 174–177, 2010.

[9] M. Kruatrachue, S. Sirisinha, P. Pacharee, D. Chandarayingyong, and P. Wasi, "An association between thalassaemia and autoimmune haemolytic anaemia (AIHA)," *Scandinavian Journal of Haematology*, vol. 25, no. 3, pp. 259–263, 1980.

[10] F. Argiolu, G. Diana, M. Arnone, M. G. Batzella, P. Piras, and A. Cao, "High-dose intravenous immunoglobulin in the management of autoimmune hemolytic anemia complicating thalassemia major," *Acta Haematologica*, vol. 83, no. 2, pp. 65–68, 1990.

[11] G. Meny, "Review: transfusing incompatible RBCs-clinical aspects," *Immunohematology*, vol. 20, no. 3, pp. 161–166, 2004.

[12] D. Mukhopadhyay, K. Saha, M. Sengupta, S. Mitra, C. Datta, and P. K. Mitra, "Spectrum of hemoglobinopathies in West Bengal, India: a CE-HPLC Study on 10407 subjects," *Indian Journal of Hematology and Blood Transfusion*, vol. 31, no. 1, pp. 98–103, 2015.

[13] S. M. Coles, H. G. Klein, and P. V. Holland, "Alloimmunization in two multitransfused patient populations," *Transfusion*, vol. 21, no. 4, pp. 462–466, 1981.

[14] J. Economidou, M. Constantoulakis, O. Augoustaki, and M. Adinolfi, "Frequency of antibodies to various antigenic determinants in polytransfused patients with homozygous thalassaemia in Greece," *Vox Sanguinis*, vol. 20, no. 3, pp. 252–258, 1971.

[15] A. G. M. A. Gader, A. K. Al Ghumlas, and A. K. M. Al-Momen, "Transfusion medicine in a developing country—alloantibodies to red blood cells in multi-transfused patients in Saudi Arabia," *Transfusion and Apheresis Science*, vol. 39, no. 3, pp. 199–204, 2008.

[16] C. K. Cheng, C. K. Lee, and C. K. Lin, "Clinically significant red blood cell antibodies in chronically transfused patients: a survey of Chinese thalassemia major patients and literature review," *Transfusion*, vol. 52, no. 10, pp. 2220–2224, 2012.

[17] A. M. Ahmed, N. S. Hasan, S. H. Ragab, S. A. Habib, N. A. Emara, and A. A. Aly, "Red cell alloimmunization and autoantibodies in Egyptian transfusion-dependent thalassaemia patients," *Archives of Medical Science*, vol. 6, no. 4, pp. 592–598, 2010.

[18] N. Guirat-Dhouib, M. Mezri, H. Hmida et al., "High frequency of autoimmunization among transfusion-dependent Tunisian thalassaemia patients," *Transfusion and Apheresis Science*, vol. 45, no. 2, pp. 199–202, 2011.

[19] B. Thakral, K. Saluja, R. R. Sharma, and N. Marwaha, "Red cell alloimmunization in a transfused patient population: a study from a tertiary care hospital in north India," *Hematology*, vol. 13, no. 5, pp. 313–318, 2008.

[20] R. Sood, R. N. Makroo, V. Riana, and N. L. Rosamma, "Detection of alloimmunization to ensure safer transfusion practice," *Asian Journal of Transfusion Science*, vol. 7, no. 2, pp. 135–139, 2013.

[21] H. K. Dhawan, V. Kumawat, N. Marwaha et al., "Alloimmunization and autoimmunization in transfusion dependent thalassemia major patients: study on 319 patients," *Asian Journal of Transfusion Science*, vol. 8, no. 2, pp. 84–88, 2014.

[22] A. Dogra, M. Sidhu, R. Kapoor, and D. Kumar, "Study of red blood cell alloimmunization in multitransfused thalassemic children of Jammu region," *Asian Journal of Transfusion Science*, vol. 9, no. 1, p. 78, 2015.

[23] C. A. Tormey, J. Fisk, and G. Stack, "Red blood cell alloantibody frequency, specificity, and properties in a population of male military veterans," *Transfusion*, vol. 48, no. 10, pp. 2069–2076, 2008.

[24] W. F. Rosse, D. Gallagher, T. R. Kinney et al., "Transfusion and alloimmunization in sickle cell disease. The cooperative study of sickle cell disease," *Blood*, vol. 76, no. 7, pp. 1431–1437, 1990.

[25] J. Poole and G. Daniels, "Blood group antibodies and their significance in transfusion medicine," *Transfusion Medicine Reviews*, vol. 21, no. 1, pp. 58–71, 2007.

[26] A. S. El Danasoury, D. G. Eissa, R. M. Abdo, and M. S. Elalfy, "Red blood cell alloimmunization in transfusion-dependent Egyptian patients with thalassemia in a limited donor exposure program," *Transfusion*, vol. 52, no. 1, pp. 43–47, 2012.

[27] J. E. Hendrickson, M. Desmarets, S. S. Deshpande et al., "Recipient inflammation affects the frequency and magnitude of immunization to transfused red blood cells," *Transfusion*, vol. 46, no. 9, pp. 1526–1536, 2006.

[28] E. G. Reisner, D. D. Kostyu, G. Phillips, C. Walker, and D. V. Dawson, "Alloantibody responses in multiply transfused sickle cell patients," *Tissue Antigens*, vol. 30, no. 4, pp. 161–166, 1987.

[29] D. A. Saied, A. M. Kaddah, R. M. Badr Eldin, and S. S. Mohaseb, "Alloimmunization and erythrocyte autoimmunization in transfusion-dependent Egyptian thalassemic patients," *Journal of Pediatric Hematology/Oncology*, vol. 33, no. 6, pp. 409–414, 2011.

[30] R. Yousuf, S. Abdul Aziz, N. Yusof, and C. F. Leong, "Incidence of red cell alloantibody among the transfusion recipients of

Universiti Kebangsaan Malaysia medical centre," *Indian Journal of Hematology and Blood Transfusion*, vol. 29, no. 2, pp. 65–70, 2013.

[31] S. Guastafierro, F. Sessa, C. Cuomo, and A. Tirelli, "Delayed hemolytic transfusion reaction due to anti-S antibody in patient with anti-Jk^a autoantibody and multiple alloantibodies," *Annals of Hematology*, vol. 83, no. 5, pp. 307–308, 2004.

[32] M. N. Haslina, N. Ariffin, I. I. Hayati, and H. Roseline, "Red cell alloimmunization in multiply transfused malay thalassemic patients," *The Southeast Asian Journal of Tropical Medicine and Public Health*, vol. 37, pp. 1015–1020, 2006.

[33] R. Ameen, O. Al-Eyaadi, S. Al-Shemmari, R. Chowdhury, and A. Al-Bashir, "Frequency of red blood cell alloantibody in Kuwaiti population," *Medical Principles and Practice*, vol. 14, no. 4, pp. 230–234, 2005.

[34] B. Aygun, S. Padmanabhan, C. Paley, and V. Chandrasekaran, "Clinical significance of RBC alloantibodies and autoantibodies in sickle cell patients who received transfusions," *Transfusion*, vol. 42, no. 1, pp. 37–43, 2002.

[35] S. M. Castellino, M. R. Combs, S. A. Zimmerman, P. D. Issitt, and R. E. Ware, "Erythrocyte autoantibodies in paediatric patients with sickle cell disease receiving transfusion therapy: frequency, characteristics and significance," *British Journal of Haematology*, vol. 104, no. 1, pp. 189–194, 1999.

23

A Preliminary Study of the Suitability of Archival Bone Marrow and Peripheral Blood Smears for Diagnosis of CML Using FISH

Alice Charwudzi,[1] Edeghonghon E. Olayemi,[2] Ivy Ekem,[2] Olufunmilayo Olopade,[3] Mariann Coyle,[3] Amma Anima Benneh,[4] and Emmanuel Alote Allotey[5]

[1] *Department of Chemical Pathology, University of Cape Coast School of Medical Sciences, Cape Coast, Ghana*
[2] *Department of Haematology, University of Ghana Medical School, Accra, Ghana*
[3] *Department of Medicine, University of Chicago, 929 East 57th Street, Chicago, IL 60637, USA*
[4] *Department of Haematology, Korle-Bu Teaching Hospital, Accra, Ghana*
[5] *Haematology Unit, Tamale Teaching Hospital, Tamale, Ghana*

Correspondence should be addressed to Alice Charwudzi; achawogi@yahoo.com

Academic Editor: Abdulkareem Almomen

Background. FISH is a molecular cytogenetic technique enabling rapid detection of genetic abnormalities. Facilities that can run fresh/wet samples for molecular diagnosis and monitoring of neoplastic disorders are not readily available in Ghana and other neighbouring countries. This study aims to demonstrate that interphase FISH can successfully be applied to archival methanol-fixed bone marrow and peripheral blood smear slides transported to a more equipped facility for molecular diagnosis of CML. *Methods.* Interphase FISH was performed on 22 archival methanol-fixed marrow (BM) and 3 peripheral blood (PB) smear slides obtained at diagnosis. The BM smears included 20 CML and 2 CMML cases diagnosed by morphology; the 3 PB smears were from 3 of the CML patients at the time of diagnosis. Six cases had known *BCR-ABL* fusion results at diagnosis by RQ-PCR. Full blood count reports at diagnosis were also retrieved. *Result.* 19 (95%) of the CML marrow smears demonstrated the *BCR-ABL* translocation. There was a significant correlation between the *BCR-ABL* transcript detected at diagnosis by RQ-PCR and that retrospectively detected by FISH from the aged BM smears at diagnosis ($r = 0.870$; $P = 0.035$). *Conclusion.* Archival methanol-fixed marrow and peripheral blood smears can be used to detect the *BCR-ABL* transcript for CML diagnosis.

1. Background

Fluorescent in situ hybridization (FISH) is a sensitive molecular cytogenetic technique that enables rapid detection of chromosomal abnormalities in pathological samples for accurate diagnosis, detection of submicroscopic deletions, risk stratification, detection of minimal residual disease, and assessment of response to therapy. Unlike conventional cytogenetic techniques which require metaphase nuclei (dividing cells), FISH can be applied to nondividing interphase nuclei; hence, uncultured cells can be used [1, 2]. This makes it a useful tool in most fields for studying neoplastic disorders such as chronic myeloid leukaemia (CML). The various chromosomal abnormalities can be detected in interphase nuclei using the appropriate DNA FISH probe set [3].

A wide range of specimens such as peripheral blood and bone marrow aspirate for metaphase cell preparation; uncultured interphase cells from archival bone marrow and blood smears, paraffin-embedded tissue sections or disaggregated cells from paraffin blocks, frozen tissue, cells from lymph node aspirates or solid tumours can all be used for the analysis [3–6]. Previous studies had proved interphase FISH as a valuable and reliable contemporary approach for retrospective studies especially when fresh samples are not available, more so when additional investigative information is required to determine an underlying molecular transformation for both diagnostic and research purposes [4].

Currently, medical laboratory practice in Ghana, like other West African countries, focuses more on the diagnosis of common infectious diseases such as HIV/AIDS, malaria, and tuberculosis due to their overwhelming burden coupled with their associated social and economic challenges [7]. The underfunding of public laboratories in Ghana due to the social and economic constraints makes it difficult to develop and apply current molecular technologies for diagnosis; as a result, laboratory practitioners depend largely on morphology to diagnose malignancies using various stains. Molecular techniques such as FISH, real-time quantitative polymerase chain reaction (RQ-PCR), and flow cytometry are generally not available for routine clinical use. However, recent WHO (World Health Organization) classification of tumours especially haemopoietic and lymphoid neoplasms requires the detection of chromosomal abnormalities for accurate diagnosis and management [8].

Chronic myeloid leukaemia is a haematologic malignancy associated with a balanced reciprocal translocation between the Abelson leukaemia virus gene (ABL) on chromosome 9 and the break-point cluster region gene (BCR) on chromosome 22 forming the BCR-ABL fusion gene. The product of the BCR-ABL gene (the bcr-abl protein) is a constitutively active tyrosine kinase, which is responsible for the pathogenesis of CML [9]. Detection and monitoring of the BCR-ABL transcripts are essential for CML diagnosis and evaluation of patient's response to treatment with tyrosine kinase inhibitors such as Imatinib [10]. The t(9;22) chromosomal abnormality occurs in more than 95% of cases. Interphase FISH is useful in confirming the presence of the translocation [2]. In Ghana, CML accounts for 12.8% of all cases of adult leukaemia but there was no standardized method for molecular diagnosis and monitoring for minimal residual disease at the time of this study [11]. In resource-constrained countries, there is a diagnostic vacuum when it is not possible to carry out these diagnostic procedures due to lack of resources; fresh samples have to be transported to more resourced countries for analysis at great cost. This study therefore sought to determine the usefulness of transporting archival methanol fixed bone marrow and peripheral blood smears to a well-resourced country for molecular diagnosis of CML.

2. Methods

The study was retrospective. Ethical approval was obtained from the Ethical and Protocol Review Committee of the University of Ghana Medical School. Twenty-two (22) archival methanol-fixed bone marrow (BM) and 3 peripheral blood (PB) smear slides at diagnosis from the haematology laboratory of Korle-Bu Teaching Hospital, Ghana, were retrieved. Completely air-dried and well labelled BM and PB smears with monolayers were fixed in absolute methanol by immersion for 1 minute and allowed to air dry. Each patient's methanol-fixed smears (about 4–6 smears) were wrapped in "non-woven instrument wrap paper", labelled with the patient's unique identification number for easy retrieval. It was then packed into a box for storage in the laboratory at room temperature. The BM smears were made up of 20 CML and 2 CMML cases diagnosed between February 2007 and January 2011; the 3 PB smears were from 3 of the CML

patients at the time of diagnosis; the slides had been stored for between 10 and 48 months. The corresponding full blood count (FBC) report at diagnosis was also retrieved. Initial diagnosis for these patients was made on the basis of clinical findings and morphological examination of Leishman stained peripheral blood and bone marrow aspirate smears. Six of the CML cases had known BCR-ABL fusion results (using fresh peripheral blood) at diagnosis made by RQ-PCR outside Ghana. Fisher exact test was used to determine the correlation between the BCR-ABL transcript detected by RQ-PCR at diagnosis and that detected by FISH from the aged smears at diagnosis. The statistical significance was set at $P \leq 0.05$. Metaphase FISH was performed on control cells; in addition, direct blood smears were prepared from the peripheral blood control for interphase FISH analysis.

2.1. Tissue Culture on Control Cells. Commercially prepared BCR-ABL fusion positive cell line in blast crisis (BV173) and a peripheral blood from a single BCR-ABL transcript negative volunteer were used as control. Tissue culture was performed in RPMI 1640 medium [12].

2.2. Pretreatment of Smears and Dropped Cells. The direct smear slides were pretreated by immersion in methanol for 1 minute, incubated in 2x standard saline citrate (2x SSC) at room temperature (RT) for 5 minutes, and digested in 0.05 mg/mL pepsin/10 mmol/HCl at 37°C for 5–10 minutes. It was then incubated in 2x SSC for 5 minutes rinsed in double distilled water and observed under a phase contrast microscope to ensure adequate lysis of the red blood cells. If red blood cells remained, an additional pepsin treatment was repeated. At this point, the desired areas for hybridization with the least amount of cell clumps were selected as previously described [4]. Glacial acetic acid: methanol fixative (1 : 3 ratios) was used to lyse red cell for direct peripheral blood control smears aged less than 3 weeks as well as two BM and one of the PB smear. Smears were then fixed in 1% formaldehyde, rinsed in 1x phosphate buffered saline (PBS), and dehydrated in 70%, 80%, and absolute ethanol [4].

2.3. FISH. FISH was performed using Vysis *LSI BCR/ABL* Dual Color, Dual Fusion Translocation DNA Probe (Downers Grove, IL, USA). The probe was validated by standard procedure. Hybridization and posthybridization wash conditions followed the manufacturer's protocol. Finally, the cells were counterstained with DAPI II.

Hybridized cells were examined through a Zeiss Axio fluorescence microscope using Vysis filter sets: DAPI/Spectrum Orange dual bandpass and DAPI/Spectrum Green dual bandpass, and images were captured using Axio Imager Z2 Vision 4.0 software. A total of one hundred (100) interphase nuclei were analysed per slide. The cut-off value for a positive signal was 1% [13]. Cells lacking BCR-ABL translocation displayed two red (R) signals, corresponding to the ABL probe, and two green (G) signals, corresponding to the BCR probe. Thus, a normal cell had 2R2G signal pattern. Cells with a balanced BCR-ABL translocation displayed two fusions (F) of red and green signals as well as one green and one red signal. Thus, a typical positive signal pattern for the *BCR-ABL* fusion showed 2F1R1G. The degree of positivity for *BCR-ABL* transcript was scored for each slide as percentages.

3. Results

3.1. Peripheral Blood Features at Diagnosis. The CML cases comprised of 5 females and 15 males, and the median age at diagnosis was 36 yrs (Range: 20–67 yrs). All the subjects showed marked leukocytosis in the range of $20.7–636.8 \times 10^9/L$ and anaemia, shown in Table 1. Anaemia, defined as haemoglobin level less than 12 g/dL [14], was observed in all the subjects. The platelet count was normal $(150–450 \times 10^9/L)$ in 8 (40%) subjects, low (less than $150 \times 10^9/L$) in two (10%) subjects, and high (greater than $450 \times 10^9/L$) in 10 (50%) subjects.

3.2. Interphase FISH. Interphase FISH analysis was carried out in 20 CML and 2 CMML patients. Nineteen (95%) out of the 20 CML bone marrow slides at diagnosis demonstrated the *BCR-ABL* translocation. The percentage means score ± SD for the *BCR-ABL* positive smears at diagnosis was 89.5 ± 6.5 (Range: 70.0–98.0%). The two CMML subjects were *BCR-ABL* negative. The major scoring signal patterns obtained for the *BCR-ABL* positive smears were categorized into 3 groups: 1 ($n = 17$) showed the classical 2F1R1G (Figure 1(d)); group 2 ($n = 1$) showed one fusion, one red, and two green (1F1R2G) indicating *ABL* deletion; group 3 ($n = 1$) showed one fusion, two red, and one green 1F2R1G (Figure 1(e)) indicating *BCR* deletion. There was a significant correlation between the *BCR-ABL* transcript detected at diagnosis by RQ-PCR using fresh peripheral blood and that retrospectively detected by FISH from the aged bone marrow smears at diagnosis ($r = 0.870$; $P = 0.035$ by fisher exact test). Two of the PB smears showed the *BCR-ABL* translocation, and the major scoring signal was the classical 2F1R1G, with 2F1R (Figure 1(f)) as a minor scoring signal in one of the PB smears, a similar signal was seen in its corresponding BM smear. The third PB smear was negative (Figure 1(c)) (it's corresponding BM smear was also *BCR-ABL* negative).

4. Discussion

With the discovery of molecular markers for some neoplastic disorders, accurate assessment of the genetic characteristics of these malignancies is the hallmark for decisions on prognosis and clinical management especially with regard to targeted molecular therapies [4]. The need to identify and correlate these individual tumor features becomes a challenge when fresh pathological samples are not available or when it is not possible to carry out diagnostic procedure due to lack of resources. In resource-constrained countries, these samples may have to be transported to more resourced countries for analysis. Fresh peripheral blood samples or bone marrow aspirates that are normally relied on in the field of haematology often possess transportation challenges due to sample degradation.

TABLE 1: Pretreatment full blood count profile of study population.

Parameter	Study subject, $N = 20$ Median	Ranges
Leucocyte count $(\times 10^9/L)$	253.1	20.7–636.8
Platelet count $(\times 10^9/L)$	446.2	46.0–1051.0
Haemoglobin (g/dL)	8.2	5.2–11.5
Neutrophils (%)**	67.6	45.7–89.3
Eosinophils (%)**	2.2	0.1–12.3
Basophils (%)**	4.5	0.0–25.0

Table 1 shows the full blood count profile of the 20 subjects at diagnosis. NB: % = percentage. **Absolute values for the differential counts were not available for majority of subjects at diagnosis; hence, percentage differential count was used.

Previous studies had revealed an excellent agreement in the detection and quantitation of the *BCR-ABL* translocation from results obtained from interphase cells of cultured bone marrow aspirate and peripheral blood [1]. This study was performed to determine the usefulness of interphase FISH as a reliable, reproducible, and quantitative molecular diagnostic technique on methanol fixed archival bone marrow and peripheral blood smears stored at room temperature which can be transported to a better equipped laboratory without fear of sample degradation.

The data obtained shows that the majority (89%) of the subjects showed the classical *BCR-ABL* dual fusion (2F1R1G) pattern at diagnosis. Approximately 11% demonstrated the unusual signal patterns 1F1R2G suggesting *ABL* deletion and 1F2R1G suggesting *BCR* deletion. Such deletions have been reported in 10–15% of patients and may confer a poor prognosis in CML patients in the advanced phase [15, 16]. There was a significant correlation between the *BCR-ABL* transcripts levels detected at diagnosis by RQ-PCR in six CML patients using fresh peripheral blood samples prior to commencement of treatment and their corresponding archival bone marrow smears at diagnosis using interphase FISH. This implies that aged methanol fixed bone marrow smear specimens are as reliable as fresh blood specimens, for quantification of the leukaemia burden at diagnosis. Hence, methanol fixed bone marrow and peripheral blood smears can conveniently be used for the diagnosis of CML using FISH technique. This study demonstrated that *BCR-ABL* transcript could be detected by FISH using aged bone marrow and peripheral blood smears.

Interphase FISH technique was applied directly without tissue culture to methanol fixed bone marrow and peripheral blood smears (stored at room temperature) retrieved from the haematology laboratory. This makes this technique rapid, simple, and less expensive since culture and other logistics will not be required.

However, thin films (smears) with monolayer sections treated with glacial acetic acid/methanol fixative for red cell lysis gave a better result, and although some red cells are not lysed, all the white cells remain intact. Also, the pepsin digestion step has to be monitored since overdigestion can lead to loss of all the cells on the slide.

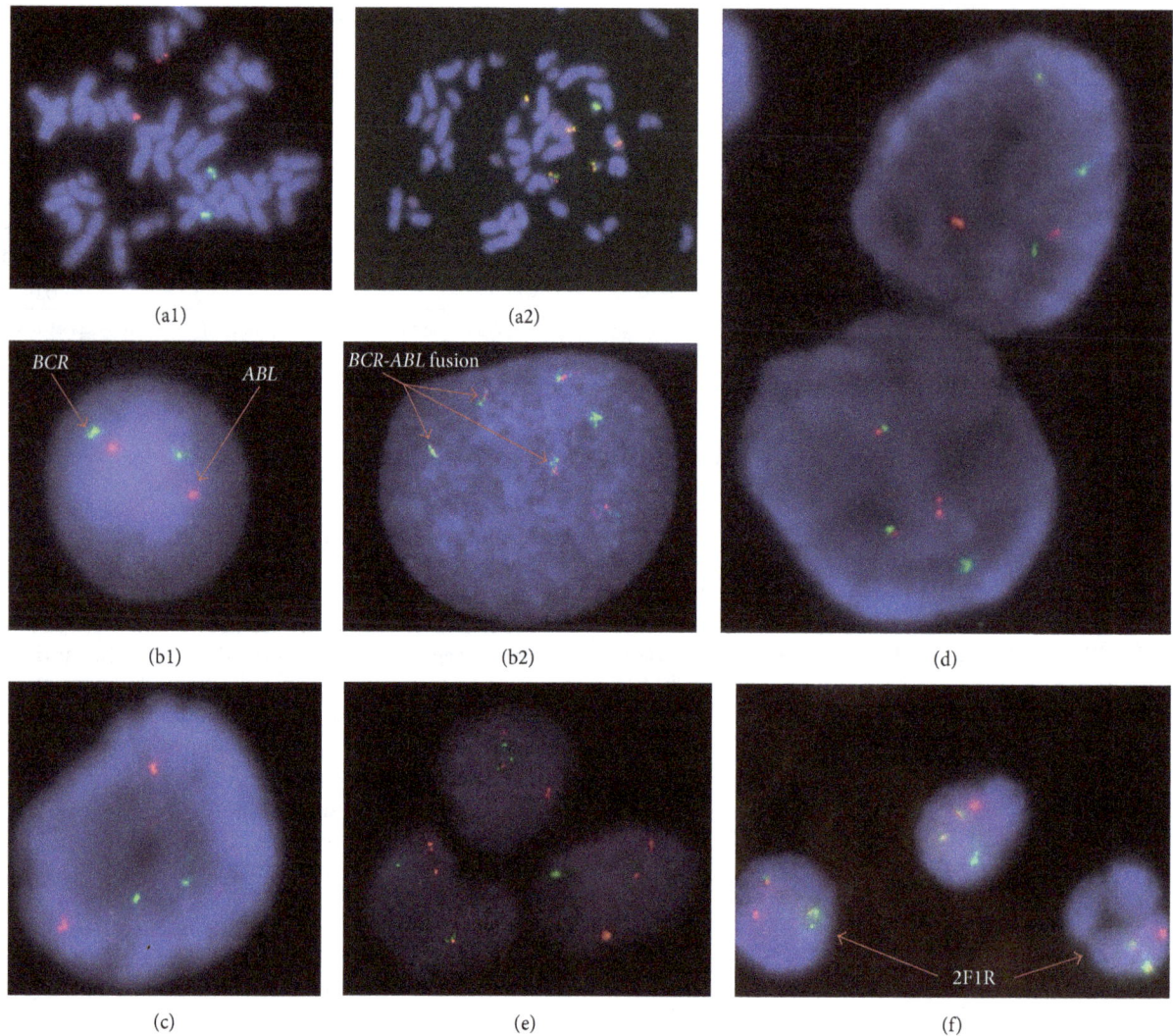

(a1)

(a2)

(b1)

(b2)

(d)

(c)

(e)

(f)

FIGURE 1: *BCR-ABL* dual colour, dual fusion translocation probe hybridized to controls, and subject's bone marrow and peripheral blood smears. ((a1) and (b1)) Two red, two green (2R2G), negative control in a metaphase cell and an interphase cell, respectively; ((a2) and (b2)) five fusion, one green (5F1G), positive control in a metaphase and an interphase cell, respectively. (c) *BCR-ABL* negative FISH signal in a subject's peripheral blood smears. (d) 2F1R1G signals in a *BCR-ABL* positive subject BM smear. (e) 1F2R1G signals in a *BCR-ABL* positive subject marrow smear. (f) 2F1R in a *BCR-ABL* positive subject's peripheral blood (red cells lysed in glacial acetic acid: methanol fixative). Negative control is from a single *BCR-ABL* negative peripheral blood donor, and BV 173 is from a *BCR-ABL* positive cell line in blastic phase. Images were taken with ×100 oil immersion objective lens.

5. Conclusions

The result confirms that archival bone marrow and peripheral blood smears can successfully be used to detect and quantify the *BCR-ABL* transcript to diagnose CML. The *BCR-ABL* fusion was reliably detected. This has significant implications for the setting-up of regional diagnostic centres of excellence in the main referral hospital, in Ghana as well as in the African continent. Since it may not be feasible in the near future to establish well-equipped medical laboratories in all regional hospitals, samples from the other regions in Ghana and even neighbouring countries can be collected, fixed, and sent to these centres, where molecular diagnosis will be made and the results relayed promptly via the internet. This will greatly improve the diagnosis, treatment, and monitoring of

response to treatment of many malignant diseases on the continent. We recommend carrying further studies with a larger sample size to determine how long methanol fixed marrow and peripheral smears can be stored at room temperature before degradation set in.

Abbreviations

CML: Chronic myeloid leukaemia
CMML: Chronic myelomonocytic leukaemia
FISH: Fluorescent in situ hybridization
RQ-PCR: Real-time quantitative polymerase chain reaction
BCR: Break-point cluster region gene
ABL: Abelson leukaemia virus gene.

Conflict of Interests

The authors declare that they have no competing interests.

Authors' Contribution

Ivy Ekem, Edeghonghon E. Olayemi, Alice Charwudzi, and Olufunmilayo Olopade planned the study. Alice Charwudzi, Mariann M. Coyle, Amma Anima Benneh, and Emmanuel Allote Allotey conducted the pilot study and the initial literature review. Alice Charwudzi, Olufunmilayo Olopade, and Mariann M. Coyle implemented the study. Olufunmilayo Olopade and Alice Charwudzi provided financial support. All authors commented on the paper. All authors read and approved the final paper. All authors contributed equally to this work.

Acknowledgments

The authors are extremely grateful to the Union for International Cancer Control, Geneva, for providing a training grant, staff of Professor Olopade's laboratory for financial support and training, the late Professor Janet Rowley's laboratory for providing BV173 cell line, and the Cytogenetics laboratory for their support, all of the University of Chicago. Special thanks are due to Mr. Ekow Aidoo who stored the smear slides used and Mr. Christopher Nyimba for assisting in the retrieval of the smear slides, all of the Haematology Department of Korle-Bu Teaching Hospital.

References

[1] S. Le Gouill, P. Talmant, N. Milpied et al., "Fluorescence in situ hybridization on peripheral-blood specimens is a reliable method to evaluate cytogenetic response in chronic myeloid leukemia," *Journal of Clinical Oncology*, vol. 18, no. 7, pp. 1533–1538, 2000.

[2] G. W. Dewald, "Interphase FISH studies of chronic myeloid leukemia," in *Molecular Cytogenetic*, Y. S. Fan, Ed., pp. 311–342, Humana Press, Totowa, NJ, USA, 2003.

[3] D. J. Wolff, A. Bagg, L. D. Cooley et al., "Guidance for fluorescence in situ hybridization testing in hematologic disorders," *Journal of Molecular Diagnostics*, vol. 9, no. 2, pp. 134–143, 2007.

[4] V. Bedell, S. J. Forman, K. Gaal, V. Pullarkat, L. M. Weiss, and M. L. Slovak, "Successful application of a direct detection slide-based sequential phenotype/genotype assay using archived bone marrow smears and paraffin embedded tissue sections," *Journal of Molecular Diagnostics*, vol. 9, no. 5, pp. 589–597, 2007.

[5] P. L. Nguyen, D. C. Arthur, C. E. Litz, and R. D. Brunning, "Fluorescence in situ hybridization (FISH) detection of trisomy 8 in myeloid cells in chronic myeloid leukemia (CML): a study of archival blood and bone marrow smears," *Leukemia*, vol. 8, no. 10, pp. 1654–1662, 1994.

[6] S. F. Paternoster, S. R. Brockman, R. F. McClure, E. D. Remstein, P. J. Kurtin, and G. W. Dewald, "A new method to extract nuclei from paraffin-embedded tissue to study lymphomas using interphase fluorescence in situ hybridization," *The American Journal of Pathology*, vol. 160, no. 6, pp. 1967–1972, 2002.

[7] O. A. Adeyi, "Pathology services in developing countriesthe West African experience," *Archives of Pathology and Laboratory Medicine*, vol. 135, no. 2, pp. 183–186, 2011.

[8] J. W. Vardiman, J. Thiele, D. A. Arber et al., "The 2008 revision of the World Health Organization (WHO) classification of myeloid neoplasms and acute leukemia: rationale and important changes," *Blood*, vol. 114, no. 5, pp. 937–951, 2009.

[9] M. W. Deininger, J. M. Goldman, and J. V. Melo, "The molecular biology of chronic myeloid leukemia," *Blood*, vol. 96, no. 10, pp. 3343–3356, 2000.

[10] H. Kantarjian, C. Schiffer, D. Jones, and J. Cortes, "Monitoring the response and course of chronic myeloid leukemia in the modern era of BCR-ABL tyrosine kinase inhibitors: practical advice on the use and interpretation of monitoring methods," *Blood*, vol. 111, no. 4, pp. 1774–1780, 2008.

[11] I. Ekem, "Haematological malignancies in Korle Bu teaching hospital," *Turkish Journal of Hematology*, supplement 22, p. 330, 2005.

[12] A. D. White, B. M. Jones, R. E. Clark, and A. Jacobs, "Chromosome aberrations following cytotoxic therapy in patients in complete remission from lymphoma," *Carcinogenesis*, vol. 13, no. 7, pp. 1095–1099, 1992.

[13] N. Testoni, G. Marzocchi, S. Luatti et al., "Chronic myeloid leukemia: a prospective comparison of interphase fluorescence in situ hybridization and chromosome banding analysis for the definition of complete cytogenetic response: a study of the GIMEMA CML WP," *Blood*, vol. 114, no. 24, pp. 4939–4943, 2009.

[14] F. S. Asobayire, P. Adou, L. Davidsson, J. D. Cook, and R. F. Hurrell, "Prevalence of iron deficiency with and without concurrent anemia in population groups with high prevalences of malaria and other infections: a study in Côte d'Ivoire1-3," *The American Journal of Clinical Nutrition*, vol. 74, no. 6, pp. 776–782, 2001.

[15] P. B. Sinclair, E. P. Nacheva, M. Leversha et al., "Large deletions at the t(9;22) breakpoint are common and may identify a poor-prognosis subgroup of patients with chronic myeloid leukemia," *Blood*, vol. 95, no. 3, pp. 738–744, 2000.

[16] A. Quintás-Cardama, H. Kantarjian, J. Shan et al., "Prognostic impact of deletions of derivative chromosome 9 in patients with chronic myelogenous leukemia treated with nilotinib or dasatinib," *Cancer*, vol. 117, no. 22, pp. 5085–5093, 2011.

24

Procoagulant Phospholipids and Tissue Factor Activity in Cerebrospinal Fluid from Patients with Intracerebral Haemorrhage

Patrick Van Dreden,[1] **Guy Hue,**[2] **Jean-François Dreyfus,**[3] **Barry Woodhams,**[4] **and Marc Vasse**[5]

[1] *Diagnostica Stago, 125 Avenue Louis Roche, 92635 Gennevilliers Cedex, France*

[2] *Biochemistry Department, IBC, Rouen University Hospital, 76031 Rouen Cedex, France*

[3] *Clinical Research Unit, Hôpital Foch, University of Versailles, 92151 Suresnes Cedex, France*

[4] *HaemaCon Ltd, Bromley, Kent CT18 7TW, UK*

[5] *Clinical Biology Department & EA 4531, Hospital Foch, 40 rue Worth, 92151 Suresnes Cedex, France*

Correspondence should be addressed to Marc Vasse; marc.vasse@u-psud.fr

Academic Editor: David Varon

Brain contains large amounts of tissue factor, the major initiator of the coagulation cascade. Neuronal apoptosis after intracerebral haemorrhage (ICH) leads to the shedding of procoagulant phospholipids (PPLs). The aim of this study was to investigate the generation of PPL, tissue factor activity (TFa), and D-Dimer (D-Di) in the cerebrospinal fluid (CSF) at the acute phase of ICH in comparison with other brain diseases and to examine the relationship between these factors and the outcome of ICH. CSF was collected from 112 patients within 48 hours of hospital admission. Thirty-one patients with no neurological or biochemical abnormalities were used to establish reference range in the CSF ("controls"). Thirty had suffered an ICH, and 51 other neurological diagnoses [12: ventricular drainage following brain surgery, 13: viral meningitis, 15: bacterial meningitis, and 11 a neurodegenerative disease (NDD)]. PPL was measured using a factor Xa-based coagulation assay and TFa by one home test. PPL, D-Di, and TFa were significantly higher ($P < 0.001$) in the CSF of patients with ICH than in controls. TFa levels were significantly ($P < 0.05$) higher in ICH than in patients with meningitides or NDD. Higher levels ($P < 0.05$) of TFa were observed in patients with ICH who died than in survivors. TFa measurement in the CSF of patients with ICH could constitute a new prognostic marker.

1. Introduction

Intracerebral haemorrhage (ICH) is a type of stroke caused by bleeding within the brain tissue itself. Primary ICH accounts for ~80% of all incidences of ICH and is more likely to result in death or major disability than ischemic stroke or subarachnoid haemorrhage. ICH has a higher incidence among populations with a higher frequency of hypertension, including African Americans and Asian populations, possibly due to environmental factors (e.g., a diet rich in fish oils) and/or genetic factors [1]. In contrast to the declining incidence of ischaemic stroke in high-income countries, the incidence of ICH has been constant [2]. The 1-month fatality rate after ICH does not appear to have changed over the last few decades with rates of 25–35% in high-income countries and 30–48% in low-/middle-income countries [3].

Computed tomography (CT) is now widely available in the developed world and has become the diagnostic test of choice in ICH to determine the site of the haemorrhage and estimate the volume of the haematoma [4]. The ability of CT scans to detect ICH depends on the length of time between the bleed and the scan. However, up to 5% of subarachnoid haemorrhage (SAH) will have a negative CT scan.

Over the past decade, numerous studies have reported a positive correlation between S100B levels in blood or CSF and impaired neurological function. S100B is a calcium-binding protein concentrated in glial cells (although it has also been detected in definite extraneural cell types) and serum S100B is considered as a relevant diagnostic and prognostic tool in acute spontaneous ICH. However, a recent study in patients with ICH suggested that its sensitivity and specificity were not as high as previously described at least in patients with traumatic brain injury [5] and considerable evidence indicates that S100B is not a specific biomarker for brain damage [6].

During stroke, the blood-brain barrier (BBB) is compromised by endothelial cell death. Cytosolic contents released from injured brain tissues have the potential to cross the barrier. We hypothesise that the measurement of molecules which are expressed in high concentration in the brain but in trace amount in normal CSF could be used to monitor ICH severity and prognosis. As the brain is a major source of tissue factor (TF), the main coagulation cascade activator [7] and rich in phospholipids [8], we investigated the activity of procoagulant phospholipids (PPL) and the activity of tissue factor (TFa) in the CSF of patients with ICH. We compared the levels of these parameters in ICH and in other pathologies [bacterial or viral meningitis, patients with a ventricular drainage (VD) following brain surgery and patients with neurodegenerative diseases]. In addition, we examined the CSF levels of D-Dimer (D-Di) and tissue factor pathway inhibitor (TFPI) and analyzed the prognostic value of these parameters.

2. Patients and Methods

2.1. Patients. Fresh CSF was collected from 112 hospitalised patients by lumbar puncture in the first 2 days after admission (i.e., the early stage of events). Among these, 31 patients that had been admitted to the emergency ward with suspected meningitis or subarachnoid haemorrhage but were found to had no CSF biochemical abnormalities and normal neurological explorations were considered as controls. Of the remaining patients, 30 had suffered a cerebral haemorrhage, and 51 had other neurological disorders: 13 with confirmed viral meningitis, 15 with bacterial meningitis, and 11 with a neurodegenerative disease (NDD) Alzheimer's type; 12 were treated with ventricular drainage (VD) following brain surgery. ICH patients, defined as an acute and persisting focal neurological deficit, were to be admitted to the neurological department within six hours after symptom onset. No patients received intrathecal fibrinolytic therapy, antiplatelet agents, or prophylactic calcium channel blockers before sample collection. Informed consent was obtained from all appropriate family members.

The CSF was immediately placed on ice to prevent enzyme activation and transported to the laboratory where each was centrifuged at 1,000 ×g for 15 min to remove cells and debris. A small number of CSF samples were bloody and were additionally centrifuged for 15 minutes. Medical treatment was started soon after the lumber puncture when cranial CT had proved the existence of ICH.

2.2. Analytical Determinations. PPLs in the CSF were measured on a STA-R analyser using a factor Xa-based coagulation assay (STA Procoag-PPL—Diagnostica Stago, Asnières, France). The test consists of the measurement of clotting time in the presence of CSF, in a system in which a phospholipid-depleted substrate plasma makes the test dependent on the PPL of the test sample. Bovine factor Xa triggers the coagulation cascade downstream from factor Xa, thus eliminating the influence of coagulation factors acting upstream [9]. A shortening of clotting times is associated with increased levels of PPL activity. The effect of contamination with red blood cell (RBC) on the PPL determination was evaluated by adding a varying number of RBC to normal CSF after baseline PPL activity determination. The addition of RBC up to 55×10^9/L in normal CSF did not change the time of PPL determination, while CSF specimens included in this study contain less than 45×10^9 RBC/L.

TFa was measured by a one-stage kinetic chromogenic method [10]. This assay measures the ability of TF-FVIIa to activate factor X to factor Xa. The CSF samples were mixed with human factor VII and factor X and fibrin polymerisation inhibitor and incubated at 37°C allowing for the formation of TF/Factor VIIa complex. The secondary generation of factor Xa was measured by adding a specific factor Xa chromogenic substrate. Inter- and intra-assay coefficients of variation for this kit were 3.8% and 4.2%, respectively.

Free tissue factor pathway inhibitor (f-TFPI) was determined by ELISA (Asserachrom Free TFPI, Diagnostica Stago). D-Dimer (D-Di) was measured on a STA-R analyser by latex immunoassay (STA-Liatest D-Di, Diagnostica Stago) according to the manufacturer's instructions.

CSF proteins, glucose, chloride, and lactate measurements were done using the routine laboratory techniques (Cobas 6000, Roche Diagnostics, Meylan, France).

2.3. Statistics. All statistical calculations were done using NCSS, version 9 (NCSS LLC, Kaysville, UI, USA) and R statistical Package, version 3.0.2 (The R Statistical Foundation, Wien, Austria). Data are presented as median (1st and 3rd quartiles). Since all tests showed significant departure from normal distribution, between—group comparisons of continuous variables between different subgroups were performed using Kruskal—Wallis non parametric analysis of variance. When this led to global significance, pairwise comparisons were done between all groups and control and all groups and ICH, using Dunn's test. The Bonferronni-Simes correction was used to preserve the nominal significance level. Coefficients of correlation (*r*) were calculated using Spearman's rank test. A two-sided *P* value <0.05 was considered significant. For survivors to nonsurvivors comparison, a Mann-Whitney test was used. Receiver operating characteristic (ROC) analysis was performed to calculate cut-off values discriminating survivors and nonsurvivors.

3. Results

3.1. Variations of PPL, TFa, D-Di, and Routine Biochemical Parameters in the CSF of Patients and Controls. Clotting time in the PPL assay and levels of TFa and D-Di, in the CSF of the controls and patients are shown in Table 1. PPL (inversely related to clotting time), TFa, and D-Di were significantly

TABLE 1: Levels of procoagulant phospholipids (PPLs), tissue factor activity (TFa), D-Dimer (D-Di), and classical biochemical parameters in the cerebrospinal fluid of different groups of patients with central nervous system pathologies.

Variable ($P^\S$)	Controls	ICH	Bacterial meningitis	Viral meningitis	VD	NDD
n	31	30	15	13	12	11
Clotting time for PPL assay (sec.) ($P < 0.00001$)	164 (158–174)[*]	125 (93–147)[***]	144 (136–165)[*+]	151 (141–155)[*+]	134 (132–147)[***]	142 (135–156)[*]
TFa (pM/L) ($P < 0.00001$)	0.74 (0.60–0.89)[ε]	2.36 (1.67–3.21)[***]	0.76 (0.68–0.83)[+++]	0.84 (0.74–0.92)[+++]	1.33 (1.12–1.60)	0.78 (0.62–0.89)[+++]
D-Di (mg/L) ($P < 0.00001$)	0.40 (0.17–0.58)[β]	0.82 (0.52–0.98)[***]	0.51 (0.43–0.59)[+]	0.44 (0.36–0.51)[β++]	0.54 (0.44–0.62)[***]	0.36 (0.23–0.52)[+++]
Protein (g/L) ($P = 0.0006$)	0.39 (0.24–0.48)	0.62 (0.44–0.85)[β***]	0.58 (0.38–0.83)[*]	0.61 (0.55–0.88)[***]	0.28 (0.18–0.71)	0.45 (0.44–0.52)
Glucose (mmol/L) ($P < 0.00001$)	3.4 (3.2–3.9)	4.8 (4.1–5.4)[***]	3.1 (2.1–3.8)[+++]	2.8 (2.6–3.4)[+++]	4.0 (3.5–5.2)	3.6 (3.5–3.7)[+]
Chloride (mmol/L) ($P = 0.57$)	125 (124–128)	126 (120–132)	124 (117–132)	122 (120–132)	128 (125–132)	126 (123–128)
Lactate (mmol/L) ($P < 0.00001$)	1.67 (1.40–2.16)[φ]	2.93 (2.18–3.21)[***]	2.60 (2.10–3.76)[Γ*]	2.77 (2.36–2.88)[δ*]	2.66 (1.71 −3.87)[*]	1.34 (1.30–1.44)[α+++]

Values are medians (1st and 3rd quartiles); n = number of patients enrolled.
§Global P for Kruskal-Wallis test [*]$P < 0.05$, [***]$P < 0.001$ versus controls; [+]$P < 0.05$, [++]$P < 0.01$, [+++]$P < 0.001$ versus ICH Missing values: α: 5, β: 1, Γ:8, δ: 4, ε: 2, φ: 4.
ICH: intracerebral haemorrhage VD: ventricular drainage; NDD: neurodegenerative disease.

higher in CSF from patients with ICH than in controls ($P < 0.001$). PPL was also significantly increased in comparison with controls in the different groups of patients analyzed, even in patients with NDD. PPL in patients with ICH was also significantly higher when compared to the different pathological groups, except in patients with VD and NDD.

When compared to controls, TFa was significantly increased only in patients with ICH. D-Di was significantly increased in patients with ICH and in patients with VD.

Compared to controls, CSF proteins, glucose, and lactates were significantly increased in patients with ICH. Significantly higher levels of CSF glucose were found in ICH patients when compared to patients with both types of meningitis and NDD and of CSF lactates when compared to NDD.

The levels of f-TFPI in the CSF of control and in patient CSF of the different groups were below the detection level (0.5 μg/L, data not shown).

In the CSF of controls, a significant positive correlation ($P < 0.001$, $\rho = 0.643$) was found only between TFa and D-Di. In the CSF of patients with ICH, clotting time in the PPL assay was significantly inversely correlated ($P = 0.005$; $\rho = -0.53$) with CSF lactate levels, which means that the quantity of PPL increases with the lactate level. In the CSF of patients with bacterial meningitis, a significant positive correlation ($P = 0.02$, $\rho = 0.637$) was found between TFa and D-Di and an inverse correlation between TFa and chloride ($P = 0.02$, $\rho = -0.614$). In CSF of patients with VD, a positive correlation was found between glucose and lactate ($P = 0.01$, $\rho = 0.761$).

3.2. Prognostic Values of PPL, TFa, and D-Di in the CSF of Patients with ICH. Significantly higher levels of TFa were observed in the CSF of patients with ICH who died compared with the survivors ($P < 0.05$). There was no significant difference in CSF D-Di levels ($P = 0.48$) and PPL ($P = 0.07$). ROC curve analysis indicated PPL to be more sensitive but less specific than TFa (Table 2).

4. Discussion

ICH has a mortality rate of 50%, and survivors may have significant neurological morbidity. Given the catastrophic consequences of missing the diagnosis and that both mortality and morbidity increase with delays in treatment, early diagnosis is essential and new approaches are needed to facilitate diagnosis. In addition to CT, identification of new biomarkers that denote the presence of ICH and contribute to an early diagnosis is welcome. They could have additional value if they can be used as a predictor of clinical outcome. Plasma S100B was previously shown to be increased in ICH and have a prognostic value [5, 11]. Increased levels of S100B in blood is however not specific for ICH, as increases occur in other neuropathologies including traumatic brain injury and extracranial malignancies and has been shown to represent ongoing neurogeneration [6]. Moreover, contradictory data interpretation exists with regard to the contribution of an altered blood-brain barrier to S100B serum levels [12].

The most frequent pathophysiologic mechanism of ICH seems to be a degenerative vessel wall change and consequently rupture of small penetrating arteries and arterioles. Recently it was shown that the plasma and the CSF of patients suffering from traumatic brain injury contain phosphatidylserine (PS) mainly of platelet and endothelial origin [13]. In this study, using a rapid assay [9] we found that PPL levels were significantly elevated in the CSF of

TABLE 2: Procoagulant phospholipids (PPLs), tissue factor activity (TFa) and D-Dimers (D-Di) in the CSF of survivor and nonsurvivor patients with ICH.

		Intracerebral haemorrhage				
	Survivors	Nonsurvivors	Cut-off	AUC	Sensitivity	Specificity
n	19	11				
TFa (pM) $P = 0.016$	1.85 (1.26–2.65)	3.21 (2.26–3.65)*	2.36	0.77	73.7	72.7
PPL (sec.) $P = 0.07$	143 (107–155)	100 (78–126)	106.6	0.70	78.9	63.6
D-Di (mg/L) $P = 0.48$	0.78 (0.51–0.98)	0.87 (0.62–1.23)	ND	ND	ND	ND

*$P < 0.05$, ICH survivors compared with ICH nonsurvivors, Mann-Whitney test.
Values are medians (1st and 3rd quartiles). n = number of patients.
AUC: area under the curve, ND: not determined.

patients with ICH in comparison with controls or other CNS pathologies and associated with a poor prognosis. The absence of correlation between PPL in the CSF and CSF proteins suggests that PPL appears in CSF, not because of changes in the BBB permeability but primarily because cells are damaged. This hypothesis is strengthened by the correlation between CSF lactate and PPL in this group of patients. In traumatic injury it has been shown that there is a difference in CSF phospholipid composition and the time of appearance of these phospholipids in patients with a poor outcome. In patients who died, phosphatidylserine (PS) and phosphatidylethanolamine were higher in the 48-hour time period following the traumatic injury [14]. Using a different methodology, based on the capture by annexin V of PS expressing microparticules, a similarly poor prognostic value associated with high levels of PS had been previously observed in patients with basal ganglia haemorrhage [15]. In our study, there was a trend for higher levels of PPL in the CSF of patients who died, but it did not reach a statistical significance. This can be due to a too weak number of patients in each group.

It was beyond the scope of this study, but it would, in future studies, be of interest to identify the origin of these cells in the different groups of patients tested in this study, since CSF PPL levels were significantly increased in each group, where different physiopathological mechanisms are suspected.

The brain is rich in TF. The cellular sources of TF are the astrocytes in the parenchyma, glia limitans, and arachnoid cells, with the latter two being in contact with the CSF [7, 16]. However little information is available on TF in the CSF of patients with diseases of the CNS in comparison with normal subjects. An increase in TF detected immunologically (TF : Ag) has been previously reported in patients after a subarachnoid haemorrhage [17, 18] and in patients with bacterial meningitis [19]. In this study, we used a functional TF assay. In normal CSF, TFa levels (0.73 pM/L) were higher than in plasma from healthy donors (0.25 pM/L) [10], which are similar to values obtained using an immunological assay (165 ± 139 pg/mL in plasma versus 868 ± 721 pg/mL in CSF) [20]. As observed by others [18], we could not detect f-TFPI in CSF from controls or from patients with subarachnoid haemorrhage. This TF-TFPI imbalance in normal and pathological CSF would tend to make it more procoagulant as the TFa cannot be neutralised. We also observed a significant increase in TFa in ICH patients, but in contrast with a previous study [19] not in patients with bacterial meningitis. This discrepancy between the two studies could be due to the proteolysis of TF by proteases secreted by bacteria, leading to the loss of TF activity, whereas the degraded/inactive TF is still recognised by antibodies used in the assay. TFa concentrations were higher in the CSF of patients with a poor outcome compared with those who survived. As TF is the major initiator of the coagulation cascade, it can be hypothesised that high CSF TFa levels are associated with generation of thrombin which is capable of releasing potent vasoconstrictors such as endothelin-1, serotonin, and platelet derived growth factor inducing a vasospasm [17]. In agreement with the hypothesis of an increased thrombin generation, elevated levels of prothrombin F1+2 and thrombin-antithrombin complexes were observed in the CSF of patients with ICH [17, 18]. It was suggested that elevation of CSF TF was predictive of vasospasm in subarachnoid haemorrhage and therefore associated with a poor prognosis [17]. However, this was not confirmed on a small series of patients [21] and has no prognostic value (independently of the appearance of a vasospasm). In our study, the prognostic value of the increase in TFa is higher than the increase in PPL, and it is clear that it deserves further investigation with a greater number of patients.

The third parameter studied was D-Di. In agreement with previous studies [22, 23], we observed increased D-Di levels in the CSF of patients with ICH compared with controls but did not identify any prognostic value for this parameter and were unable to find any previous studies in the literature evaluating the value of D-Di in CSF. Most studies investigated whether the presence of D-Di in the CSF can rapidly distinguish between a traumatic tap and ICH, but all with inconclusive results [22–24]. These discrepancies and the absence of prognostic value in our study can possibly be explained by the lack of specificity of CSF D-Di, since increased levels of D-Di were shown in the CSF of patients with different pathologies [24].

In conclusion, PPL and TFa assays presented in this study are rapid tests which can be performed in an emergency context of ICH and can provide useful diagnostic information. Further studies are required to better assess the relation between these markers and the occurrence of cerebral vasospasm or oedema formation and to evaluate whether the time-course of these factors may be helpful in predicting patient complications. The limitations of our study are the small sample size and relatively small number of patients included in each group. This makes it difficult to draw firm conclusions. These assays should be compared to new parameters such as copeptin or resistin which were recently described as having a prognostic value in ICH [25, 26].

Conflict of Interests

The authors declare that there is no conflict of interests regarding the publication of this paper.

References

[1] H. S. Pedersen, G. Mulvad, K. N. Seidelin, G. T. Malcom, and D. A. Boudreau, "N-3 fatty acids as a risk factor for haemorrhagic stroke," *The Lancet*, vol. 353, no. 9155, pp. 812–813, 1999.

[2] C. J. van Asch, M. J. Luitse, G. J. Rinkel, I. van der Tweel, A. Algra, and C. J. Klijn, "Incidence, case fatality, and functional outcome of intracerebral haemorrhage over time, according to age, sex, and ethnic origin: a systematic review and meta-analysis," *The Lancet Neurology*, vol. 9, no. 2, pp. 167–176, 2010.

[3] C. E. Lovelock, G. J. Rinkel, and P. M. Rothwell, "Time trends in outcome of subarachnoid hemorrhage: population-based study and systematic review," *Neurology*, vol. 74, no. 19, pp. 1494–1501, 2010.

[4] J. Broderick, S. Connolly, E. Feldmann et al., "Guidelines for the management of spontaneous intracerebral hemorrhage in adults: 2007 update," *Stroke*, vol. 38, no. 6, pp. 2001–2023, 2007.

[5] A. Dilek, H. Alacam, F. Ulger et al., "Comparison of predictive powers of S100B and cell-free plasma DNA values in intensive care unit patients with intracranial hemorrhage," *Journal of Critical Care*, vol. 28, no. 5, pp. 883.e1–883.e7, 2013.

[6] F. Michetti, V. Corvino, M. C. Geloso et al., "The S100B protein in biological fluids: more than a lifelong biomarker of brain distress," *Journal of Neurochemistry*, vol. 120, no. 5, pp. 644–659, 2012.

[7] R. A. Fleck, L. V. Rao, S. I. Rapaport, and N. Varki, "Localization of human tissue factor antigen by immunostaining with monospecific, polyclonal anti-human tissue factor antibody," *Thrombosis Research*, vol. 59, no. 2, pp. 421–437, 1990.

[8] L. Svennerholm, "Distribution and fatty acid composition of phosphoglycerides in normal human brain," *Journal of Lipid Research*, vol. 9, no. 5, pp. 570–579, 1968.

[9] P. van Dreden, A. Rousseau, S. Fontaine, B. J. Woodhams, and T. Exner, "Clinical evaluation of a new functional test for detection of plasma procoagulant phospholipids," *Blood Coagulation & Fibrinolysis*, vol. 20, no. 7, pp. 494–502, 2009.

[10] P. van Dreden, A. Rousseau, A. Savoure, B. Lenormand, S. Fontaine, and M. Vasse, "Plasma thrombomodulin activity, tissue factor activity and high levels of circulating procoagulant phospholipid as prognostic factors for acute myocardial infarction," *Blood Coagulation & Fibrinolysis*, vol. 20, no. 8, pp. 635–641, 2009.

[11] P. Delgado, J. A. Sabin, E. Santamarina et al., "Plasma S100B level after acute spontaneous intracerebral hemorrhage," *Stroke*, vol. 37, no. 11, pp. 2837–2839, 2006.

[12] A. Kleindienst, C. Schmidt, H. Parsch, I. Emtmann, Y. Xu, and M. Buchfelder, "The passage of S100B from brain to blood is not specifically related to the blood-brain barrier integrity,"

Cardiovascular Psychiatry and Neurology, vol. 2010, Article ID 801295, 8 pages, 2010.

[13] N. Morel, O. Morel, L. Petit et al., "Generation of procoagulant microparticles in cerebrospinal fluid and peripheral blood after traumatic brain injury," *Journal of Trauma*, vol. 64, no. 3, pp. 698–704, 2008.

[14] A. E. Pasvogel, P. Miketova, and I. M. Moore, "Differences in CSF phospholipid concentration by traumatic brain injury outcome," *Biological Research for Nursing*, vol. 11, no. 4, pp. 325–331, 2010.

[15] M. Huang, Y.-Y. Hu, and X.-Q. Dong, "High concentrations of procoagulant microparticles in the cerebrospinal fluid and peripheral blood of patients with acute basal ganglia hemorrhage are associated with poor outcome," *Surgical Neurology*, vol. 72, no. 5, pp. 481–489, 2009.

[16] M. Eddleston, J. C. de la Torre, M. B. A. Oldstone, D. J. Loskutoff, T. S. Edgington, and N. Mackman, "Astrocytes are the primary source of tissue factor in the murine central nervous system. A role for astrocytes in cerebral hemostasis," *The Journal of Clinical Investigation*, vol. 92, no. 1, pp. 349–358, 1993.

[17] Y. Hirashima, S. Nakamura, M. Suzuki et al., "Cerebrospinal fluid tissue factor and thrombin-antithrombin III complex as indicators of tissue injury after subarachnoid hemorrhage," *Stroke*, vol. 28, no. 9, pp. 1666–1670, 1997.

[18] M. Suzuki, A. Kudo, Y. Otawara, Y. Hirashima, A. Takaku, and A. Ogawa, "Extrinsic pathway of blood coagulation and thrombin in the cerebrospinal fluid after subarachnoid hemorrhage," *Neurosurgery*, vol. 44, no. 3, pp. 487–493, 1999.

[19] M. Weisfelt, R. M. Determann, J. de Gans et al., "Procoagulant and fibrinolytic activity in cerebrospinal fluid from adults with bacterial meningitis," *Journal of Infection*, vol. 54, no. 6, pp. 545–550, 2007.

[20] J. Fareed, D. D. Callas, D. Hoppensteadt, and E. W. Bermes Jr., "Tissue factor antigen levels in various biological fluids," *Blood Coagulation & Fibrinolysis*, vol. 6, no. 1, pp. S32–S36, 1995.

[21] S. P. Lad, H. Hegen, G. Gupta, F. Deisenhammer, and G. K. Steinberg, "Proteomic biomarker discovery in cerebrospinal fluid for cerebral vasospasm following subarachnoid hemorrhage," *Journal of Stroke & Cerebrovascular Diseases*, vol. 21, no. 1, pp. 30–41, 2012.

[22] D. T. Lang, L. B. Berberian, S. Lee, and M. Ault, "Rapid differentiation of subarachnoid hemorrhage from traumatic lumbar puncture using the D-dimer assay," *American Journal of Clinical Pathology*, vol. 93, no. 3, pp. 403–405, 1990.

[23] M. L. Juliá-Sanchis, P. L. Estela-Burriel, F. J. Lirón-Hernández, and A. Guerrero-Espejo, "Rapid differential diagnosis between subarachnoid hemorrhage and traumatic lumbar puncture by D-dimer assay," *Clinical Chemistry*, vol. 53, no. 5, article 993, 2007.

[24] V. Eclache, T. Vu, and G. Le Roux, "D-dimer levels in the cerebrospinal fluid: a marker of central nervous system involvement in neoplastic disease," *Nouvelle Revue Francaise d'Hematologie*, vol. 36, no. 4, pp. 321–324, 1994.

[25] C. Zweifel, M. Katan, P. Schuetz et al., "Copeptin is associated with mortality and outcome in patients with acute intracerebral hemorrhage," *BMC Neurology*, vol. 10, article 34, 2010.

[26] X.-Q. Dong, Y.-Y. Hu, W.-H. Yu, and Z.-Y. Zhang, "High concentrations of resistin in the peripheral blood of patients with acute basal ganglia hemorrhage are associated with poor outcome," *Journal of Critical Care*, vol. 25, no. 2, pp. 243–247, 2010.

25

Profiling β Thalassemia Mutations in Consanguinity and Nonconsanguinity for Prenatal Screening and Awareness Programme

Ravindra Kumar,[1] Vandana Arya,[2] and Sarita Agarwal[3]

[1]Central Research Laboratory, Sri Aurobindo Medical College and PG Institute, Indore, Madhya Pradesh 453111, India
[2]Department of Molecular Hematology, Sir Ganga Ram Hospital, New Delhi 110060, India
[3]Department of Genetics, Sanjay Gandhi Post Graduate Institute of Medical Sciences, Lucknow, Uttar Pradesh 226014, India

Correspondence should be addressed to Ravindra Kumar; ravindrachhabra@gmail.com

Academic Editor: Elvira Grandone

Mutation spectrum varies significantly in different parts and different ethnic groups of India. Social factors such as preference to marry within the community and among 1st degree relatives (consanguinity) play an important role in impeding the gene pool of the disease within the community and so in society by and large. The present paper discusses the role of consanguinity in profiling of beta thalassemia mutation, and thus the approach for prenatal screening and prevention based awareness programme. Clinically diagnosed 516 cases of beta thalassemia were screened at molecular level. A detailed clinical Proforma was recorded with the information of origin of the family, ethnicity, and consanguinity. The present study reports that subjects originating from Uttar Pradesh, Uttarakhand, Bihar, and Jharkhand have c.92+5G>C and c.124_127delTTCT mutation as the commonest mutation compared to the subjects hailing from Madhya Pradesh and Chhattisgarh and Nepal where sickle mutation was found more common. In 40 consanguineous unions more common and specific beta mutations with higher rate of homozygosity have been reported. This consanguinity-based data helps not only in deciding target oriented prenatal diagnostic strategies but also in objective based awareness programmes in prevention of thalassemia major birth.

1. Introduction

Thalassemia is a heterogeneous group of hemoglobin disorders in which the production of normal hemoglobin is partly or completely suppressed as a result of the defective synthesis of one or more globin chains [1]. Thalassemia presents a significant health problem in 71% of 229 countries, and these 71% of countries include 89% of all births worldwide. It has been estimated that approximately 7% of the world population are carriers of thalassemia and about 56,000 have a major thalassemia, including at least 30,000 who need regular transfusions to survive and 5,500 who die perinatally due to α thalassemia major [2].

This increase of thalassemia birth might be due to lack of prevention and awareness programs running in India. Awareness strategies need intervention at two levels, that is, among medical practitioners and population in mass.

Awareness programs are usually less popular in mass as there exist variable ethnic groups and various customs pertaining to their marriage pattern within the community itself prevent their exposure to wide society and prevent them from coming out of the traditions existing within the community. This by and large affects their decision in making mating pattern. The marriage within the community or relatives is relatively more or less dictated by their religious gurus and then it becomes very hard to overcome rituals, as education also becomes a limiting factor to understand the facts of life with quality. As a result, the country gets overburdened with the genetic disorders and family faces the social, mental, and economical trauma due to limited medical facilities available in the state.

Prevention of the disease by genetic counseling and prenatal diagnosis has an ultimate option in those parts of the world where limited resources for the medical care persist.

Pattern of mutations varies significantly between different geographical regions and community/ethnic groups; however each population and ethnic group has its own sets of common mutations [3–6]. This knowledge of spectrum of mutations enables medical fratinity and nongovernment organizations (NGOS) to create awareness programs, genetic counseling, and target oriented prenatal diagnosis to avoid long awaited trauma to the high risk couples [7].

In India the social factors such as preference to marry within the community and among 1st degree relatives (consanguinity) is quite prevailing and thus plays an important role in increasing the gene pool of the mutation responsible for disease within the community [5, 8, 9]. In that scenario target oriented prenatal diagnosis helps early detection of the fetus status.

Therefore, our aim of study is to first dissect the regional and ethnic profiling of beta thalassemia mutation and further look into the angle of the implication of consanguinity on spectrum of mutation in the state of Uttar Pradesh which is the second largest state of the country and where social and casts based marriages are very common.

2. Material and Methods

Total 516 clinically and molecularly diagnosed cases of beta thalassemia were included in the present study. The data pertaining to origin of the family, ethnicity, and consanguinity were evaluated for making reasonable and sizable group for including in the study. All the patients were grouped according to their origin and community. For beta thalassemia mutation detection analysis, 2 mL of blood was drawn and collected in EDTA coated vials from each individual. DNA was extracted from peripheral blood leucocytes by commercial available DNA extraction kit (Qiagen). Mutation detection was done using ARMS-PCR as described previously by Agarwal et al. 2000 [3]. Data was entered in Microsoft Excel 2007 and spectrum of mutation was identified in different groups.

3. Results

These 516 cases were grouped according to their native place. The 419 subjects were from Uttar Pradesh (UP) and Uttarakhand, 46 were from Bihar and Jharkhand, 25 were from Madhya Pradesh (MP) and Chhattisgarh, and 15 were the natives of Nepal. The remaining 11 cases were from other states. Spectrum analysis in different neighboring states or country shows quite different patterns from each other. Interestingly, the high frequency of sickle mutation (c.20A>T) was found in the subjects who had family origin from MP and Chhattisgarh and Nepal (Figure 1).

Total 674 chromosomes from 516 individuals were analyzed to find out molecular lesions of beta globin gene. To assess the mutation pattern among Hindus and Non-Hindus communities as their marriage rituals differ from each other, we have divided subjects into two groups (Table 1). A quite variable pattern was observed in both the groups. c.48C>T

TABLE 1: Spectrum of mutation in Hindu and Non-Hindu groups.

Mutations	Chromosomes	
	Non-Hindus [% prevalence]	Hindus [% prevalence]
c.92+5G>C	36 [31.8]	216 [38.5]
c.124_127delTTCT	12 [10.6]	57 [10.1]
c.27_28insG	13 [11.5]	40 [7.1]
c.92+1G>T	1 [0.9]	22 [3.9]
NG_000007.3:g.71609_72227del619	1 [0.9]	35 [6.2]
c.51delC	5 [4.4]	31 [5.5]
c.91G>C	5 [4.4]	21 [3.7]
c.-50A>T	2 [1.7]	15 [2.6]
c.48C>T	10 [8.8]	11 [1.9]
c.92+1G>A	1 [0.9]	2 [0.3]
c.-138C>T	—	4 [0.7]
c.79G>A	15 [13.2]	46 [8.1]
c.20A>T	11 [9.7]	64 [11.4]
	113	561

mutation was found with high frequency of 8.8% in Non-Hindus compared to 1.9% in Hindus.

Since the marriage pattern and the customs prevailing within the community are different and so is the pattern of mutation, we have divided the group into two, depending upon the consanguinity and nonconsanguinity in the family. Table 2 summarizes the pattern of beta mutations in consanguineous versus nonconsanguineous group. Since we have not observed any consanguinity in sickle cell (c.20A>T) and HbE (c.79G>A) group, we have excluded those 126 variant cases from Table 2.

This present compiled data showed 40 consanguineous families. Interestingly only 7 beta mutations covered the whole consanguineous group; however, 11 beta mutations are attributed to the nonconsanguineous group (Table 2).

c.92+5G>C was the most common mutation in both the groups. In consanguineous group c.27_28insG, c.48C>T, and c.124_127delTTCT followed it whereas in nonconsanguineous group c.124_127delTTCT, c.51delC, 619 bp, and c.27_28insG mutations were common after c.92+5G>C. Approximately 80% of the chromosomes from consanguineous category were covered by only 3 mutations whereas 8 mutations are needed to screen the nonconsanguineous group. A more heterogeneity in the nonconsanguineous group was found as compared to consanguineous group (Table 2).

In order to find out the homozygosity pattern for these mutations, we observed an increased rate of homozygosity (15%) in consanguineous group as compared to nonconsanguineous group (6.3%) (Table 3).

4. Discussion

Prevention of β thalassemia by genetic counseling and prenatal diagnosis is an important health issue in India. One of the

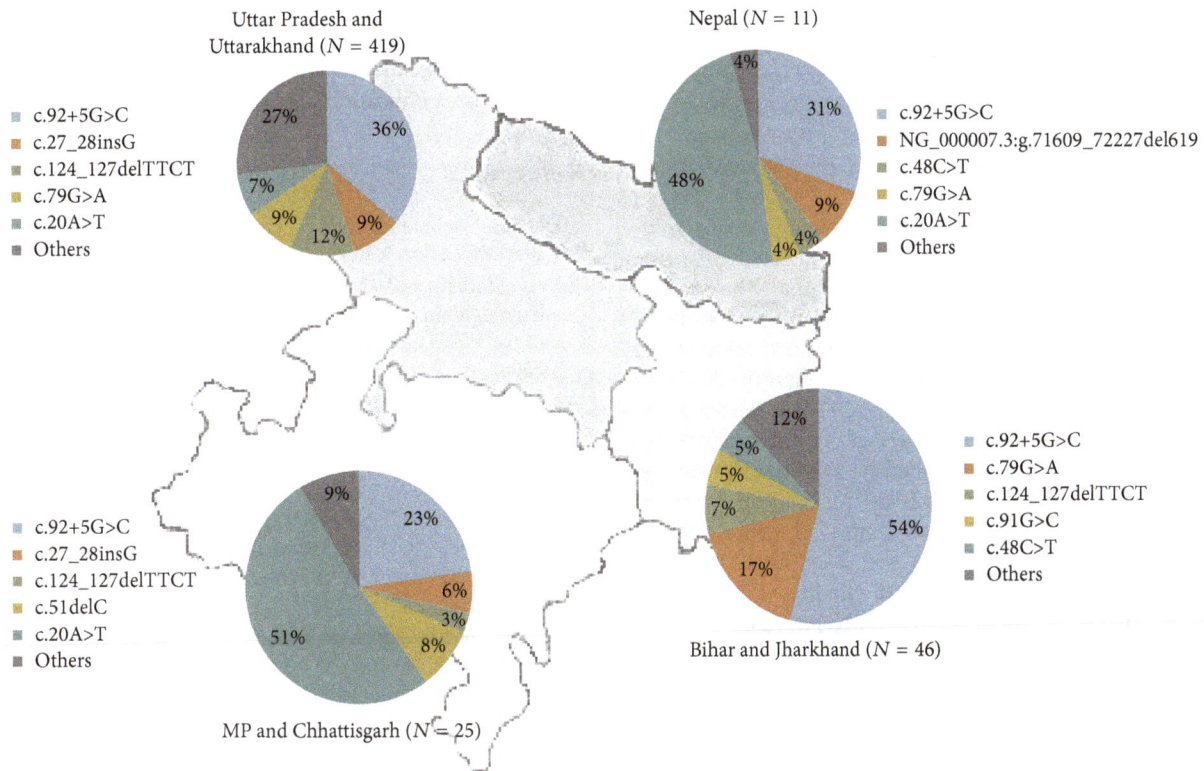

FIGURE 1: Spectrum of beta mutations.

TABLE 2: Status of the β mutation in consanguineous and nonconsanguineous group.

Mutations	Consanguineous [ch = 52] [%]	Nonconsanguineous [ch = 388] [%]
c.92+5G>C	19 [36.5]	168 [43.3]
c.124_127delTTCT	5 [9.6]	49 [12.6]
c.27_28insG	15 [28.8]	29 [7.5]
c.48C>T	7 [13.4]	12 [3.1]
c.51delC	—	44 [11.3]
c.92+1G>T	1 [1.9]	16 [4.1]
NG_000007.3:g.71609_72227del619	3 [5.7]	30 [7.7]
c.91G>C	—	23 [5.9]
c.-50A>T	2 [3.8]	10 [2.6]
c.92+1G>A	—	3 [0.7]
c.-138C>T	—	4 [1.0]

ch = chromosomes.

TABLE 3: Homozygosity versus compound heterozygosity in two groups.

	Consanguineous [9]	Nonconsanguineous [85]
Homozygous	6 (15%)	23 (6.3%)
Compound heterozygous	3 (7.5%)	62 (17.1%)

approaches for community control of β thalassemia, outlined by the World Health Organization (WHO), is documentation

of molecular heterogeneity of the disease. The knowledge of the geographic profiling of mutation in the population has proved to be the best strategy in diagnosis of the disease at prenatal level.

Several previous reports from North India have emphasized the need for regular evaluation of the mutation, as the shift in the frequencies of the mutation is very high [5, 6, 8, 9]. Thereby we have analyzed the spectrum of mutation in different neighboring states or country. This data indicates that few mutations are common in different parts of the country, though the frequency differs (Figure 1). In Uttar Pradesh and

Uttarakhand, Bihar and Jharkhand the c.92+5G>C mutation was found in 36% and 54%, respectively. The HbS, a common Hb variant, was found more frequently in Madhya Pradesh (51%) and Nepal (48%). Surprisingly c.92+1G>T, one of the common mutations reported in Punjabis by Garewal and Das in 2003 [10], was found to be absent in Madhya Pradesh, Bihar and Jharkhand, and Nepal.

This study clearly indicates that consanguineous marriages have a higher risk of producing affected offspring than general populations due to high gene pool. The consanguineous marriages are frequently present in South India as compared to North India [11, 12]. However no specific report related to the overall prevalence of consanguinity in India has been reported so far; Bittles in 2002 has reported the prevalence of consanguineous marriages in different parts of India which was basically compiled by National Family and Health Survey (IIPS 1995) in 1992-93 [13].

As our centre is the referral centre for genetic disorders, the majority of the cases are from Uttar Pradesh, Uttarakhand, Bihar and Jharkhand, Madhya Pradesh and Chhattisgarh, and neighboring country Nepal. In our hospital based study we have found that consanguinity is 7.9% in Uttar Pradesh and Uttarakhand, while in Madhya Pradesh and Chhattisgarh it is 1.6% and 4.3% in Bihar and Jharkhand. The present data supports the findings of Bittles as they have reported the rate of consanguineous marriages to be 7.5, 4.1, and 5% in Uttar Pradesh and Uttarakhand, Madhya Pradesh and Chhattisgarh, and Bihar and Jharkhand, respectively [13].

When focusing on consanguinity rate by religion, Bittles has reported a remarkably higher frequency in Muslims (59.6%) than in Hindus (1.7%) and other religious groups [13, 14]. In our data we have not observed the consanguinity in other religions like Christians, Buddhists, and nonbelievers.

The highest rates of consanguineous marriage in North Central part of India are usually reported from rural areas and among the economically weak and least educated groups. Considerable attention is paid to the role of consanguineous marriages as a causative factor in the high prevalence of genetic disorders [15–17]. At the same time the potential influence of this community endogamy on disease type, its severity, and the approach towards management has not been noticed properly and has been underestimated.

The probability of homozygosity rate in consanguineous marriages is higher than that of unrelated parents; this may be due to the limited gene pool and thus more expression of recessive alleles. The statement is supported by the present study as homozygosity was found significantly higher (15%) in consanguineous group as compared to nonconsanguineous group (6.3%).

Thus consanguinity causes clustering of mutations within the community, which increases the risk of a thalassemic child to be born.

This study shows that in a consanguineous group the specific set of mutations accounts for nearly 80% of subjects. This prompted the molecular geneticist to extend the approach for the early and rapid prenatal diagnosis and development of diagnostic kit with few selected mutations for the consanguineous unions on the one hand and strategy of awareness programmes for NGOs on the other hand.

Conflict of Interests

The authors declare that there is no conflict of interests regarding the publication of this paper.

References

[1] D. J. Weatherall and B. Clegg, *The Thalassemia Syndromes*, Blackwell Science, Oxford, UK, 4th edition, 2001.

[2] B. Modell and M. Darlison, "Global epidemiology of haemoglobin disorders and derived service indicators," *Bulletin of the World Health Organization*, vol. 86, no. 6, pp. 480–487, 2008.

[3] S. Agarwal, M. Pradhan, U. R. Gupta, S. Samai, and S. S. Agarwal, "Geographic and ethnic distribution of β-thalassemia mutations in Uttar Pradesh, India," *Hemoglobin*, vol. 24, no. 2, pp. 89–97, 2000.

[4] E. S. Edison, R. V. Shaji, S. G. Devi et al., "Analysis of β globin mutations in the Indian population: presence of rare and novel mutations and region-wise heterogeneity," *Clinical Genetics*, vol. 73, no. 4, pp. 331–337, 2008.

[5] R. Kumar, K. Singh, I. Panigrahi, and S. Agarwal, "Genetic heterogeneity of beta globin mutations among Asian-Indians and importance in genetic counselling and diagnosis," *Mediterranean Journal of Hematology and Infectious Diseases*, vol. 5, no. 1, Article ID e2013003, 2013.

[6] D. Mohanty, R. B. Colah, A. C. Gorakshakar et al., "Prevalence of β-thalassemia and other haemoglobinopathies in six cities in India: a multicentre study," *Journal of Community Genetics*, vol. 4, no. 1, pp. 33–42, 2013.

[7] A. Cao and R. Galanello, "Effect of consanguinity on screening for thalassemia," *The New England Journal of Medicine*, vol. 347, no. 15, pp. 1200–1202, 2002.

[8] R. Colah, A. Gorakshakar, A. Nadkarni et al., "Regional heterogeneity of β-thalassemia mutations in the multi ethnic Indian population," *Blood Cells, Molecules, and Diseases*, vol. 42, no. 3, pp. 241–246, 2009.

[9] S. Sinha, A. Kumar, V. Gupta, S. Kumar, V. P. Singh, and R. Raman, "Haemoglobinopathies: thalassaemias and abnormal haemoglobins in eastern Uttar Pradesh and adjoining districts of neighbouring states," *Current Science*, vol. 87, no. 6, pp. 775–780, 2004.

[10] G. Garewal and R. Das, "Spectrum of β-thalassemia mutations in punjabis," *International Journal of Human Genetics*, vol. 3, no. 4, pp. 217–219, 2003.

[11] N. Appaji Rao, H. S. Savithri, and A. H. Bittles, "A genetic perspective on the South Indian tradition of consanguineous marriage," in *Austral-Asian Encounters*, C. Vanden Driesen and S. Nandan, Eds., pp. 326–341, Prestige Books, New Delhi, India, 2002.

[12] N. Audinarayana and S. Krishnamoorthy, "Contribution of social and cultural factors to the decline in consanguinity in South India," *Social Biology*, vol. 47, no. 3-4, pp. 189–200, 2000.

[13] A. H. Bittles, "Endogamy, consanguinity and community genetics," *Journal of Genetics*, vol. 81, no. 3, pp. 91–98, 2002.

[14] A. H. Bittles and R. Hussain, "An analysis of consanguineous marriage in the Muslim population of india at regional and state levels," *Annals of Human Biology*, vol. 27, no. 2, pp. 163–171, 2000.

[15] M. I. El Mouzan, A. A. Al Salloum, A. S. Al Herbish, M. M. Qurachi, and A. A. Al Omar, "Consanguinity and major genetic disorders in Saudi children: a community-based cross-sectional

study," *Annals of Saudi Medicine*, vol. 28, no. 3, pp. 169–173, 2008.

[16] A. H. Bittles and I. Egerbladh, "The influence of past endogamy and consanguinity on genetic disorders in northern Sweden," *Annals of Human Genetics*, vol. 69, no. 5, pp. 549–558, 2005.

[17] R. Mokhtari and A. Bagga, "Consanguinity, genetic disorders and malformations in the Iranian population," *Acta Biologica Szegediensis*, vol. 47, no. 1–4, pp. 47–50, 2003.

26

Protein Kinase CK2: A Targetable BCR-ABL Partner in Philadelphia Positive Leukemias

Alessandro Morotti,[1] Giovanna Carrà,[1] Cristina Panuzzo,[1] Sabrina Crivellaro,[1] Riccardo Taulli,[2] Angelo Guerrasio,[1] and Giuseppe Saglio[1]

[1]*Department of Clinical and Biological Sciences, University of Turin, 10043 Orbassano, Italy*
[2]*Department of Oncology, University of Turin, 10043 Orbassano, Italy*

Correspondence should be addressed to Alessandro Morotti; alessandro.morotti@unito.it

Academic Editor: Estella M. Matutes

BCR-ABL-mediated leukemias, either Chronic Myeloid Leukemia (CML) or Philadelphia positive Acute Lymphoblastic Leukemia (ALL), are the paradigm of targeted molecular therapy of cancer due to the impressive clinical responses obtained with BCR-ABL specific tyrosine kinase inhibitors (TKIs). However, BCR-ABL TKIs do not allow completely eradicating both CML and ALL. Furthermore, ALL therapy is associated with much worse responses to TKIs than those observed in CML. The identification of additional pathways that mediate BCR-ABL leukemogenesis is indeed mandatory to achieve synthetic lethality together with TKI. Here, we review the role of BCR-ABL/protein kinase CK2 interaction in BCR-ABL leukemias, with potentially relevant implications for therapy.

1. Introduction

The t(9;22) chromosomal translocation (also known as Philadelphia chromosome, or Ph$^+$) is the genetic hallmark of Chronic Myeloid Leukemia (CML) and characterizes one quarter of adult Acute Lymphoblastic Leukemia (ALL) and less than 5% of pediatric ALL [1–4]. CML is sustained by the p210-BCR-ABL isoform, while Ph$^+$-ALL is driven by a shorter p190-BCR-ABL isoform [5]. BCR-ABL leukemias are the paradigm of cancer targeted therapy, due to the successful development of BCR-ABL specific tyrosine kinase inhibitors (TKIs). However, CML and Ph$^+$-ALL still challenge clinicians and biologists. Clinicians are facing the fact that CML is still an uncurable disease [6]. Even if CML is effectively targeted by TKIs with astonishing responses rates, most of those patients that discontinue TKI therapy eventually relapse [7] due to the persistence of TKI resistant CML stem cells [8–11]. The second, Ph$^+$-ALL, is associated with much worse responses to TKI than those observed in CML [1, 12] and therefore requires additional targets to achieve synthetic lethality together with TKI. Furthermore, clinicians have also

to address the issue of TKI resistance due to the development of BCR-ABL point mutations [13]. Therefore, the definition of those pathways that are necessary for the maintenance of Ph$^+$ leukemias could identify novel targets to achieve synthetic lethality together with TKI. Here, we will review the role of protein kinase CK2 (Casein Kinase 2, CK2 from here on) as a BCR-ABL substrate.

2. Protein Kinase CK2

2.1. Biological Characterization. CK2 is an ubiquitously expressed serine-threonine kinase [14–21]. It is composed of two catalytic and two regulator subunits. The catalytic units are represented by the isoforms CK2α and CK2α'; the regulatory unit is composed of the CK2β isoform. Each subunit is the product of different genes. The relevance of CK2 in biological processes is highlighted by the phenotype of CK2 knockout mice. In particular, both CK2α [22, 23] and CK2β [24] knockout mice are lethal with multiple embryonic alterations; however, knockout mice of CK2α' are viable [25], although sterile, suggesting some grade of

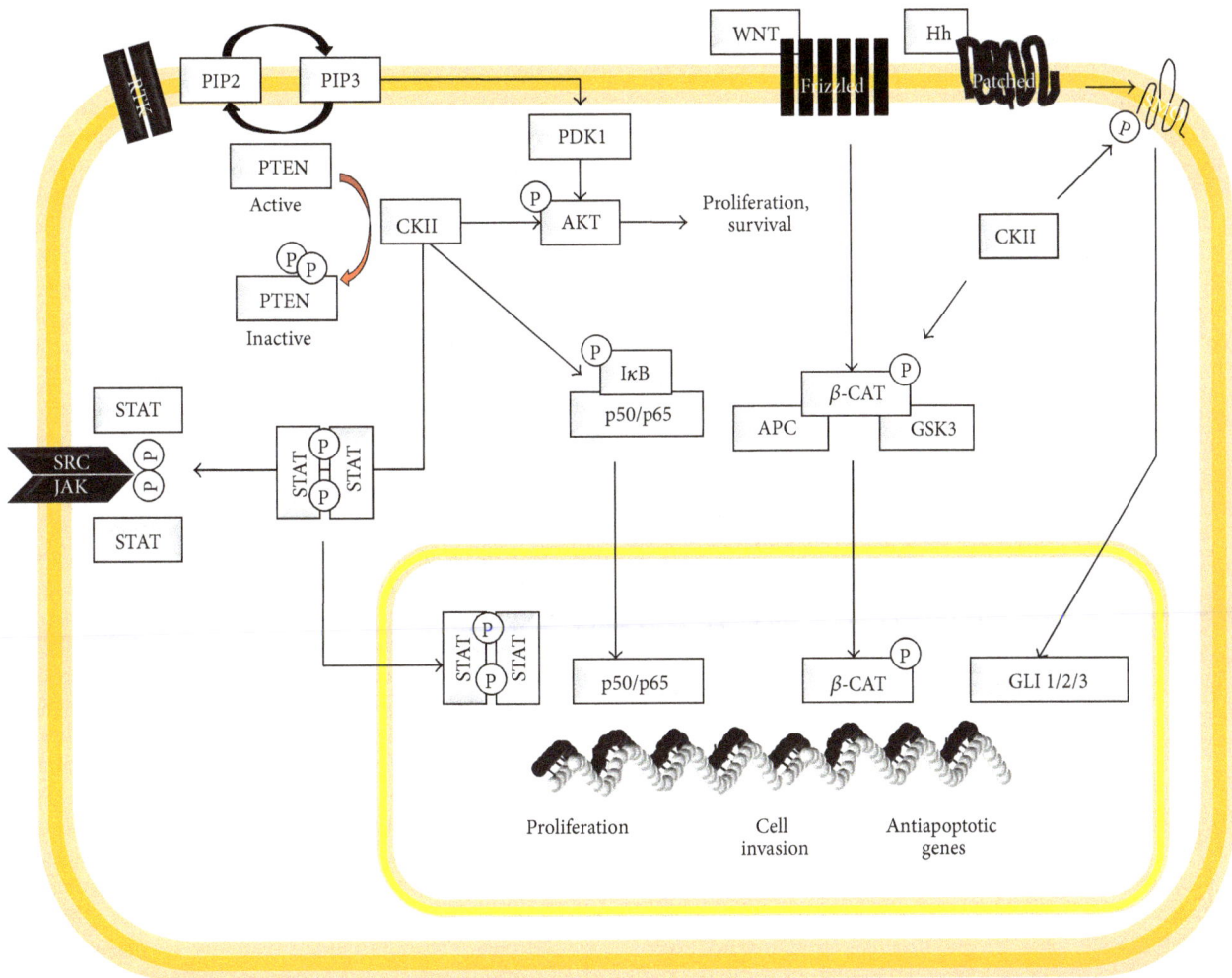

FIGURE 1: Protein kinase CK2 targets. This figure summarizes major CK2 targets.

compensations among the CK2 catalytic subunits. The CK2β subunit is highly conserved among species and is involved in the assembly of the tetrameric complex with the catalytic subunits and in the modulation of substrate recognition. Two CK2β interact with two identical (two CK2α or two CK2α') or nonidentical (one CK2α and one CK2α') catalytic subunits. The CK2 kinase is able to phosphorylate serine or threonine residues in proteins bearing a minimal consensus sequence that contains an acidic residue (Glu, Asp, pSer, or pTyr). CK2 is a unique kinase in that it can utilize GTP as well as ATP as the phosphate donor [19]. CK2 was often referred to as a constitutively active kinase, although several reports suggested different chances of kinase modulation [26]. In particular, it was extensively reviewed that CK2 activity can be modulated by changes in the subunit assembly, interaction with different regulatory elements, and protein interaction and finally even through different levels of phosphorylation/autophosphorylation [16, 19, 26, 27]. Several phosphorylation residues have indeed been identified both in the catalytic and regulatory subunits. Even if these phosphorylation sites did not appear to directly affect the kinase activity, these sites could affect the stability of the tetramer and therefore regulate substrate phosphorylation.

2.2. CK2 Targets. Beside the complex mechanisms of CK2 regulation and activation, which still require further investigations, it is well documented that CK2 phosphorylates several different targets, as extensively reviewed [18, 28]. CK2 was discovered in each cellular compartment, from the membrane to the nucleus, suggesting that it can interact and regulate the function of several proteins in every cellular compartment. In particular, CK2 is known to regulate cellular proliferation and apoptosis, DNA damage repair and gene expression, regulation of cell structure, and other cellular processes. Figure 1 shows some of the cancer associated targets, such as AKT, IkB-α, STAT5, and β-catenin.

2.3. CK2 Inactivates PTEN. PTEN is a tumor suppressor that negatively regulates the PI3K-AKT pathway, therefore counteracting one of the major signaling transduction networks involved in cancer pathogenesis [29, 30]. PTEN function is regulated by several posttransductional modifications such as serine/threonine-phosphorylation, acetylation, ubiquitination, and sumoylation [30]. Notably, the C-terminal domain of PTEN contains six serine/threonine residues (Thr-366; Ser-370; Ser-380; Thr-382; Thr-383 and Ser-385) that regulate the activity of the phosphatase PTEN, cellular compartmentalization, and protein stability [31–35]. Even if Ser-370 and Ser-385 were identified by mass-spectrometry as the mostly phosphorylated sites in PTEN [36, 37], all these residues have been described as CK2 substrates. Notably, CK2-mediated PTEN tail phosphorylation was clearly shown to play a role in different Philadelphia chromosome negative leukemias [38–42].

3. CK2 Inhibitors

Several CK2 inhibitors have been developed with different grades of selectivity and potency, as extensively reported [17, 43–54]. CK2 inhibitors have already been tested in hematological cancers. In particular, Chronic Lymphocytic Leukemia has been extensively studied for its high sensitiveness to CK2 inhibitors [41, 55]. Similarly, CK2 inhibitors appeared to display important effects in T-ALL [56]. Currently, some clinical trials are ongoing and will assess the relevance of CK2 inhibitors in the setting of hematological and solid cancers.

4. CK2 in Philadelphia Positive Leukemias

An original report showed that CK2 is highly expressed in proliferating CML myeloid progenitors [57]. Later, it was shown that BCR-ABL is able to physically interact with CK2α in K562 cell line, via the ABL portion of the chimeric protein [58]. Similarly, CK2α was shown to interact with c-Abl in NIH3T3 cells. Furthermore, BCR-ABL appeared to phosphorylate CK2α on tyrosine residues. Notably, in this first report, BCR-ABL was shown to inhibit the function of CK2α [58]. BCR-ABL/CK2α interaction was also investigated by another group [59], who demonstrated that CK2α strongly interacts with the BCR region between amino acids 242 and 413. Oppositely to the first report, CK2α was shown to positively mediate BCR-ABL signaling in both CML and Ph+-ALL [59]. Treatment with CK2α inhibitor 4,5,6,7-tetrabromo-2-benzotiazole was indeed shown to inhibit the growth of both p210- and p190-BCR-ABL transformed cells and BCR-ABL positive cells. Notably, the inhibition of BCR-ABL with TKI is also associated with the reduction of CK2α serine/threonine kinase activity. These original observations offer important implications for the therapeutical approach of BCR-ABL-positive CML/ALL and for the definition of CK2 regulation mechanisms. In particular, while CK2 has always been referred to as a constitutively active kinase, this work demonstrated that BCR-ABL regulates CK2 kinase activity, even if through a complex yet unknown mechanism. Another report further highlights the utility of targeting CK2 in the setting of BCR-ABL-mediated leukemias and in particular p190-BCR-ABL ALL cells [60]. A great step forward in the understanding of the role of BCR-ABL/CK2 complex was carried out by the group of Donella-Deana [61]. In particular,

while the first two reports lead to opposite conclusions, probably due to different cellular context, the last report confirmed that BCR-ABL interacts with CK2α in CML cells and that this interaction promotes cellular proliferation. Furthermore, this work provided additional insights on the mechanisms of CK2α regulation by BCR-ABL. In particular, authors have shown that CK2, both CK2α and CK2β, may be upregulated in imatinib-resistance CML cell lines with a consequent increase in the CK2 kinase activity [61]. Notably, no changes on the mRNA levels were observed, clearly suggesting upstream CK2 regulation. This observation, and the previous observation that CK2α tyrosine phosphorylation by BCR-ABL affects the CK2 kinase activity, suggests that in CML CK2 not only is just a constitutively active kinase but also can be somehow regulated. To further investigate the mechanisms of interaction, authors have also confirmed that BCR-ABL tyrosine phosphorylates CK2 and that this event is not required for the interaction between the two kinases. However, inhibition of CK2 abrogates the interaction. Although these data did not shed light on the complex mechanism of CK2 regulation, it is clear that BCR-ABL is able to force CK2 to modulate proliferation/survival in Ph+ leukemias. The authors have indeed clearly confirmed that CK2 inhibitor CX-4945 is able to promote cell death [61]. All these works did not link BCR-ABL/CK2α interaction with specific CK2α targets [58–60]. Recently, we have demonstrated that BCR-ABL/CK2α promotes serine phosphorylation of PTEN tail [62] (Figure 2). PTEN is found mostly in the cytosol of CML progenitor cells [63] where it is highly phosphorylated by CK2. PTEN tail phosphorylation inhibits its phosphatase activity both in cellular models and in primary CML cells. Interestingly, PTEN mutants, unable to be phosphorylated by CK2α, restored the phosphatase activity and were able to promote strong apoptosis induction in CML cells. Altogether, these works demonstrate that BCR-ABL interacts with CK2α which is in turn tyrosine phosphorylated [58, 59, 61]; BCR-ABL somehow "activates" CK2α towards substrates that are involved in the regulation of proliferation and survival. Lastly, BCR-ABL/CK2α interaction promotes the phosphorylation of PTEN with consequent inactivation of its phosphatase activity [62].

5. Conclusions

Since the discovery of the t(9;22) translocation, the Philadelphia chromosome, as the hallmark of CML, this disease has been the paradigm of precision medicine. However, BCR-ABL targeting with TKI did not allow eradicating both CML and Ph+-ALL, therefore highlighting the need of combinational therapies. In this review, we have summarized the role of CK2 as an essential mediator of BCR-ABL oncogenic signal. The BCR-ABL/CK2 complex is indeed responsible for mediating BCR-ABL induced cellular proliferation and survival. Targeting CK2 with specific inhibitors has been clearly shown to achieve synthetic lethality together with TKI, suggesting that a combinatorial therapy could help in eradicating Ph+ leukemias. Finally, the intriguing role of BCR-ABL/CK2 complex as being able to functionally inactivate the tumor suppressor PTEN may point to a highly effective

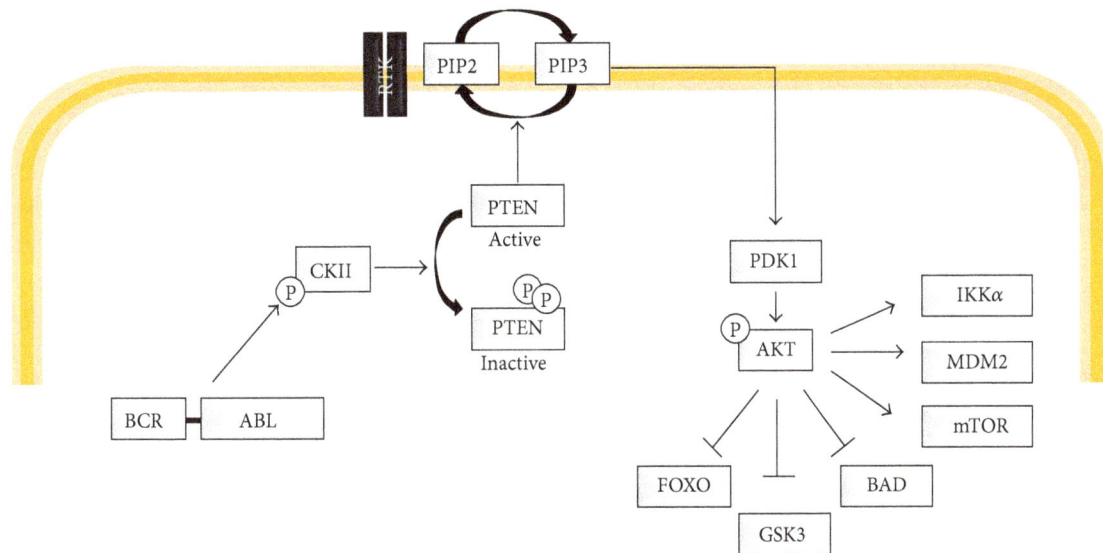

FIGURE 2: BCR-ABL/CK2/PTEN pathway. This figure describes the BCR-ABL/CK2/PTEN pathway.

proapoptotic therapy even in those cases characterized by TKI resistance due to BCR-ABL mutations.

Conflict of Interests

The authors have no conflict of interests regarding this work.

Authors' Contribution

Alessandro Morotti wrote the paper; Giovanna Carrà generated the figures; Giovanna Carrà, Cristina Panuzzo, Sabrina Crivellaro, Riccardo Taulli, Angelo Guerrasio, and Giuseppe Saglio reviewed the paper and provided insights.

Acknowledgments

The authors thank all the members of Professor Saglio laboratory and clinical division and Professor Pier Paolo Pandolfi for insights. This work has been supported by Giovani Ricercatori, GR-2010-2312984, from the Ministero della Salute, Ricerca Finalizzata, to Alessandro Morotti.

References

[1] E. Maino, R. Sancetta, P. Viero et al., "Current and future management of Ph/BCR-ABL positive ALL," *Expert Review of Anticancer Therapy*, vol. 14, no. 6, pp. 723–740, 2014.

[2] G. Saglio, A. Morotti, G. Mattioli et al., "Rational approaches to the design of therapeutics targeting molecular markers: the case of chronic myelogenous leukemia," *Annals of the New York Academy of Sciences*, vol. 1028, pp. 423–431, 2004.

[3] A. Morotti, C. Fava, and G. Saglio, "Milestones and monitoring," *Current Hematologic Malignancy Reports*, vol. 10, no. 2, pp. 167–172, 2015.

[4] J. V. Melo and D. J. Barnes, "Chronic myeloid leukaemia as a model of disease evolution in human cancer," *Nature Reviews Cancer*, vol. 7, no. 6, pp. 441–453, 2007.

[5] K. M. Bernt and S. P. Hunger, "Current concepts in pediatric Philadelphia chromosome-positive acute lymphoblastic leukemia," *Frontiers in Oncology*, vol. 4, article 54, 2014.

[6] E. Jabbour and H. Kantarjian, "Chronic myeloid leukemia: 2014 update on diagnosis, monitoring, and management," *American Journal of Hematology*, vol. 89, no. 5, pp. 547–556, 2014.

[7] K. Sweet and V. Oehler, "Discontinuation of tyrosine kinase inhibitors in chronic myeloid leukemia: when is this a safe option to consider?" *Hematology/the Education Program of the American Society of Hematology*, vol. 2013, no. 1, pp. 184–188, 2013.

[8] A. Morotti, C. Panuzzo, C. Fava, and G. Saglio, "Kinase-inhibitor-insensitive cancer stem cells in chronic myeloid leukemia," *Expert Opinion on Biological Therapy*, vol. 14, no. 3, pp. 287–299, 2014.

[9] F. Pellicano, L. Mukherjee, and T. L. Holyoake, "Concise review: cancer cells escape from oncogene addiction: Understanding the mechanisms behind treatment failure for more effective targeting," *Stem Cells*, vol. 32, no. 6, pp. 1373–1379, 2014.

[10] A. Hamilton, G. V. Helgason, M. Schemionek et al., "Chronic myeloid leukemia stem cells are not dependent on Bcr-Abl kinase activity for their survival," *Blood*, vol. 119, no. 6, pp. 1501–1510, 2012.

[11] A. S. Corbin, A. Agarwal, M. Loriaux, J. Cortes, M. W. Deininger, and B. J. Druker, "Human chronic myeloid leukemia stem cells are insensitive to imatinib despite inhibition of BCR-ABL activity," *Journal of Clinical Investigation*, vol. 121, no. 1, pp. 396–409, 2011.

[12] A. Hochhaus and H. Kantarjian, "The development of dasatinib as a treatment for Chronic Myeloid Leukemia (CML): from initial studies to application in newly diagnosed patients," *Journal of Cancer Research and Clinical Oncology*, vol. 139, no. 12, pp. 1971–1984, 2013.

[13] K. Yang and L.-W. Fu, "Mechanisms of resistance to BCR-ABL TKIs and the therapeutic strategies: a review," *Critical Reviews in Oncology/Hematology*, vol. 93, no. 3, pp. 27–292, 2015.

[14] M. Ruzzene and L. A. Pinna, "Addiction to protein kinase CK2: a common denominator of diverse cancer cells?" *Biochimica et*

Biophysica Acta—Proteins and Proteomics, vol. 1804, no. 3, pp. 499–504, 2010.

[15] A. Venerando, M. Ruzzene, and L. A. Pinna, "Casein kinase: the triple meaning of a misnomer," *Biochemical Journal*, vol. 460, no. 2, pp. 141–156, 2014.

[16] M. Montenarh, "Cellular regulators of protein kinase CK2," *Cell and Tissue Research*, vol. 342, no. 2, pp. 139–146, 2010.

[17] L. A. Pinna, "Protein kinase CK2: a challenge to canons," *Journal of Cell Science*, vol. 115, part 20, pp. 3873–3878, 2002.

[18] F. Piazza, S. Manni, M. Ruzzene, L. A. Pinna, C. Gurrieri, and G. Semenzato, "Protein kinase CK2 in hematologic malignancies: Reliance on a pivotal cell survival regulator by oncogenic signaling pathways," *Leukemia*, vol. 26, no. 6, pp. 1174–1179, 2012.

[19] D. W. Litchfield, "Protein kinase CK2: structure, regulation and role in cellular decisions of life and death," *Biochemical Journal*, vol. 369, no. 1, pp. 1–15, 2003.

[20] R. Battistutta and G. Lolli, "Structural and functional determinants of protein kinase CK2α: facts and open questions," *Molecular and Cellular Biochemistry*, vol. 356, no. 1-2, pp. 67–73, 2011.

[21] J. S. Duncan and D. W. Litchfield, "Too much of a good thing: the role of protein kinase CK2 in tumorigenesis and prospects for therapeutic inhibition of CK2," *Biochimica et Biophysica Acta*, vol. 1784, no. 1, pp. 33–47, 2008.

[22] D. C. Seldin, D. Y. Lou, P. Toselli, E. Landesman-Bollag, and I. Dominguez, "Gene targeting of CK2 catalytic subunits," *Molecular and Cellular Biochemistry*, vol. 316, no. 1-2, pp. 141–147, 2008.

[23] D. Y. Lou, I. Dominguez, P. Toselli, E. Landesman-Bollag, C. O'Brien, and D. C. Seldin, "The alpha catalytic subunit of protein kinase CK2 is required for mouse embryonic development," *Molecular and Cellular Biology*, vol. 28, no. 1, pp. 131–139, 2008.

[24] T. Buchou, M. Vernet, O. Blond et al., "Disruption of the regulatory β subunit of protein kinase CK2 in mice leads to a cell-autonomous defect and early embryonic lethality," *Molecular and Cellular Biology*, vol. 23, no. 3, pp. 908–915, 2003.

[25] X. Xu, P. A. Toselli, L. D. Russell, and D. C. Seldin, "Globozoospermia in mice lacking the casein kinase II α' catalytic subunit," *Nature Genetics*, vol. 23, no. 1, pp. 118–121, 1999.

[26] D. W. Litchfield, G. Dobrowolska, and E. G. Krebs, "Regulation of casein kinase II by growth factors: a reevaluation," *Cellular and Molecular Biology Research*, vol. 40, no. 5-6, pp. 373–381, 1994.

[27] K. Niefind and O.-G. Issinger, "Conformational plasticity of the catalytic subunit of protein kinase CK2 and its consequences for regulation and drug design," *Biochimica et Biophysica Acta—Proteins and Proteomics*, vol. 1804, no. 3, pp. 484–492, 2010.

[28] O. Filhol and C. Cochet, "Protein kinase CK2 in health and disease: cellular functions of protein kinase CK2: a dynamic affair," *Cellular and Molecular Life Sciences*, vol. 66, no. 11-12, pp. 1830–1839, 2009.

[29] Y. Shi, B. E. Paluch, X. Wang, and X. Jiang, "PTEN at a glance," *Journal of Cell Science*, vol. 125, no. 20, pp. 4687–4692, 2012.

[30] M. S. Song, L. Salmena, and P. P. Pandolfi, "The functions and regulation of the PTEN tumour suppressor," *Nature Reviews Molecular Cell Biology*, vol. 13, no. 5, pp. 283–296, 2012.

[31] S. J. Miller, D. Y. Lou, D. C. Seldin, W. S. Lane, and B. G. Neel, "Direct identification of PTEN phosphorylation sites," *FEBS Letters*, vol. 528, no. 1–3, pp. 145–153, 2002.

[32] F. Vazquez, S. R. Grossman, Y. Takahashi, M. V. Rokas, N. Nakamura, and W. R. Sellers, "Phosphorylation of the PTEN tail acts as an inhibitory switch by preventing its recruitment into a protein complex," *The Journal of Biological Chemistry*, vol. 276, no. 52, pp. 48627–48630, 2001.

[33] F. Vazquez, S. Ramaswamy, N. Nakamura, and W. R. Sellers, "Phosphorylation of the PTEN tail regulates protein stability and function," *Molecular and Cellular Biology*, vol. 20, no. 14, pp. 5010–5018, 2000.

[34] M.-M. Georgescu, K. H. Kirsch, T. Akagi, T. Shishido, and H. Hanafusa, "The tumor-suppressor activity of PTEN is regulated by its carboxyl-terminal region," *Proceedings of the National Academy of Sciences of the United States of America*, vol. 96, no. 18, pp. 10182–10187, 1999.

[35] J. Torres and R. Pulido, "The tumor suppressor PTEN is phosphorylated by the protein kinase CK2 at its C terminus. Implications for PTEN stability to proteasome-mediated degradation," *Journal of Biological Chemistry*, vol. 276, no. 2, pp. 993–998, 2001.

[36] F. Cordier, A. Chaffotte, E. Terrien et al., "Ordered phosphorylation events in two independent cascades of the PTEN C-tail revealed by NMR," *Journal of the American Chemical Society*, vol. 134, no. 50, pp. 20533–20543, 2012.

[37] L. Odriozola, G. Singh, T. Hoang, and A. M. Chan, "Regulation of PTEN activity by its carboxyl-terminal autoinhibitory domain," *The Journal of Biological Chemistry*, vol. 282, no. 32, pp. 23306–23315, 2007.

[38] A. Silva, J. A. Yunes, B. A. Cardoso et al., "PTEN posttranslational inactivation and hyperactivation of the PI3K/Akt pathway sustain primary T cell leukemia viability," *Journal of Clinical Investigation*, vol. 118, no. 11, pp. 3762–3774, 2008.

[39] A. Silva, P. Y. Jotta, A. B. Silveira et al., "Regulation of PTEN by CK2 and Notch1 in primary T-cell acute lymphoblastic leukemia: Rationale for combined use of CK2- and γ-secretase inhibitors," *Haematologica*, vol. 95, no. 4, pp. 674–678, 2010.

[40] A. M. Gomes, M. V. D. Soares, P. Ribeiro et al., "Adult B-cell acute lymphoblastic leukemia cells display decreased PTEN activity and constitutive hyperactivation of PI3K/Akt pathway despite high PTEN protein levels," *Haematologica*, vol. 99, no. 6, pp. 1062–1068, 2014.

[41] L. R. Martins, Y. Perera, P. Lúcio, M. G. Silva, S. E. Perea, and J. T. Barata, "Targeting chronic lymphocytic leukemia using CIGB-300, a clinical-stage CK2-specific cell-permeable peptide inhibitor," *Oncotarget*, vol. 5, no. 1, pp. 258–263, 2014.

[42] M. Shehata, S. Schnabl, D. Demirtas et al., "Reconstitution of PTEN activity by CK2 inhibitors and interference with the PI3-K/Akt cascade counteract the antiapoptotic effect of human stromal cells in chronic lymphocytic leukemia," *Blood*, vol. 116, no. 14, pp. 2513–2521, 2010.

[43] I. M. Hanif, I. M. Hanif, M. A. Shazib, K. A. Ahmad, and S. Pervaiz, "Casein Kinase II: an attractive target for anti-cancer drug design," *International Journal of Biochemistry and Cell Biology*, vol. 42, no. 10, pp. 1602–1605, 2010.

[44] G. Cozza, L. A. Pinna, and S. Moro, "Kinase CK2 inhibition: an update," *Current Medicinal Chemistry*, vol. 20, no. 5, pp. 671–693, 2013.

[45] G. Cozza, L. A. Pinna, and S. Moro, "Protein kinase CK2 inhibitors: a patent review," *Expert Opinion on Therapeutic Patents*, vol. 22, no. 9, pp. 1081–1097, 2012.

[46] G. Cozza, S. Zanin, S. Sarno et al., "Design, validation and efficacy of bisubstrate inhibitors specifically affecting ecto-CK2 kinase activity," *Biochemical Journal*, vol. 471, no. 3, pp. 415–430, 2015.

[47] C. Girardi, D. Ottaviani, L. A. Pinna, and M. Ruzzene, "Different persistence of the cellular effects promoted by protein kinase CK2 inhibitors CX-4945 and TDB," *BioMed Research International*, vol. 2015, Article ID 185736, 9 pages, 2015.

[48] E. Iori, M. Ruzzene, S. Zanin, S. Sbrignadello, L. A. Pinna, and P. Tessari, "Effects of CK2 inhibition in cultured fibroblasts from Type 1 Diabetic patients with or without nephropathy," *Growth Factors*, vol. 33, no. 4, pp. 259–266, 2015.

[49] G. Cozza, A. Venerando, S. Sarno, and L. A. Pinna, "The selectivity of CK2 inhibitor quinalizarin: a reevaluation," *BioMed Research International*, vol. 2015, Article ID 734127, 9 pages, 2015.

[50] A. Siddiqui-Jain, D. Drygin, N. Streiner et al., "CX-4945, an orally bioavailable selective inhibitor of protein kinase CK2, inhibits prosurvival and angiogenic signaling and exhibits antitumor efficacy," *Cancer Research*, vol. 70, no. 24, pp. 10288–10298, 2010.

[51] V. Moucadel, R. Prudent, C. F. Sautel et al., "Antitumoral activity of allosteric inhibitors of protein kinase CK2," *Oncotarget*, vol. 2, no. 12, pp. 997–1010, 2011.

[52] B. Guerra, J. Hochscherf, N. B. Jensen, and O. Issinger, "Identification of a novel potent, selective and cell permeable inhibitor of protein kinase CK2 from the NIH/NCI Diversity Set Library," *Molecular and Cellular Biochemistry*, vol. 406, no. 1-2, pp. 151–161, 2015.

[53] B. Guerra, T. D. L. Rasmussen, A. Schnitzler et al., "Protein kinase CK2 inhibition is associated with the destabilization of HIF-1α in human cancer cells," *Cancer Letters*, vol. 356, no. 2, pp. 751–761, 2015.

[54] B. Guerra, M. Fischer, S. Schaefer, and O. Issinger, "The kinase inhibitor D11 induces caspase-mediated cell death in cancer cells resistant to chemotherapeutic treatment," *Journal of Experimental & Clinical Cancer Research*, vol. 34, no. 1, article 125, 2015.

[55] R. C. Prins, R. T. Burke, J. W. Tyner, B. J. Druker, M. M. Loriaux, and S. E. Spurgeon, "CX-4945, a selective inhibitor of casein kinase-2 (CK2), exhibits anti-tumor activity in hematologic malignancies including enhanced activity in chronic lymphocytic leukemia when combined with fludarabine and inhibitors of the B-cell receptor pathway," *Leukemia*, vol. 27, no. 10, pp. 2094–2096, 2013.

[56] F. Buontempo, E. Orsini, L. R. Martins et al., "Cytotoxic activity of the casein kinase 2 inhibitor CX-4945 against T-cell acute lymphoblastic leukemia: targeting the unfolded protein response signaling," *Leukemia*, vol. 28, no. 3, pp. 543–553, 2014.

[57] F. Phan-Dinh-Tuy, J. Henry, C. Boucheix, J. Y. Perrot, C. Rosenfeld, and A. Kahn, "Protein kinases in human leukemic cells," *American Journal of Hematology*, vol. 19, no. 3, pp. 209–218, 1985.

[58] J.-K. Hériché and E. M. Chambaz, "Protein kinase CK2α is a target for the Abl and Bcr-Abl tyrosine kinases," *Oncogene*, vol. 17, no. 1, pp. 13–18, 1998.

[59] S. Mishra, A. Reichert, J. Cunnick et al., "Protein kinase CKIIα interacts with the Bcr moiety of Bcr/Abl and mediates proliferation of Bcr/Abl-expressing cells," *Oncogene*, vol. 22, no. 51, pp. 8255–8262, 2003.

[60] S. Mishra, V. Pertz, B. Zhang et al., "Treatment of P190 Bcr/Abl lymphoblastic leukemia cells with inhibitors of the serine/threonine kinase CK2," *Leukemia*, vol. 21, no. 1, pp. 178–180, 2007.

[61] C. Borgo, L. Cesaro, V. Salizzato et al., "Aberrant signalling by protein kinase CK2 in imatinib-resistant chronic myeloid leukaemia cells: biochemical evidence and therapeutic perspectives," *Molecular Oncology*, vol. 7, no. 6, pp. 1103–1115, 2013.

[62] A. Morotti, C. Panuzzo, S. Crivellaro et al., "BCR-ABL inactivates cytosolic PTEN through Casein Kinase II mediated tail phosphorylation," *Cell Cycle*, vol. 14, no. 7, pp. 973–979, 2015.

[63] A. Morotti, C. Panuzzo, S. Crivellaro et al., "BCR-ABL disrupts PTEN nuclear-cytoplasmic shuttling through phosphorylation-dependent activation of HAUSP," *Leukemia*, vol. 28, no. 6, pp. 1326–1333, 2014.

27

Results of a Prospective Study of High-Dose or Conventional Anthracycline-Cyclophosphamide Regimen Plus Radiotherapy for Localized Adult Non-Hodgkin's Primary Bone Lymphoma

A. Schmidt-Tanguy,[1] R. Houot,[2] S. Lissandre,[3] J. F. Abgrall,[4] P. Casassus,[5] P. Rodon,[6] B. Desablens,[7] J. P. Marolleau,[7] R. Garidi,[8] T. Lamy,[2] M.-P. Moles-Moreau,[1] and G. Damaj[7,9]

[1] *Hematology Department of the University of Angers, Angers, France*
[2] *Hematology Department of the University of Rennes, Rennes, France*
[3] *Hematology Department of the University of Tours, Tours, France*
[4] *Hematology Department of the University of Brest, Brest, France*
[5] *Hematology Department of the University of Bobigny, Bobigny, France*
[6] *Hematology Department of the Hospital of Blois, Blois, France*
[7] *Hematology Department of the University of Amiens, Amiens, France*
[8] *Hematology Department, St. Quentin General Hospital, St. Quentin, France*
[9] *University Hospital of Amiens, Department of Clinical Haematology, Avenue Laennec, 80054 Amiens, France*

Correspondence should be addressed to G. Damaj; damaj.gandhi@chu-amiens.fr

Academic Editor: Giuseppe G. Saglio

Background. Primary bone lymphoma (PBL) is a rare entity that has only been reviewed in one prospective and small retrospective studies, from which it is difficult to establish treatment guidelines. We prospectively evaluated high-dose or conventional anthracycline-cyclophosphamide dose and radiotherapy for PBL. *Patients and Methods*. The GOELAMS prospective multicenter study (1986–1998) enrolled adults with localized high-grade PBL according to age and performance status (PS). Patients <60 years received a high-dose CHOP regimen (VCAP) and those ≥60 years a conventional anthracycline-cyclophosphamide regimen (VCEP-bleomycin); all received intrathecal chemotherapy and local radiotherapy. *Results*. Among the 26 patients included (VCAP: 19; VCEP-bleomycin: 7), 39% had poor PS ≥2. With a median follow-up of 8 years, overall survival, event-free survival, and relapse-free survival were 64%, 62%, and 65%, respectively, with no significant difference between treatment groups. Poor PS was significantly associated with shorter OS and EFS. *Conclusions*. Our results confirm the efficacy of our age-based therapeutic strategy. High-doses anthracycline-cyclophosphamide did not improve the outcome. VCEP-bleomycin is effective and well tolerated for old patients. The intensification must be considered for patients with PS ≥2, a poor prognostic factor.

1. Introduction

Primary bone lymphoma (PBL) is a rare clinicopathological entity accounting for about 3% of malignant bone tumors, 1% of non-Hodgkin lymphomas (NHL), and 5% of extranodal NHL [1–4]. In most cases, histology is diffuse large B-cell lymphoma (DLBCL). Whether or not PBL requires specific treatment guidelines has to be determined. Since the 1960s, management of limited stage I-II PBL has usually consisted of radiotherapy to the involved bone and adjacent lymph nodes inducing at least a good local control [2, 5]. Then, adjunction of chemotherapy has systematically been recommended to counter the relatively high rates of relapse occurring outside the original location after radiation alone. For advanced cases, corresponding to disease with multiple bones localizations, treatment can only be based on this combined-modality with generally very good prognosis [1, 6, 7].

To date, PBL has primarily been reviewed in several small retrospective studies and only one prospective study [1, 4, 8–10]. Our prospective study aimed to evaluate overall survival (OS), event-free survival (EFS), and relapse-free survival (RFS) after high-dose or conventional anthracycline-cyclophosphamide regimen for adults with localized non-Hodgkin's PBL before rituximab era.

2. Patients and Methods

2.1. Study Design and Patient Eligibility. Patients 17–75 years old with localized high-grade PBL were enrolled in a prospective, multicenter GOELAMS study. These patients accounted for 9.3% of the 305 NHL included in the 02 and 03 GOELAMS trials between March 1986 and May 1998 and gave their written informed consent to participate. The histological diagnosis was confirmed on an excision biopsy, in accordance with the previous working formulation criteria [11].

Staging procedures included performance status (PS), differential white blood-cell counts, biochemical analyses (serum lactate dehydrogenase (LDH) and hepatic and renal function tests), thoracic-abdominal-pelvic computed tomography scan, bone-marrow biopsy, and cerebrospinal fluid cytology. Human immunodeficiency virus-positive patients were excluded. The stage was determined according to the Ann Arbor criteria. Bulky disease was defined as a lesion exceeding >5 cm.

2.2. Treatment Protocol. Patients <60 years old (GOELAMS 02 trial) received three cycles of the high-dose CHOP regimen (VCAP), as follows: eldisine i.v. 3 mg/m^2 on day 1, doxorubicin i.v. 60 mg/m^2 on day 1, cyclophosphamide i.v. 1500 mg/m^2 on day 1, and oral prednisone 80 mg/m^2/d on days 1–5. Patients ≥60 years old (GOELAMS 03 trial) received three cycles of a conventional anthracycline-cyclophosphamide regimen (VCEP-bleomycin), as follows: eldisine i.v. 3 mg/m^2 on day 1, farmorubicin i.v. 80 mg/m^2 on day 1, cyclophosphamide i.v. 750 mg/m^2 on day 2, oral prednisone 50 mg/m^2/d on days 1–7, and bleomycin 10 mg on days 1 and 5.

For both trials, each course was repeated every 21 days and intrathecal chemotherapy (methotrexate 15 mg) was administered with each cycle. Since January 1990, all patients have been given granulocyte-colony-stimulating factor between chemotherapy cycles.

One month after completing chemotherapy, every patient received involved-field radiotherapy (total dose: 40 Gy delivered in 20 fractions, 2 Gy/day) over 4 weeks.

2.3. Response Assessment and Follow-Up Evaluation. Treatment response was determined by physical examination and biological and radiological workup. In the GOELAMS prospective multicenter study, complete response (CR) was defined as the complete disappearance of all clinical, biological, and radiological evidence of disease (absence of progressive bone lesions). The follow-up included clinical and radiological evaluation every six months.

Survival analyses included OS, EFS, and RFS. OS was calculated from the time of diagnosis until death from any cause. EFS was calculated from time of diagnosis (i.e., study entry) until disease progression, relapse, second malignancy, and death from any cause. RFS was calculated as survival after achievement of CR until relapse or death.

2.4. Statistical Methods. Results are expressed as median (range), mean ± SD, or number (%).

Survival curves were calculated using the actuarial Kaplan-Meier method. Log-rank analysis was used to assess the significance of differences between curves for patients groups. Patients' characteristics were subjected to univariate analysis using log-rank test, before being entered into Cox proportional hazards (multivariate analyses) regression models, to determine prognostic factors (two sided). A $P = 0.05$ was considered significant. The studied prognostic factors are the gender, the sex, the stage, the B symptoms, the site, the LDH level, the bulky disease, the PS, and the epidural involvement.

All statistical analyses were conducted with the statistical package for social sciences (SPSS Inc., Chicago, IL).

3. Results

Twenty-six patients with PBL were included in GOELAMS 02 (19/26 patients, 73%) and 03 (7/26 patients, 37%) trials from 1986 to 1998 and their characteristics are summarized in Table 1.

Their median age was 46 years (range 17–69) (19 patients) and 70 years (range 65–75) (7 patients) in the GOELAMS 02 and 03 trials (cutoff of 60 years), respectively. Three patients between 63 and 69 years old but with excellent PS were included in the GOELAMS 02 trial by the investigators. Overall male/female ratio was 1.6.

The main PBL site was the axial skeleton. Two patients had bifocal bones lesions (axial and peripheral skeleton bone lesions). Skin and subcutaneous tissues were also involved in two patients. According to the Ann Arbor classification, 81% of patients were stage I and 19% were stage II. Six patients of the GOELAMS 02 trial had epidural involvement, revealed by paraplegia which may largely explain why PS was ≥2 for 35% of the patients. Predominant histological subtypes were diffuse, small cleaved cell lymphoma and diffuse, mixed small and large cell according to the Working Formulation, which correspond to DLBCL in the Working Health Organization classification.

Except for age and bulky disease, the two trials were comparable for histological type, site, Ann Arbor classification, B symptoms, and LDH (Table 1). All but one patient achieved CR (96%). A 63-year-old patient with VCAP-resistant costal disease died of progressive disease after 15 months. Eight (30%) relapses occurred at a median of 2.3 years (range 0.4–6.5) after CR: two relapses in the group of the 7 older patients and 6 in this of the 19 younger patients, which also included 65- and 69-year-old patients. Two out of the 8 relapses occurred at the initial PBL site.

Bulky disease was observed in nine patients and four of them relapsed. Four relapses occurred less than 2 years after CR, three between 2.1 and 5 years and one 6.5 years after CR. Among the six patients with epidural involvement, three relapsed (50%) and three were in sustained CR: two of these three relapses occurred *in situ*.

With median follow-up of 8 years (range 1.2–17), OS, EFS, and RFS were 64% ± 12, 62% ± 10, and 65% ± 10 years, respectively. OS, EFS, and RFS in the GOELAM 02 and 6 03 trials were, respectively, 66% ± 13, 59% ± 21, 62% ± 12 and 64% ± 21, 71% ± 14, 71% ± 17 with no significant difference between the two study groups (Table 2).

According to univariate and multivariate analysis, poor PS (≥2) was associated with significantly shorter OS and EFS (Figure 1 and Table 2).

4. Discussion

This report summarizes the results of a prospective study that evaluated the long-term outcome of 26 non-Hodgkin's PBL in adults after high-dose or conventional anthracycline-cyclophosphamide regimen combined with radiotherapy. Because of PBL rarity [1–4] and the heterogeneity of clinical procedure applied for diagnosis, staging, and treatment, controversies persist and no specific guidelines have been established.

The predominant histological profile of diffuse large B-cell lymphomas observed herein is consistent with published data [9, 10, 12]. No significant survival difference among between PLB subtypes has been observed in the literature [12, 13]. The median age was slightly higher than those reported previously (45–50 years) [3, 9, 14], which may reflect inclusion criteria. Unlike the majority of reports [1, 13, 15, 16], age did not influence the survival parameters (response rate, relapses, OS, RFS, progression, or EFS) of our patients. Indeed, the relatively good tolerance of treatment probably reflects the modulation of the chemotherapy dose according to age. Moreover, no radiotherapy complications were observed, certainly because of the low radiation dose delivered.

PBL was mostly diagnosed at stages I and II [9] except in one study with more stage IV with vertebral localization [17]. The stage appeared as the most important prognostic variable [1, 6, 8, 18]. The standard staging procedures (including bone radiographic, bone scan, and bone magnetic resonance imaging) may have underestimated the Ann Arbor staging. They do not allow an evaluation of the entire skeleton which is now optimately performed by using positron emission tomography [19]. Indeed stage IV is a factor of poor prognosis and probably requires an intensified treatment. An undervaluation of the stage leads to an insufficient treatment.

Peripheral skeleton is the most common site of PBL. However, one previous study reported high frequency of axial skeleton locations [20], which is a remarkable characteristic of our patients. Nevertheless PBL site did not influence OS and EFS in our study. However, some discrepancies concerning the definition of the axial involvement in the literature make it difficult to distinguish between the prognoses of axial skeleton versus limb involvement [2, 20].

Bulky disease was observed in 9 patients (all included in the VCAP group), 3 of whom having paraplegia. A pejorative impact of paraplegia has been suggested once [21]. Our univariate analysis identified a significantly unfavorable

TABLE 1: Characteristics of 26 adults with non-Hodgkin primary bone lymphoma.

	No.	%
Trial		
02	19	73
03	7	27
Gender		
Male	16	61
Female	10	39
Stage		
I	21	81
II	5	19
B symptoms		
No	21	81
Yes	5	19
Site		
Axial skeleton	20	59
Spine	13	50
Pelvis	5	19
Rib	2	7
Peripheral skeleton	10	28
Limbs	6	23
Tibia	1	4
Humerus	1	4
Scapula	2	8
Radius/ulna	1	4
Finger	1	4
Skull	4	12
Mandible	3	12
Occipital	1	4
Histology		
Diffuse, mixed, small, large	4	15
Diffuse, large cleaved or not	18	69
Large cell immunoblastic	3	12
Anaplastic large-cell ANA Ki+	1	4
Immunophenotyping		
B cells	14	54
T cells	1	4
ANA Ki+	1	4
Nonassessable	10	38
LDH > N	7/21	33
PS		
0	6	23
1	11	42
2	6	23
3	3	12
IPI score		
0	5	19
1	11	42
2	3	11

TABLE 1: Continued.

	No.	%
3	2	7
Non-assessable	5	19

LDH: lactatedehydrogenase; N: normal; PS: performance status; IPI: international prognostic index.
Except for age and bulky disease, the two trials were comparable (no statistical significance). Bulky disease was observed in 9 patients, all included in the trial 02 ($P = 0.02$).
Six patients of the GOELAMS 02 trial had epidural involvement, revealed by paraplegia.

impact of PS $\geq$2 (OS, EFS). Our multivariate analysis retained poor PS but not epidural extension as being significantly associated with shorter EFS and OS. This observation is probably explained by relative redundancy between epidural extension and PS, since, quite frequently in neoplasic situations, paraplegic patients had PS $\geq$2.

Once, the standard treatment for localized disease primarily consisted of radiotherapy alone that is, from 40–60 Gy delivered within 4–6 weeks. Radiotherapy achieved high levels of local control (80–100%) but was followed by a high late relapse rate (50%) [5]. Then different CMT schedules of chemotherapy and radiotherapy were proposed [7, 15, 16, 22, 23]. It has been shown that anthracycline-based therapy improves the response rate and prolongs OS of patients with localized lymphomas [23]. In combination with radiotherapy is superior to radiotherapy regarding RFS and OS. this is may be explained by less relapse in the combined treatment group [23]. Thus, the general PBL reputation of poor prognosis no longer seems justified compared to other extranodal lymphomas [2, 4, 9, 10, 24]. Notably, the OS of disseminated PBL, that is, PBL with multiple locations treated with CMT, was higher than for localized-stage disease in some studies [15, 16, 25].

Our results confirmed the efficacy of CMT. The 96% CR rate is excellent, and mean 5- and 10-year OS reached 79% $\pm$ 8 (22 patients) and 63% $\pm$ 12 (19 patients), respectively. The 5- and 10-RFS at 70% $\pm$ 9 and 64% $\pm$ 10, respectively, were similar for both GOELAMS trials. These outcomes are not worse than those for 325 localized aggressive NHL that were treated in another GOELAMS trial [26] and confirm data suggested by comparable—although generally not randomized—published studies [6, 7, 13, 15, 16, 23]. We did not observe any significant difference between the stages I and II or normal versus high LDH levels. However, some prognostic criteria for localized aggressive NHL do not apply to PBL [2]. In our study, modulation of the anthracycline-cyclophosphamide dose did not significantly influence survival parameters (response, relapses, death, OS, RFS, progression, or EFS) for either group.

We observed a 30% relapse rate. Among them, seven relapses concerned pelvic localization, including three patients with paraplegia. A higher relapse rate of axial localization was reported previously [14, 27], leading once to a poor OS [14]. Although local control appears to be good, we think that systemic treatment can be further improved. Because of the period of recruitment, the potential benefit of

TABLE 2: Univariate and multivariate analyses of characteristics affecting survival of adults with non-Hodgkin primary bone lymphoma.

Characteristics	Univariate analysis		Multivariate analysis
	mean $\pm$ SD	P	P
10-year OS, %			
Trial			
02	66 $\pm$ 13	ns	ns
03	64 $\pm$ 21		
Epidural extension			
No	75 $\pm$ 11	ns	ns
Yes	33 $\pm$ 25		
PS $\geq$2			
No	86 $\pm$ 10	0.046	ns
Yes	28 $\pm$ 21		
10-year EFS, %			
Trial			
02	59 $\pm$ 21	ns	ns
03	71 $\pm$ 14		
Epidural extension			
No	66 $\pm$ 11	ns	ns
Yes	50 $\pm$ 20		
PS $\geq$2			
No	79 $\pm$ 11	0.038	0.018
Yes	33 $\pm$ 17		

OS: overall survival; PS: performance status; EFS: event-free survival; ns: not significant.
Other studied factors (gender, stage, B symptoms, site, lactatedehydrogenase level, and bulky disease) do not have significantly statistical prognosis.

adding an anti-CD20 monoclonal antibody, which seemed to be advantageous against PBL in one study [28], could not be tested here. Increasing the number of chemotherapy cycles alternating regimen cycles is another option.

The high paraplegia rate (6 patients, 23%) observed in our population merits attention. Epidural localization with paraplegia was associated with shorter OS (33% $\pm$ 25) but not statistically significant (OS of patients without paraplegia 75% $\pm$ 11, $P = 0.18$). However, of the seven deaths recorded, three were of patients with paraplegia. Among the six patients with paraplegia, three relapsed and two of these three relapses occurred *in situ*. Only 25% of the patients without epidural involvement relapsed. The poor prognosis of epidural PBL was reported in several studies [13, 29] with only one exception [30].

In summary, our results confirmed the efficacy of CMT against localized PBL. The systemic arm of CMT remains insufficient, in light of the high late relapse rate. The two schedules, the conventional VCEP-b and the high dose VCAP chemotherapy, are different in terms of drug dosages and for the type of anthracycline and the absence of bleomycin. VCEP-bleomycin regimen is effective, tolerated for older patients and high-dose anthracycline-cyclophosphamide did not improve the outcome.

But because of the period of recruitment of our prospective study, the potential benefit of an anti-CD20 monoclonal

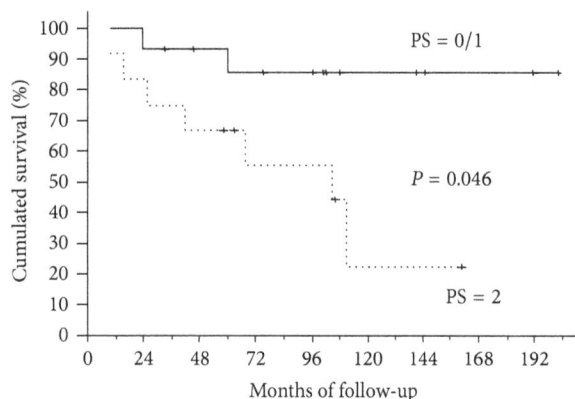

FIGURE 1: Overall survival curves of adults with non-Hodgkin primary bone lymphoma as a function of their performance status (PS).

antibody is not tested. However the majority of PBL histology is B phenotype. Since 10 years, in these situations, the standard of chemotherapy included an anti-CD20 monoclonal antibody. The management of limited stage I-II PBL probably consists of 3 to 4 cycles of chemotherapy adding an anti-CD20 monoclonal antibody. More chemotherapy cycles should be considered for the patients with a high IPI score, even if the impact of IPI score is not yet validated in PBL. Radiotherapy is valid for local control and intensification remains discussed in the localized stages. But the staging must be precise. The staging procedure should now include positron emission tomography (PET) to see the entire skeleton, what it is not the case of our study. Furthermore, for bone lymphoma, the assessment of CR with CT scan is one major problem, the use of the PET allowed to solve.

On the other hand, epidural disease and PS ≥2 are factors of poor prognosis. New therapeutic strategies should be considered for these patients: addition of anti-CD20 monoclonal antibody, more chemotherapy cycles, and/or their alternation and intensification.

5. Clinical Practice Point

(1) Treatment guidelines do not exist in PBL, because it is a rare entity and thus randomized prospective clinical trials are lacking. Nevertheless, combined chemotherapy and radiotherapy strategies have improved the management of PBL in particular in cases of advanced disease.

(2) In this study, we review the clinical outcome of 26 patients with previously untreated PBL, all receiving anthracycline-cyclophosphamide containing regimen and consolidative radiation therapy. With median follow-up of 8 years, overall survival, event-free survival, and relapse-free survival were, respectively, 64%, 62%, and 65%. Poor PS was associated with shorter OS and EFS. High dose anthracycline-cyclophosphamide did not improve outcome.

(3) In our opinion, combined chemotherapy and radiotherapy, nowadays probably in association with monoclonal anti-CD20 infusion, are efficace treatment for PBL. Intensified treatment must be considered for patients with PS ≥2. Moreover, new staging procedure including positron emission tomography should be now included.

Conflict of Interests

The authors declare that there is no conflict of interests regarding the publication of this paper.

References

[1] F. H. Heyning, P. C. W. Hogendoorn, M. H. H. Kramer et al., "Primary non-Hodgkin's lymphoma of bone: a clinicopathological investigation of 60 cases," *Leukemia*, vol. 13, no. 12, pp. 2094–2098, 1999.

[2] J. M. Horsman, J. Thomas, R. Hough, and B. W. Hancock, "Primary bone lymphoma: a retrospective analysis," *International Journal of Oncology*, vol. 28, no. 6, pp. 1571–1575, 2006.

[3] E. Misgeld, A. Wehmeier, O. Krömeke, and N. Gattermann, "Primary non-Hodgkin's lymphoma of bone: three cases and a short review of the literature," *Annals of Hematology*, vol. 82, no. 7, pp. 440–443, 2003.

[4] N. G. Mikhaeel, "Primary Bone Lymphoma," *Clinical Oncology*, vol. 24, no. 5, pp. 366–370, 2012.

[5] D. E. Dosoretz, G. F. Murphy, and A. K. Raymond, "Radiation therapy for primary lymphoma of bone," *Cancer*, vol. 51, no. 1, pp. 44–46, 1983.

[6] K. Beal, L. Allen, and J. Yahalom, "Primary bone lymphoma: treatment results and prognostic factors with long-term follow-up of 82 patients," *Cancer*, vol. 106, no. 12, pp. 2652–2656, 2006.

[7] P. L. Zinzani, G. Carrillo, S. Ascani et al., "Primary bone lymphoma: experience with 52 patients," *Haematologica*, vol. 88, no. 3, pp. 280–285, 2003.

[8] C. Brousse, E. Baumelou, and P. Morel, "Primary lymphoma of bone: a prospective study of 28 cases," *Joint Bone Spine*, vol. 67, no. 5, pp. 446–451, 2000.

[9] A. Alencar, D. Pitcher, G. Byrne Jr., and I. S. Lossos, "Primary bone lymphoma the university of miami experience," *Leukemia and Lymphoma*, vol. 51, no. 1, pp. 39–49, 2010.

[10] C. Pellegrini, L. Gandolfi, F. Quirini et al., "Primary bone lymphoma: evaluation of chemoimmunotherapy as front-line treatment in 21 patients," *Clinical Lymphoma, Myeloma and Leukemia*, vol. 11, no. 4, pp. 321–325, 2011.

[11] S. A. Rosenerg, C. W. Berand, and B. W. Brown Jr., "National Cancer Institute sponsored study of classifications of non-Hodgkin's lymphomas. Summary and description of a working formulation for clinical usage," *Cancer*, vol. 49, no. 10, pp. 2112–2135, 1982.

[12] P. Kitsoulis, M. Vlychou, A. Papoudou-Bai et al., "Primary lymphomas of bone," *Anticancer Research*, vol. 26, no. 1 A, pp. 325–337, 2006.

[13] A. J. Rathmell, M. K. Gospodarowicz, S. B. Sutcliffe, and R. M. Clark, "Localised lymphoma of bone: prognostic factors and treatment recommendations," *British Journal of Cancer*, vol. 66, no. 3, pp. 603–606, 1992.

[14] O. P. de Camargo, T. M. dos Santos Machado, A. T. Croci et al., "Primary bone lymphoma in 24 patients treated between 1955 and 1999," *Clinical Orthopaedics and Related Research*, no. 397, pp. 271–280, 2002.

[15] R. K. Fairbanks, J. A. Bonner, C. Y. Inwards et al., "Treatment of stage IE primary lymphoma of bone," *International Journal of Radiation Oncology Biology Physics*, vol. 28, no. 2, pp. 363–372, 1994.

[16] P. Fidias, I. Spiro, M. L. Sobczak et al., "Long-term results of combined modality therapy in primary bone lymphomas," *International Journal of Radiation Oncology Biology Physics*, vol. 45, no. 5, pp. 1213–1218, 1999.

[17] D. Maruyama, T. Watanabe, Y. Beppu et al., "Primary bone lymphoma: a new and detailed characterization of 28 patients in a single-institution study," *Japanese Journal of Clinical Oncology*, vol. 37, no. 3, pp. 216–223, 2007.

[18] M. E. Stein, A. Kuten, E. Gez et al., "Primary lymphoma of bone: a retrospective study. Experience at the Northern Israel Oncology Center (1979–2000)," *Oncology*, vol. 64, no. 4, pp. 322–327, 2003.

[19] M. E. Juweid, S. Stroobants, O. S. Hoekstra et al., "Use of positron emission tomography for response assessment of lymphoma: consensus of the imaging subcommittee of international harmonization project in lymphoma," *Journal of Clinical Oncology*, vol. 25, no. 5, pp. 571–578, 2007.

[20] C. Charousset, A. Anract, B. Carlioz et al., "Les lymphomes osseux primitifs. Etude rétrospective sur 22 cas avec étude immuno-histochimique récente et homogène," *Revue de Chirurgie Orthopédique*, vol. 88, pp. 439–448, 2002.

[21] E. Barbieri, S. Cammelli, F. Mauro et al., "Primary non-Hodgkin's lymphoma of the bone: treatment and analysis of prognostic factors for Stage I and Stage II," *International Journal of Radiation Oncology Biology Physics*, vol. 59, no. 3, pp. 760–764, 2004.

[22] O. C. G. Baiocchi, G. W. B. Colleoni, C. A. Rodrigues et al., "Importance of combined-modality therapy for primary bone lymphoma [3]," *Leukemia and Lymphoma*, vol. 44, no. 10, pp. 1837–1839, 2003.

[23] D. R. Ford, D. Wilson, S. Sothi, R. Grimer, and D. Spooner, "Primary bone lymphoma: treatment and outcome," *Clinical Oncology*, vol. 19, no. 1, pp. 50–55, 2007.

[24] S. J. Horning, E. Weller, K. Kim et al., "Chemotherapy with or without radiotherapy in limited-stage diffuse aggressive non-Hodgkin's lymphoma: eastern Cooperative Oncology Group Study 1484," *Journal of Clinical Oncology*, vol. 22, no. 15, pp. 3032–3038, 2004.

[25] P. Gill, D. E. Wenger, and D. J. Inwards, "Primary lymphomas of bone," *Clinical Lymphoma and Myeloma*, vol. 6, no. 2, pp. 140–142, 2005.

[26] M. Bernard, G. Cartron, P. Rachieru et al., "Long-term outcome of localized high-grade non-Hodgkin's lymphoma treated with high dose CHOP regimen and involved field radiotherapy: results of a GOELAMS study," *Haematologica*, vol. 90, no. 6, pp. 802–809, 2005.

[27] M. L. Ostrwoski, K. K. Unni, and P. M. Banks, "Malignant lymphoma of bone," *Cancer*, vol. 58, no. 12, pp. 2646–2655, 1986.

[28] K. M. Ramadan, T. Shenkier, L. H. Sehn, R. D. Gascoyne, and J. M. Connors, "A clinicopathological retrospective study of 131 patients with primary bone lymphoma: a population-based study of successively treated cohorts from the British Columbia Cancer Agency," *Annals of Oncology*, vol. 18, no. 1, pp. 129–135, 2007.

[29] M. Salvati, L. Cervoni, M. Artico, A. Raco, P. Ciappetta, and R. Delfini, "Primary spinal epidural non-Hodgkin's lymphomas: a clinical study," *Surgical Neurology*, vol. 46, no. 4, pp. 339–344, 1996.

[30] V. Monnard, A. Sun, R. Epelbaum et al., "Primary spinal epidural lymphoma: patients' profile, outcome, and prognostic factors: a multicenter Rare Cancer Network study," *International Journal of Radiation Oncology Biology Physics*, vol. 65, no. 3, pp. 817–823, 2006.

28

Predictors of Outcome and Severity in Adult Filipino Patients with Febrile Neutropenia

Marc Gregory Y. Yu, Ralph Elvi M. Villalobos, Ma. Jasmin Marinela C. Juan-Bartolome, and Regina P. Berba

Department of Medicine, Philippine General Hospital, Taft Avenue, Ermita, 1000 Manila, Philippines

Correspondence should be addressed to Marc Gregory Y. Yu; marcgreggy@yahoo.com

Academic Editor: Helen A. Papadaki

Aim. The study aimed to describe the profile of Filipino febrile neutropenia patients and to determine parameters associated with severe outcomes. *Methods.* This is a retrospective study of Filipino febrile neutropenia patients admitted to the Philippine General Hospital. Patients were described in terms of clinical presentation and stratified according to the presence or absence of severe outcomes. Prognostic factors were then identified using regression analysis. *Results.* 115 febrile episodes in 102 patients were identified. Regression analysis yielded prolonged fever >7 days prior to admission (OR 2.43; 95% CI, 0.77–7.74), isolation of a pathogen on cultures (OR 2.69; 95% CI, 1.04–6.98), and nadir absolute neutrophil count (ANC) < 100 during admission (OR 1.96; 95% CI, 0.75–5.12) as significant predictors of poor outcome. Factors that significantly correlated with better outcome were granulocyte colony-stimulating factor (G-CSF) use (OR 0.31; 95% CI, 0.11–0.85) and completeness of antibiotic therapy (OR 0.26; 95% CI, 0.10–0.67). *Conclusion.* Prolonged fever >7 days prior to admission, positive pathogen on cultures, and nadir ANC < 100 during admission predicted severe outcomes, whereas G-CSF use and complete antibiotic therapy were associated with better outcomes. These prognostic variables might be useful in identifying patients that need more intensive treatment and monitoring.

1. Introduction

Febrile neutropenia refers to the presentation of fever in a neutropenic patient, commonly with an uncontrolled neoplasm of the bone marrow, or in a patient undergoing cytotoxic treatment [1]. Around 50% of patients with solid tumors and 80% of those with hematologic malignancies will develop concomitant fever and neutropenia [2]; despite advances in diagnostics and therapy, these patients still face a mortality rate of 5–21.5% [3–5]. This is partly explained by the fact that neutropenic patients who develop fever have a 60% chance of being infected. Infections arise from defects caused by the underlying disease, those induced by cytotoxic drugs, and those associated with invasive procedures [6, 7]. With newer, more potent agents and dose-dense chemotherapy schedules, patients are faced with more severe and prolonged degrees of neutropenia leading to more complications and higher healthcare costs [8].

Gram negative organisms traditionally predominated as the most common causative pathogens in patients with febrile

neutropenia [9, 10], although there is a rising incidence of Gram positive organisms among Western patients [11, 12]. In the Philippines, a retrospective study showed Gram negative bacilli (51.5%) as the most frequently isolated pathogen [3]; in another study involving pediatric patients with malignancy and febrile neutropenia, the most common organisms were *Streptococcus viridans*, Gram negative bacilli, *Staphylococcus epidermidis*, *Candida* sp., and *Salmonella* sp. [13].

The standard management of patients with febrile neutropenia includes cultures, hospitalization and close observation, and intravenous broad-spectrum antibiotics [14]. However, these patients comprise a heterogeneous group and possess different risks of developing severe infections and complications [15]. Models such as those developed by Talcott et al. [16] and the Multinational Association of Supportive Care in Cancer (MASCC) attempted to aid practitioners in classifying patients into low- and high-risk groups [17–19]. Using these models, poor prognostic variables identified in Western studies included a MASCC score <21, an Eastern Cooperative Oncology Group (ECOG) performance status score ≥2, chronic bronchitis and heart failure, a monocyte count <200 mm³, and stress hyperglycemia, among others [20]. In Korea, prognostic indicators included hypotension, previous and invasive fungal infection, recovery from neutropenia, median days to fever, pneumonia, and total febrile days [21, 22].

There is presently no such study in the Philippines. Being a third-world country with limited health resources, the study aims to provide Filipino data on prognostic factors associated with adverse outcomes and mortality and thereby recognize patients that need more intensive treatment and monitoring.

2. Materials and Methods

This retrospective study involved adult febrile neutropenia patients, regardless of cause, admitted to the Philippine General Hospital from January 2010 to October 2014. The inclusion criteria consisted of patients >19 years old with a suspected or documented risk factor for febrile neutropenia (hematologic malignancy, bone marrow failure state, or solid-organ tumor after myelosuppressive chemotherapy) who developed fever coexistent with or during the neutropenic episode; patients with existing severe infection prior to the onset of neutropenia were excluded. Patients were stratified into the "complicated group" if they developed severe outcomes, defined by any of the following: hypotension (systolic blood pressure < 90 mmHg and/or diastolic blood pressure < 60 mmHg), respiratory failure (arterial oxygen pressure < 60 mmHg on room air or need for mechanical ventilation), congestive heart failure, uncontrolled arrhythmia, hepatic or renal failure requiring treatment, severe bleeding requiring transfusion, altered sensorium, intensive care unit admission, and death; and they were stratified into the "noncomplicated group" if they did not manifest any severe outcome. Patients who left prior to recommended discharge were assumed to have developed severe outcomes and were categorized under the complicated group.

Clinical, laboratory, and microbiologic data were expressed as frequencies and percentages. Stepwise logistic regression with backward selection strategy was employed on specific variables; the significance of the main effects of the different independent variables on severe outcomes was determined by univariate analysis to establish the strength of association of each independent variable and outcome variable. Univariate test of any variable resulting in a p value ≤ 0.25 was considered a candidate for the multivariable model. Since some of the variables did not reach significance level p value ≤ 0.25 in the univariate analysis, a model that included significant variables was constructed. The variables included in the model were then subjected to multivariate analysis.

3. Results

3.1. Patient Characteristics. 115 febrile episodes in 102 neutropenic patients were documented. Of these, 58 patients (50.4%) were classified under the complicated group and 57 (49.6%) fell under the noncomplicated group. There was no significant difference in the mean age and sex ratio of the patients between both groups. The overall mortality rate was 19.1%.

Almost half of the sample population had leukemia ($n = 56$, 48.7%) as the primary underlying disease, followed by solid-organ tumors ($n = 27$, 23.45%). In addition, 21 patients (18.26%) did not have a primary hematologic disorder or malignancy as the underlying disease; these included systemic lupus erythematosus (SLE), liver cirrhosis, HIV/AIDS, and drug-induced agranulocytosis. Majority of patients ($n = 84$, 73.04%) had no comorbidities. In those with comorbidities, cardiovascular disease ($n = 21$, 18.26%) had the highest frequency.

More patients in the complicated group did not receive treatment and/or had relapse of their underlying disease ($n = 26$, 44.83%). This nontreatment or relapse status significantly correlated with poor outcomes in the univariate analysis (OR 2.28; 95% CI, 1.04–4.98; $p = 0.040$). Similarly, prolonged duration of fever >7 days prior to admission ($n = 16$, 27.6%), nonrecovery from neutropenia ($n = 41$, 70.7%), and prolonged duration of neutropenia >7 days during admission ($n = 31$, 53.4%) were also seen more in the complicated group. However, only the last two variables (OR 2.17; 95% CI, 1.01–4.68; $p = 0.048$; OR 3.24; 95% CI, 1.16–9.01; $p = 0.024$, resp.) were significantly associated with poor outcomes in the univariate analysis. In contrast, more patients in the noncomplicated group received G-CSF ($n = 23$, 40.3%) but this did not reach statistical significance in the univariate analysis. The baseline characteristics of the study patients are summarized in Table 1 while the results of the univariate analysis for clinical variables are shown in Table 4.

3.2. Laboratory Characteristics. More subjects in the complicated group were observed to have ANC counts <100 on admission ($n = 19$, 32.8%) as well as nadir ANC counts <100 during the entire admission ($n = 36$, 62.1%). Likewise, more patients in this group had hemoglobin levels ≤ 80 g/L, platelet counts ≤ 50,000/μL, peak BUN >20 mg/dL, peak creatinine >177 μmol/L, nadir bicarbonate ≤ 21 mmol/L, nadir albumin ≤ 30 g/L, and peak AST and ALT levels > 40 IU/L. Among these factors, however, only severe thrombocytopenia showed significant prognostic correlation with poor outcomes in the univariate analysis (OR 3.45; 95% CI, 1.52–7.84; $p = 0.003$). The laboratory parameters of the study patients are summarized in Table 2 while the results of the univariate analysis are included in Table 4.

3.3. Microbiologic Characteristics. Of the 115 febrile episodes included in the study, 79 (68.7%) were clinically defined infections (CDI), 32 (27.83%) were microbiologically defined infections (MDI), and four (3.48%) had fever of unknown origin (FUO). A greater number of patients in the complicated group had MDI ($n = 20$, 34.5%). The most common site of infection was the respiratory tract ($n = 58$, 50.43%) in both groups, followed by the genitourinary tract ($n = 13$, 22.4%) in the complicated group and the oral cavity ($n = 15$, 26.3%) in the noncomplicated group. The overall bacteremia

TABLE 1: Baseline clinical characteristics of febrile neutropenia cases.

Clinical parameter	Outcome frequency (%)	
	Complicated group $n = 58$ (50.4)	Noncomplicated group $n = 57$ (49.6)
Age		
Mean (SD)	41.24 (15.99)	40 (11.89)
Median	40.5	42
Range	19–71	19–61
Sex		
Male	23 (39.7)	24 (42.1)
Female	35 (60.3)	33 (57.9)
Primary underlying disease		
Leukemia	29 (50)	27 (47.4)
Lymphoma (all sites)	1 (1.7)	1 (1.8)
Solid-organ tumor	9 (15.5)	18 (31.6)
Bone marrow failure state	6 (10.3)	3 (5.2)
Others	13 (22.4)	8 (14.0)
Comorbid		
None	41 (70.7)	43 (7.5)
Cardiovascular disease	8 (13.8)	13 (22.8)
Pulmonary disease	1 (1.7)	0
Liver disease	0	1 (1.8)
Renal disease	3 (5.2)	0
Diabetes mellitus	2 (3.4)	0
Others	3 (5.2)	0
Outcome		
Discharged improved	32 (60.3)	57 (100.0)
Expired	22 (37.9)	0
Left against advice	4 (6.9)	0
Status of treatment		
Treated/on treatment	32 (55.2)	40 (70.2)
Remission	0	2 (3.5)
Relapse	3 (5.2)	3 (5.3)
Not on treatment	23 (39.7)	12 (21)
Type of treatment		
Chemotherapy	26 (44.8)	28 (49.1)
Combination therapy	6 (10.3)	17 (29.8)
None	26 (44.8)	12 (21.1)
G-CSF use		
Yes	16 (27.6)	23 (40.3)
No	42 (72.4)	34 (59.7)
Duration of fever prior to admission		
≤7 days	42 (72.4)	51 (89.5)
>7 days	16 (27.6)	6 (10.5)
Duration of neutropenia during admission		
≤7 days	27 (46.6)	35 (61.4)
>7 days	31 (53.4)	22 (39.6)
Recovery from neutropenia		
Yes	17 (29.3)	27 (47.4)
No	41 (70.7)	30 (52.6)

TABLE 2: Laboratory parameters of febrile neutropenia cases.

Laboratory parameter	Outcome frequency (%)	
	Complicated group	Noncomplicated group
ANC on admission (mm^{-3})		
≤100	19 (32.8)	13 (22.8)
>100	39 (67.2)	44 (77.2)
Nadir ANC during admission (mm^{-3})		
≤100	36 (62.1)	26 (45.6)
>100	22 (37.9)	31 (54.4)
Nadir hemoglobin (g/L)		
>80	18 (31)	23 (40.4)
≤80	40 (69)	34 (59.6)
Nadir platelet count (μL^{-3})		
≤50,000	46 (79.3)	30 (52.6)
>50,000	12 (20.7)	27 (47.4)
Peak serum BUN (mg/dL)		
>20	3 (5.2)	0
≤20	35 (60.3)	29 (50.9)
No data	20 (34.5)	28 (49.1)
Peak serum creatinine (μmol/L)		
>177	9 (15.5)	2 (3.5)
≤177	45 (81.8)	47 (82.5)
No data	4 (6.9)	8 (14)
Nadir serum bicarbonate (mmol/L)		
≤21	15 (25.9)	0
>21	5 (8.6)	5 (8.8)
No data	38 (65.5)	52 (91.2)
Nadir serum albumin (g/L)		
≤30	33 (56.9)	20 (35.1)
>30	10 (17.2)	6 (10.5)
No data	15 (25.9)	31 (54.4)
Peak serum AST (IU/L)		
>40	21 (36.2)	17 (29.8)
≤40	17 (29.3)	17 (29.8)
No data	20 (34.5)	23 (40.4)
Peak serum ALT (IU/L)		
>40	22 (37.9)	18 (31.6)
≤40	18 (31)	16 (28.1)
No data	18 (31)	23 (40.3)

rate was 13.04%, but this did not show statistical significance in the univariate analysis.

Pseudomonas aeruginosa ($n = 9$, 7.83%) was the most commonly isolated organism, followed by *Escherichia coli* ($n = 7$, 6.09%). As a whole, Gram negative bacteria comprised the predominant isolate in the complicated group. Isolation of a pathogen in cultures, however, was not significantly associated with poor outcomes in the univariate analysis. In contrast, complete antibiotic therapy significantly predicted

TABLE 3: Microbiologic profiles of febrile neutropenia cases.

Microbiologic parameter	Outcome frequency (%)	
	Complicated group	Noncomplicated group
Infection type		
MDI	20 (34.5)	12 (21.1)
CDI	36 (62.1)	43 (75.4)
FUO	2 (3.4)	2 (3.5)
Site of infection		
Oral cavity	2 (3.4)	15 (26.3)
Respiratory tract	33 (56.9)	25 (43.9)
GI tract/intra-abdominal	4 (6.9)	2 (3.5)
Genitourinary tract	13 (22.4)	6 (10.5)
Skin and soft tissue	4 (6.9)	6 (10.5)
Unknown	1 (1.7)	0
Others	1 (1.7)	3 (5.6)
Bacteremia		
Yes	7 (12.1)	8 (14)
No	51 (87.9)	49 (86)
Isolated organism		
Gram positive bacteria, non-MDRO	3 (12)	0
Gram positive bacteria, MDRO	3 (12)	1 (6.7)
Gram negative bacteria, non-MDRO	8 (32)	4 (26.7)
Gram negative bacteria, MDRO	7 (28)	4 (26.7)
Fungus	4 (16)	4 (26.7)
TB	0	2 (13.3)
Antibiotic use		
Complete	21 (36.2)	39 (68.4)
Incomplete	37 (64.8)	18 (31.2)

*MDRO: multi-drug-resistant organism.

TABLE 4: Prognostic factors related to severe outcomes based on univariate analysis.

Variable	OR (95% CI)	p value
Age	1.00 (0.98–1.03)	0.635
Sex		
Male		
Female	1.11 (0.53–2.33)	0.789
Primary underlying disease		
Hematologic disease	1.37 (0.65–2.87)	0.405
Others		
Status of treatment		
Treated		
Not treated	2.28 (1.04–4.98)	0.040
G-CSF use		
Yes	0.56 (0.26–1.23)	0.150
No		
Comorbid		
Yes	1.27 (0.56–2.91)	0.566
No		
Duration of fever prior to admission		
≤7 days		
>7 days	3.24 (1.16–9.01)	0.024
ANC on admission (mm^{-3})		
≤100	1.65 (0.72–3.77)	0.236
>100		
Nadir ANC during admission (mm^{-3})		
≤100	1.95 (0.93–4.10)	0.078
>100		
Duration of neutropenia during admission		
≤7 days		
>7 days	1.83 (0.87–3.84)	0.112
Recovery from neutropenia		
Yes		
No	2.17 (1.01–4.68)	0.048
Nadir hemoglobin (g/L)		
≤80	1.50 (0.70–3.24)	0.298
>80		
Nadir platelet count (μL^{-3})		
≤50,000	3.45 (1.52–7.84)	0.003
>50,000		
Peak serum creatinine (μmol/L)		
≤177		
>177	4.70 (0.96–22.95)	0.056
Bacteremia		
Yes	0.84 (0.28–2.49)	0.754
No		
Isolated organism		
Unknown		
Known	2.12 (0.97–4.65)	0.061
Antibiotic use		
Complete	0.26 (0.12–0.57)	0.001
Incomplete		

better outcomes in the univariate analysis (OR 0.26; 95% CI, 0.12–0.57; $p = 0.001$) with Piperacillin-Tazobactam being the most commonly administered antibiotic ($n = 57$, 49.57%).

The microbiologic profiles of the study patients are summarized in Table 3 while the results of the univariate analysis are displayed in Table 4.

3.4. Multivariate Analysis. Significant variables in the univariate analysis resulting in a p value ≤ 0.25 were considered candidates for the multivariable model. Since some variables did not reach significance level p value ≤ 0.25 in the univariate analysis, a model that included significant variables was constructed. Results of the multivariate analysis showed prolonged fever >7 days prior to admission (OR 2.43; 95% CI, 0.77–7.74) being associated with a significant risk for poorer outcomes. In the same manner, isolation of a known pathogen on cultures (OR 2.69; 95% CI, 1.04–6.98) and profound ANC < 100 during admission (OR 1.96; 95% CI, 0.75–5.12) were

TABLE 5: Prognostic factors related to severe outcomes based on multivariate analysis.

Variable	OR (95% CI)	Standard error
G-CSF use		
Yes	0.31 (0.11–0.85)	0.16
No		
Duration of fever prior to admission		
≤7 days		
>7 days	2.44 (0.77–7.74)	1.44
Nadir ANC during admission (mm^{-3})		
≤100	1.96 (0.75–5.11)	0.96
>100		
Isolated organism		
Unknown		
Known	2.69 (1.04–6.98)	1.31
Antibiotic use		
Complete	0.26 (0.11–0.67)	0.12
Incomplete		

also found to be significant predictors of poor outcome. The factors that significantly correlated with better outcome, on the other hand, were G-CSF use (OR 0.31; 95% CI, 0.11–0.85) and completeness of antibiotic therapy (OR 0.26; 95% CI, 0.10–0.67). The results of the multivariate analysis are shown in Table 5.

4. Discussion

This is the first Philippine study dealing with prognostic variables in patients with febrile neutropenia. Our results generally show that febrile neutropenia confers a significant morbidity and mortality rate: 58 patients (50.4%) developed severe outcomes, with 22 (19.1%) of these eventually succumbing. This is consistent with the 5–21.5% mortality rate documented in the literature [3–5]. Leukemia was found to be the most common primary underlying disease, also consistent with the findings of earlier studies [3]. The nature of hematologic malignancies, plus the intensity of myelosuppressive treatment, predisposes these patients to a more rapid development of neutropenia and consequent infection, as compared to patients with solid tumors [19, 22].

Of the different clinical variables examined, prolonged fever >7 days prior to admission and G-CSF use both showed prognostic importance in the multivariate analysis. In contrast, our results did not consider the presence of comorbidities as significant indicators, as opposed to other studies [20–22]. This can be explained by the relatively small number of study patients with comorbid diseases. In terms of laboratory findings, multivariate analysis yielded a nadir ANC < 100 during admission as an indicator of adverse outcome. Since neutropenia is the main defect in host defense after chemotherapy, variables associated with neutropenia are closely related to infection susceptibility and are therefore likely to affect

prognosis [21]. However, many of the study patients had incomplete workup (lacking, e.g., albumin, bicarbonate, and liver enzyme levels) and no data on levels of promising prognostic markers (procalcitonin, erythrocyte sedimentation rate, and C-reactive protein) [23, 24], thereby precluding the use of these variables for logistic regression analysis.

The predominance of the respiratory tract as the most common site of infection among study patients, as well as the isolation of *Pseudomonas* and *E. coli* as the most frequently implicated organisms, conformed with the results of previous studies [3, 21, 22]. In particular, the predominance of Gram negative bacteria in the complicated group affirms the reemergence of these pathogens as a result of more intensive chemotherapy regimens and the decreased use of quinolone prophylaxis [25].

A unique microbiologic profile observed in the study was the presence of tuberculosis in two cases, which was not observed in the literature. This can be explained by the unusually high prevalence of the disease in the country. Furthermore, no viral infection was documented in the study. As the main defect in host immunity after chemotherapy is in the innate rather than adaptive immunity, viral infections following chemotherapy do not seem to be common. The rarity of fungal infections, too, can be explained by the difficulty in confirming fungal infections as the condition of febrile neutropenic patients seldom permits invasive diagnostic procedures [21].

The study was limited by a small sample size and involvement of only one tertiary medical center and hence may have led to underestimation or overestimation of projections. It was also conducted in a resource-limited setting and was thereby constrained by the unavailability of full workup and ideal treatment in many patients, precluding these from further analyses. Finally, the data might not have been completely independent because several febrile episodes were assessed in the same patients. Thus, the presence of confounding factors, despite the use of an appropriate statistical model, cannot be fully excluded in multivariate analysis. This is a common difficulty encountered in retrospective studies [22].

5. Conclusion and Recommendations

Adult Filipino febrile neutropenia patients with prolonged fever >7 days prior to admission, known pathogen on cultures, and nadir ANC < 100 during admission were at significant risk of developing worse outcomes, whereas those with G-CSF use and complete antibiotic therapy were significantly associated with better outcomes. These variables might help identify patients with an increased risk of developing complications, thereby needing more intensive treatment and monitoring. The completeness of antibiotic therapy cannot be overemphasized and could lead to improved drug procurement policies for indigent patients. We recommend, however, bigger studies to further validate and strengthen our study findings.

Conflict of Interests

There was no conflict of interests.

References

[1] E. Braunwald, A. S. Fauci, D. L. Kasper et al., *Harrison's Principles of Internal Medicine*, McGraw-Hill, 18th edition, 2008.

[2] J. Crawford, D. C. Dale, and G. H. Lyman, "Chemotherapy-induced neutropenia," *Cancer*, vol. 100, no. 2, pp. 228–237, 2004.

[3] K. Billote, M. Mendoza, and H. Baylon, "Infections in febrile neutropenia and possible prognostic factors associated with mortality," *Philippine Journal of Microbiology and Infectious Diseases*, vol. 26, no. 2, pp. 55–59, 1997.

[4] N. M. Kuderer, D. C. Dale, J. Crawford, L. E. Cosler, and G. H. Lyman, "Mortality, morbidity, and cost associated with febrile neutropenia in adult cancer patients," *Cancer*, vol. 106, no. 10, pp. 2258–2266, 2006.

[5] G. H. Lyman, S. L. Michels, M. W. Reynolds, R. Barron, K. S. Tomic, and J. Yu, "Risk of mortality in patients with cancer who experience febrile neutropenia," *Cancer*, vol. 116, no. 23, pp. 5555–5563, 2010.

[6] H. Giamarellou, "Empiric therapy for infections in the febrile, neutropenic, compromised host," *Medical Clinics of North America*, vol. 79, no. 3, pp. 559–580, 1995.

[7] A. E. Brown, "Neutropenia, fever, and infection," *The American Journal of Medicine*, vol. 76, no. 3, pp. 421–428, 1984.

[8] N. Lathia, N. Mittmann, C. DeAngelis et al., "Evaluation of direct medical costs of hospitalization for febrile neutropenia," *Cancer*, vol. 116, no. 3, pp. 742–748, 2010.

[9] N. Hiransuthikul, T. Tantawichien, P. Suwangool, and T. Nuchprayoon, "Febrile neutropenia in Chulalongkorn Hospital during 1994-1995," *Chulalongkorn Medical Journal*, vol. 40, pp. 781–799, 1996.

[10] N. Voravud and V. Sriuranpong, "Febrile neutropenia after chemotherapy in patients with non-hematologic malignancies," *Chulalongkorn Medical Journal*, vol. 47, pp. 151–161, 2003.

[11] R. Feld, "Bloodstream infections in cancer patients with febrile neutropenia," *International Journal of Antimicrobial Agents*, vol. 32, supplement 1, pp. S30–S33, 2008.

[12] H. Wisplinghoff, H. Seifert, R. P. Wenzel, and M. B. Edmond, "Current trends in the epidemiology of nosocomial bloodstream infections in patients with hematological malignancies and solid neoplasms in hospitals in the United States," *Clinical Infectious Diseases*, vol. 36, no. 9, pp. 1103–1110, 2003.

[13] A. Isais-Agdeppa and L. Bravo, "A five-year retrospective study on the common microbial isolates and sensitivity pattern on blood culture of pediatric cancer patients admitted at the Philippine General Hospital for febrile neutropenia," *Philippine Journal of Microbiology and Infectious Diseases*, vol. 9, no. 2, 2005.

[14] A. G. Freifeld, E. J. Bow, K. A. Sepkowitz et al., "Clinical practice guideline for the use of antimicrobial agents in neutropenic patients with cancer: 2010 update by the infectious diseases society of America," *Clinical Infectious Diseases*, vol. 52, no. 4, pp. e56–e93, 2011.

[15] M. Paesmans, "Risk factors assessment in fabrile neutropenia," *International Journal of Antimicrobial Agents*, vol. 16, no. 2, pp. 107–111, 2000.

[16] J. A. Talcott, R. D. Siegel, R. Finberg, and L. Goldman, "Risk assessment in cancer patients with fever and neutropenia: a prospective, two-center validation of a prediction rule," *Journal of Clinical Oncology*, vol. 10, no. 2, pp. 316–322, 1992.

[17] J. Klastersky, M. Paesmans, E. B. Rubenstein et al., "The multinational association for supportive care in cancer risk index: a multinational scoring system for identifying low-risk febrile neutropenic cancer patients," *Journal of Clinical Oncology*, vol. 18, no. 16, pp. 3038–3051, 2000.

[18] A. Uys, B. L. Rapoport, and R. Anderson, "Febrile neutropenia: a prospective study to validate the Multinational Association of Supportive Care of Cancer (MASCC) risk-index score," *Supportive Care in Cancer*, vol. 12, no. 8, pp. 555–560, 2004.

[19] S. Ahn, Y.-S. Lee, Y.-H. Chun et al., "Predictive factors of poor prognosis in cancer patients with chemotherapy-induced febrile neutropenia," *Supportive Care in Cancer*, vol. 19, no. 8, pp. 1151–1158, 2011.

[20] A. Carmona-Bayonas, J. Gómez, E. González-Billalabeitia et al., "Prognostic evaluation of febrile neutropenia in apparently stable adult cancer patients," *British Journal of Cancer*, vol. 105, no. 5, pp. 612–617, 2011.

[21] J.-H. Yoo, S. M. Choi, D.-G. Lee et al., "Prognostic factors influencing infection-related mortality in patients with acute leukemia in Korea," *Journal of Korean Medical Science*, vol. 20, no. 1, pp. 31–35, 2005.

[22] Y. Park, D. S. Kim, S. J. Park et al., "The suggestion of a risk stratification system for febrile neutropenia in patients with hematologic disease," *Leukemia Research*, vol. 34, no. 3, pp. 294–300, 2010.

[23] L. Persson, P. Engervall, A. Magnuson et al., "Use of inflammatory markers for early detection of bacteraemia in patients with febrile neutropenia," *Scandinavian Journal of Infectious Diseases*, vol. 36, no. 5, pp. 365–371, 2004.

[24] M. Ortega, M. Rovira, M. Almela, J. P. de la Bellacasa, E. Carreras, and J. Mensa, "Measurement of C-reactive protein in adults with febrile neutropenia after hematopoietic cell transplantation," *Bone Marrow Transplantation*, vol. 33, no. 7, pp. 741–744, 2004.

[25] S. Gençer, T. Salepçi, and S. Özer, "Evaluation of infectious etiology and prognostic risk factors of febrile episodes in neutropenic cancer patients," *Journal of Infection*, vol. 47, no. 1, pp. 65–72, 2003.

29

Real-World Assessment of Clinical Outcomes in Patients with Lower-Risk Myelofibrosis Receiving Treatment with Ruxolitinib

Keith L. Davis,[1] **Isabelle Côté,**[2] **James A. Kaye,**[3] **Estella Mendelson,**[2] **Haitao Gao,**[2] **and Julian Perez Ronco**[4]

[1]*RTI Health Solutions, Research Triangle Park, NC 27709, USA*
[2]*Novartis Pharmaceuticals Corporation, East Hanover, NJ 07936, USA*
[3]*RTI Health Solutions, Waltham, MA 02451, USA*
[4]*Novartis Pharma AG, 4056 Basel, Switzerland*

Correspondence should be addressed to Keith L. Davis; kldavis@rti.org

Academic Editor: Elvira Grandone

Few trial-based assessments of ruxolitinib in patients with lower-risk myelofibrosis (MF) have been conducted, and no studies have made such assessments in a real-world population. We assessed changes in spleen size and constitutional symptoms during ruxolitinib treatment using a retrospective, observational review of anonymized US medical record data of patients diagnosed with IPSS low-risk ($n = 25$) or intermediate-1-risk ($n = 83$) MF. The majority of patients were male (low risk, 60%; intermediate-1 risk, 69%). Most patients (92% and 77%) were still receiving ruxolitinib at the medical record abstraction date (median observation/exposure time, 8 months). The proportion of patients with moderate or severe palpable splenomegaly (≥ 10 cm) decreased from diagnosis (56%) to best response (12%). Fatigue was reported in 47% of patients and was the most common constitutional symptom. For most symptoms in both risk groups, shifts in the distribution of severity from more to less severe from diagnosis to best response were observed. Both patients with low-risk and intermediate-1-risk MF experienced a substantial decrease in spleen size with ruxolitinib treatment in real-world settings. For most symptoms examined, there were distinct improvements in the distribution of severity during ruxolitinib treatment. These findings suggest that patients with lower-risk MF may benefit clinically from ruxolitinib treatment.

1. Introduction

Myelofibrosis (MF) is a myeloproliferative neoplasm (MPN) characterized by cytopenias, splenomegaly, constitutional symptoms (e.g., fatigue, early satiety, weight loss, night sweats, fever, bone pain, and pruritus), and progressive bone marrow fibrosis [1]. It is a chronic disease that reduces life expectancy and quality of life [2]. MF is rare, with an incidence in the United States of 0.2 per 100,000 persons [3]. Survival in patients with MF is highly variable [4, 5], depending on the presence of specific prognostic factors such as those incorporated in the International Prognostic Scoring System (IPSS; Table 1). Median survival has been estimated at 11 years for patients with IPSS low-risk MF, 8 years for intermediate-1-risk MF, 4 years for intermediate-2-risk MF, and 2 years for high-risk MF [4].

Until recently, medical and surgical options for patients with MF have been limited [6]. Most pharmacotherapies were palliative [7], and their effect on spleen size and symptoms was minimal and generally of short duration [8, 9]. Splenectomy may be considered for patients with substantial spleen enlargement and/or refractory splenic symptoms that have not responded to pharmacotherapy [10]; however, mortality and morbidity rates associated with splenectomy (9% and 31%, resp.) are significant and limit its therapeutic use [11]. For patients with symptomatic splenomegaly who are not candidates for surgery, splenic irradiation may be offered; however, its benefit (mainly palliative) is often short lived and patients may experience significant toxicities [10]. Although allogeneic stem cell transplant is the only treatment with curative potential [12], it carries significant risks of morbidity and mortality [13], particularly in older patients; therefore,

TABLE 1: International Prognostic Scoring System.

Variable (1 point each)	Risk group
Age > 65 years	Low risk: 0 points
Constitutional symptoms	Intermediate-1 risk: 1 point
Hemoglobin < 10 g/dL	Intermediate-2 risk: 2 points
Leukocyte count > 25×10^9/L	High risk: ≥ 3 points
Circulating blasts ≥ 1%	

few patients with MF are suitable candidates for this approach [7].

The recent identification of mutations associated with the Janus kinase (JAK)/signal transducer and activator of transcription (STAT) pathway and a new appreciation of the role of cytokines signaled through JAK1 and JAK2 in the pathogenesis of MPNs [14–16] has resulted in new treatment strategies for these diseases. Based on this new knowledge, a selective, orally available JAK inhibitor (ruxolitinib) has been developed for the treatment of MF. Randomized clinical trials of ruxolitinib demonstrated reductions in splenomegaly and MF-related symptoms that led to US regulatory approval of the drug [8, 17] for patients with IPSS intermediate- and high-risk MF [4] and European market authorization for patients with MF-related splenomegaly or symptoms.

To date, few trial-based assessments of ruxolitinib in patients with lower-risk MF have been conducted, and no studies have made such assessments in a real-world setting. In this study, we sought to understand whether symptomatic patients with lower-risk MF would also benefit from ruxolitinib treatment, as was seen in patients with intermediate-2- and high-risk disease studied in the registration trials, by retrospectively assessing changes in spleen size and disease-related symptoms in routine clinical practice.

2. Methods

This was a retrospective, observational review of anonymized medical record data collected in January 2014 by 49 hematologists and oncologists in the United States. Participating physicians were recruited from an existing research panel maintained by All Global, Ltd. Data were collected with secure, online case report forms (CRFs) administered to the selected physicians who had treated ≥2 patients with MF with ruxolitinib since November 2011 (US launch date for the drug). Patient inclusion criteria were as follows: (1) being diagnosed with lower-risk MF (IPSS score of 0 [low risk] or 1 [intermediate-1 risk]); (2) being first treated with ruxolitinib ≥3 months before the medical record abstraction date; (3) being ≥18 years of age at ruxolitinib initiation; (4) having a medical history from MF diagnosis until the medical record abstraction date; and (5) never being enrolled in an MF-related interventional trial. Minimum quotas of 25 and 50 were set for patients with low- and intermediate-1-risk disease, respectively, with a predetermined maximum of 110 patients in the combined total. To increase generalizability of the sample, each physician was limited to 3 patient entries (although most physicians entered only 2). Furthermore, when >3 patient records were available for a physician,

patients with birth months nearest to a birth month randomly generated by the electronic CRF were selected.

Spleen size and constitutional symptoms were the key measures, retrospectively extracted at MF diagnosis, at ruxolitinib initiation, and at best response while receiving ruxolitinib treatment. Symptoms of interest included those described in the validated Myeloproliferative Neoplasm Symptom Assessment Form (MPN-SAF) [18], which were categorized as mild, moderate, or severe based on medical notes recorded at each time point. Symptom data were collected only to the extent that they were documented in the patient medical records; patients were not contacted by their physicians or other study personnel to obtain this information. For this analysis, we present findings on the 7 most commonly observed MPN-SAF symptoms in our sample (full tabular results on all 17 MPN-SAF symptoms are available upon request). Spleen size was captured using predefined categories of no splenomegaly present (spleen not palpable), very mild or mild splenomegaly (<10 cm palpated), moderate splenomegaly (10–20 cm palpated), or severe splenomegaly (>20 cm palpated).

Although this study was not designed as a safety evaluation of ruxolitinib, we additionally report the frequency of thrombocytopenia and anemia, which are the 2 most common adverse events associated with ruxolitinib (as expected based on the drug's mechanism of action), as well as the proportion of patients who required a change in ruxolitinib treatment (i.e., dose reduction, temporary therapy interruption, or therapy discontinuation) as a result of an adverse reaction. Following previous safety reporting from the ruxolitinib COMFORT-I trial [17], we specifically report the proportion of patients experiencing grade ≥3 thrombocytopenia (platelet count <50×10^9/L) or grade ≥3 anemia (hemoglobin <8 g/dL) as measured at any point after ruxolitinib initiation through last ruxolitinib dose.

All statistical analyses were carried out using SAS (version 9.3; SAS Institute Inc., Cary, NC, USA) statistical software. Because this study was exploratory in nature with no proposed hypotheses to test, only descriptive analyses were implemented. These analyses entailed the tabular display of means, SDs, medians, and value ranges for continuous variables and the frequency distribution of categorical variables. Conduct of this study was approved by an authorized institutional review board (Research Triangle Institute Committee for the Protection of Human Subjects, Federal Wide Assurance #3331) and carried out in accordance with the 1996 Helsinki Declaration regarding the ethical conduct of human subject research. Because anonymized retrospective patient data were collected, an informed consent waiver was granted.

3. Results

A total of 49 physicians were recruited for the data abstraction, of whom 82% specialized in hematology/oncology. Mean (SD) duration of practice experience was 12.7 (5.9) years, and the majority (73%) of the physicians practiced in community-based group clinics. A total of 108 patients were included (25 with low-risk and 83 with intermediate-1-risk disease) in this study (Table 2 shows summarized data on key

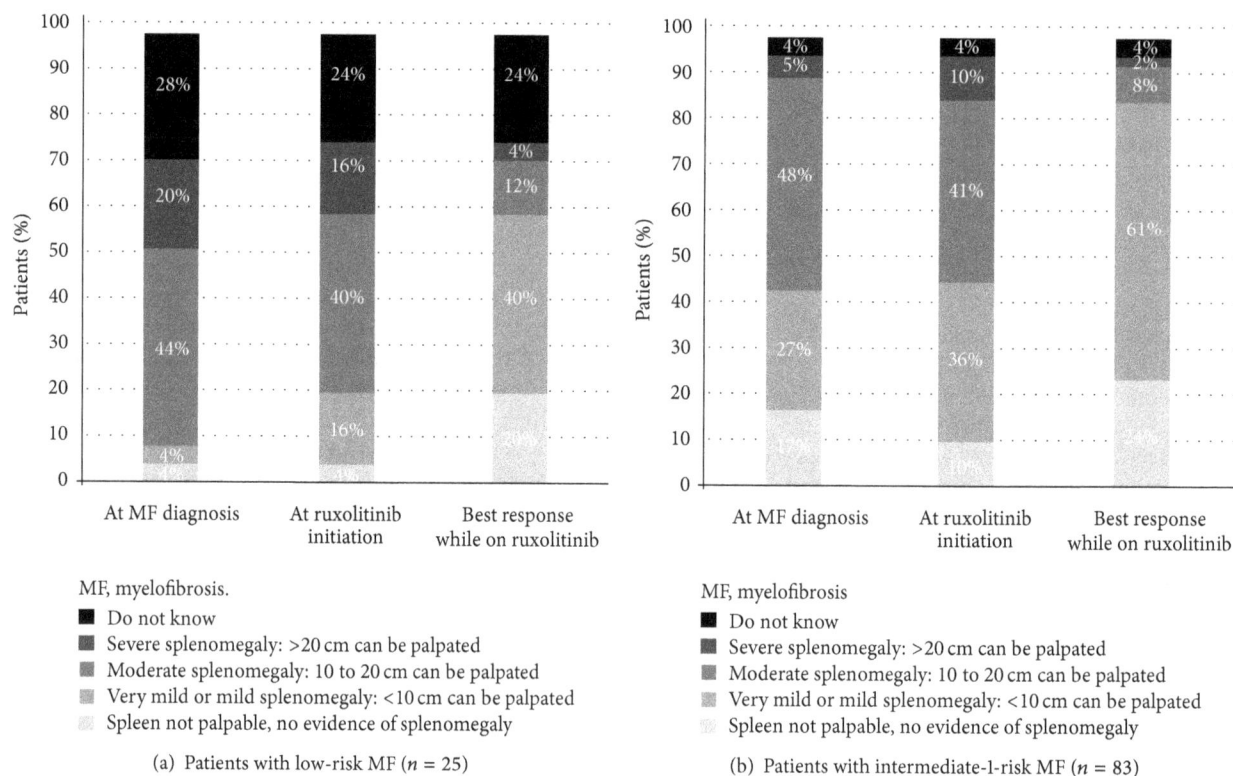

MF, myelofibrosis.

■ Do not know
■ Severe splenomegaly: >20 cm can be palpated
■ Moderate splenomegaly: 10 to 20 cm can be palpated
▨ Very mild or mild splenomegaly: <10 cm can be palpated
░ Spleen not palpable, no evidence of splenomegaly

(a) Patients with low-risk MF (*n* = 25)

MF, myelofibrosis

■ Do not know
■ Severe splenomegaly: >20 cm can be palpated
■ Moderate splenomegaly: 10 to 20 cm can be palpated
▨ Very mild or mild splenomegaly: <10 cm can be palpated
░ Spleen not palpable, no evidence of splenomegaly

(b) Patients with intermediate-1-risk MF (*n* = 83)

FIGURE 1: Spleen size distribution.

characteristics of these patients). All 25 patients with low-risk and nearly 80% of those with intermediate-1-risk MF were aged ≤65 years. The majority of patients in both risk groups were male (60% for low risk and 69% for intermediate-1 risk). Most patients in both risk groups (80% for low risk and 82% for intermediate-1 risk) had primary MF at initial diagnosis. A substantially higher proportion of the patients with intermediate-1-risk disease were positive for the *JAK2* V617F mutation (72%) compared with patients with low-risk disease (56%). The prevalence of comorbidities in the selected patients appeared to be consistent with that in the general population, with diabetes and hypertension the most common conditions recorded at ruxolitinib initiation. Finally, most patients in both risk groups (92% for low risk and 77% for intermediate-1 risk) were still receiving ruxolitinib treatment at the time of data abstraction or last available follow-up.

3.1. Spleen Size. Based on patients' best treatment response, Figure 1 shows that patients with low-risk disease experienced a substantial improvement in spleen size during ruxolitinib treatment compared with the recorded spleen size at MF diagnosis and at ruxolitinib initiation. Specifically, the combined proportion of patients with low-risk MF with moderate or severe splenomegaly decreased from 64% at MF diagnosis to 16% at best response during ruxolitinib treatment. Likewise, the combined proportion of patients with low-risk disease with either no evidence of splenomegaly or mild splenomegaly increased from 8% at MF diagnosis to 60% at best response during ruxolitinib treatment. Overall, 78% of

patients with low-risk disease had a decrease in spleen size from MF diagnosis to best response during ruxolitinib treatment, and 68% of patients had a decrease from ruxolitinib initiation to best response. Similar findings were obtained for patients with intermediate-1-risk MF: the combined proportion of patients with intermediate-1-risk disease with moderate or severe splenomegaly decreased from 53% at MF diagnosis to 10% at best response during ruxolitinib treatment, whereas the combined proportion of patients with either no evidence of splenomegaly or only mild splenomegaly increased from 44% at MF diagnosis to 85% at best response during ruxolitinib treatment. Similar to the low-risk population, 55% of patients with intermediate-1-risk disease had a decrease in spleen size from MF diagnosis to best response during ruxolitinib treatment, and 55% of those patients had a decrease from ruxolitinib initiation to best response.

3.2. Symptoms. In general, for both risk groups, a distinct shift was observed in the distribution of symptom severity toward a more favorable profile (i.e., less severe) from MF diagnosis to the time of best response during ruxolitinib treatment (Figure 2). Among patients with low-risk MF with fatigue, for example, the proportion with moderate or severe fatigue decreased from 90% at MF diagnosis to 37% at best ruxolitinib response; in patients with intermediate-1-risk disease, the decrease was from 76% at MF diagnosis to 42% at best response. However, the number of patients still experiencing each symptom, even though experiencing it in a less severe form for the majority of the symptoms, did not decrease for all symptoms examined. For patients

TABLE 2: Patient characteristics.

| | All patients | | IPSS category | | | |
| | | | Low risk | | Intermediate-1 risk | |
	n	%	n	%	n	%
Total patients	108	100.00	25	100.00	83	100.00
Age						
≤65 years	91	84.26	25	100.00	66	79.52
>65 years	17	15.74	0	0.00	17	20.48
Sex						
Male	72	66.67	15	60.00	57	68.67
Female	36	33.33	10	40.00	26	31.33
Race or ethnicity						
White	79	73.15	21	84.00	58	69.88
Black	16	14.81	2	8.00	14	16.87
Hispanic	10	9.26	0	0.00	10	12.05
Other	2	1.85	1	4.00	1	1.20
Do not know	1	0.93	1	4.00	0	0.00
Primary insurance type at ruxolitinib initiation						
Commercial	43	39.81	10	40.00	33	39.76
Medicare	47	43.52	9	36.00	38	45.78
Medicaid	9	8.33	2	8.00	7	8.43
Uninsured	0	0.00	0	0.00	0	0.00
Other	2	1.85	0	0.00	2	2.41
Do not know	7	6.48	4	16.00	3	3.61
MF type at diagnosis						
Primary MF	88	81.48	20	80.00	68	81.93
Postpolycythemia vera MF	10	9.26	3	12.00	7	8.43
Postessential thrombocythemia MF	9	8.33	2	8.00	7	8.43
Do not know	1	0.93	0	0.00	1	1.20
JAK2 V617F mutation test result						
Positive	74	68.52	14	56.00	60	72.29
Negative	21	19.44	7	28.00	14	16.87
Test not done	3	2.78	1	4.00	2	2.41
Do not know	10	9.26	3	12.00	7	8.43
Charlson comorbidities at ruxolitinib initiation						
Hypertension	35	32.41	6	24.00	29	34.94
Diabetes (overall)	17	15.74	2	8.00	15	18.07
Diabetes (without end organ damage)	15	13.89	1	4.00	14	16.87
Chronic pulmonary disease	9	8.33	1	4.00	8	9.64
Liver disease (overall)	7	6.48	1	4.00	6	7.23
Depression	7	6.48	0	0.00	7	8.43
Mild liver disease	6	5.56	1	4.00	5	6.02
Cerebrovascular disease	5	4.63	1	4.00	4	4.82
Connective tissue disease	4	3.7	1	4.00	3	3.61
Dementia	3	2.78	0	0.00	3	3.61
Malignant solid tumor	3	2.78	1	4.00	2	2.41
HIV/AIDS	2	1.85	0	0.00	2	2.41
Hemiplegia	2	1.85	0	0.00	2	2.41
Myocardial infarction	2	1.85	0	0.00	2	2.41

TABLE 2: Continued.

| | All patients | | IPSS category | | | |
| | | | Low risk | | Intermediate-1 risk | |
	n	%	n	%	n	%
Diabetes (with end organ damage)	2	1.85	1	4.00	1	1.20
Malignant lymphoma	1	0.93	0	0.00	1	1.20
Moderate or severe liver disease	1	0.93	0	0.00	1	1.20
Peripheral vascular disease	1	0.93	0	0.00	1	1.20
Ulcer disease	1	0.93	1	4.00	0	0.00
Congestive heart failure	0	0	0	0.00	0	0.00
None of these	36	33.33	11	44.0	25	30.12
Other	0	0.00	0	0.0	0	0.00
Do not know	8	7.41	4	16.0	4	4.82
Ruxolitinib doses utilized						
Starting median daily dose, mg (min, max)	30 (2, 56)		30 (4, 56)		30 (2, 50)	
Dose range observed over entire treatment duration, n (min, max)	2, 60		4, 60		2, 50	
Still on ruxolitinib at last available follow-up?						
Yes	87	80.60	23	92.00	64	77.10
No	15	13.90	2	8.00	13	15.70
Do not know	6	5.60	0	0.00	6	7.20

IPSS, International Prognostic Scoring System; JAK2, Janus kinase 2; MF, myelofibrosis.

with low-risk disease, general fatigue, night sweats, and early satiety were the 3 most common symptoms, experienced by one-third to nearly one-half of patients, depending on the observation point and symptom examined. For patients with intermediate-1-risk disease, general fatigue, night sweats, and weight loss were the 3 most common symptoms, reported in approximately one-half to two-thirds of patients.

3.3. Adverse Events. Grade $\geq$ 3 thrombocytopenia was observed in 7% of all patients at some point during ruxolitinib treatment (12% of low-risk patients and 6% of intermediate-1-risk patients); grade $\geq$ 3 anemia was observed in 22% of patients (20% of low-risk patients and 23% of intermediate-1-risk patients) (Table 3). A reduction in ruxolitinib dose due to an adverse reaction was documented in 18% of all patients (12% of low-risk patients and 19% of intermediate-1-risk patients). Temporary therapy interruption and/or discontinuation were rare, only 1 reported case of each event (both events were observed in low-risk patients).

4. Conclusions

In light of robust trial data showing that ruxolitinib improved both splenomegaly-related and non-splenomegaly-related constitutional symptoms in patients with intermediate-2-risk and high-risk MF [8, 17], the present study sought to explore whether patients with MF in lower-risk prognostic categories may also benefit from treatment with ruxolitinib in a routine clinical setting. Our findings indicated that patients with lower-risk MF may indeed benefit from ruxolitinib,

particularly with regard to splenomegaly reduction and improvement in both splenomegaly-related and constitutional symptoms. Based on patients' best treatment response, both patients with low-risk MF and those with intermediate-1-risk MF experienced a substantial improvement in spleen size during ruxolitinib treatment compared with the recorded spleen size at MF diagnosis and at ruxolitinib initiation. It is important to note that the reductions in spleen size reported here may be a conservative estimate of the maximum spleen size reduction each patient experienced during ruxolitinib treatment because the majority of patients were still on ruxolitinib at last follow-up; with longer follow-up, it is possible that an even more favorable response would have been observed, but additional research in patients with longer ruxolitinib exposure is needed to evaluate this. Furthermore, for most commonly occurring symptoms, we observed a distinct shift in the severity distribution toward a more favorable profile (i.e., less severe) from MF diagnosis to the time of best response during the observed duration of treatment.

To our knowledge, only 1 previous study [19] sought to assess in a clinical trial setting the possible therapeutic benefits of ruxolitinib in patients with lower-risk MF. These data from the ROBUST trial (ClinicalTrials.gov NCT01558739) in the United Kingdom showed that half of the patients with intermediate-1-risk MF treated with ruxolitinib achieved a reduction in spleen size of $\geq$50% at week 48 (versus baseline) after initiation of ruxolitinib. Mead et al. [19] also reported improvements in disease-related symptoms, as assessed using the Myelofibrosis Symptom Assessment Form (MF-SAF), for more than half (57%) of patients with intermediate-1-risk

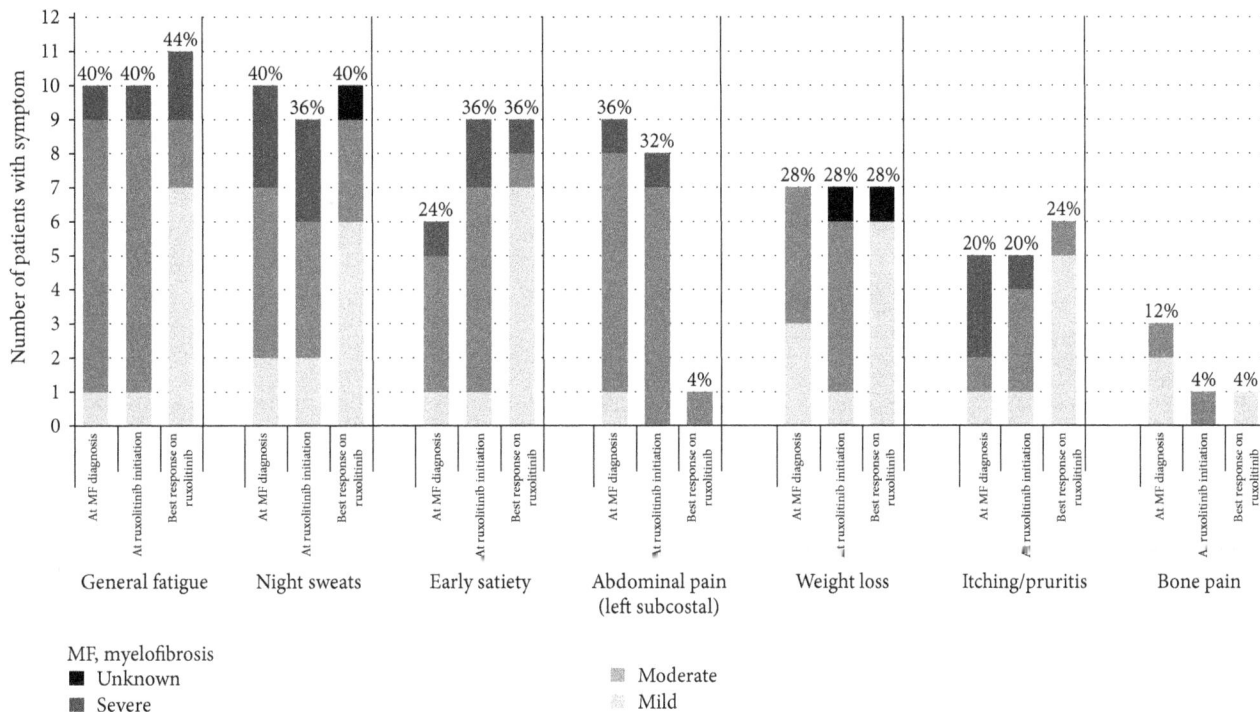

(a) Patients with low-risk MF (n = 25)

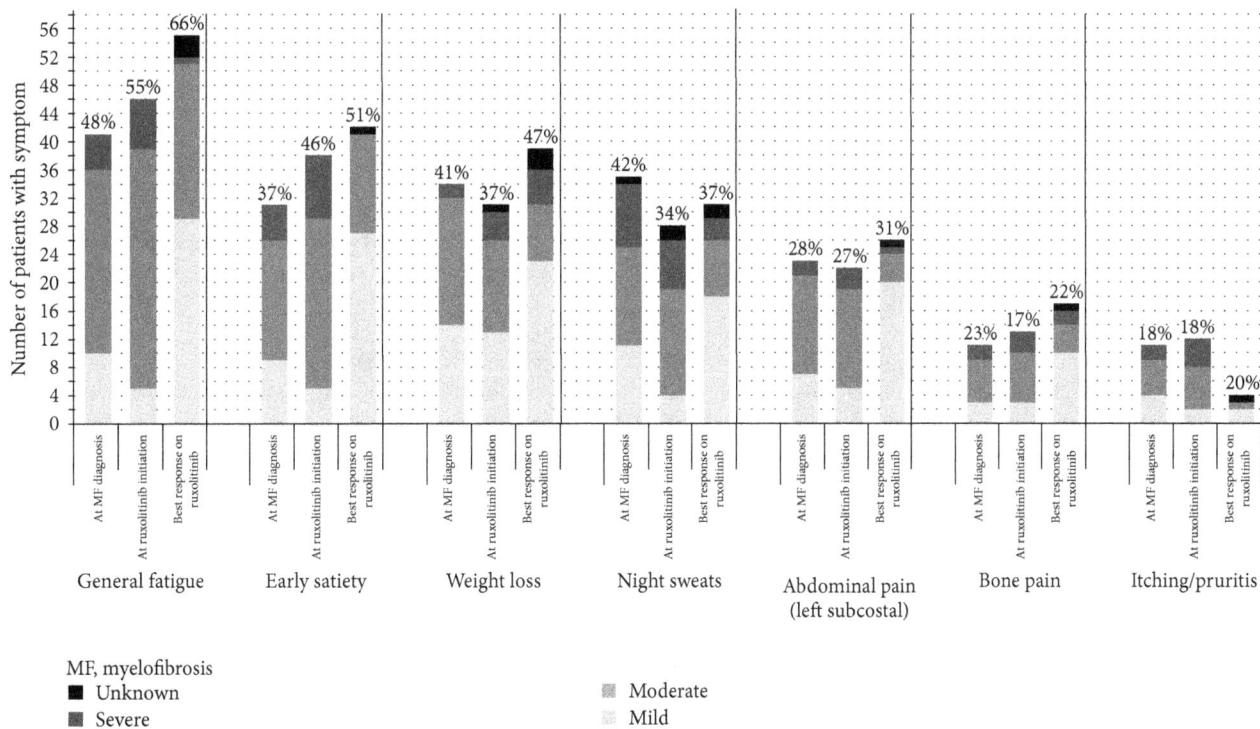

(b) Patients with intermediate-1-risk MF (n = 83)

FIGURE 2: Symptom frequency and severity distribution.

TABLE 3: Specific adverse events during ruxolitinib treatment.

| | All patients | | IPSS category | | | |
| | | | Low risk | | Intermediate-1 risk | |
	n	%	n	%	n	%
Total patients	108	100.00	25	100.00	83	100.00
Grade 3 or higher thrombocytopenia[a]	8	7.41	3	12.00	5	6.02
Grade 3 or higher anemia[b]	24	22.22	5	20.00	19	22.89
Ruxolitinib treatment changes due to adverse reactions						
Dose reduction	19	17.59	3	12.00	16	19.28
Temporary therapy interruption	1	0.93	1	4.00	0	0.00
Therapy discontinuation	1	0.93	1	4.00	0	0.00

IPSS, International Prognostic Scoring System.
[a]Defined as a platelet count $< 50 \times 10^9$/L at any point after ruxolitinib initiation through last ruxolitinib dose.
[b]Defined as hemoglobin < 8 g/dL at any point after ruxolitinib initiation through last ruxolitinib dose.

disease treated with ruxolitinib. Taken together, these findings are consistent with those reported for the routine clinical setting from which our study data were collected.

Although the study by Mead et al. [19] represents the only trial-based assessment to date of the clinical benefits of ruxolitinib in patients with lower-risk MF, our study remains, to our knowledge, the only such reporting from a clinical practice setting that stratified lower-risk patients based on the IPSS classification system. One previous study [20] reported on symptom improvement in the first month of ruxolitinib therapy for a small cohort of patients ($n = 6$) without splenomegaly at MF diagnosis. To the extent that absence of splenomegaly is a proxy for lower-risk MF, a comparison of findings on symptom improvement between that study and ours may be useful. Benjamini et al. [20] found a significant improvement in fatigue in all patients. Drenching night sweats (2 patients), itching (2 patients), and bone pain and skin rash thought to be paraneoplastic (1 patient) were also observed to resolve. As in that study, we observed improvements in fatigue, night sweats, itching, and bone pain for patients with intermediate-1-risk disease; we did not directly evaluate skin rash. Another study reporting the first postmarketing clinical experience with ruxolitinib ($N = 28$) found substantial improvements in constitutional symptoms and in spleen size [21]. However, although more than half of the patients in this study were intermediate-1 risk, the study did not present results by risk category, and no patients with low-risk MF were included in the analysis.

In our study sample, we also found that more than half (53%) of patients with intermediate-1-risk MF had moderate to severe splenomegaly (palpable spleen > 10 cm) at MF diagnosis. Two previous medical record reviews [22, 23] also indicated the possibility of a considerable rate of moderate to severe splenomegaly, even in patients with lower-risk MF. These studies, however, examined pooled cohorts of patients with both lower-risk (low and intermediate-1 risk) and higher-risk (intermediate-2 and high risk) patients and did not stratify splenomegaly frequency by risk category at diagnosis. Nonetheless, in the pooled cohorts ($n = 74$ in

Benites et al. [22] and $n = 1000$ in Tefferi et al. [23]), at least moderate splenomegaly was found in 42% [22] and 21% [23] of patients. Because these samples comprised both patients with higher- and lower-risk disease, our finding of a 53% moderate to severe splenomegaly rate in patients with intermediate-1-risk MF (the rate was 66% in our small sample of patients with low-risk disease) might seem high. However, as previously noted, our study's data collection effort targeted hematologists and oncologists with experience prescribing ruxolitinib, and therefore we may inadvertently have studied a patient population that may have been inherently more complex (i.e., with higher rates of splenomegaly and constitutional symptoms) or more thoroughly evaluated than the patients seen in more general hematology/oncology practice settings. Despite this caveat, our findings, combined with those of the noted studies by Benites et al. [22] and Tefferi et al. [23], indicated that some degree of symptomatic splenomegaly was present in many patients with MF of all risk categories, which further supports the conclusion that ruxolitinib may address an unmet medical need in patients with lower-risk disease, as well as those for whom ruxolitinib treatment is currently indicated.

Our findings on the 2 most common adverse events associated with ruxolitinib (thrombocytopenia and anemia) were consistent with safety data reported in the ruxolitinib COMFORT-I trial [17], in which rates of grade ≥3 thrombocytopenia peaked at 6% at week 8 of treatment and those of grade ≥3 anemia peaked at 26% at week 8. In our study, we found that approximately 7% of patients had ≥1 occurrence of grade ≥3 thrombocytopenia at any point during ruxolitinib treatment, while 22% had ≥1 occurrence of anemia during treatment. Although assessments of these adverse events in the COMFORT-I study were protocol driven in that they were made at frequent predefined intervals, findings from our study (in which assessments were likely made less frequently and not at predefined intervals) appear to be consistent with the COMFORT-I results. In line with the anticipated occurrences of thrombocytopenia and anemia, we observed that nearly 18% of patients had a reduction in ruxolitinib dose due to an adverse reaction; complete discontinuation of ruxolitinib treatment due to an adverse reaction occurred in only 1 patient. Moreover, 12% of patients in our study received a red blood cell transfusion during ruxolitinib treatment to treat anemia (tabular data available upon request). These findings indicate, as described in a recent review article by Mesa and Cortes [24] in the context of a trial-based population, that hematologic events in real-world settings in patients treated with ruxolitinib can be successfully managed with dose modifications and red blood cell transfusions (in the case of anemia) and, importantly, are seldom reason for permanent treatment discontinuation.

This study is subject to several limitations. As in many retrospective medical record abstraction studies, patients selected for inclusion represent a convenience sample. Our study findings therefore may not be generalizable to the overall low- or intermediate-1-risk MF populations in the United States, and although participating physicians were recruited from all geographic regions, it was not possible to construct sampling weights that allowed for generalization to the national population. Only physicians who agreed to participate in the study contributed data; these physicians therefore may not be representative of all physicians treating low-risk or intermediate-1 MF in the United States. Finally, although no time limit was imposed on physicians for the completion of individual CRFs, the CRF was designed to limit physicians' time burden to help ensure full and accurate responses. Therefore, the scope of information that could be collected in this study was limited, and it is possible that additional information could have contributed further context to the study findings.

Despite the noted limitations, findings from this study indicated that patients with lower-risk MF in routine clinical practice may benefit from ruxolitinib treatment, specifically for spleen size reduction and improved splenomegaly-related and constitutional symptoms. Furthermore, ruxolitinib has been shown to prolong overall survival in patients with intermediate-2 or high-risk MF and to reduce the risk of death among high-risk patients receiving ruxolitinib to that of intermediate-2-risk patients receiving placebo or best available therapy [25]. These results suggest a potential to alter the clinical course of patients with MF and strongly support further evaluation of the effect of ruxolitinib in patients with intermediate-1 or low-risk MF. Data presented in this study, in conjunction with additional clinical trials, may also be useful in economic (e.g., cost-effectiveness) assessments of ruxolitinib use in patients with lower-risk MF.

Conflict of Interests

Keith L. Davis and James A. Kaye are employees of RTI Health Solutions, an independent contract research organization that received research funding from Novartis Pharmaceuticals Corporation to conduct this study. Isabelle Côté, Haitao Gao, and Estella Mendelson are employees of Novartis Pharmaceuticals Corporation, and Julian Perez Ronco is an employee of Novartis Pharma AG, which markets ruxolitinib outside of the United States and is conducting clinical research in patients with myelofibrosis. Final decisions regarding paper's content were made jointly by the authors.

References

[1] R. A. Mesa, J. Niblack, M. Wadleigh et al., "The burden of fatigue and quality of life in myeloproliferative disorders (MPDs): an international internet-based survey of 1179 MPD patients," *Cancer*, vol. 109, no. 1, pp. 68–76, 2007.

[2] C. N. Harrison, R. A. Mesa, J.-J. Kiladjian et al., "Health-related quality of life and symptoms in patients with myelofibrosis treated with ruxolitinib versus best available therapy," *British Journal of Haematology*, vol. 162, no. 2, pp. 229–239, 2013.

[3] S. J. Swaim, "Ruxolitinib for the treatment of primary myelofibrosis," *American Journal of Health-System Pharmacy*, vol. 71, no. 6, pp. 453–462, 2014.

[4] F. Cervantes, B. Dupriez, A. Pereira et al., "New prognostic scoring system for primary myelofibrosis based on a study of the International Working Group for Myelofibrosis Research and Treatment," *Blood*, vol. 113, no. 13, pp. 2895–2901, 2009.

[5] M. Hultcrantz, S. Y. Kristinsson, T. M.-L. Andersson et al., "Patterns of survival among patients with myeloproliferative neoplasms diagnosed in Sweden from 1973 to 2008: a population-based study," *Journal of Clinical Oncology*, vol. 30, no. 24, pp. 2995–3001, 2012.

[6] N. Gangat, D. Caramazza, R. Vaidya et al., "DIPSS plus: a refined dynamic international prognostic scoring system for primary myelofibrosis that incorporates prognostic information from karyotype, platelet count, and transfusion status," *Journal of Clinical Oncology*, vol. 29, no. 4, pp. 392–397, 2011.

[7] A. Quintás-Cardama and S. Verstovsek, "Spleen deflation and beyond: the pros and cons of Janus kinase 2 inhibitor therapy for patients with myeloproliferative neoplasms," *Cancer*, vol. 118, no. 4, pp. 870–877, 2012.

[8] C. Harrison, J.-J. Kiladjian, H. K. Al-Ali et al., "JAK inhibition with ruxolitinib versus best available therapy for myelofibrosis," *The New England Journal of Medicine*, vol. 366, no. 9, pp. 787–798, 2012.

[9] R. A. Mesa, S. Verstovsek, F. Cervantes et al., "Comparison of the efficacy of placebo and best available therapy for the treatment of myelofibrosis in the COMFORT studies," *Blood*, vol. 118, article 1753, 2011.

[10] R. A. Mesa, "How I treat symptomatic splenomegaly in patients with myelofibrosis," *Blood*, vol. 113, no. 22, pp. 5394–5400, 2009.

[11] A. Tefferi, R. A. Mesa, D. M. Nagorney, G. Schroeder, and M. N. Silverstein, "Splenectomy in myelofibrosis with myeloid metaplasia: a single- institution experience with 223 patients," *Blood*, vol. 95, no. 7, pp. 2226–2233, 2000.

[12] T. Barbui, G. Barosi, G. Birgegard et al., "Philadelphia-negative classical myeloproliferative neoplasms: critical concepts and management recommendations from European LeukemiaNet," *Journal of Clinical Oncology*, vol. 29, no. 6, pp. 761–770, 2011.

[13] K. K. Ballen, S. Shrestha, K. A. Sobocinski et al., "Outcome of transplantation for myelofibrosis," *Biology of Blood and Marrow Transplantation*, vol. 16, no. 3, pp. 358–367, 2010.

[14] E. J. Baxter, L. M. Scott, P. J. Campbell et al., "Acquired mutation of the tyrosine kinase JAK2 in human myeloproliferative disorders," *The Lancet*, vol. 365, no. 9464, pp. 1054–1061, 2005.

[15] R. Kralovics, F. Passamonti, A. S. Buser et al., "A gain-of-function mutation of JAK2 in myeloproliferative disorders," *The New England Journal of Medicine*, vol. 352, no. 17, pp. 1779–1790, 2005.

[16] R. L. Levine, M. Wadleigh, J. Cools et al., "Activating mutation in the tyrosine kinase JAK2 in polycythemia vera, essential thrombocythemia, and myeloid metaplasia with myelofibrosis," *Cancer Cell*, vol. 7, no. 4, pp. 387–397, 2005.

[17] S. Verstovsek, R. A. Mesa, J. Gotlib et al., "A double-blind, placebo-controlled trial of ruxolitinib for myelofibrosis," *The New England Journal of Medicine*, vol. 366, no. 9, pp. 799–807, 2012.

[18] R. Scherber, A. C. Dueck, P. Johansson et al., "The Myeloproliferative Neoplasm Symptom Assessment Form (MPN-SAF): international prospective validation and reliability trial in 402 patients," *Blood*, vol. 118, no. 2, pp. 401–408, 2011.

[19] A. J. Mead, D. Milojkovic, S. Knapper et al., "Response to ruxolitinib in patients with intermediate-1, intermediate-2 and high-risk myelofibrosis: results of the UK ROBUST Trial," *British Journal of Haematology*, vol. 170, no. 1, pp. 29–39, 2015.

[20] O. Benjamini, P. Jain, Z. Estrov, H. M. Kantarjian, and S. Verstovsek, "Therapeutic effects of ruxolitinib in patients with myelofibrosis without clinically significant splenomegaly," *Blood*, vol. 120, no. 13, pp. 2768–2769, 2012.

[21] H. Geyer, K. Cannon, E. Knight et al., "Ruxolitinib in clinical practice for therapy of myelofibrosis: single USA center experience following Food and Drug Administration approval," *Leukemia and Lymphoma*, vol. 55, no. 1, pp. 195–197, 2014.

[22] B. D. Benites, C. S. Costa Lima, I. Lorand-Metze et al., "Primary myelofibrosis: risk stratification by IPSS identifies patients with poor clinical outcome," *Clinics*, vol. 68, no. 3, pp. 339–343, 2013.

[23] A. Tefferi, T. L. Lasho, T. Jimma et al., "One thousand patients with primary myelofibrosis: the Mayo Clinic experience," *Mayo Clinic Proceedings*, vol. 87, no. 1, pp. 25–33, 2012.

[24] R. A. Mesa and J. Cortes, "Optimizing management of ruxolitinib in patients with myelofibrosis: the need for individualized dosing," *Journal of Hematology and Oncology*, vol. 6, article 79, 2013.

[25] A. M. Vannucchi, H. M. Kantarjian, J. J. Kiladjian et al., "A pooled analysis of overall survival in COMFORT-I and COMFORT-II, 2 randomized phase III trials of ruxolitinib for the treatment of myelofibrosis," *Haematologica*, vol. 100, no. 9, pp. 1139–1145, 2013.

30

Comparison of Bone Mineral Density in Thalassemia Major Patients with Healthy Controls

Mahesh Chand Meena,[1] Alok Hemal,[1] Mukul Satija,[1] Shilpa Khanna Arora,[1] and Shahina Bano[2]

[1]*Department of Pediatrics, PGIMER and Dr. RML Hospital, New Delhi 110001, India*
[2]*Department of Radiology, PGIMER and Dr. RML Hospital, New Delhi 110001, India*

Correspondence should be addressed to Shilpa Khanna Arora; drshilpakhanna@yahoo.co.in

Academic Editor: Meral Beksac

Chronic hemoglobinopathies like thalassemia are associated with many osteopathies like osteoporosis. *Methods*. This observational study was carried out to compare the bone mineral density (BMD) in transfusion dependent thalassemics with that of healthy controls. Thirty-two thalassemia patients, aged 2–18 years, and 32 age and sex matched controls were studied. The bone mineral concentration (BMC) and BMD were assessed at lumbar spine, distal radius, and neck of femur. Biochemical parameters like serum calcium and vitamin D levels were also assessed. *Results*. The BMC of neck of femur was significantly low in cases in comparison to controls. We also observed significantly lower BMD at the lumbar spine in cases in comparison to controls. A significantly positive correlation was observed between serum calcium levels and BMD at neck of femur. *Conclusion*. Hence, low serum calcium may be used as a predictor of low BMD especially in populations where incidence of hypovitaminosis D is very high.

1. Introduction

The management of patients with thalassemia has improved markedly over the past few decades with the use of optimized transfusion programs and chelating therapy. There has been a considerable improvement in the life expectancy and the quality of life of these patients. With prolongation in the life expectancy, it has been observed that this hemoglobinopathy is associated with a variety of bone disorders like deformities, bone pains, delayed bone age, growth failure, rickets, scoliosis, spinal deformities, nerve compression, pathologic fractures, osteopenia, and osteoporosis [1]. Apart from disease process per se, high-dose iron chelating therapy with desferrioxamine may also contribute to osteopenia and osteoporosis [2, 3].

Osteoporosis is a significant cause of morbidity in these patients [4]. It is characterized by low bone mass and disruption of bone architecture, resulting in reduced bone strength and increased risk of fractures [5, 6]. Though many techniques are available for quantitative assessment of the degree of osteoporosis and total bone mass, bone density measurement by Dual Energy X-Ray Absorptiometry (DEXA) of lumbar spine, femoral neck, and distal radius is considered a very reliable and noninvasive technique [7].

This study was carried out to evaluate the bone mineral density (BMD) in children with thalassemia major by DEXA and to compare with healthy controls.

2. Methods

This cross-sectional observational study was conducted in a tertiary care center in Delhi from November 2011 to January 2013. Clearance was taken from the institutional ethical committee. The primary objective of the study was to compare the BMD of thalassemia major patients with that of age and sex matched controls. The sample size was calculated considering a power of 80% using a 2-sided Student's t-test and α-error = 5%. Assuming mean BMD to be $0.63 \pm 0.076 \, \text{g/cm}^2$ in patients and $0.78 \pm 0.3 \, \text{g/cm}^2$ in controls, the sample size was calculated to be 32 in each group.

Thalassemia patients, aged 2–18 years, attending the thalassemia clinic of the hospital, were enrolled consecutively. The patients who were taking medicines like antiepileptic drugs, oral calcium, vitamin D, and so forth that affect bone mineral density were excluded. A total of 32 patients and 32 age and sex matched healthy controls were recruited after an informed written consent was obtained from the parents. Assent was taken from children older than 7 years.

The details of all the subjects were recorded including age, sex, weight, height, and body mass index (BMI). In addition, details like duration of disease, blood transfusion, chelation, and other treatment histories were recorded for the patients. The biochemical assessment included determination of serum calcium, phosphorus, and 25-hydroxy vitamin D levels.

All the subjects underwent DEXA scan using HOLOGIC (Discovery QDR series) bone densitometer. Bone Mineral Content (BMC), areal bone mineral density (aBMD), and volumetric bone mineral density (vBMD) were obtained at lumbar spine, femoral neck, and distal radius. BMC was expressed in gram, aBMD in gram/cm^2, and volumetric BMD in gram/cm^3. The "T score" and the "Z score" were also calculated at these 3 sites after DEXA scan. The T score refers to the number of standard deviations above or below the mean for a healthy 30-year-old adult of the same sex and ethnicity as the patient. A T score of −1.0 or higher is considered normal. Osteopenia has been defined as a "T score" between −1.0 and −2.5 while osteoporosis has been defined as score of −2.5 or lower. T score does not have clinical utility in children and adolescents. Z score is the preferred parameter in children which is calculated as the number of standard deviations above or below the mean for the patient's age, sex, and ethnicity. The diagnosis of osteoporosis and osteopenia in childhood is not made on densitometric data alone especially in absence of a clinically significant fracture history.

Statistical analysis was performed by the SPSS program for Windows, version 17.0. Normally distributed continuous variables were compared using the unpaired t-test, whereas the Mann-Whitney U test was used for those variables that were not normally distributed. Categorical variables were analyzed using either the chi square test or Fisher's exact test. Spearman's correlation was also performed between BMD, age, sex, body mass index (BMI), chelation, ferritin, calcium, and vitamin D in cases and controls. $P < 0.05$ was considered statistically significant.

3. Results

A total of 32 thalassemic patients (21 male, 11 female) between 5 to 16 years of age (mean ± SD = 10.03 ± 3.03) were studied along with 32 age and sex matched controls. The mean height (133.84 ± 13.40 cm), weight (32.28 ± 10.25 kg), and BMI (17.70 ± 3.86 kg/m^2) of cases were lower in comparison to controls but only weight ($P = 0.023$) and BMI ($P = 0.030$) were statistically significant. The mean age of receiving first blood transfusion in the patients was 3.72 ± 1.14 years (range = 2–6 years). The mean serum ferritin value of the

thalassemia patients was 3349 ± 2012.9 ng/mL (range = 1082–9002 ng/mL). The mean value of total serum iron in children was 459.13 ± 119.47 μg/dL (range = 320–765 μg/dL).

Comparison of biochemical profile in the two groups revealed a significantly lower mean serum calcium level in cases (8.69 ± 1.04 mg/dL) (range = 7–10.4 mg/dL) in comparison to the controls (9.44 ± 0.61 mg/dL) (range = 8.3–10.8 mg/dL) ($P = 0.001$). The mean serum phosphorus levels were 3.97 ± 0.53 mg/dL (range = 3.1–4.9 mg/dL) in cases and 3.73 ± 0.60 mg/dl (range = 2.5–4.9 mg/dL) in controls and the difference was not statistically significant ($P = 0.094$). The mean serum alkaline phosphatase values were 241.54 ± 89.30 IU/L (range = 112–432 IU/L) in cases and 287 ± 101.94 IU/L (range = 112–607 IU/L) in controls and it was not statistically significant ($P = 0.056$). The mean levels of vitamin D were 19.74 ± 10.71 nmol/L (range = 12–63.4 nmol/L) in cases and 23.21 ± 11.10 nmol/L (range = 11.4–63.4 nmol/L) in controls and the difference was not statistically significant ($P = 0.144$). Analysis of serum 25-hydroxy vitamin D demonstrated that none of the subjects in both groups had levels in the normal range (>75 nmol/L) and there was no significant difference in the mean values between the two. Majority (59.4%) of the cases demonstrated moderate 25-OH Vit D deficiency (12.5 to 25 nmol/L), 21.9% were severely deficient (<12.5 nmol/L), and the rest had levels in the minor deficiency (25–50 nmol/L) or insufficient range (50–75 nmol/L).

The BMC and BMD were assessed at lumbar spine, distal radius, and neck of femur and the values are depicted in Table 1. The BMC of neck of femur was significantly low in cases (1.87 ± 0.51 gm) in comparison to controls (14.13 ± 12.23 gm) ($P < 0.001$). The mean BMC at lumbar spine (LS) as well as distal radius (DR) was also lower for the cases (LS, 20.55 ± 8.22 gm; DR, 3.711 ± 2.24 gm) in comparison to controls (LS, 20.98 ± 6.48 gm; DR, 4.60 ± 2.68 gm) but the difference was not statistically significant (LS, $P = 0.818$; DR, $P = 0.143$). The mean BMD for thalassemia cases (0.48 ± 0.17 gm/cm^3) at lumbar spine was significantly low in comparison to controls (0.568 ± 0.110 gm/cm^3) ($P = 0.013$) but the difference was not statistically significant at distal radius ($P = 0.933$) and neck of femur ($P = 0.495$). The difference in mean BMD at lumbar spine was more marked in children aged more than 10 years.

Correlation of bone mineral density at all three sites with calcium and other parameters was done for the patients as depicted in Table 2. A positive correlation was found between calcium level and BMD at all three sites, namely, lumbar spine ($r = 0.116$, $P = 0.526$), distal radius ($r = 0.063$, $P = 0.733$), and neck of femur ($r = 0.392$, $P = 0.026$). However, the difference was statistically significant only at neck of femur. A positive correlation was also observed between vitamin D level and BMD at all the three sites but the difference was not statistically significant (Table 2).

Bone mineral density at all the sites showed a negative correlation with age although the difference was not statistically significant as depicted in Table 2. No significant correlation was seen for BMI, serum ferritin, and chelation with the BMD at any of the sites. There was no significant

TABLE 1: Bone mineral content (BMC) and bone mineral density (BMD) in cases and control at lumbar spine (LS), distal radius (DR), and neck of femur (NF).

	Controls		Cases		P value
	Mean ± SD	Min–max	Mean ± SD	Min–max	
BMC_LS (gm)	20.98 ± 6.48	13.28–38.18	20.55 ± 8.22	13.28–38.18	0.818
BMD_LS (gm/cm^3)	0.568 ± 0.110	0.379–0.821	0.48 ± 0.17	0.211–0.791	0.013
BMC_DR (gm)	4.60 ± 2.68	0.60–10.01	3.711 ± 2.24	1.06–10.81	0.143
BMD_DR (gm/cm^3)	0.323 ± 0.06	0.218–0.441	0.324 ± 0.99	0.110–0.560	0.933
BMC_NF (gm)	14.13 ± 12.23	1.2–37.3	1.87 ± 0.51	1.2–2.9	<0.001
BMD_NF (gm/cm^3)	0.496 ± 0.17	0.321–0.869	0.464 ± 0.198	0.230–0.907	0.495

TABLE 2: Correlation of bone mineral density at lumbar spine (LS), distal radius (DR), and neck of femur (NF) in cases.

		BMD_LS	BMD_DR	BMD_NF
Age	r	−0.052	−0.289	−0.066
	P value	0.776	0.109	0.718
Sex	r	−0.078	0.011	−0.153
	P value	0.670	0.954	0.402
BMI	r	0.393	0.003	0.039
	P value	0.026	0.987	0.832
S. ferritin	r	0.201	0.043	0.180
	P value	0.270	0.817	0.325
Chelation	r	−0.065	−0.208	−0.064
	P value	0.726	0.254	0.728
Ca	r	0.116	0.063	0.392
	P value	0.526	0.733	0.026
Vit D levels	r	0.086	0.236	0.236
	P value	0.641	0.193	0.194

difference between BMD of male and BMD of female thalassemia patients.

4. Discussion

During the last decade, osteopenia or osteoporosis has been reported in approximately 40–50% of well treated thalassemia major patients in different studies and is major cause of morbidity in these patients [8, 9]. Bone changes in thalassemic patients are due to increased marrow erythropoiesis and extensive iron deposition resulting in expansion of bone marrow cavities and reduced trabecular bone volume, leading to decreased bone tissue and osteoporosis [4, 10]. Chelation is another important risk factor for causing osteoporosis in these patients as high dose desferrioxamine therapy causes decrease in the differentiation and proliferation of bone-forming cells, decreases collagen formation, and increases osteoblast programmed cell death. Chelation also leads to deficiency of vitamins and minerals like vitamin D and zinc, which in turn worsen the bone health [2, 3]. Presence of other endocrinopathies like hypothyroidism, hypoparathyroidism, diabetes mellitus, and hypogonadism also contributes to bone disease.

The present study observed significantly lower BMD at the lumbar spine which is in accordance with previous studies suggesting that the lumbar spine is more affected in thalassemia patients in comparison to the other sites of BMD assessment [5].

In this study, the mean weight and body mass index of cases were significantly lower than controls. The mean height of cases was also lower though the difference was not statistically significant. These changes can be explained due to chronic illness and endocrinal changes due to iron overload.

Vitamin D deficiency was observed in almost all the cases of thalassemia in the present study. The main causes of vitamin D deficiency in thalassemic patients are nutritional deficiency and defective hydroxylation of vitamin D in liver due to hemochromatosis. But there was no significant difference in vitamin D levels between cases and controls. This could be due to vitamin D deficiency being a common finding in the general population in India.

Hypocalcemia is a common finding in thalassemic patients. In our study, serum calcium level <8 mg/dL was found in 31.3% of the cases, while none in the control group had serum calcium value <8 mg/dL. There was a statistically significant difference in serum calcium value between cases and controls. This suggests that factors other than vitamin D deficiency also play a role in causing hypocalcemia in thalassemics.

In this study, there was a significant difference in bone mineral density at lumbar spine between cases and controls ($P = 0.013$) but at distal radius and neck of femur in cases and controls it was not statistically significant ($P = 0.933$). It is likely that the differences in the BMD of cases and controls would have been more striking if the control population had normal serum Vit D levels. This is a limitation of the present study that the majority of the control group too had vitamin D deficiency. We also observed that the bone mineral density was most affected at lumbar spine which is in accordance with a previous study by Jensen et al. [7].

Bone mineral density at all the sites showed a negative correlation, though not statistically significant, with age. This suggests that BMD decreases with advancing age, as previously observed in a study of Indian thalassemia children between 10 and 25 years of age [6]. We also observed a positive correlation between BMD and vitamin D levels but it was not statistically significant. Similarly, positive correlation was found between calcium level and BMD at all three sites but the difference was statistically significant only at neck of femur. A statistically significant positive correlation might have become evident at other sites as well if a larger number of cases were evaluated in this study. Thus, the present study suggests that not only low serum vitamin D levels but also low serum calcium levels can be an important predictor of low bone mineral density in thalassemics.

Thalassemia International Federation [11] suggests annual BMD assessment in these patients, starting in adolescence. The availability and affordability of DEXA are a major limitation in many poor as well as developing nations. This study observed that serum calcium and vitamin D deficiency and low BMD are widely present in thalassemic children. Low serum calcium may be used as predictor for low BMD, more so in populations where incidence of hypovitaminosis D is very high. Thus, in regions with poor availability of DEXA, serum calcium and vitamin D levels must be routinely monitored in thalassemics especially after the age of 10 for evaluation of bone health.

Disclosure

The paper has been read and approved by all the authors and requirement for authorship of this document has been met. Each author believes that the paper represents honest work.

Conflict of Interests

The authors declare that there is no conflict of interests.

Acknowledgment

The authors wish to acknowledge the contribution of late Dr. Sachchida Nand Yadav in this study. This study could not have been possible without his guidance and support.

References

[1] P. Mahachoklertwattana, V. Sirikulchayanonta, A. Chuansumrit et al., "Bone histomorphometry in children and adolescents with β-thalassemia disease: iron-associated focal osteomalacia," *Journal of Clinical Endocrinology and Metabolism*, vol. 88, no. 8, pp. 3966–3972, 2003.

[2] S. Perrotta, M. D. Cappellini, F. Bertoldo et al., "Osteoporosis in β-thalassaemia major patients: analysis of the genetic background," *British Journal of Haematology*, vol. 111, no. 2, pp. 461–466, 2000.

[3] P. Pennisi, G. Pizzarelli, M. Spina, S. Riccobene, and C. E. Fiore, "Quantitative ultrasound of bone and clodronate effects in thalassemia-induced osteoporosis," *Journal of Bone and Mineral Metabolism*, vol. 21, no. 6, pp. 402–408, 2003.

[4] K. H. Ehlers, P. J. Giardina, M. L. Lesser, M. A. Engle, and M. W. Hilgartner, "Prolonged survival in patients with beta-thalassemia major treated with deferoxamine," *The Journal of Pediatrics*, vol. 118, no. 4, pp. 540–545, 1991.

[5] M. Karimi, A. F. Ghiam, A. Hashemi, S. Alinejad, M. Soweid, and S. Kashef, "Bone mineral density in beta-thalassemia major and intermedia," *Indian Pediatrics*, vol. 44, no. 1, pp. 29–32, 2007.

[6] R. Merchant, A. Udani, V. Puri, V. D'cruz, D. Patkar, and A. Karkera, "Evaluation of osteopathy in thalassemics by bone mineral densitometry and biochemical indices," *Indian Journal of Pediatrics*, vol. 77, pp. 987–991, 2010.

[7] C. E. Jensen, S. M. Tuck, I. E. Agnew et al., "High incidence of osteoporosis in thalassaemia major," *Journal of Pediatric Endocrinology and Metabolism*, vol. 11, no. 3, pp. 975–977, 1998.

[8] M. Yildiz and D. Canatan, "Soft tissue density variations in thalassemia major: a possible pitfall in lumbar bone mineral density measurements by dual-energy X-ray absorptiometry," *Pediatric Hematology and Oncology*, vol. 22, no. 8, pp. 723–726, 2005.

[9] E. B. Fung, "Nutritional deficiencies in patients with thalassemia," *Annals of the New York Academy of Sciences*, vol. 1202, pp. 188–196, 2010.

[10] M. G. Vogiatzi, E. A. Macklin, E. B. Fung et al., "Bone disease in thalassemia: a frequent and still unresolved problem," *Journal of Bone and Mineral Research*, vol. 24, no. 3, pp. 543–557, 2009.

[11] E. Voskaridou and E. Terpos, "Osteoporosis," in *Guidelines for the Management of Transfusion Dependent Thalassemics*, M. D. Cappellini, A. Cohen, J. Porter, A. Taher, and V. Viprakasit, Eds., pp. 170–176, Thalassemia International Federation, Nicosia, Cyprus, 3rd edition, 2014.

31

Determinants of Overall and Progression-Free Survival of Nigerian Patients with Philadelphia-Positive Chronic Myeloid Leukemia

Anthony A. Oyekunle,[1,2] **Rahman A. Bolarinwa,**[1,2] **Adesola T. Oyelese,**[2] **Lateef Salawu,**[1,2] **and Muheez A. Durosinmi**[1,2]

[1]*Department of Hematology and Immunology, Obafemi Awolowo University, Ile-Ife 234-220005, Nigeria*
[2]*Department of Hematology and Blood Transfusion, Obafemi Awolowo University Teaching Hospital Complex, Ile-Ife 234-220005, Nigeria*

Correspondence should be addressed to Anthony A. Oyekunle; oyekunleaa@yahoo.co.uk

Academic Editor: Estella M. Matutes

Objective. The tyrosine kinase inhibitors have markedly changed the disease course for patients with Ph$^+$ and/or *BCR-ABL1*$^+$ chronic myeloid leukemia (CML). This study was embarked upon to assess the long-term effects of imatinib therapy on survival in adult Nigerian patients with CML. *Methods.* All adult patients on imatinib (400–600 mg) seen from July 2003 to December 2010 were assessed. Male/female distribution was 171/101, with a median age of 38 (range, 20–75) years. Overall survival (OS) and progression-free survival (PFS) were determined using the Kaplan-Meier techniques. *Results.* Of all the 272 patients, 205 were in chronic phase, 54 in accelerated phase, and five in blastic phase, at commencement of imatinib. As at December 2010, 222 were alive. OS at 1 and 5 years was 94% and 63%, while PFS was 89% and 54%, respectively. Similarly, amongst the 205 patients in chronic phase, OS at 1 and 5 years was 97% and 68%, while PFS was 92% and 57%. *Conclusion.* Imatinib's place as first-line therapy in the treatment of CML has further been reinforced in our patients, with improved survival and reduced morbidity, comparable with outcomes in other populations.

1. Introduction

Chronic myeloid leukemia (CML) is a myeloproliferative neoplasm caused by the *BCR-ABL1*, a chimeric gene generated as a result of a reciprocal translocation [t(9;22)(q34;q11)], cytogenetically visible as the Philadelphia chromosome (Ph) that places sequences from the *ABL* gene from chromosome 9 downstream of the *BCR* gene on chromosome 22 [1, 2]. CML occurs with an incidence of one to two cases per 100,000 people per year and accounts for 15% of adult leukemias [3]. CML may affect any age group; the peak incidence is between 40 and 60 years with the median age at diagnosis being 53 years in the Western world [4]. However, patients with CML in Nigeria and other African countries, with similar demographic pattern, have a median age of about 38 years [5–8]. Clinically, CML is a bi- or triphasic disease. The chronic phase (present at diagnosis in approximately 85% of patients) is easily controlled with conventional chemotherapy, followed by an unstable accelerated phase and terminating in a blastic phase [9]. Until the 1980s, CML was regarded as incurable and thus inexorably fatal, with effective treatment limited to a minority of patients [10]. The treatment of CML has greatly evolved through the years, with the use of chemotherapeutic agents like interferon (IFN), cytarabine, hydroxyurea, and in some stem cell transplantation being the modality of treatment. However, the discovery of the tyrosine kinase inhibitors, the first being imatinib, which has shown significant activity in all phases of the disease, has altered the course of the disease drastically [11–13]. Imatinib is now recognized as the first-line drug in the treatment of CML, especially in patients in the chronic phase [12, 14, 15]. CML patients in Nigeria, since 2003, like in some other

African counties have continued to access imatinib freely through the collaborative efforts of Novartis Pharmaceutical, Axios International, and The Max Foundation. This review is intended to take a look at the long-term survival outcomes of patients with Philadelphia chromosome or *BCR-ABL1*-positive CML on imatinib over a 7-year period.

2. Patients and Methods

The study was carried out in accordance with the ethical standards of our institutional ethics review board. All patients were treated according to the Helsinki Declaration of 1975, as revised in Edinburgh 2000. All patients reviewed in this study were originally part of a prospective cohort for the clinical postapproval use of imatinib in Nigeria, and all gave written informed consent after appropriate counselling. All 272 Philadelphia chromosome and/or *BCR-ABL1*-positive CML patients enrolled under the Nigerian arm of the GIPAP programme and receiving imatinib since July 2003 to December 2010 were reviewed. Clinical and haematological parameters considered included organomegaly, complete blood counts, and percentage peripheral blasts. The interval between diagnosis and commencement of imatinib was noted and ranged from 0 to 1673 days. Unfortunately, access to cytogenetic and molecular testing in Nigeria at the time of this study was rather limited, and a significant number of these patients did not take these follow-up tests at the prescribed time. Consequently, molecular testing data was excluded from this study.

Collection of data was in MS Excel spreadsheets (Microsoft 2007, USA) and statistical analysis was done using SPSS 17 package (SPSS Inc., 2008, USA). Data cleaning and validation was done in MS Excel, where it was examined for accuracy, correctness, and consistency and cleaned appropriately.

For the purpose of this analysis, only patients in chronic phase, presenting within 3 months of diagnosis and with complete data, were assessed for risk status using the Sokal and Hasford scoring systems.

Survival analysis was done using the Kaplan-Meier method. For the survival studies, overall survival (OS) was calculated as the time interval between the date of commencement of imatinib and the date of last follow-up (for living patients) or the date of death from any cause. Progression-free survival (PFS) was calculated from the date of starting imatinib to the date of documented disease progression to accelerated or blastic phase or to the date of death, whichever was earlier.

3. Results

3.1. Survival Outcomes for All 272 Patients. Over the period of review, 272 patients were enrolled with 205, 54, and 5 of them in chronic, accelerated, and blastic phases, respectively, at diagnosis. Of these, 171 (63%) and 101 (37%) were male and female, respectively. Median age was 38 (range, 20–75) years and median follow-up duration was 81 months. Table 1 shows a summary of patient characteristics at diagnosis.

TABLE 1: Summary of clinical parameters of all 272 patients at diagnosis.

Variables	Number	Median	(Range)
Age, years: patient	272	38	(20–75)
Gender: male/female (%)	171/101	(63/37)	
Splenomegaly (cm, BCM)	207	12	(2–38)
Time from diagnosis to imatinib (days)	272	56	(0–2308)
Percent peripheral blasts (%)	112	3	(1–20)
Hematocrit (%)	269	32	(13–49)
WBC ($\times 10^9$/L)	265	83.2	(2.1–710.0)
Platelet count ($\times 10^9$/L)	254	247	(10–1173)
Sokal* score (low/intermediate/high)	78/205	(28/30/20)	
Hasford* score (low/intermediate/high)	73/205	(35/33/5)	

*Sokal and Hasford scores were applicable only for the 205 patients in chronic phase, presenting within 3 months of diagnosis.

Overall survival at 1, 2, and 5 years was 94%, 84%, and 63%, respectively, and correspondingly PFS was 89%, 77%, and 54% (Table 2). At the time of this analysis, median OS and PFS were not yet reached. Using the log-rank statistical test (Mantel-Cox) regression model, with the variables as individual predictors of OS and PFS, revealed that chronic phase disease at diagnosis ($p = 0.030$) and male gender ($p = 0.041$) were associated with significantly better OS (Table 3). Significantly better PFS was associated with the male gender ($p = 0.005$), haematocrit >0.30 ($p = 0.009$), and splenic enlargement of <10 cm at diagnosis ($p = 0.048$). A multivariable Cox regression model using disease phase at diagnosis and gender as predictors for OS revealed that disease phase at diagnosis was the sole significant predictor of OS ($p = 0.035$, OR = 1.995, and 95% CI = 1.049–3.793). Similarly, using gender, hematocrit (>0.30 versus <0.30), and spleen size (>10 versus <10 cm) as predictors for PFS, in a multivariable model, revealed that gender was the sole predictor that attained statistical significance ($p = 0.019$, OR = 1.789, and 95% CI = 1.100–2.911).

3.2. Survival Outcomes for 205 Patients in Chronic Phase. Based on the outcomes of the multivariate analysis, we embarked on a more detailed analysis of patients presenting in the chronic phase. Of the 205 patients in chronic phase, 132 were males and 73 were females. Only 78 of these (38%) and 73 (34%), respectively, could be assessed for risk status using the Sokal and Hasford scoring systems (Table 1). After a median follow-up period of 82 months, OS at 1, 2, and 5 years was 97%, 87%, and 68%, respectively, while correspondingly PFS was 92%, 79%, and 57%, respectively. Expectedly, the median OS and PFS for this subgroup (performing better than the whole cohort) were not yet reached at the time of analysis.

Univariate log-rank statistical test of the impact of variables on survival revealed that patients younger than 42 years and those who achieved complete haematologic remission (CHR) within 30 days of commencing imatinib had better

TABLE 2: Overall and progression-free survival (OS and PFS) of all 272 patients and of 205 patients in chronic phase (CP).

(a)

Variables*	p values, for all 272 adult patients			
Survival statistics	OS	SE	PFS	SE
At 1 year	94%	0.016	89%	0.020
At 2 years	84%	0.027	77%	0.030
At 5 years	63%	0.052	54%	0.053
Median survival	*Not reached yet			

(b)

Variables*	p values, for 205 CP adult patients			
Survival statistics	OS	SE	PFS	SE
At 1 year	97%	0.013	92%	0.020
At 2 years	87%	0.029	79%	0.030
At 5 years	68%	0.059	57%	0.053
Median survival	*Not reached yet			

TABLE 3: Univariate analysis of all 272 patients' characteristics as predictors of overall and progression-free survival.

Parameters at recruitment	Number	OS	PFS
Sex: male/female	171/101	**0.041**	**0.005**
Age (years)			
≤30/>30	68/204	ns	ns
≤38/>38	134/138	ns	ns
≤50/>50	207/65	ns	ns
Hematocrit at diagnosis (%)			
≤30/>30	110/162	0.069	**0.009**
≤35/>35	165/107	0.078	**0.022**
WBC at diagnosis (×10⁹/L)			
≤100/>100	144/128	ns	ns
Platelet count (×10⁹/L)			
≤250/>250	144/128	ns	ns
≤350/>350	187/85	ns	ns
Disease phase at diagnosis			
CP/AP/BP	205/54/5	0.078	ns
CP/Adv	205/59	**0.030**	ns
Spleen (cm, BCM)			
≤10/>10	113/159	ns	**0.048**

p values in bold type are significant; those in regular type are close to significance. The variables with better outcomes are written first. OS, overall survival; PFS, progression-free survival; BCM, below the costal margin; ns, not significant; NA, not applicable.

OS (p = 0.011 and <0.001, resp.) and PFS (p = 0.013 and 0.002, resp.). Additionally, patients presenting with anaemia (haematocrit < 0.30) and hepatomegaly also had worse PFS (p = 0.022 and 0.035; Table 4). Multivariable Cox regression analysis using CHR within 30 days and age (≤42 versus >42 years) as predictors revealed that both variables remained significantly predictive for OS (p < 0.001 and p = 0.015, resp.). Similarly, multivariable analysis of CHR within 30 days, age (≤42 versus >42 years), anaemia (haematocrit ≤0.30 versus >0.30), and hepatomegaly as predictors of PFS

TABLE 4: Univariate analysis of all 205 chronic phase patients' characteristics as predictors of overall and progression-free survival.

Parameters at recruitment	Number	OS	PFS	Number	CCR
Sex: male/female	132/73	ns	0.077	65/39	ns
Age (years)					
≤35/>35	70/135	**0.035**	ns	37/67	ns
≤40/>40	102/103	**0.035**	0.056	54/50	ns
≤42/>42	111/94	**0.011**	**0.013**	60/44	ns
Hematocrit at diagnosis (%)					ns
≤30/>30	76/129	0.098	**0.022**	37/67	ns
≤35/>35	120/85	ns	0.067	58/46	ns
WBC at diagnosis (×10⁹/L)					ns
≤100/>100	144/128	ns	ns	61/43	ns
Platelet count (×10⁹/L)					ns
≤250/>250	144/128	ns	ns	62/42	**0.045**
≤350/>350	187/85	ns	ns		ns
Time-to-imatinib (days)					
>30/≤30	68/137	ns	ns	32/72	ns
>60/≤60	109/96	ns	0.083	49/55	0.083
Time-to-CHR (days)					
≤30/>30	79/126	**<0.001**	**0.002**	16/88	ns
≤90/>90	125/80	**0.010**	**0.049**	50/54	ns
Spleen (cm, BCM)					
Spleen: no/yes	50/155	ns	ns	23/81	ns
≤5/>5	58/147	ns	ns	28/76	ns
≤10/>10	93/112	ns	ns	48/56	ns
Liver (cm, BCM)					
Liver: no/yes	140/65	ns	**0.035**	72/32	ns
≤5/>5	155/50	ns	ns	82/22	ns

p values in bold type are significant; those in regular type are close to significance. The variables with better outcomes are written first. OS, overall survival; PFS, progression-free survival; BCM, below the costal margin; ns, not significant; NA, not applicable; CHR, complete haematologic remission; CCR, complete cytogenetic remission.

revealed that the former three variables remained statistically significant (p = 0.001, 0.010, and 0.012, resp.).

Only 104 of the 205 patients (50.7%) had carried out cytogenetic studies as frequently as desired and could be assessed for complete cytogenetic response (CCR). Only 52 (50%) of these had achieved CCR at any time during therapy. Log-rank regression analysis of factors predicting attainment of CCR revealed that platelet count (≤250 versus >250 × 10⁹/L) was the only variable that was significantly predictive (p = 0.045).

4. Discussion

The results presented have further proven the efficacy of imatinib in the treatment of CML in Nigerians. In terms of demographics, the median age of 38 years is comparable with reports from other sub-Saharan populations and significantly differs from populations in the developed parts of the world [8, 16]. The younger age at presentation remains a controversial issue, as researchers are divided on whether this is a mere reflection of the country demographics or a true difference in population genetics or disease biology.

Expectedly, the survival pattern of patients presenting in chronic phase is better than those in more advanced stages of disease. In our previous report on part of this cohort, when we reviewed the first 98 patients, after a 4-year follow-up, the OS at 2 years was 81%, compared to 84% in the present larger cohort after a 7-year follow-up [7]. The 5-year OS of the patients in chronic phase in this study (68%) is also more accurate, given that the actual follow-up already exceeds 60 months. When compared to our historical cohort [6], this 5-year survival estimate is impressive, though it is significantly inferior to what has been reported from studies in several Western countries [17–19]. In 2008, Hochhaus et al. [17] reported a 6-year OS of 76% among a cohort of 532 late CP-CML patients, managed on imatinib after interferon. Similarly, in their review of 1148 CP-CML patients in 2012, Kantarjian et al. [19] reported an 8-year survival of 87%, among those patients managed during the imatinib era (i.e., after 2001). It is also noteworthy that there has been a significant reduction in the duration of time from diagnosis to commencement of imatinib (median, 56 days) in our patients. In our previous review [7], it was 100 days, while in a recent study by Koffi et al. [8], a duration of 282 days was reported.

Though our patients are younger than their counterparts in the developed world, survival was not adversely affected, especially if imatinib was commenced in the chronic phase of disease. Patients' survival has also improved due to this difference. The availability of other ancillary investigative tools particularly the detection of BCR-ABL1 transcript by PCR can also be said to have impacted positively on when patients are commenced on imatinib.

However, in face of these significant improvements in patient's survival, certain challenges cannot be ignored; our hospital remains the only referral centre in the country for patients to access imatinib freely and many of our patients are domiciled at distant places, making follow-up difficult for some of them. Similarly, access to cytogenetic and molecular testing facilities remains markedly limited. This makes deeper disease monitoring more challenging in this cohort.

In conclusion, imatinib has indeed come to stay as the first-line drug of choice in the management of chronic myeloid leukemia, particularly patients in the chronic phase.

Conflict of Interests

We declare that none of the authors have a conflict of interests.

References

[1] H. Kantarjian, C. Sawyers, A. Hochhaus et al., "Hematologic and cytogenetic responses to imatinib mesylate in chronic myelogenous leukemia," The New England Journal of Medicine, vol. 346, no. 9, pp. 645–652, 2002.

[2] J. V. Melo, T. P. Hughes, and J. F. Apperley, "Chronic myeloid leukemia," The American Society of Hematology, pp. 132–152, 2003.

[3] S. Faderl, H. M. Kantarjian, and M. Talpaz, "Chronic myelogenous leukemia: update on biology and treatment," Oncology, vol. 13, no. 2, pp. 169–180, 1999.

[4] C. L. Sawyers, "Chronic myeloid leukemia," The New England Journal of Medicine, vol. 340, no. 17, pp. 1330–1340, 1999.

[5] C. C. Okany and O. O. Akinyanju, "Chronic leukaemia: an African experience," Medical Oncology and Tumor Pharmacotherapy, vol. 6, no. 3, pp. 189–194, 1989.

[6] P. O. Boma, M. A. Durosinmi, I. A. Adediran, N. O. Akinola, and L. Salawu, "Clinical and prognostic features of Nigerians with chronic myeloid leukemia," The Nigerian Postgraduate Medical Journal, vol. 13, no. 1, pp. 47–52, 2006.

[7] M. A. Durosinmi, J. O. Faluyi, A. A. Oyekunle et al., "The use of Imatinib mesylate (Glivec) in Nigerian patients with chronic myeloid leukemia," Cellular Therapy and Transplantation, vol. 1, no. 2, pp. 58–62, 2008.

[8] K. G. Koffi, D. C. Nanho, E. N'Dathz et al., "The effect of imatinib mesylate for newly diagnosed philadelphia chromosome-positive, chronic-phase myeloid leukemia in sub-saharan african patients: the experience of côte d'ivoire," Advances in Hematology, vol. 2010, Article ID 268921, 6 pages, 2010.

[9] J. E. Sokal, E. B. Cox, M. Baccarani et al., "Prognostic discrimination in 'good-risk' chronic granulocytic leukemia," Blood, vol. 63, no. 4, pp. 789–799, 1984.

[10] J. M. Goldman, "Treatment of chronic myeloid leukaemia lessons and challenges," International Journal of Hematology, vol. 76, supplement 2, pp. 189–192, 2002.

[11] S. G. O'Brien, F. Guilhot, R. A. Larson et al., "Imatinib compared with interferon and low-dose cytarabine for newly diagnosed chronic-phase chronic myeloid leukemia," The New England Journal of Medicine, vol. 348, no. 11, pp. 994–1004, 2003.

[12] B. J. Druker, F. Guilhot, S. G. O'Brien et al., "Long-term benefits of imatinib (IM) for patients newly diagnosed with chronic myelogenous leukemia in chronic phase (CML-CP): the 5-year update from the IRIS study," Journal of Clinical Oncology, vol. 24, no. 18, supplement, abstract 6506, 2006.

[13] A. Oyekunle, E. Klyuchnikov, S. Ocheni et al., "Challenges for allogeneic hematopoietic stem cell transplantation in chronic myeloid Leukemia in the era of tyrosine kinase inhibitors," Acta Haematologica, vol. 126, no. 1, pp. 30–39, 2011.

[14] B. J. Druker, F. Guilhot, S. G. O'Brien et al., "Five-year follow-up of patients receiving imatinib for chronic myeloid leukemia," The New England Journal of Medicine, vol. 355, no. 23, pp. 2408–2417, 2006.

[15] C. Gambacorti-Passerini, L. Antolini, F.-X. Mahon et al., "Multicenter independent assessment of outcomes in chronic myeloid leukemia patients treated with imatinib," Journal of the National Cancer Institute, vol. 103, no. 7, pp. 553–561, 2011.

[16] A. M. Mendizabal, P. Garcia-Gonzalez, and P. H. Levine, "Regional variations in age at diagnosis and overall survival among patients with chronic myeloid leukemia from low and middle income countries," Cancer Epidemiology, vol. 37, no. 3, pp. 247–254, 2013.

[17] A. Hochhaus, B. Druker, C. Sawyers et al., "Favorable long-term follow-up results over 6 years for response, survival, and safety with imatinib mesylate therapy in chronic-phase chronic myeloid leukemia after failure of interferon-α treatment," Blood, vol. 111, no. 3, pp. 1039–1043, 2008.

[18] B. Hanfstein, M. C. Müller, R. Hehlmann et al., "Early molecular and cytogenetic response is predictive for long-term progression-free and overall survival in chronic myeloid leukemia (CML)," *Leukemia*, vol. 26, no. 9, pp. 2096–2102, 2012.

[19] H. Kantarjian, S. O'Brien, E. Jabbour et al., "Improved survival in chronic myeloid leukemia since the introduction of imatinib therapy: a single-institution historical experience," *Blood*, vol. 119, no. 9, pp. 1981–1987, 2012.

32

RhD Specific Antibodies Are Not Detectable in HLA-DRB1*1501 Mice Challenged with Human RhD Positive Erythrocytes

Lidice Bernardo,[1,2] **Gregory A. Denomme,**[3] **Kunjlata Shah,**[4] **and Alan H. Lazarus**[1,2,5]

[1] *The Canadian Blood Services, Canada*

[2] *Department of Laboratory Medicine and the Keenan Research Centre in the Li Ka Shing Knowledge Institute of St. Michael's Hospital, 30 Bond Street, Toronto, ON, Canada M5B 1W8*

[3] *Immunohematology Reference Laboratory, BloodCenter of Wisconsin, Milwaukee, WI 53226, USA*

[4] *Department of Transfusion Medicine, St. Michael's Hospital, Toronto, ON, Canada M5B 1W8*

[5] *Departments of Medicine and Laboratory Medicine & Pathobiology, University of Toronto, Toronto, ON, Canada*

Correspondence should be addressed to Alan H. Lazarus; lazarusa@smh.ca

Academic Editor: Thomas Kickler

The ability to study the immune response to the RhD antigen in the prevention of hemolytic disease of the fetus and newborn has been hampered by the lack of a mouse model of RhD immunization. However, the ability of transgenic mice expressing human HLA DRB1*1501 to respond to immunization with purified RhD has allowed this question to be revisited. In this work we aimed at inducing anti-RhD antibodies by administering human RhD$^+$ RBCs to mice transgenic for the human HLA DRB1*1501 as well as to several standard inbred and outbred laboratory strains including C57BL/6, DBA1/J, CFW(SW), CD1(ICR), and NSA(CF-1). DRB1*1501 mice were additionally immunized with putative extracellular immunogenic RhD peptides. DRB1*1501 mice immunized with RhD$^+$ erythrocytes developed an erythrocyte-reactive antibody response. Antibodies specific for RhD could not however be detected by flow cytometry. Despite this, DRB1*1501 mice were capable of recognizing immunogenic sequences of Rh as injection with Rh peptides induced antibodies reactive with RhD sequences, consistent with the presence of B cell repertoires capable of recognizing RhD. We conclude that while HLA DRB1*1501 transgenic mice may have the capability of responding to immunogenic sequences within RhD, an immune response to human RBC expressing RhD is not directly observed.

1. Introduction

The RhD antigen is a clinically important human blood group that can be a primary target in hemolytic disease of the fetus and newborn (HDFN) as well as some cases of autoimmune hemolytic anemia. Antibodies to RhD (anti-D) have been used for many years to prevent HDFN. The ability to manipulate and study the immune response to the RhD antigen in the prevention of HDFN has been hampered by the lack of a murine model to study this antigen. Although never formally published, it has been generally considered that standard laboratory mice do not make an immune response to the RhD antigen [1]. However, the more recent ability of creating transgenic mice expressing functional human HLA antigens has allowed this question to be revisited in a murine model.

The Aberdeen group has successfully induced an immune response to solubilized RhD protein in humanized mice that express the human HLA-DRB1*1501 allele [1]. Human HLA class II DR has been found as a major restricting element for human T-helper cells specific for RhD protein [2], and the HLA-DRB1*1501 allele is significantly overrepresented in RhD negative donors who have produced anti-RhD antibodies in response to RhD-positive RBCs [3]. In particular, the expression of the HLA DRB1*1501 transgene was found to confer on mice the ability to respond to immunization with purified RhD protein [1].

In addition to being able to stimulate an immune response, T cell epitopes derived from RhD protein sequences were also shown to induce oral tolerance to the RhD antigen in the HLA-DRB1*1501 murine model. While an immune response to purified RhD protein is of interest, the ability of

TABLE 1: Amino acid sequence and properties of the RhD peptides synthesized.

Peptide #	Amino acids	Sequence	M.W.	Sequence identity with RhCE	Net charge (pH 7)
1	34–46	YDASLEDQKGLVAC*	1510.68	100%	−1
2	228–238	LRSPIERKNAVC*	1384.66	82%	3
3	350–358	DTVGAGNGMRRC*a	1235.40	67%	2
4	97–111	FLSQFPSGKVVITLFC*	1785.17	93%	2

*A cysteine was added at the C-terminus for conjugation purposes.
aTwo arginines (R) were added to peptide 3 to increase its solubility.

an immune response to be generated to naturally expressed RhD on the surface of red cells is needed to move forward with relevant murine models. Thus far, an immune response to RhD expressed on the surface of erythrocytes in mice expressing HLA-DRB1*1501 has not yet been addressed.

In this work we aimed at inducing an anti-RhD antibody response by administering human RBCs expressing RhD in mice expressing HLA DRB1*1501 [4]. It is important to mention that the HLA DRB1*1501 mouse strain used here is different from the one used by Hall and his collaborators in 2005. Specifically, the HLA DRB1*1501 mice used in our study lack the expression of functional murine MHC class II, forcing the restricting element for immune responses through HLA DRB1*1501 [4]. In addition, conventional inbred and outbred mouse strains were also challenged with human RhD-positive RBCs to formally assess if standard strains of mice can generate anti-RhD specific antibody responses.

The results showed that when HLA DRB1*1501 transgenic mice are challenged with RhD positive RBC under a variety of conditions, despite the development of an immune response to the red cells, no antibodies to RhD were detected by flow cytometry. However, the results of the peptide studies were consistent with the presence of a B cell repertoire capable of recognizing each of the three immunogenic sequences evaluated. We conclude that while HLA DRB1*1501 transgenic mice have the capability of responding to sequences from RhD, an immune response specific for human RBC expressing RhD is not directly observed.

2. Materials and Methods

2.1. Mice. HLA-DRB1*1501 transgenic mice expressing the human HLA-DRB1*1501 allele, without endogenous class II molecules, were kindly provided by Dr. Chella David (Mayo Medical School, Rochester, MN, USA) [4]. The only functional class II molecules on DRB1*1501 antigen-presenting cells are the human class II molecules. C57BL/6 and DBA1/J mouse strains were purchased from Jackson Laboratory (Bar Harbor, ME. USA). Outbred mouse strains CFW(SW) and CD1(ICR) were purchased from Charles River (Montreal, QC, Canada) while NSA(CF-1) was bought from Harlan Sprague Dawley Inc. (Indianapolis, IN, USA). All mouse work was approved by the St Michael's Hospital animal care committee and mice were housed in the St Michael's Hospital Research Vivarium.

2.2. Immunization of Mice with Human Red Blood Cells. Whole blood and fully leukoreduced RBC units were obtained from The Canadian Blood Services Network Centre for Applied Development (NetCAD) and the work was approved by The Canadian Blood Services Research Ethics Board. Before immunization, RBCs taken from the units were washed three times in phosphate-buffered saline (PBS), pH 7.2, and counted using Guava EasyCyte Mini System cell analyzer (Guava Technologies, Hayward, CA, USA). Mice were challenged with one dose of 10^8 human RhD positive RBCs (DRB1*1501n = 4, C57BL/6 n = 3, DBA1/J n = 2, CFW(SW) n = 3, CD1(ICR) n = 4, NSA(CF-1) n = 4). DRB1*1501 mice were additionally immunized with 10^8 human RhD positive RBCs in the presence of CpG ODN adjuvant (Magic Mouse Adjuvant, Creative Diagnostics, NY, USA) (n = 2), or with two doses of 10^8 human RhD positive RBCs administered 21 days apart without adjuvant (n = 2). Untreated mice were used as negative controls (n = 2). All the mice were bled for serum fifteen days after the first or seven days after the second challenge.

2.3. RhD Peptide Design and Immunization. Peptides were designed and selected according to the human RhD sequence published in gene bank (accession number L08429). Putative linear epitopes were predicted using the antibody epitope prediction tool of the Immune Epitope Data Base (IEDB) Analysis Resource (http://tools.immunee-pitope.org/tools/bcell/iedb_input). Four peptides that theoretically correspond to extracellular regions of the human RhD protein and that are different in sequence from mouse RhD [5] were selected (Table 1, Figure 1). Peptides were synthesized by Peptides International and shipped lyophilized (Louisville, Kentucky, USA). Peptides 1 to 3 were successfully solubilized in 1 M ammonium bicarbonate. Unfortunately, peptide 4 was not soluble in up to 10% organic solvent and was therefore not used. Peptides 1 to 3 were successfully linked to Keyhole Limpet Haemocyanin (KLH) (Sigma-Aldrich, St Louis, MO, USA) using a cysteine added at the C-terminus and Sulfo-SMCC (4-(N-Maleimidomethyl) cyclohexane-1-carboxylic acid 3-sulfo-N-hydroxysuccinimide ester sodium salt) (Sigma-Aldrich, St Louis, MO, USA) used as a cross-linker. The coupling efficiency of the cysteine containing peptides to KLH was determined by a cysteine assay using 5,5′-Dithiobis(2-nitrobenzoic acid) (DTNB or Ellman's reagent) which reacts with sulfhydryl groups at pH 8.0 to produce

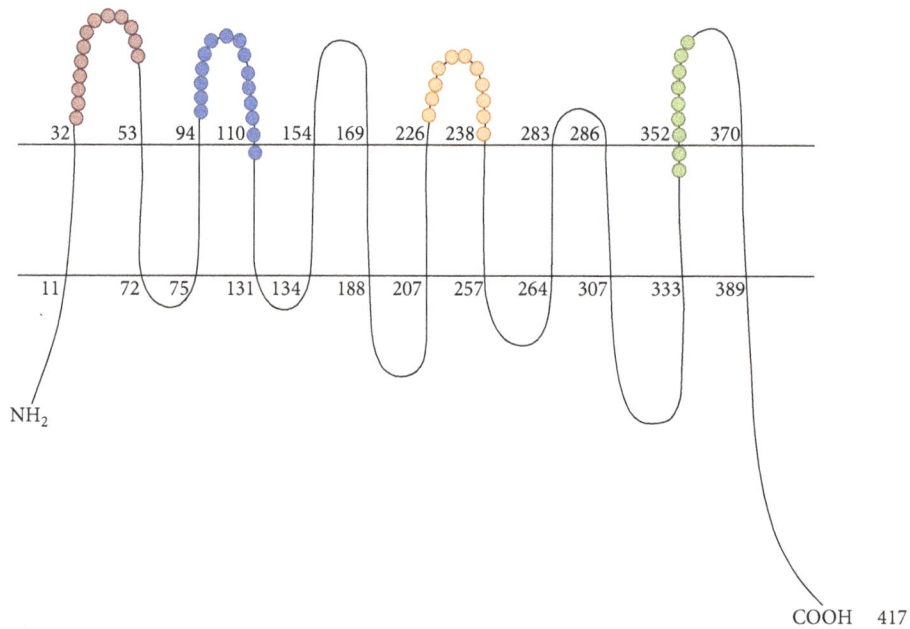

(a)

(b)

FIGURE 1: Predicted topographic features of the RhD protein (a) [5, 13] and alignment of human RHD, human RHCE, and mouse RHD sequences (b). Peptides 1–4 are highlighted in colors. Peptide 1: red; Peptide 2: orange; Peptide 3: green; Peptide 4: blue.

a chromophore with maximum absorption at 412 nm. The coupling efficiency was then calculated by measuring the concentration of the initial and residual cysteine-peptide in the assay mixture from a standard curve of cysteine (Sigma-Aldrich, St Louis, MO, USA). DRB1*1501 mice were separately immunized with three doses of 50 μg of peptide 1, 2, or 3 coupled to KLH and emulsified in Freund's adjuvant (complete Freund's adjuvant for the first dose and incomplete for the second and third) (Sigma-Aldrich, St Louis, MO,

USA), administered 14 days apart (2 mice per peptide). Mice were bled via the saphenous vein at the indicated times and serum was collected for detecting anti-peptide, anti-KLH, and anti-human RBC antibodies.

2.4. Analysis of the Antibody Response to RhD Peptides. To detect antibodies against the synthetic peptides themselves, ELISA plates (Cat # 07-200-35, Thermo Fisher Scientific Inc.,

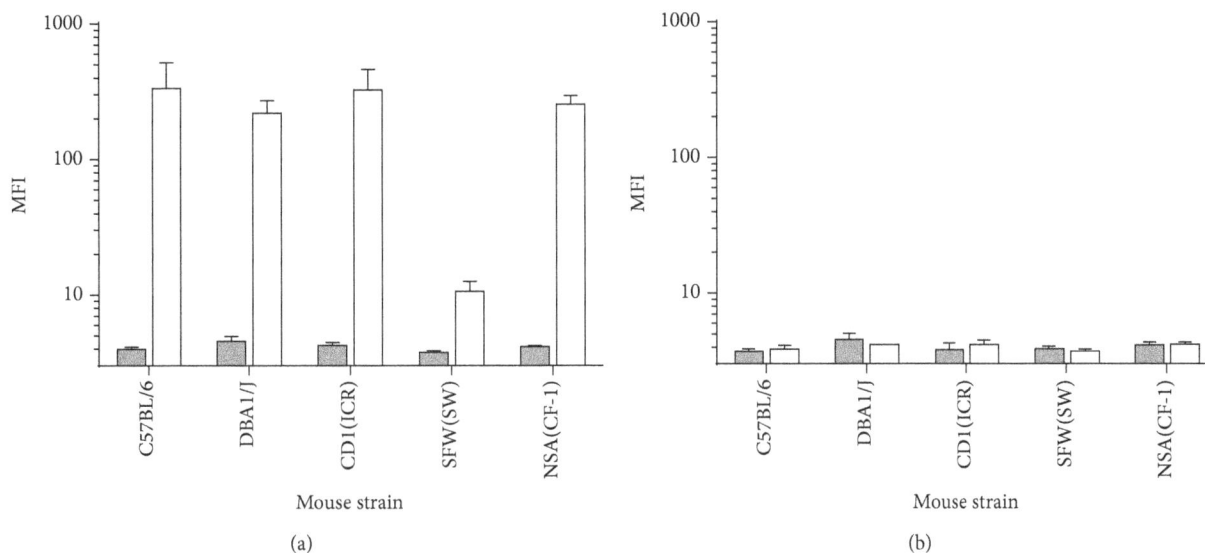

FIGURE 2: Immunization of standard laboratory mice with human RhD positive RBC induces RBC-reactive but not RhD-specific IgG as detected by flow cytometry. Conventional inbred and outbred mice were immunized with a single dose of 10^8 RhD positive RBC (blood group A) (white bars) (C57BL/6 $n = 3$, DBA1/J $n = 2$, CFW(SW) $n = 3$, CD1(ICR) $n = 4$, NSA(CF-1) $n = 4$). Untreated mice were used as negative controls (grey bars) ($n = 2$). (a) Antibodies reactive with human RhD positive RBC (blood group A). (b) Antibody binding to RhD positive RBC after adsorbing the sera with human RhD$^-$ cells (blood group A). MFI: mean fluorescence intensity.

MA, USA) were coated with 10 μg/mL of the corresponding peptide in PBS. After overnight incubation at 4°C, plates were washed with 0.05% Tween 20 in PBS and blocked with 2% (wt/vol) bovine serum albumin (BSA) (Sigma-Aldrich, St Louis, MO, USA) in PBS for 2 hours at 22°C. After washing, serum samples (end point dilutions) were then added and incubated at 22°C for 1.5 hours. The plates were then washed and incubated with alkaline phosphatase F(ab')$_2$ fragment goat anti-mouse IgG, Fcγ fragment specific (Jackson Immunoresearch Laboratories, IN, USA). After 1 hour of incubation at 22°C, plates were washed again and 1 mg/mL p-nitrophenyl phosphate (Sigma-Aldrich, St Louis, MO, USA) in 0.001 mol/L MgCl$_2$, 9.7% diethanolamine, pH 9.6, was added to the plates. Plates were read by an ELISA reader at 405 nm after 15 to 30 minutes. Antibody titers were defined as the highest serum dilution that showed a positive value.

2.5. Analysis of the RBC-Specific Antibody Response. Sera from mice challenged with human RhD positive RBC were tested for antibodies using RhD positive and RhD negative RBC by flow cytometry [6]. RBCs were washed three times in PBS, pH 7.2, and 2×10^6 cells incubated with 20 μL of serum diluted to 1/100 at 22°C for 1 hour, followed by 2.5 μg/mL goat F(ab')$_2$ anti-mouse IgG (FITC conjugated) before analyzing by a Guava EasyCyte Mini System cell analyzer. To selectively detect RhD specific antibodies, the sera were first adsorbed with RhD negative RBC followed by an assessment of binding to RhD positive RBC. Serum adsorptions were performed by incubating packed RhD negative RBC with sera at 22°C for 1 hour under shaking conditions. Tubes were then centrifuged and the supernatant containing the serum dilutions was collected. A second adsorption cycle was also done at 4°C.

Adsorbed serum dilutions were assessed against human RhD positive RBC as above. Human polyclonal anti-D serum (WINRHO, Cangene bioPharma Inc., MD, USA) was used as a positive control.

3. Results

3.1. Response of Selected Standard Mice to Immunization with Human RhD Positive Red Blood Cells. Although it has been considered that standard laboratory mice do not make an immune response to the RhD antigen [1], there is no published data that we are aware of regarding the immune response to the RhD antigen when mice are challenged with human RBCs. To address this, some of the most commonly used inbred and outbred (Swiss and non-Swiss origin) mouse strains were challenged with human RhD positive RBCs and the antibodies reactive with human RBC as well as RhD specific antibodies were evaluated by flow cytometry. With the exception of SFW(SW), all the mouse strains tested [C57BL/6 (H2^b), DBA/1J (H2^q), CD1(ICR), and NSA(CF-1)] developed high levels of IgG antibodies reactive with human RhD positive RBC (Figure 2(a)). However, reactivity against human RhD positive RBC was not detected when sera were first adsorbed with RhD negative RBCs (Figure 2(b)), indicating that significant levels of RhD specific antibodies could not be detected.

The antibody response of SFW(SW) mice to human RBCs was particularly low. A potential explanation is that this strain contains a deletion in the promoter region of *H2-Ea* (which encodes the alpha chain of the MHC class II E$\alpha\beta$ heterodimer), which strongly contributes to setting the ratio of CD4+ and CD8+ lymphocytes [7].

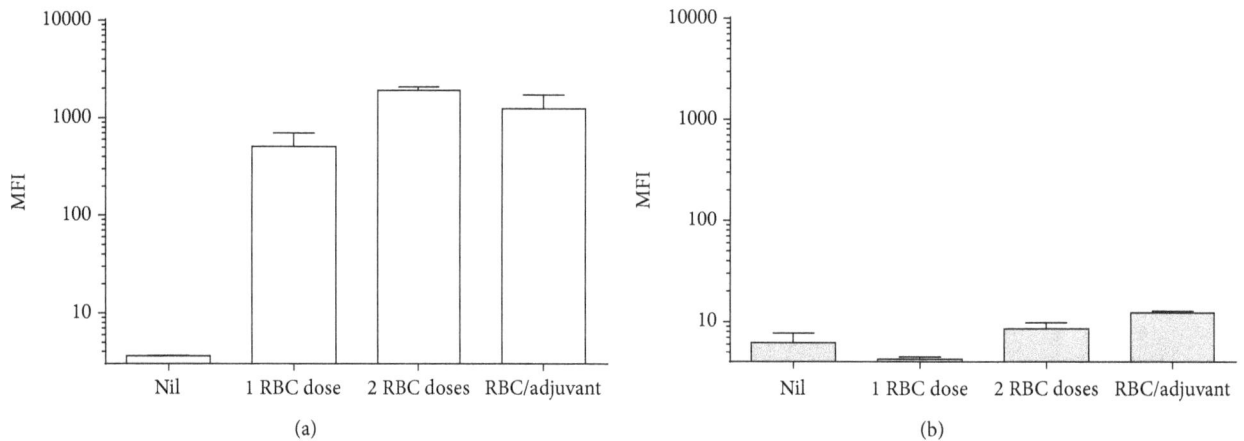

FIGURE 3: Immunization of DRB1*1501 mice with human RhD positive RBCs induces RBC-reactive but not RhD-specific IgG as detected by flow cytometry. DRB1*1501 mice were challenged with one ($n = 4$) or two doses of 10^8 RhD positive RBC ($n = 2$) or 1 dose of 10^8 RhD positive RBC emulsified in CpG ODN adjuvant ($n = 2$). Untreated mice were used as negative controls (Nil) ($n = 2$). (a) Detection of IgG reactive with human RhD positive RBC. (b) Detection of IgG reactive with human RhD positive RBC after adsorbing the sera with RhD negative cells. MFI: mean fluorescence intensity.

3.2. Immunization of HLA-DRB1*1501 Transgenic Mice with Human RhD Positive Red Blood Cells.

Considering that the expression of the HLA DRB1*1501 transgene was previously found to confer on mice the ability to respond to immunization with purified RhD protein [1], we examined HLA DRB1*1501 transgenic mice for an immune response by challenging these mice with human RhD positive RBC. Mice were challenged with one or two doses of 10^8 human RhD positive RBC administered 21 days apart, or the same number of cells in the presence of the CpG ODN adjuvant. HLA-DRB1*1501 mice developed antibodies reactive with human RBC after challenge and the administration of two immunizations or the use of adjuvant increased the magnitude of the antibody response (Figure 3(a)). However, when sera produced from these mice were first adsorbed with RhD negative RBCs, antibodies specific for RhD could not be detected (Figure 3(b)).

3.3. Immunization of HLA-DRB1*1501 Transgenic Mice with Synthetic Peptides Corresponding to Human RhD Sequences.

As in no case was there evidence that HLA-DRB1*1501 mice were capable of making a humoral immune response specific for the RhD antigen on the surface of red cells, we performed experiments with peptides from putative immunogenic regions of RhD to evaluate if these mice possess an appropriate B cell repertoire reactive with human RhD. Based on the predicted structure of the RhD protein on the RBC membrane (Figure 1), we synthesized four peptides that contain putative extracellular immunogenic regions of RhD. It is important to note that peptide 1 is identical between both Rh gene loci (RHD and RHCE) while peptides 2 and 3 displayed 82% and 67% sequence identity between RHD and RHCE, respectively. HLA-DRB1*1501 transgenic mice were then challenged with three doses of peptide 1, 2, or 3 conjugated to KLH. The fourth peptide was insoluble

in buffers compatible for KLH conjugation and was not evaluated.

Anti-peptide antibodies were successfully raised in HLA-DRB1*1501 mice from the sera collected 28 and 35 days after immunization; as detected by ELISA, using the immunizing peptides as antigens (Figure 4).

4. Discussion

Our studies provide evidence that selected inbred and outbred laboratory mice do not make an antibody response specific for naturally expressed human RhD. When we challenged standard inbred ($H2^b$ and $H2^q$) and outbred mice with human RhD positive RBC, the mice responded to the human RBC but antibodies specific for RhD protein were not observed from any of the mouse strains tested, despite using multiple RBC exposures or the addition of adjuvant to potentiate the immune response. Different incubation temperatures were also evaluated (data not shown). To the best of our knowledge, this is the first published study to show that selected conventional mice injected with human RBC do not develop antibodies specific to RhD protein detectable by flow cytometry.

An important consideration for the immunogenicity of the human RhD protein in mice is the degree of sequence homology with the mouse Rh protein. In the mouse, Rh protein is encoded by a single RH gene on chromosome 4 and exhibits only 60% sequence identity to the human proteins [8], which does not explain the lack of responsiveness to human Rh proteins. For instance, human RhD and RhCE are homologous proteins that have more than 90% sequence identity and still exposure to RhD can result in a potent immune response in a D-negative individual (RhC positive) [9–11].

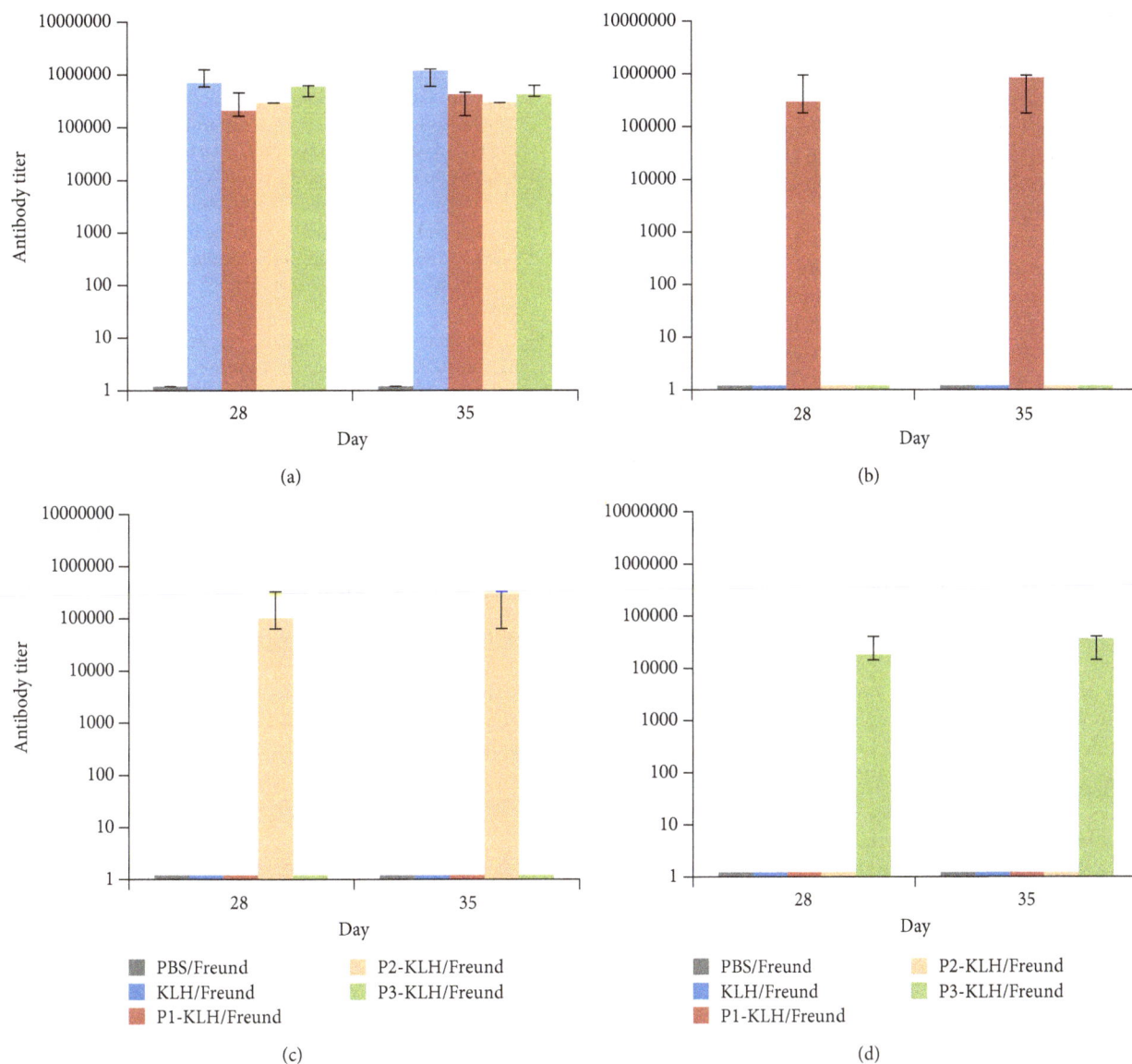

FIGURE 4: Immunization of DRB1*1501 mice with KLH-conjugated synthetic RhD peptides induces peptide specific IgG. Mice were immunized with each peptide (P) conjugated to KLH in Freund's adjuvant as indicated in Materials and Methods (2 mice per peptide). Detection of IgG specific for KLH (a), peptide 1 (b), peptide 2 (c), or peptide 3 (d) was assessed by ELISA. The sera tested were collected at days 28 and 35 (i.e., 14 days after 2nd and 7 days after the 3rd immunization, resp.).

A likely explanation could be that standard mice do not have the proper B or T cell repertoire to respond to the RhD protein. However, it has been previously demonstrated that mice transgenic for HLA DRB1*1501 respond to immunization with RhD purified protein [1], demonstrating that at least these mice (capable of expressing both human HLA-DRB1*1501 and murine MHC class II) have B cells specific for RhD epitopes. Conversely, when we challenged mice expressing only human HLA-DRB1*1501 with intact human RhD positive RBCs, antibodies specific to RhD were not observed though these mice successfully developed antibodies reactive with human RBCs. It could be possible that the naturally expressed human RhD protein is not a sufficiently dominant antigen in mice to generate a response.

B or T cell lymphocyte responses are usually limited to a small proportion of the potential determinants on a protein antigen. Thus, when mice are challenged with human RBC expressing a variety of foreign proteins, the RhD protein could behave as a cryptic antigen. It is also likely that the antibody response to the RhD protein may be very low and that the flow cytometry assay is not sensitive enough to detect it. While flow cytometry has the advantage of measuring antibodies against the naturally expressed antigen on the red blood cell, it needs at least 100 molecules bound per cell to be detectable [12].

To confirm if mice expressing only HLA DRB1*1501 as a potential restricting element have the proper B cell repertoire to respond to human RhD sequences, these mice were challenged with RhD synthetic peptides. An anti-peptide specific antibody response was successfully induced after immunizing HLA DRB1*1501 mice with RhD synthetic peptides. These results are consistent with DRB1*1501 mice having a B and T cell repertoire able to recognize Rh immunogenic peptides and help demonstrate that the DRB1*1501 allele can theoretically be a restriction element for immune responses to RhD protein [1].

Although anti-D prophylaxis has been used to prevent HDFN in clinical medicine for more than four decades, the mechanism of action is still unclear. The lack of a mouse model of anti-D immunization has limited the study of HDFN to the RhD antigen as well as the protective mechanism of anti-D. However, naturally expressed human RhD proved to be poorly immunogenic in mice and, as a result, there remains a need for a relevant murine model.

A better understanding of the antigenic properties of RhD in mice will be helpful in designing future experiments to study the immune response to Rh. We have demonstrated herein that neither selected wild-type nor DRB1*1501 transgenic mice produce significant levels of anti-RhD specific antibodies in response to immunization with human RhD positive RBC, though these mice possess the B cell repertoire necessary for a response. The contribution of antigen dominance to RhD immunization may be a hurdle to overcome and would be a worthy next step to be addressed in detail.

Conflict of Interests

The authors declare that there is no conflict of interests regarding the publication of this paper.

Acknowledgments

The authors thank Dr. Chella David (Mayo Clinic, Rochester, MN, USA) for kindly providing the DRB1*1501 transgenic mice. They also thank the Canadian Blood Services Network Centre for Applied Development (NetCAD) staff and blood-for-research donor volunteers for providing the red blood cell units. All authors contributed significantly to the design of the experiments, the analysis of the data, and the writing and criticism of the paper. This work was supported by a grant from the Canadian Blood Services, Canadian Institutes of Health Research Request for Proposals program to Alan H. Lazarus. Lidice Bernardo is supported by a postdoctoral fellowship from the Canadian Blood Services. The views expressed herein do not necessarily represent the view of the federal government of Canada.

References

[1] A. M. Hall, L. S. Cairns, D. M. Altmann, R. N. Barker, and S. J. Urbaniak, "Immune responses and tolerance to the RhD blood group protein in HLA-transgenic mice," *Blood*, vol. 105, no. 5, pp. 2175–2179, 2005.

[2] L.-M. Stott, R. N. Barker, and S. J. Urbaniak, "Identification of alloreactive T-cell epitopes on the Rhesus D protein," *Blood*, vol. 96, no. 13, pp. 4011–4019, 2000.

[3] S. J. Urbaniak, "Alloimmunity to human red blood cell antigens," *Vox Sanguinis*, vol. 83, supplement s1, pp. 293–297, 2002.

[4] M. Khare, A. Mangalam, M. Rodriguez, and C. S. David, "HLA DR and DQ interaction in myelin oligodendrocyte glycoprotein-induced experimental autoimmune encephalomyelitis in HLA class II transgenic mice," *Journal of Neuroimmunology*, vol. 169, no. 1-2, pp. 1–12, 2005.

[5] C. L. van Kim, I. Mouro, B. Cherif-Zahar et al., "Molecular cloning and primary structure of the human blood group RhD polypeptide," *Proceedings of the National Academy of Sciences of the United States of America*, vol. 89, no. 22, pp. 10925–10929, 1992.

[6] J. Freedman and A. H. Lazarus, "Applications of flow cytometry in transfusion medicine," *Transfusion Medicine Reviews*, vol. 9, no. 2, pp. 87–109, 1995.

[7] B. Yalcin, J. Nicod, A. Bhomra et al., "Commercially available outbred mice for genome-wide association studies," *PLoS Genetics*, vol. 6, no. 9, Article ID e1001085, 2010.

[8] Z. Liu and C. H. Huang, "The mouse Rh11 and Rhag genes: Sequence, organization, expression, and chromosomal mapping," *Biochemical Genetics*, vol. 37, no. 3-4, pp. 119–138, 1999.

[9] C. M. Westhoff, "The structure and function of the Rh antigen complex," *Seminars in Hematology*, vol. 44, no. 1, pp. 42–50, 2007.

[10] S. Simsek, C. A. de Jong, H. T. Cuijpers et al., "Sequence analysis of cDNA derived from reticulocyte mRNAs coding for Rh polypeptides and demonstration of E/e and C/c polymorphisms," *Vox Sanguinis*, vol. 67, no. 2, pp. 203–209, 1994.

[11] W. A. Flegel, "Molecular genetics of RH and its clinical application," *Transfusion Clinique et Biologique*, vol. 13, no. 1-2, pp. 4–12, 2006.

[12] H. Zola, "High-sensitivity immunofluorescence/flow cytometry: detection of cytokine receptors and other low-abundance membrane molecules," in *Current Protocols in Cytometry*, Chapter 6: Unit 3, 2004.

[13] M. A. Arce, E. S. Thompson, S. Wagner, K. E. Coyne, B. A. Ferdman, and D. M. Lublin, "Molecular cloning of RhD cDNA derived from a gene present in RhD-positive, but not RhD-negative individuals," *Blood*, vol. 82, no. 2, pp. 651–655, 1993.

33

Update on Edoxaban for the Prevention and Treatment of Thromboembolism: Clinical Applications Based on Current Evidence

Ali Zalpour[1] and Thein Hlaing Oo[2]

[1]*University of Texas MD Anderson Cancer Center, 1400 Pressler Avenue, Unit 1465, FCT 13.5021, Houston, TX 77030, USA*
[2]*Section of Thrombosis & Benign Hematology, The University of Texas MD Anderson Cancer Center, Houston, TX, USA*

Correspondence should be addressed to Ali Zalpour; azalpour@mdanderson.org

Academic Editor: Elvira Grandone

Vitamin K antagonists (VKA) and heparins have been utilized for the prevention and treatment of thromboembolism (arterial and venous) for decades. Targeting and inhibiting specific coagulation factors have led to new discoveries in the pharmacotherapy of thromboembolism management. These targeted anticoagulants are known as direct oral anticoagulants (DOACs). Two pharmacologically distinct classes of targeted agents are dabigatran etexilate (Direct Thrombin Inhibitor (DTI)) and rivaroxaban, apixaban, and edoxaban (direct oral factor Xa inhibitors (OFXaIs)). Emerging evidence from the clinical trials has shown that DOACs are noninferior to VKA or low-molecular-weight heparins in the prevention and treatment of thromboembolism. This review examines the role of edoxaban, a recently approved OFXaI, in the prevention and treatment of thromboembolism based on the available published literature. The management of edoxaban in the perioperative setting, reversibility in bleeding cases, its role in cancer patients, the relevance of drug-drug interactions, patient satisfaction, financial impacts, and patient education will be discussed.

1. Introduction

Unfractionated heparin (UFH), a highly sulfated naturally occurring glycosaminoglycan, was discovered in Howell's laboratories in the early 1920s. Sweet clover disease or hemorrhagic disease of the cattle in Wisconsin led to the discovery of coumarin. Since then, warfarin has become one of the mostly used antithrombotic agents [1]. Low-molecular-weight heparin (LMWH) was also discovered in the late 1970s and early 1980s as clinicians sought longer acting heparins with a more predicable pharmacokinetic profile. UFH requires frequent monitoring and administration in a hospital setting and carries a risk of heparin-induced thrombocytopenia (HIT). Warfarin demonstrates unpredictable pharmacodynamic (PD) and pharmacokinetic (PK) properties and numerous drug-drug and drug-food interactions and requires frequent international normalized ratio (INR) monitoring. In the past decade, an injectable factor Xa inhibitor, fondaparinux, was introduced. LMWH and fondaparinux exhibit a more predictable PK and PD profile, but patients are subjected to injections that can be burdensome [2].

Advances in pharmacology and drug design therapy have led to the development and introduction of DOACs such as dabigatran, rivaroxaban, apixaban, and edoxaban [3–5]. DOACs have been approved for the prevention of stroke in nonalular atrial fibrillation (NVAF) and the prevention and treatment of venous thromboembolism (VTE). Numerous trials have shown noninferiority of DOACs compared to standard-of-care (SOC) anticoagulants. DOACs have eased the burden of frequent monitoring and painful injections, curtailed food and drug interactions, reduced cost, and achieved higher degree of patient satisfaction [6, 7].

2. Physiology of Hemostasis and Pharmacology of Edoxaban

Coagulation cascade is a multistep interaction characterized by the sequential activation of coagulation factor proteins and

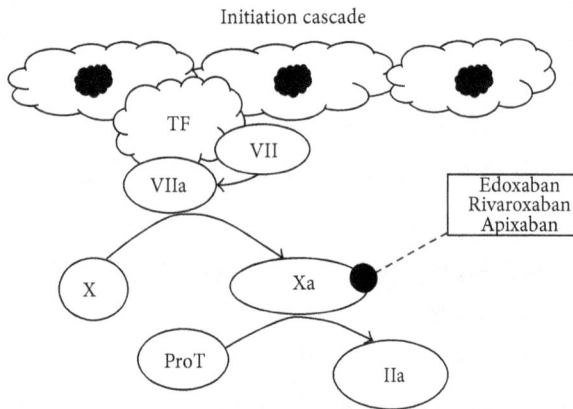

FIGURE 1: Adapted with permission: Zalpour and Oo [8]. Abbreviations: TF, tissue factor; VII, factor VII; VIIa, activated factor VII; X, factor X; Xa, activated factor X; ProT, prothrombin; IIa, thrombin; IX, factor IX; IXa, activated factor IX; Xa, activated factor X; Va, activated factor V; VIIIa, activated factor VIII; vWF, Von Willebrand factor.

their interactions with platelets [9]. Preserving hemostasis is an intricate process following the activation of intrinsic (contact activation) or extrinsic (tissue factor) pathways [10, 11]. The initiation phase of the coagulation involves the generation of tissue factor (TF) which subsequently leads to the activation of factors FVIIa and FXa and the generation of FIIa (thrombin). In the amplification and propagation phases, thrombin activates platelets and, in sequence, factors VIIIa and IXa. Platelet activation induces a surge in thrombin generation leading to the clot formation within the vasculature [12]. The vitamin K antagonist inhibits factors II, VII, XI, and X and proteins C, S, and Z [13]. Heparins inactivate FIIa and FXa via binding their saccharide chain to antithrombin (AT) [14]. FXa is considered a great target for inhibition, as one molecule of FXa can generate approximately 1,000 molecules of thrombin [15]. Edoxaban inhibits thrombin generation by actively inhibiting free and bound FXa in the prothrombinase complex. This inhibition leads to halting of positive feedback loop existing between FXa and FIIa (Figures 1 and 2). The capability of edoxaban to penetrate into the thrombus and rendering free and bound FXa inactive is proven to be beneficial, for the need for AT-drug complex is diminished [12].

3. Pharmacodynamics and Pharmacokinetics of Edoxaban

Edoxaban (molecular weight 838.274 gram/mol) exhibits a high affinity (>10,000-fold) to inhibit FXa without the need of binding to antithrombin and has a low affinity for FIIa [16]. Edoxaban is 55% protein bound and not completely removed by dialysis. The absorption of edoxaban from the gastrointestinal tract is about 60% and food has minimal effect on systemic exposure of area under the curve (AUC) [17]. Edoxaban reaches a maximum concentration in 1-2

hours and has a low volume of distribution of ~19.9 liters. In a phase 1 PK study of edoxaban, the $T_{1/2}$ was 5.71 to 10.7 hours after a single dose administration ranging from 10 mg to 150 mg and 8.75 to 9.75 hours after multiple doses of edoxaban ranging from 90 mg to 120 mg daily [18]. The mean elimination half-life of edoxaban is estimated in the range of 10–14 hours and reaches a steady state concentration in 72 hours. Edoxaban is metabolized via hydrolysis with minimal enzymatic pathways of liver (CYP metabolism is less than 4%). Human carboxylesterase 1 (hCE-1) forms M4, a major metabolite of edoxaban, which is pharmacologically active. M4 reaches less than 10% of the exposure of the parent compound in healthy subjects. Exposure to the other metabolites of edoxaban is less than 5%. Edoxaban elimination is 50% via renal route and 50% via biliary and intestinal route [19]. Age has no direct effect on the PK of edoxaban; however, in patients with body weight less than 60 kilograms, there is an increase in exposure [20]. In a PK simulation study of 278 patients from phase 1 trials, the bioavailability (F) was estimated to be 67.2% in a dose ranging from 10 to 30 mg. Female patients exhibited 13.1% lower clearance (CL) than males. AUC_{∞} in females was higher than that in males as the dose of edoxaban increased from 10 mg to 180 mg; for example, in the edoxaban 90 mg, AUC_{∞} is 3,385 (ng*h/mL) in male patients and 3,893 (ng*h/mL) in female patients, respectively. The clinical significance of these findings has not been validated in clinical trials (Table 1) [21].

3.1. Pharmacodynamics and Pharmacokinetics of Edoxaban in Patients with Liver Dysfunction. The presence of encephalopathy or ascites (clinical parameters) along with serum albumin, serum bilirubin, and prothrombin time (laboratory parameters) collectively classifies patients into three distinct groups of liver diseases: Child-Pugh A (mild), Child-Pugh B (moderate), and Child-Pugh C (severe). Patients with Child-Pugh C class are typically excluded from the clinical trials involving anticoagulation due to excess bleeding risk [39]. In a hepatic impairment study (Child-Pugh A, n = 8; Child-Pugh B, n = 8) matched for healthy patients (n = 16), after the administration of single oral dose of edoxaban 15 mg, compared to healthy subjects, the AUC_{∞} decreased by 4.2% in subjects with Child-Pugh A and 4.8% in subjects with Child-Pugh B. The peak serum concentration (C_{max}) decreased by 10% and 32% in patients with Child-Pugh A and Child-Pugh B, respectively [40]. Currently, no PK data exists for edoxaban use in patients with Child-Pugh C and the use of edoxaban in patients with moderate or severe hepatic impairment (Child-Pugh B and Child-Pugh C) is not recommended as these patients may have intrinsic coagulation abnormalities [17].

3.2. Pharmacodynamics and Pharmacokinetics of Edoxaban in Patients with Renal Dysfunction. Patients with end stage renal disease (ESRD) are typically excluded from the edoxaban clinical trials, because of increased bleeding risk. For patients with ESRD who may require anticoagulation, VKA and UFH are the anticoagulants of choice [41]. All OFX-aIs have some degree of renal elimination: apixaban 27%,

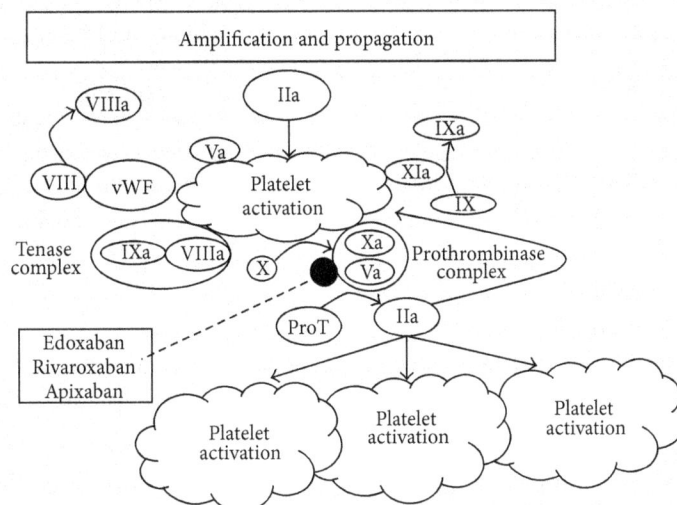

FIGURE 2: Adapted with permission: Zalpour and Oo [8]. Abbreviations: TF, tissue factor; VII, factor VII; VIIa, activated factor VII; X, factor X; Xa, activated factor X; ProT, prothrombin; IIa, thrombin; IX, factor IX; IXa, activated factor IX; Xa activated factor X; Va, activated factor V; VIIIa, activated factor VIII; vWF, Von Willebrand factor.

TABLE 1: Edoxaban pharmacodynamics and pharmacokinetics [16–21].

Drug/mechanism of action	Edoxaban/direct oral factor Xa inhibitor (FXa-I) without antithrombin III
Indication and dosing guidelines	(1) Treatment of nonvalvular atrial fibrillation (NVAF) (i) 60 mg orally daily for CrCl greater than 50 to less than or equal to 95 mL/min (ii) 30 mg orally daily for CrCl 15–50 mL/min (iii) Do not use if CrCl is greater than 95 mL/min (Black Box Warning) (2) Treatment of venous thromboembolism (VTE) (i) 60 mg orally daily (ii) 30 mg orally daily if CrCl is 15–50 mL/min or body weight is less than 60 Kg or patient is on P-gp inhibitor
Protein binding/removed by dialysis	55%/No
F (%)	62% absorption in gastrointestinal tract Food does not affect the systemic exposure No data available for administration via feeding tube
T_{max} (h)	1-2
Vd (L)	19.9
$T_{1/2}$ (h)	10–14 with steady state reached in 72 hours
Metabolism	Minimal hepatic, undergoes biotransformation to various metabolites, the most abundant of which [M4] is formed through hydrolysis
Effect of P-gp/ABCG2 on metabolism	Minimal
Renal excretion (%)	50%
Biliary-intestinal excretion (%)	50%
Pregnancy category	C

Bioavailability, F; creatinine clearance, cytochrome P450 3A4 (CYP3A4/5), CrCl; half-life, $T_{1/2}$; P-glycoprotein/ABCG2, P-gp/ABCG2; volume of distribution, Vd, time to reach maximum concentration in hours (h), T_{max}.

rivaroxaban 33%, and edoxaban 50%. OFXaIs are excluded in clinical trials enrolling patients with CrCl < 25–30 mL/min [42]. The safety and PK of edoxaban (15 mg, 30 mg, and 60 mg) daily for 12 weeks in patients with normal or mild renal insufficiency (CrCl ≥ 50 mL/min) and severe renal insufficiency (CrCl ≥ 15 to < 30 mL/min) in 92 patients have been evaluated. Patients on hemodialysis or at high risk for bleeding were excluded. The dose of edoxaban was decreased by 50% in patients with normal or mild renal insufficiency who weigh less than 60 kg or who are on verapamil or quinidine. The bleeding complication rates in patients with severe renal impairment (edoxaban 15 mg group) and normal or mild renal insufficiency (edoxaban 30 mg or edoxaban 60 mg group) were 20%, 23.8%, and 22.7%, respectively. This study showed that edoxaban 15 mg might be appropriate for patients with severe renal insufficiency [43].

In a PK study of 10 patients with ESRD on dialysis, patients received a single dose of edoxaban 15 mg in 2 different schemes: on-dialysis days, 2 hours before, and off-dialysis days between hemodialysis sessions. Patients with history of bleeding, major trauma, or major surgical procedure, peptic ulcer, or gastrointestinal bleeding within the past 6 months or those who use any drugs that are strong inhibitors or inducers of CYP3A4 or P-gp within the past 4 weeks were excluded. $T_{1/2}$ was 10.6 ± 3.13 hours in on-dialysis group and 10.4 ± 2.72 in off-dialysis group. T_{max} on-dialysis and off-dialysis was 2.3 and 2.0 hours accordingly. The C_{max} was 53.3 ± 15.14 nanograms/milliliter (ng/mL) in on-dialysis group and 56.3 ± 23.25 ng/mL in off-dialysis group. The AUC_{∞} (ng∗L/hr) was 676.2 ± 220.86 in on-dialysis group versus 691.7 ± 149.84 in off-dialysis group. Clearance measured in (CL/h) was 24.7 ± 7.07 and 22.5 ± 4.50 in on-dialysis and in off-dialysis groups, respectively. These results showed that hemodialysis did not alter the PK of edoxaban. Mean percent of edoxaban protein binding remained ~60% in on- and off-dialysis groups. The effect of dialysis on M-4 (active metabolite of edoxaban) on C_{max} in on-dialysis and off-dialysis was 9.8 ± 7.05 ng/mL and 10.2 ± 4.98 ng/mL, respectively. The T_{max} was prolonged in off-dialysis group to 4 hours versus 2.1 hours in on-dialysis group and the AUC_{∞} was lower in off-dialysis group versus on-dialysis group, 151.9 ± 101.843 (ng∗L/hr) versus 193.3 ± 255.48 (ng∗L/hr). The $T_{1/2}$ was prolonged at 8.05 to 17.95 hours in on-dialysis group versus 7.52 to 15.08 hours in off-dialysis group. There was no bleeding, death, or any serious adverse reactions. This study showed that dialysis has no effect on the removal of edoxaban [44]. Currently, there are no clinical trials comparing different does of edoxaban in patients with renal insufficiency; however, a recent metaregression analysis was undertaken to examine the safety and efficacy of DOACs versus warfarin in patients with various degrees of renal function. The hazard ratio (HR) of bleeding in patients with moderate renal impairment (CrCl 25–49 mL/min), mild renal impairment (CrCl 50–79 mL/min), and nonrenal impairment (CrCl > 80 mL/min) has been estimated for edoxaban 30 mg versus warfarin as HR: 0.31 (95% Confidence Interval (CI): 0.23–0.42) in moderate renal impairment, not reported in mild renal impairment, and HR: 0.55 (95% CI: 0.46–0.65) for nonrenal impairment patients. Comparing edoxaban 60 mg against warfarin resulted in HR: 0.63 (95% CI: 0.50–0.81) in moderate renal impairment, not reported in mild renal impairment, and HR: 0.88 (95% CI: 0.76–1.03) in nonrenal impairment. In patients with CrCl 25–49 mL/min, indirect comparison between DOACs showed less major bleeding with apixaban compared to dabigatran, rivaroxaban, and edoxaban 60 mg, but not edoxaban 30 mg. Edoxaban 30 mg demonstrated less major bleeding in all comparisons to other DOACs. The HR of major bleeding for edoxaban 30 mg versus edoxaban 60 mg was estimated as 0.49 (95% CI: 0.33–0.72). In patients with CrCl 50–79 mL/min, edoxaban 30 mg offered a lower major bleeding profile compared to other DOACs. Edoxaban 30 mg versus edoxaban 60 mg showed HR of bleeding as 0.63 (95% CI: 0.50–0.79) [45]. The PK differences such as T_{max}, $T_{1/2}$, F, and various degrees of renal elimination could potentially confound the results of this metaregression. A recent

multicenter, open-label, 3-parallel-group, phase 3 study in Japanese patients undergoing lower limb replacement has evaluated the safety of edoxaban administered for 11 to 14 days. Patients with mild renal insufficiency or CrCl ≥ 50 to ≤ 80 mL/min received oral edoxaban 30 mg once daily. Patients with severe renal insufficiency or CrCl > 20 to < 30 mL/min were randomized to receive edoxaban 15 mg once daily or fondaparinux 1.5 mg daily. Patients with severe renal insufficiency or CrCl ≥ 15 to ≤ 20 mL/min received edoxaban 15 mg daily. Edoxaban was given 12–24 hours after surgery. Patients undergoing hemodialysis, high risk of bleeding, risk of thromboembolism, hepatic dysfunction, spinal anesthesia, inability to take oral medication, and abnormal bleeding after surgery were excluded. There was no major bleeding in any groups; and clinically relevant bleeding occurred at a rate of 6.7% in mild renal insufficiency (CrCl ≥ 50 to ≤ 80 mL/min on edoxaban 30 mg), 3.4% in severe renal insufficiency (CrCl ≥ 15 to < 30 mL/min on edoxaban 15 mg), 0% in patients in severe renal insufficiency on edoxaban 15 mg, 4.5% in severe renal insufficiency (CrCl ≥ 20 to ≤ 30 mL/min on edoxaban 15 mg), and 5% in severe renal insufficiency (CrCl ≥ 20 to < 30 mL/min on fondaparinux 1.5 mg). There was no VTE reported in any treatment groups. This study demonstrated that edoxaban 15 mg is safe in patients with severe renal impairment [46]. The limited number of patients in a subpopulation of Asian patients makes the applicability of data restrictive. The manufacturer recommends dose reduction by 50% in patients with CrCl 15–50 mL/min [17].

4. Edoxaban in Venous Thromboembolism (VTE) Trials

4.1. Primary Thromboprophylaxis after Knee Surgery. The incidence of 42%–57% for deep vein thrombosis (DVT) on screening, and 0.1%–2.0% for pulmonary embolism (PE), without the use of pharmacologic prophylaxis within 2 weeks in patients undergoing total hip arthroplasty (THA) has been described. In total knee arthroplasty (TKA) setting, incidence of DVT climbs to 41%–85% and prevalence of PE could be as high as 0.1%–1.7%. In hip fracture surgery (HFS), the incidence of DVT is estimated at 40%–60% and prevalence for PE at 0.3%–7.5% [47, 48]. In patients undergoing major orthopedic surgery (TKA or THA), the American College of Chest Physicians (ACCP) recommends utilizing one of the following pharmacological antithrombotics rather than no antithrombotic prophylaxis: LMWH, fondaparinux, dabigatran, apixaban, rivaroxaban, low-dose unfractionated heparin (LDUFH), adjusted-dose VKA, aspirin, or an intermittent pneumatic compression device (IPCD) for a minimum of 10 to 14 days. For HFS, the ACCP guidelines do not recommend utilizing DOACs for thromboprophylaxis. These guidelines suggest the use of LMWH in preference to the other agents and adding an IPCD during the hospital stay and suggest extending thromboprophylaxis for up to 35 days. In patients who decline injections, guidelines recommend using apixaban or dabigatran [49]. In the setting of TKA, a dose ranging study of edoxaban (5 mg, 15 mg, 30 mg, and 60 mg) once daily (first dose 6–24 hours after surgery) versus placebo in 523 patients has been conducted in a randomized, double-blind, placebo-controlled fashion for 11–14 days. Importantly, patients at high risk for bleeding, that is, history of intracranial bleeding, gastrointestinal bleeding, intraocular bleeding, peptic ulcer disease, elevated prothrombin time (PT), or activated partial thromboplastin time (aPTT) above the upper normal limit (UNL), hemoglobin (Hgb) < 9 g/dL or platelets of < 100,000/mm^3, systolic blood pressure (SBP) > 160 mmHg or diastolic blood pressure (DBP) > 100 mmHg, inherited coagulation abnormality, history of VTE, myocardial infarction, cerebral infarction, or transient ischemic attack (TIA), body weight < 40 kg, concurrent antiplatelet therapy, pregnancy, and clinically significant hepatic dysfunction, that is, liver enzymes (LFTs) or total bilirubin above 1.5 times upper limit of normal (UNL). The incidence of thromboembolic complications (DVT, PE) or primary endpoint in placebo and edoxaban (5 mg, 15 mg, 30 mg, 60 mg) was 48.3%, 29.5%, 26.1%, 12.5%, and 9.1%, respectively, P < 0.001, for all comparisons (placebo versus edoxaban). No major bleeding was observed in placebo and in only 1/106 (0.9%) in edoxaban 60 mg daily, all statistically nonsignificant. The clinically relevant nonmajor bleeding (CRNM) was 3.9% in placebo, 1.9% in edoxaban 5 mg, 3.8% in edoxaban 15 mg, 3.9% in edoxaban 30 mg, and 3.8% in edoxaban 60 mg groups accordingly. Notably, the incidence of treatment-related bleeding increased with higher doses of edoxaban (P = 0.004). There were no elevations in liver enzymes associated with edoxaban therapy. Additionally, single doses of edoxaban (5–60 mg) resulted in dose-dependent increases in anti-FXa activity, demonstrating target-specific effect versus placebo [50]. Nonpharmacological thromboprophylaxis (21–28% IPC and 72% elastic stockings) was used in addition to edoxaban, but no stratified analysis was provided on their effect on the outcomes. The effect of anti-FXa on clinical outcomes was not measured. This study confirmed the higher degree of bleeding with higher doses of edoxaban. A retrospective study of 300 patients undergoing TKA analyzed the safety and efficacy of edoxaban 15 mg daily for the prevention of DVT administered for 14 days. This study compared edoxaban 15 mg daily versus enoxaparin 20 mg twice daily versus fondaparinux 1.5 mg daily. The incidence of total DVT in enoxaparin, fondaparinux, and edoxaban was 28%, 28%, and 22% accordingly, not statistically significant, and no PE was noted. Hemoglobin levels were lower in patients with edoxaban than in patients with enoxaparin and fondaparinux on postoperative days; however, the difference was not statistically significant. Finally, the incidence of hepatic dysfunction was lower in patients with edoxaban than in patients with enoxaparin and fondaparinux [51]. Applying the results of a retrospective study into clinical practice poses many challenges. This study provided very limited information of patient's baseline characteristics, that is, renal function, concomitant use of IPCS, and comorbidities. Utilization of different doses of fondaparinux (1.5 mg) and enoxaparin (20 mg twice daily) is questionable in western countries as such doses are not recommended. Finally, no conclusion can be drawn for the efficacy and safety of edoxaban 30 mg

daily. In a randomized double-blind, double-dummy trial of TKA patients (n = 716), the safety and efficacy of edoxaban 30 mg (first dose given 6–24 hours after surgery) were compared to enoxaparin 20 mg twice daily (first dose 6–24 hour after surgery) for 11–14 days. Patients at high risk for bleeding, high risk for VTE, body weight < 40 Kg, CrCl < 30 mL/min, hepatic dysfunction, concomitant antiplatelet, or thrombolytic agents or pregnant patients were excluded. Patients in whom epidural catheter could not be removed by 2 hours prior to the initiation of study were not enrolled as well. The primary efficacy outcome (thromboembolic events) occurred in 7.4% and 13.9% patients in the edoxaban and enoxaparin groups, respectively (relative risk reduction = 46.8%), demonstrating noninferiority (P < 0.001) and superiority (P = 0.010) of edoxaban over enoxaparin. In the edoxaban and enoxaparin groups, the major bleeding (primary safety outcome) occurred in 1.1% versus 0.3% of patients (P = 0.373). Major or CRNM bleeding occurred in 6.2% versus 3.7% patients (P = 0.129), accordingly. There was no report of drug-induced liver injury. It is important to note that in each group approximately 22% were permitted to use IPCD and 62% elastic stockings as nonpharmacological prophylaxis measures [32]. Evidence has shown that addition of IPCD to pharmacological methods further decreased the incidence of VTE in orthopedic surgical patients; however, no analysis was conducted to examine the effect of covariates such as use of IPCD. Together, all of edoxaban data in TKA trials may not be applicable to patients in western countries as weight-based dosing of pharmacological thromboprophylaxis and methods of diagnosis may differ.

4.2. Primary Thromboprophylaxis after Hip Surgery. Edoxaban has been studied in total hip replacement (THR) trial for prevention of VTE. A randomized double-blind dose response of edoxaban on 903 patients undergoing THR has been conducted. In this trial, THR patients were randomized to edoxaban (15 mg, 30 mg, 60 mg, and 90 mg) versus dalteparin (2,500 units initially then 5,000 units) daily thereafter for 7 days. Patients were excluded if they have known or suspected bleeding or coagulation disorder, hemorrhagic stroke, nonhemorrhagic stroke within the past three months, intraocular hemorrhage, intracranial malignancy, gastrointestinal bleeding, or documented peptic ulcer within the past three months, if they are expected to receive epidural catheter, if they have received spinal or epidural anesthesia with traumatic tap, if they have abnormal PT and aPTT time, positive serology for hepatitis A, B, and C, known drug or alcohol dependence within the past 12 months, estimated survival of less than 12 months, liver function tests greater than 1.5 times UNL, systolic and diastolic blood pressure > 180/110 mmHg, Hgb < 9 g/dL, platelet count < 100,000/mm^3, if they receive aspirin > 100 mg per day or required concomitant clopidogrel or dipyridamole or nonsteroidal anti-inflammatory drugs, and if they received therapeutic dose of VKA or fibrinolytics within the past 10 days. Primary efficacy result, incidence of venographically proven VTE, was reported as 43.5% (dalteparin), 28.2% ((edoxaban 15 mg) versus dalteparin P = 0.005), 21.2% ((edoxaban 30 mg) versus dalteparin; $P < 0.001$), 15.2% ((edoxaban 60 mg) versus dalteparin; $P < 0.001$), and 10.6% ((edoxaban 90 mg) versus dalteparin; $P < 0.001$). Primary safety results, incidence of all bleeding, were reported as 0.6% (dalteparin), 2.1% (edoxaban 15 mg versus dalteparin; $P = 0.250$), 1.8% (edoxaban 30 mg versus dalteparin; $P = 0.122$), 4.9% (edoxaban 60 mg versus dalteparin), and 4.0% (edoxaban 90 mg versus dalteparin). There was no report of edoxaban induced liver injury. This study showed that edoxaban was effective in reduction of VTE in patients undergoing THR. This study was conducted in a patient population that had a different population PK than patients in North America, and generalizability is limited. No information was provided on the addition of nonpharmacological thromboprophylaxis [33]. A population PK based study of 1,795 patients enrolled in 10 phase 1 studies of edoxaban has been published for patients undergoing THR. Range of plasma concentration of edoxaban (15 mg, 30 mg, 60 mg, and 90 mg) was reported as $C_{max,ss}$ (200–300 ng/mL), AUC_{ss} (2000–3000 ng*h/mL), and $C_{min,ss}$ (20–50 ng/mL) and there was a significant predictor of decreasing incidence of VTE in patients undergoing THR: $P < 0.005$ for all variables; and no relationship was identified between edoxaban exposure and bleeding [34]. The applicability of these pharmacometric analyses might be to guide the future clinical trials in dosing and monitoring edoxaban in patients undergoing orthopedic surgery. Edoxaban 15 or 30 mg daily versus enoxaparin 20 mg twice daily has been studied for the prevention of VTE in patients undergoing THA in a randomized, active controlled, double-blind, phase II trial of 264 patients. Patients who required revision of THA and had history of intracranial bleeding, history of intraocular bleeding, intracranial tumor, gastrointestinal bleeding or peptic ulcer disease within the past 90 days, or history of symptomatic VTE, patients weighing < 40 kg and using antithrombotics, CrCl < 30 mL/min, and patients with evidence of hepatic dysfunction (LFTs > 2 times UNL and total bilirubin > 1.5 times UNL) were excluded. Edoxaban was started 6–24 hours after surgery and enoxaparin 24–36 hours after surgery for 11–14 days at which patients underwent venography. The primary endpoint (composite of asymptomatic VTE or symptomatic DVT) occurred in 3.8% of edoxaban 15 mg, 2.8% in edoxaban 30 mg group (incidence difference of 1.1%), and 4.1% in enoxaparin group. The incidence difference was −0.2% and −1.3% in edoxaban 15 mg and 30 mg versus enoxaparin, respectively ($P = 1.000$). There were no VTE-related deaths. The incidence of overall bleeding was 18% in edoxaban 15 mg, 21.2% in edoxaban 30 mg, and 21.8% in enoxaparin groups ($P = 1.000$). This study demonstrated that edoxaban once daily showed similar efficacy while maintaining safety as enoxaparin for the prevention of VTE after THA. Approximately 50% of patients were allowed to have IPCD therapy for sole foot, 40% IPCD for lower legs and thigh, and 80% for elastic stockings [52]. The dose of enoxaparin for prophylaxis was different than the dose recommended in the western countries; however, enoxaparin 20 mg twice daily might be appropriate for smaller frame patients. Currently, there are no large scale trials in America and Europe to compare the different doses of edoxaban and enoxaparin. Edoxaban 30 mg daily versus enoxaparin 20 mg

twice daily has also been studied for the prevention of VTE in patients undergoing THA in a randomized, double-blind, double-dummy, noninferiority phase III trial involving 610 patients. Edoxaban was started 6–24 hours after surgery and enoxaparin was initiated 24–36 hours after surgery for 11 to 14 days. VTE events occurred in 6.9% of enoxaparin group and 2.4% of edoxaban group ($P < 0.001$ for noninferiority). No symptomatic DVT or PE was noted in both treatment groups. The incidence of major and CRNM bleeding events was 3.7% versus 2.6% in the enoxaparin and edoxaban groups, respectively ($P = 0.475$). The major bleeding rates were 2.0% versus 0.7% in the enoxaparin and edoxaban groups, respectively. This study was presented as an abstract and the full paper has not been published yet [35].

4.3. Primary Thromboprophylaxis after Hip Fracture Surgery (HFS). To date, one multicenter, open-label, active comparator, phase 3 trial of 92 patients has compared edoxaban 30 mg to enoxaparin 20 mg twice daily for VTE prevention after HFS in Japanese patients for 11–14 days. First dose of edoxaban was given 6–24 hours and enoxaparin 24–36 hours after surgery. Patients were excluded if they were at increased risk of bleeding (e.g., history of intracranial bleeding and recent gastrointestinal bleeding) and patients with prior VTE, recent myocardial infarction, cerebral infarction, transient ischemic attack, body weight < 40 Kg, use of concomitant antithrombotics, CrCl < 30 mL/min, evidence of hepatic impairment, or abnormal bleeding at the site of anesthesia were also excluded. The primary endpoint of major or CRNM bleeding occurred in 3.4% (95% CI: 0.9–11.5) of edoxaban and 6.9% (95% CI: 1.9–22.0) of enoxaparin, for absolute difference of −3.5% (95% CI: −18.8–6.0). The secondary endpoint of composite VTE occurred in 6.5% of edoxaban (95% CI: 2.2–17.5) and 3.7% of enoxaparin (95% CI: 0.7–18.3), with absolute difference of 2.8% (95% CI: −12.4–14.2). There were no major adverse events such as death or liver toxicity related to treatment. This study confirmed the efficacy and safety of edoxaban for VTE prevention in high-risk postorthopedic surgical patients [36]. Patient eligibility and recruitment variations along with dosing differences for VTE prevention might impede the generalizability of these findings. Edoxaban is not indicated for the prevention of VTE postorthopedic surgery [17].

4.4. Primary Thromboprophylaxis in Acutely Ill Medical Patients. Hospitalized patients admitted for acute medical illnesses such as infection, advanced age, congestive heart failure, acute exacerbation of chronic obstructive lung disease, acute rheumatological disease, immobilization, cancer, respiratory failure, and prior history of thromboembolism are at risk for VTE [53]. Studies have shown the incidence of VTE in acutely ill hospitalized medical patients varies from 5% to 15% and this risk could be reduced by 50% to 75% with appropriate pharmacological thromboprophylaxis [54–56]. The International Medical Prevention Registry on Venous Thromboembolism (IMPROVE) registry ($n = 15,156$) showed suboptimal VTE prophylaxis rates, less than

50% [57]. The ACCP recommends pharmacological thromboprophylaxis with LMWH, LDUFH, or fondaparinux for acutely ill hospitalized medical patients at increased risk of thrombosis [58]. Currently, there are no recommendations for thromboprophylaxis with OFXaIs in medically ill hospitalized patients. Although data exists for apixaban and rivaroxaban thromboprophylaxis in this setting, to date, no published data exists for edoxaban prophylaxis in acutely ill medical patients [59, 60]. Generalizability of these data to edoxaban is not clinically advisable, for there are clear PK differences among OFXIs such as protein binding, renal clearance, hepatobiliary elimination, and prophylaxis dosing differences. Edoxaban is not indicated for the prevention of VTE in acutely ill hospitalized patients.

4.5. Initial Treatment of VTE. The overall annual incidence of VTE (DVT and PE) is estimated between 1 and 2 per 1000 of population or between 300,000 and 600,000 cases per year with average treatment cost of $7594 to $16,664 per case and 10 to 30% of all patients suffer mortality [61]. The ACCP recommendation for the VTE treatment consists of administration of either UFH or LMWH or fondaparinux for a minimum of 3 months for the first VTE; selected patients may be transitioned to warfarin [62]. OFXaIs have been studied for the initial treatment of acute VTE in several large randomized, noninferiority trials. Rivaroxaban and apixaban are considered noninferior to the standard-of-care VTE treatment in the general population [63–65]. The Hokusai-VTE investigated the role of edoxaban versus warfarin for the treatment of symptomatic VTE (DVT and PE) in a randomized, double-blind, double-dummy, noninferiority design trial. All patients were initially treated with heparins (UFH or enoxaparin) for a minimum of 5 days followed by warfarin (target INR 2-3) or edoxaban 60 mg daily unless the body weight was < 60 Kg or CrCl was 30–50 mL/min or were on potent P-glycoprotein inhibitor, in which cases edoxaban 30 mg daily was given for a minimum of 3 months in all patients and for a maximum of 12 months. The following patients were excluded: patients who required thrombectomy, insertion of a caval filter, or use of fibrinolytic agent; patients with CrCl < 30 mL/min, significant liver disease (e.g., acute hepatitis, chronic active hepatitis, positive hepatitis B antigen or hepatitis C antibody, and cirrhosis) or alanine transaminase (ALT) > 2 times UNL, total bilirubin 1.5 times UNL, active bleeding or high risk for bleeding, SBP > 170 mmHg, or DBP > 100 mmHg; pregnant patients; patients with chronic condition requiring treatment with nonsteroidal anti-inflammatory drugs (NSAIDs) including both cyclooxygenase-1 (COX-1) and cyclooxygenase-2 (COX-2) inhibitors for 4 days/week; patients requiring treatment with aspirin in a dosage of > 100 mg/per day or dual antiplatelet therapy (any two antiplatelet agents including aspirin plus any other oral or intravenous (IV) antiplatelet drug); patients requiring treatment with the potent P-gp inhibitors ritonavir, nelfinavir, indinavir, or saquinavir; however, systemic use of the strong P-gp inhibitors erythromycin, azithromycin, clarithromycin, ketoconazole, or itraconazole at the time of randomization was permitted. The primary efficacy outcome

(first recurrent VTE or VTE-related death) occurred in 3.2% in edoxaban and 3.5% in warfarin groups, HR: 0.89 (95% CI: 0.70–1.33; P < 0.01 for noninferiority). The primary safety outcome (first major or CRNM bleeding) occurred in 8.5% of edoxaban and 10.3% of warfarin groups, HR: 0.81 (95% CI: 0.71–0.94; P = 0.004 for superiority). Therapeutic INR range occurred in 65% of patients and adherence to edoxaban was 80%. Approximately 12% of patients in each arm were treated for 3 months, 26% for 3 to 6 months, 62% for greater than 6 months, and 40% for 12 months. In patients with PE, the rates of recurrent VTE occurred in 3.3% in the edoxaban group and 6.2% in the warfarin group, HR: 0.52 (95% CI: 0.28–0.98) and for those with documented right ventricular dysfunction based on computed tomography the HR of recurrent VTE was 0.42 (95% CI: 0.15–1.20) in edoxaban versus warfarin. Compared to warfarin, the rate of recurrent VTE in patients on edoxaban 30 mg was 3.0% versus 4.2%, HR: 0.73 (95% CI: 0.42–1.26). The rates of arterial thromboembolism in both arms were less than 0.6% and rates of liver injury were less than 2% in each arm [37]. The Hokusai-VTE showed noninferiority of edoxaban; however, clinicians should be aware that edoxaban was started after the initial treatment with heparins (5 days) as some patient with life-threatening VTE may require immediate procedures such as thrombectomy with or without thrombolysis. There is no subgroup analysis on edoxaban 60 mg and 30 mg to determine the dose effect on safety and efficacy outcomes. Edoxaban 60 mg orally daily is the approved dose for VTE treatment, unless CrCl is between 15 and 50 mL/min or body weight < 60 kg or patient was on concomitant Pap inhibitor in which 30 mg orally daily should be used (Table 1) [17].

4.6. Extended Treatment of VTE. The rate of VTE recurrence after discontinuation of therapy has been reported as 11.0% after 1 year, 19.6% after 3 years, and 29.1% after 5 years [66]. The risk of mortality is estimated as 3.6% for a recurrent VTE and 11.3% for a major bleed [67]. The ACCP guidelines recommend chronic anticoagulation for patients with recurrent VTE [61]. Although data is available for extended treatment for VTE with apixaban or rivaroxaban [68, 69], limited data exists for edoxaban.

4.7. Primary Thromboprophylaxis in Ambulatory Cancer Patients Receiving Chemotherapy. The association of malignancy and VTE is well described [70]. Pancreatic, brain, gastric, esophageal, and renal cell cancers and acute myelogenous leukemia confer a higher cumulative risk of VTE than breast, prostate, and melanoma malignancies [71]. In a population-based cohort of cancer patients with VTE, the cumulative incidence of VTE recurrence was 26.7 to 52.2% from the incidence of first VTE with mortality of 55.9% to 85.2% over 10 years [72]. In a study of cancer patients (n = 3,805) with VTE, risk of bleeding was 4.1% with 29% mortality. Predictive variables of bleeding were CrCl ≤ 30 mL/min, immobility ≥ 4 days, history of recent major bleeding, and metastatic cancer [73]. Predictive variables such as site of cancer, platelet count > 350,000/mm^3, hemoglobin < 10 g/dL, use of erythropoiesis-stimulating agents, leukocyte count $> 11 \times 10^9$/L, and body mass index ≥ 35 kg/m^2 may assist in identifying high-risk cancer patients for developing VTE [74]. Although randomized phase II study (tolerability trial) data exists for apixaban in this setting [75], no published data exists for edoxaban.

4.8. Initial Treatment of VTE in Cancer Patients. Enrolling cancer patients in clinical trials of DOACs has posed a challenge for investigators, due to underlying coagulopathy and thrombocytopenia and uncertain prognosis. VTE treatment trials of rivaroxaban enrolled 5 to 7% active cancer patients (acute DVT and continued treatment), 2.5% apixaban patients with active cancer, and 9% edoxaban patients [37, 63–65]. A subgroup analysis of patients enrolled in EINSTEIN-DVT and EINSTEIN-PE with active cancer (diagnosed at baseline or during treatment) has been published. Overall rivaroxaban was deemed similar in efficacy and safety to VKA in a subgroup of cancer patients [76]. Subgroup analysis may create false positive results by decreasing power, alteration of hypothesis, and generation of a mere observation. None of OFXaIs VTE treatment trials were designed to look at cancer patients as a subgroup. A systemic review of 4 randomized controlled phase III trials of 19,060 of which 759 with cancer randomized to either DOAC or SOC demonstrated efficacy (OR: 0.56 (95% CI: 0.28 to 1.13)) in DOACs versus SOC group. Safety outcomes comparing DOAC to VKA of yielded OR: 0.88 (95% CI: 0.57 to 1.35) [77]. A recent meta-analysis of six studies (two with dabigatran, two with rivaroxaban, one with edoxaban, and one with apixaban) comparing DOACs to SOC for treatment of VTE including patients with cancer demonstrated that VTE recurred in 3.9% (23/595) and 6% (32/537) of patients with cancer treated with DOACs and SOC, respectively (OR: 0.63 (95% CI: 0.37–1.10; I^2 0%)). Major bleeding occurred in 3.2% and 4.2% of patients receiving DOACs and SOC, respectively (OR: 0.77 (95% CI: 0.41–1.44; I^2 0%)) [78]. This meta-analysis, despite a high degree of homogeneity ($I^2 = 0\%$), analyzed dabigatran (DTI) in addition to OFXaIs. Dabigatran weight in this meta-analysis was 37% which might have skewed the results. Dabigatran PD/PK properties are completely different and should not be compared to OFXaI in the absence of direct comparison randomized head-to-head clinical trial in VTE setting. Currently, the American Society of Clinical Oncology (ASCO), National Comprehensive Cancer Network (NCCN), and ACCP recommend LMWH as the first line and warfarin as the second line for treatment of VTE in cancer patients. These guidelines currently do not recommend DOACs in cancer patients due to lack of randomized clinical trials [79, 80]. Another point to consider is that none of the trials with DOACs were set to analyze cancer subset data analysis. A phase III study comparing low-molecular-weight heparin versus edoxaban for the treatment of cancer-associated VTE is underway.

5. Edoxaban Studies in Acute Coronary Syndrome (ACS)

OFXaIs have been investigated in patients with recent ACS. In the ATLAS-ACS 2-TIMI 51 trial, rivaroxaban reduced the rates of death from cardiovascular causes (2.7% versus 4.1%, $P = 0.002$) and, compared with placebo, rivaroxaban increased the rates of major bleeding not related to coronary artery bypass grafting (2.1% versus 0.6%, $P < 0.001$) and intracranial hemorrhage (0.6% versus 0.2%, $P = 0.009$), without a significant increase in fatal bleeding (0.3% versus 0.2%, $P = 0.66$) [81]. In the APRAISE-2, addition of apixaban to antiplatelet therapy did not reduce the risk of cardiovascular death, myocardial infarction, or ischemic stroke versus placebo, 13.2 versus 14.0%, $P = 0.51$, but significantly increased the risk of major bleeding (2.4 versus 0.9%, $P = 0.001$) [82]. To our knowledge, there is no clinical trial published for the role of edoxaban in patients with ACS.

6. Prevention of Stroke in Nonvalvular Atrial Fibrillation (NVAF)

A three-arm, randomized, double-blind, double-dummy trial (ENGAGE AF-TIMI 48) compared once daily edoxaban (30 mg and 60 mg) with warfarin in 21,105 patients with NVAF. Patients with an estimated CrCl < 30 mL/min, high risk of bleeding, use of dual antiplatelet therapy, moderate to severe mitral stenosis, acute coronary syndromes, stroke within 30 days before randomization, and an inability to adhere to study procedures were excluded. The annual rate of the stroke or systemic embolism during treatment was 1.50% with warfarin, as compared with 1.18% with high-dose edoxaban (HR: 0.79 (97.5% CI: 0.63–0.99); $P < 0.001$ for noninferiority) and 1.61% with low-dose edoxaban (HR: 1.07 (97.5% CI, 0.87–1.31); $P = 0.005$ for noninferiority). In the intention-to-treat analysis, there was a trend favoring edoxaban 60 mg versus warfarin (HR: 0.87 (97.5% CI: 0.73–1.04); $P = 0.08$) and an unfavorable trend with edoxaban 30 mg versus warfarin (HR: 1.13 (97.5% CI: 0.96–1.34); $P = 0.10$). The annual rate of major bleeding was 3.43% with warfarin versus 2.75% with 60 mg edoxaban (HR: 0.80 (95% CI: 0.71–0.91); $P < 0.001$) and 1.61% with 30 mg edoxaban (HR: 0.47 (95% CI: 0.41–0.55); $P < 0.001$). The corresponding annual rates of death from cardiovascular causes were 3.17% versus 2.74% (HR: 0.86 (95% CI: 0.77–0.97); $P = 0.01$) and 2.71% (HR: 0.85 (95% CI: 0.76–0.96); $P = 0.008$), and the corresponding rates of the key secondary endpoint (a composite of stroke, systemic embolism, or death from cardiovascular causes) were 4.43% versus 3.85% (HR: 0.87 (95% CI: 0.78–0.96); $P = 0.005$) and 4.23% (HR: 0.95 (95% CI: 0.86–1.05); $P = 0.32$). Warfarin was within the therapeutic range in 58% of patients. This study showed noninferiority of edoxaban to SOC and significantly lower bleeding rates in prevention of stroke in patients with NVAF [38]. The subgroup analysis of patients with CrCl > 95 mL/min in ENGAGE AF-TIMI 48 showed higher rates of stroke and systemic embolism events (SEE) in edoxaban versus warfarin 1.0 versus 0.6 (HR: 1.87 (95% CI: 1.10–3.17)). The rate of ischemic stroke was higher relative to warfarin in the patients with CrCl > 95 mL/min (HR: 2.16 (95% CI: 1.17, 3.97)). The PK data indicated that patients with CrCl > 95 mL/min had lower plasma edoxaban levels, along with a lower rate of bleeding relative to warfarin than patients with CrCl ≤ 95 mL/min.

Consequently, edoxaban should not be used in patients with CrCl > 95 mL/min [17]. The dose of edoxaban for NVAF is 60 mg orally daily unless CrCl is 15–50 mL/min in which the dose should be decreased to 30 mg (Table 1) [17].

7. Thrombolysis Management in Edoxaban-Treated Patients Who Develop Acute Ischemic Stroke (AIS)

Despite edoxaban prophylaxis in NVAF, some patients develop AIS. Intravenous administration of recombinant tissue plasminogen activator (rTPA) is the only FDA-approved therapy for treatment of patients with AIS. The American Heart Association and the American Stroke Association recommend thrombolysis with rTPA in AIS patients with 3–4.5 hours of onset of stroke symptoms. Data on thrombolysis in edoxaban-treated patients with AIS are very limited. Patients who are already on edoxaban pose many challenges because of increased risk of major bleeding complications when the rTPA is concurrently administered. Unless rapidly performed PT, aPTT, and appropriate direct factor Xa activity assays are normal or the patient has not received a dose for > 2 days (assuming normal renal function), AHA/ASA guidelines do not recommend thrombolysis. Unfortunately, most of the tests are time-consuming to meet the 3–4.5-hour thrombolysis window [83].

8. Measurement of the Anticoagulant Effect of Edoxaban

The effect of edoxaban levels on coagulation parameters such as PT (prothrombin time), INR (international normalized ratio), aPTT (activated partial thromboplastin time), and factor Xa has not been extensively studied. An ex vivo study of 12 healthy volunteers assessed the antithrombotic effect of edoxaban 60 mg on coagulation parameters. Thrombin generation decreased by 28% and 10% at 1.5 hours and 10 hours. Changes in PT, INR, and anti-FXa activity correlated well with plasma drug concentrations (R^2 = 0.79, 0.78, and 0.85), but aPTT changes did not (R^2 = 0.40). Drug levels at 1.5, 5, and 12 hours after edoxaban 60 mg were 240 ± 16, 127 ± 6, and 37 ± 3 ng/mL. The effect of drug level on the thrombus size reduction was not measured [84]. Edoxaban concentration in plasma after multiple dose administration has been evaluated. Edoxaban 90 mg daily provided $C_{max/min}$ for day 1 as 451/10.2 (ng/mL) and 424/16.4 (ng/mL) on day 10. Edoxaban 60 mg twice daily achieved $C_{max/min}$ of 347/38.3 (ng/mL) on day 1 and 397/80.3 (ng/mL) on day 10. Finally, edoxaban 120 mg daily showed $C_{max/min}$ of 387/11.1 (ng/mL) on day 1 and 406/15.6 (ng/mL) on day 10 [18]. A phase 2 study on edoxaban for prevention of stroke in NVAF measured the $C_{max/min}$ of edoxaban in 1,146 patients. At steady state, the median $C_{max/min}$ was 80/10 (ng/mL) for edoxaban 10 mg daily, 175/20 (ng/mL) for edoxaban 60 mg daily, 120/40 (ng/mL) for edoxaban 30 mg twice daily, and 225/75 (ng/mL) for edoxaban 60 mg twice daily. This study showed higher bleeding rates with higher total daily doses of edoxaban. Interestingly, C_{min} correlated more closely with

bleeding; that is, frequency of bleeding was higher with edoxaban 30 mg twice daily versus edoxaban 60 mg daily. No analysis of edoxaban level on primary outcome such as stroke was evaluated [85]. A recent study has shown the significant variation is prolonged in PT and aPTT postedoxaban dose diluted to reach plasma concentrations of 50–400 ng/mL. The PT prolongation remained variable and dependent on specific reagent, but prolonged aPTT variability remained smaller; however, thrombin generation assay proved to be sensitive [86]. Differences in PK variables (T_{max}, C_{max}, and C_{min}) in edoxaban studies have been observed. There is no consensus at this point to make recommendations for monitoring edoxaban in special populations (obesity, underweight, and renal insufficiency). Lack of a standardized assay to monitor FXa poses a dilemma for clinicians assessing safety and efficacy of treatment with edoxaban.

9. Management of Bleeding Complications

Bleeding is a complication of anticoagulation therapy. Availability of antidote can prevent potential unfavorable outcomes associated with hemorrhagic events. Rates of major bleeding in edoxaban group versus warfarin group have been reported as 1.4% versus 1.6% in a VTE treatment trial [37]. In the setting of NVAF, the rates of major bleeding with high-dose edoxaban (60 mg daily) group were 2.75% per year versus 1.61% per year in low-dose edoxaban (30 mg daily) (Table 5) [38]. To date, there are not any clinical trials investigating the reversal of edoxaban in humans. In an edoxaban-anticoagulated animal study, the prothrombin complex concentrate (PCC), recombinant factor VIIa (rFVIIa), and activated prothrombin complex concentrate (aPCC) shortened PT prolonged by edoxaban. Among those, rFVIIa and aPCC showed potent activities in reversing the PT prolongation by edoxaban. rFVIIa (1 and 3 mg/kg) and aPCC (100 U/kg) significantly reversed edoxaban (1 mg/kg/h) induced prolongation of bleeding time. In venous thrombosis model, no potentiation of thrombus formation was observed when the highest dose (3 mg/kg) of rFVIIa was added to edoxaban (0.3 and 1 mg/kg/h) compared with the control. This study indicated that rFVIIa, aPCC, and PCC have the potential to be reversal agents for edoxaban [87]. In a rabbit model acute hemorrhage induced by edoxaban, blood loss was increased to 30 mL (2–44) and time to reach hemostasis was prolonged by 23 minutes (8.5–30) versus control group. Administration of 4F-PCC significantly reduced time to hemostasis to 8 minutes (6.5–14), $P < 0.0001$, versus control. In this study, PT (seconds) was 9.7 ± 0.9 in glucose saline 5% group versus 17.4 ± 1.7 in edoxaban 1,200 μg/kg saline group, $P < 0.0001$. Addition of 4F-PCC (50 IU/kg) lowered the PT (s) to 13.5 ± 0.7, $P < 0.0001$. This study confirmed that 4F-PCC effectively normalizes PT [88]. Edoxaban (500 or 1,000 ng/mL) was added to blood sample from 6 healthy volunteers followed by rFVIIa (0.8 or 1.8 μg/mL) or factor VIII inhibitor bypassing agent (FEIBA (0.75 or 1.5 U/mL)). In edoxaban-containing blood samples, reductions in measures of PT ($P < 0.0001$), aPTT ($P < 0.0001$), and anti-FXa ($P < 0.0001$) were observed when rFVIIa or aPCC was added. Intrinsic FXa activity was increased up to 20% and 31% of normal in the presence of edoxaban by rFVIIa and aPCC, accordingly. The onset of their impact on the anticoagulant effects of edoxaban was observed within 15 minutes and remained relatively unchanged. Results of this ex vivo study suggest that rFVIIa and aPCC rapidly reversed edoxaban-mediated anticoagulation effects based on PT and aPTT but had minimal effect based on intrinsic FX activity [89]. In acute overdose, if ingestion is within 3 hours, activated charcoal (50–100 gm) can be given along with fluid and red blood cell resuscitation [90]. Overall, the administration of 4-FPCC (50 units/kg) and aPCC (50 units/kg) and addition of rVIIa (90 μg/kg) in refractory cases have been shown in animal studies to normalize thrombin generation, decrease PT, and reduce bleeding time. In a recent study of 110 healthy subjects (17 in part one and 93 in part two), the effect of 4-FPCC (50, 25, and 10 IU/kg) on edoxaban (60 and 180 mg) was evaluated in a double-blind, randomized, placebo, 2-way crossover design. Patients were excluded if they were on strong inhibitors or inducers of CYP3A4 or P-gp within the past 28 days, if they had recent major or minor bleeding, and if they had history of coagulopathy. The effects of 4-FPCC on bleeding duration (BD) and bleeding volume (BV) and PT were assessed. BD (minutes) and BV (mL) were completely reversed (above 100%) by 4-FPCC (50 IU/kg); however, PT did not (less than 50%). 4-FPCC (25 IU/kg) effect on BD, BV, and PT was suboptimal (less than 75%) and 4-FPCC (10 IU/kg) had no effect on BD, BV, and PT. No death or thrombotic events were reported. 4-FPCC demonstrated complete reversal effect of edoxaban on coagulation parameters [91, 92]. Currently, there are no specific antidotes for OFXaIs; however, 2 investigational antidotes are in phase 2 clinical trials. Andexanet alfa, a modified recombinant FXa, with terminal $T_{1/2}$ of ~6 hours binds to OFXaIs specifically, thereby neutralizing its anticoagulant effects. Aripazine, a small synthetic molecule, universally targets OFXaIs, LMWHs, thrombin inhibitor (IIaI), and fondaparinux by binding them. Upcoming large scale trials should shed light onto these antidotes' safety and efficacy [93].

10. Drug-Drug Interactions with Edoxaban

Drug-drug or dietary supplement interactions with edoxaban may potentially predispose patients to bleeding or thromboembolism. Edoxaban's metabolism involves a major pathway via permeability glycoprotein (P-gp; ATP-binding cassette, subfamily B, membrane 1, or multidrug resistance-1 (MDR1)) transporter of the intestinal lining and a minor pathway of CYP3A4 [22]. Therefore, drugs that inhibit the P-gp pump can increase the level of edoxaban and drugs that induce the P-gp pump can lower the edoxaban level [23]. The addition of other antithrombotic or nonsteroidal anti-inflammatory agents to edoxaban may enhance the bleeding effect and combination should be avoided. Patients on edoxaban with recent coronary stent (on dual antiplatelet: aspirin and clopidogrel) may require lower doses of aspirin. Some inducers of P-gp transporter such as rifampin and St. John's Wort will lower the plasma concentration of edoxaban should be avoided. Cardiac medications such as verapamil

and quinidine that are P-gp inhibitors require dose adjustment of edoxaban by 50%. Potent inhibitors of P-gp such as lansoprazole, omeprazole, azithromycin, erythromycin, ketoconazole, and itraconazole require 50% dose reduction of edoxaban if coadministered. Dose reduction of edoxaban is required if concomitant use of cardiac agents such as amiodarone or dronedarone (P-gp inhibitors) is warranted. Vascular endothelial growth factor (VEGF) inhibitors such as pazopanib, lapatinib, and sorafenib could potentially increase edoxaban plasma levels via P-gp inhibition. Dietary supplements such as vitamin E (>800 units per day) and fish oil can inhibit platelet aggregation and their combination with edoxaban may predispose patient to bleeding. There are supplements that have warfarin derivatives such as sweet clover, chamomile, and horseradish that should be avoided in combination with edoxaban, Table 2 [17, 24–29]. Patients on edoxaban should be counselled on drug or dietary supplement interactions.

11. Perioperative Management of Edoxaban Therapy

Clinicians should recognize that the data for use of edoxaban in perioperative setting is limited. Unless an emergent surgery is planned, elective surgery cases for patients on edoxaban require assessment of the risk of perioperative thromboembolism and the risk of bleeding. This assessment aids in determining the need for perioperative bridging with short-acting anticoagulants in the immediate perioperative setting. Patients with atrial fibrillation (CHADS$_2$ (congestive heart failure, hypertension, age, diabetes, and stroke) score of 0 to 2, without prior history of stroke or transient ischemic attack (TIA)) and remote VTE event (history of more than 1 year in the past) are considered at low risk (less than 4% per year risk for ATE or less than 2% per month risk for VTE). This low-risk group does not require bridging. Patients with atrial fibrillation (CHADS$_2$ score of 3 or 4), VTE (within the past 3 to 12 months), recurrent VTE, nonsevere thrombophilia, and active cancer disease are considered to be at intermediate risk (4 to 10% per year risk for ATE or 4 to 10% per month risk for VTE). This group may require bridging if bleeding risk is deemed low. Finally, patients with recent (<6 months) history of stroke or TIA, atrial fibrillation (CHADS$_2$ score > 5, < 3 months history of stroke or TIA, and rheumatic valvular heart diseases), recent history of VTE ((history of < 3 months), severe thrombophilia, being positive for antiphospholipid antibodies, proteins C and S deficiency, and antithrombin deficiency) carry risk exceeding 10% per year for ATE and 10% per month for VTE. These patients require bridging with short-acting anticoagulants [30]. Once the patient was deemed an appropriate candidate for bridging, bleeding risk associated with procedure should be estimated as some procedures carry a higher risk of bleeding (major surgeries and renal biopsy) than simple dental extraction. For procedure with lower risk of bleeding, aiming for mild to moderate residual anticoagulant effect at surgery (12%–25%) or 2-3 half-lives should suffice, whereas for higher bleeding risk procedure, aiming for no or minimal

TABLE 2: Edoxaban Drug-Drug and Supplement Interactions [17, 22–29].

(a)

Interacting drugs	Effect	Clinical Implications
Rivaroxaban, apixaban, dabigatran	Enhanced bleeding via additional antithrombotic effects	Avoid combination
Enoxaparin, dalteparin, tinzaparin, fondaparinux, Unfractionated Heparin, warfarin		Avoid combination
Streptokinase, alteplase, reteplase, urokinase, TNK-tPA		Avoid combination
PAR antagonist (atopaxar, vorapaxar)		Avoid combination
GPIIb/IIIa inhibitors (abciximab, eptifibatide, tirofiban)		Avoid combination
ADP receptor antagonists (cangrelor, clopidogrel, elinogrel, prasugrel, ticagrelor)		Monitor therapy
Thromboxane inhibitors:aspirin		Monitor therapy: aspirin < 100 mg is safe
Non-Steroidal Anti-inflammatory Agents: naproxen		Monitor therapy: naproxen < 500 mg per day is safe
Cyclooxygenase inhibitor (COX-2)		Monitor therapy
Cilostazol, dipyridamole, ticlopidine		Monitor therapy
Rifampin	Decrease efficacy via P-gp induction	Avoid combination
Carbamazepine, phenobarbital, primidone,		Monitor therapy
St. John's Wort (Hypericum Perforatum)		Monitor therapy
Tipranavir		Monitor therapy
Verapamil, trandolapril, quinidine	Enhanced bleeding via P-gp inhibition	Decrease the dose of edoxaban to 30 mg daily for VTE treatment. No dose adjustment required for atrial fibrillation (AF) (i) Verapamil: ↑ AUC of edoxaban by 52.7% (ii) Quinidine: ↑ AUC of edoxaban by 76.7%
Diltiazem		Dose reduction may be necessary for treatment of Venous Thromboembolism (VTE); and monitor therapy
Azithromycin, clarithromycin, erythromycin, amoxicillin, ketoconazole, itraconazole		Decrease the dose of edoxaban to 30 mg daily for VTE treatment. No dose adjustment required for AF
Posaconazole		Dose reduction may be necessary for VTE
Lansoprazole, omeprazole		Decrease the dose of edoxaban to 30 mg daily for VTE treatment. No dose adjustment required for AF
Amiodarone (oral administration at 600 to 1600 mg per day: causes inhibition of intestinal P-gp efflux pump inhibition), dronaderone		Dose reduction may be necessary for treatment of VTE; and monitor therapy (i) Amiodarone: ↑ AUC of edoxaban by 39.8% (ii) Dronaderone ↑ AUC of edoxaban by 84.5%
Propafenone		
Atorvastatin, lovastatin, simvastatin, niacin, ezetimibe, amlodipine, carvedilol, nicardipine, nifedipine, ralonazine		
Bosutinib, cabozantinib, crizitinib, lapatinib, nilotinib, regorafenib, pazopanib, sorafenib, tamoxifen, vemurafenib,		
Canagliflozin, metformin		Dose reduction may be necessary for treatment of VTE; and monitor therapy
Cobicistat, elvitegravir, emtricitabine, tenofovir, ritonavir, lopinavir, saquinavir, aimprevir, nelfinavir, lepidasvir, sofosbuvir, etravirine, draunavir, telaprivir, cyclosporine, eliglustat, enzalutamide, iloperidone, paliperidone, ivacaftor, mefloquine, mifepristone, pirfenidone, ulipristal, testosterone		
Grapefruit		
Tolvaptan		

(b)

Interacting dietary supplements	Effect	Clinical Pearls
Thrombolytic activity: Nattokinase	Enhanced bleeding	Avoid combination
Decrease/inhibit platelet aggregation: caffeine, fish oil, fenugreek, flax seed, garlic, ginko, gingeng (panax, Siberian), willow bark, vitamin E (greater than 800 units per day), turmeric, resveratrol		
Anticoagulants: gamma Linolenic acid, glucosamine, melatonin,		
Warfarin derivatives:		
Alfalfa, celery seed, chamomile, dandelion, dong quai, horseradish, licorice root, horse chestnut, parsley, red clover, sweet clover, wild carrot, wild lettuce, nettle, passion flower, horseradish, cassia		

TABLE 3: Interruption/holding of edoxaban for procedures [17, 30, 31].

	$T_{1/2}$	Low risk or minor surgery (procedures with 2-day risk for major bleeding 0–2%) ↓ Aiming for mild to moderate residual anticoagulant effect at surgery (12%–25%) or 2-3 half-lives	High risk or major surgery (procedures with 2-day risk for major bleeding 2%–4%) ↓ Aiming for no or minimal residual anticoagulant effect (3%–6%) at surgery or 4-5 half-lives
Edoxaban	10–14 hr	24 hr	48–72 hr
Types of surgical procedures		(i) Cholecystectomy (ii) Abdominal hernia repair (iii) Abdominal hysterectomy (iv) Coronary angiography/percutaneous coronary intervention (v) Electrophysiologic testing (vi) Pacemaker/cardiac defibrillator insertion (vii) Gastrointestinal endoscopy ± biopsy, enteroscopy, biliary/pancreatic stent without sphincterotomy, and endosonography without aspiration (viii) Minor plastic surgery (carpal tunnel repair) (ix) Minor orthopedic surgery/arthroscopy (x) Minor gynecologic surgery (dilation and curettage) (xi) Minor dental procedures (extractions) (xii) Minor skin procedures (cancer excision) (xiii) Minor eye procedures (cataract)	(i) Major cardiac surgery (surgical heart valve replacement/coronary artery bypass grafting) (ii) Major neurosurgical procedures (iii) Major cancer surgery (head and neck/abdominal/thoracic) (iv) Major orthopedic surgery (joint replacement/laminectomy) (v) Major urologic surgery (prostate/bladder resection) (vi) Major vascular surgery (vii) Kidney biopsy (viii) Polypectomy, variceal treatment, biliary sphincterectomy, and pneumatic dilation (ix) Endoscopically guided fine-needle aspiration

Creatinine clearance, CrCl.

residual anticoagulant effect (3%–6%) at surgery or 4-5 half-lives should suffice; therefore, edoxaban interruption can range from 24 to 72 hours (Table 3). If the patient is unable to tolerate oral tablets (prolonged nothing by mouth state) in the immediate postoperative period, transition LMWH or UFH infusion might be appropriate. Some institutions may not carry edoxaban due to formulary restrictions; in these situations, transition to other antithrombotics could be implemented [17, 31]. In order to assure a safe and effective practice, it is prudent to develop specific institutional guidelines or clinical practice algorithms for management of DOACs in the perioperative period by a multidisciplinary group compromising internists, surgeons, nursing staffs, and pharmacists.

12. Transition to Other Anticoagulants

Currently, there is no published trial evaluating the safety and efficacy role of bridging with edoxaban in the perioperative setting or transition to other antithrombotics. Transition to and from edoxaban requires estimation of CrCl and PK parameters such as $T_{1/2}$ of each of the antithrombotics, monitoring INR and aPTT when necessary. Table 4 will provide guidance to clinicians when bridging to and from edoxaban is required. Patients should be given a complete calendar and education of transition to and from edoxaban [17].

13. Current Approval Status

Edoxaban has been approved to reduce the risk of stroke or systemic embolism in patients with NVAF and for treatment of deep vein thrombosis and pulmonary embolism in USA, European Union, and Japan. Edoxaban has been approved for prophylaxis of deep vein thrombosis following orthopedic surgery in Japan. Edoxaban should not be used in patients with mechanical heart valves as no research trial has been conducted in this population. Dabigatran, an oral DTI, has been shown to be inferior to warfarin in reducing systemic embolism in this clinical setting [94].

14. Patient Satisfaction

Curtailing the need for frequent INR monitoring and administration of oral tables rather than injections could possibly improve patient compliance and satisfaction with anticoagulant therapy. Anti-Clot Treatment Scale (ACTS: burdens score range 12–60; benefits score range 3–15) and Treatment Satisfaction Questionnaire for Medication (TSQM: effectiveness; side effects; convenience, global satisfaction score

TABLE 4: (a) Transition to edoxaban [17]. (b) Transition from edoxaban [17].

(a)

From	To	Recommendation
Warfarin		Discontinue warfarin and start edoxaban when INR ≤2.5
Rivaroxaban, apixaban Dabigatran	Edoxaban	Discontinue current oral anticoagulant and start edoxaban at the time of the next scheduled dose of the other oral anticoagulant
Low-molecular-weight heparin (LMWH) Fondaparinux		Discontinue LMWH or fondaparinux and start edoxaban at the time of the next scheduled administrastion of LMWH or fondaparinux
Heparin Intravenous Infusion (IVI)		Discontinue the infusion and start edoxaban 4 hours later

(b)

From	To	Recommendations
Edoxaban	Warfarin	(1) Oral option: (i) For patients taking 60 mg of edoxaban, reduce the dose to 30 mg and begin warfarin concomitantly. (ii) For patients receiving 30 mg of edoxaban, reduce the dose to 15 mg and begin warfarin concomitantly. (iii) INR must be measured at least weekly and just prior to the daily dose of edoxaban to minimize the influence of edoxaban on INR measurements. (iv) Once a stable INR greater or equal to 2.0 is achieved, edoxaban should be discontinued and the warfarin continued. (2) Parenteral option: (i) Discontinue edoxaban and administer a parenteral anticoagulant and warfarin at the time of the next scheduled edoxaban dose. (ii) Once a stable INR greater or equal to 2.0 is achieved, the parenteral anticoagulant should be discontinued and the warfarin continued.
	Apixaban Rivaroxaban Dabigatran	Discontinue edoxaban and start the other anticoagulant at the time of the next dose of edoxaban.
	LMWH Fondaparinux Heparin IV	Discontinue edoxaban and start the parenteral anticoagulant at the time of the next dose of edoxaban.

range 0–100) are two frequently validated tools to assess the patient's satisfaction with anticoagulation and higher score equals higher satisfaction. In EINSTEIN-PE, mean ACTS for burdens score was 55.4 in rivaroxaban group and 51.9 in SOC group, $P < 0.0001$. The mean ACTS scores for benefits were 11.9 for rivaroxaban group and 11.4 for SOC group, $P < 0.0001$. TSQM scores for effectiveness, side effects, convenience, and global satisfaction were 73.3, 86.6, 81.6, and 80.7 for rivaroxaban, versus 69.6, 82.3, 71.8, and 73.0 for SOC group, $P < 0.0001$, for all groups [95]. In EINSTEIN-DVT significant benefits in terms of ACTS and TSQM scores were observed in rivaroxaban versus warfarin, $P < 0.0001$ [96]. One could presume the same satisfaction scores or even higher for edoxaban since it is dosed once daily. Future trials should provide additional evidence for benefits of edoxaban in terms of patient satisfaction.

15. Economic Impact

Recently, the cost-effectiveness of OFXaIs in orthopedic surgery patients has been investigated in a pharmacoeconomic decision model. In THR replacement model, the average cost per patient for LMWHs and that for oral FXa-Is were $18,897 and $18,762 accordingly; and quality-adjusted life-years (QALY) were 0.932 and 0.938. In TKR model, the average cost for LMWHs and that for oral FXa-Is were $18,891 and $18,804, respectively, with QALYs of 0.931 and 0.935 for LMWHs and OFXaIs, respectively. Overall sensitivity analysis indicated cost-effectiveness of OFXAIs is greater in 98% of patients undergoing major orthopedic surgery with the assumption of willingness-to-pay threshold of $50,000/QALY. Authors concluded that OFXaIs may be economically superior to LMWHs for VTE prevention in orthopedic surgery patients [97]. A recent pharmacoeconomic study examined the cost differences between DOACs and warfarin for treatment of atrial fibrillation and treatment of VTE in a hypothetical patient population. The incidence and prevalence of primary efficacy outcomes (ischemic stroke, hemorrhagic stroke, and systemic embolism), secondary efficacy outcomes (myocardial infarction, pulmonary embolism, and deep vein thrombosis), and safety endpoints (major bleeding and clinically relevant nonmajor bleeding) were extracted from all clinical trials of DOACs (dabigatran, rivaroxaban, apixaban, and edoxaban). Total medical cost

TABLE 5: Summary of important edoxaban trials. [32–38].

Thromboprophylaxis after total knee replacement surgery

Trial	Interventions	Duration (days)	N	Total VTE (%)	Major and CRNM bleeding (%)
STARS E-3 (Phase III)	Edoxaban 30 mg QD versus Enoxaparin 20 mg BID	11–14	716	7.4 / 13.9 (P < 0.001 for NI)	6.2 / 3.7 (P = 0.129)

Thromboprophylaxis after total hip replacement surgery

Trial	Interventions	Duration (days)	N	Total VTE (%)	Major and CRNM bleeding (%)
Phase IIb	Edoxaban 15 mg QD 30 mg QD 60 mg QD 90 mg QD versus Dalteparin 2,500 IU QD followed by 5,000 IU QD	7–10	903	28.2 (P = 0.005) 21.2 (P < 0.001) 15.2 (P < 0.001) 10.6 (P < 0.001) / 43.5	3.7 / 6.2 (P = 0.129)
Phase IIb	Edoxaban 15 mg QD 30 mg QD versus Enoxaparin 20 mg BID	11–14	264	3.8 2.8 / 4.1	18 21.2 / 21.8
Phase III STARS J-V	Edoxaban 30 mg QD versus Enoxaparin 20 mg BID	11–14	610	2.4 / 6.9 (P = 0.001 for NI)	2.6 / 3.7

Thromboprophylaxis after hip fracture surgery

Trial	Intervention	Duration (days)	N	Total VTE (%)	Major and CRNM bleeding (%)
STARS J-IV (Phase III)	Edoxaban 30 mg QD versus Enoxaparin 20 mg BID	11–14	92	3.7 / 6.5	3.4 / 6.9

Treatment and secondary prevention of VTE

Trial	Interventions	Duration (months)	N	Total VTE (%)	Major and CRNM bleeding (%)
Hokusai-VTE (Phase III)	Enoxaparin or UFH/Edoxaban 60 mg QD (or reduced to 30 mg QD) versus Enoxaparin or UFH/warfarin (INR 2.0–3.0)	3–12	8,292	3.2 / 3.5 (P < 0.01 for NI)	8.5 / 10.3 (P = 0.004)

TABLE 5: Continued.

| Trial | Interventions | Prevention of stroke and systemic embolism in nonvalvular atrial fibrillation | | | |
		Duration (years)	N	Annual rate of stroke and systemic embolism (%)	Annual rate for major bleeding (%)
ENGAGE-AF-TIMI 48	Edoxaban 60 mg QD or 30 mg QD (or reduced to 15 mg QD) versus Warfarin (INR 2.0–3.0)	2.8	21,105	1.18 (P < 0.001 for NI)	2.75 (P < 0.001)
				1.61 (P = 0.005 for NI)	1.61 (P < 0.001)
				1.50	3.43

N, number of patients; NI, noninferiority; QD, once daily; BID, twice daily; VTE, venous thromboembolism; CRNM, clinically relevant nonmajor; IU, international units; mg, milligrams; UFH, unfractionated heparin; INR, international normalized ratio.

difference measured as dollars/patient-years was −$204 for dabigatran versus warfarin, −$140 for rivaroxaban versus warfarin, −$495 for apixaban versus warfarin, and −$340 for edoxaban versus warfarin [98]. These results are promising; however, one must consider the acquisition cost differences across states and institutions and payer preference based on contracts.

16. Patient Education

Clinicians should become familiar with approved indications, pharmacodynamics, and pharmacokinetic properties of OFXaIs, duration of therapy, screen for drug interactions, communicate with other providers involved when an OFXaI is prescribed, and conduct a comprehensive patient education. Patient education should include signs and symptoms of bleeding, fall and injury precautions, reminders for the exact dose (color of the pill and frequency), and education on missed doses. Instructions on periodic monitoring of renal function, hemoglobin level, and platelet counts should be given to patients with significant comorbidities. There should be a plan of action in place, if pregnancy or planned procedures that require interruption of OFXaI occur.

17. Conclusion

Edoxaban seems safe and effective for prevention and treatment of VTE and prevention of stroke in NVAF. Edoxaban might be financially cost-effective and an attractive option compared to injections or warfarin. Edoxaban might provide better patient compliance and satisfaction with antithrombotic therapy. There is clearly lack of evidence for its role in cancer patients, perioperative bridging, transition to other anticoagulants, FXa monitoring, and reversibility for bleeding cases.

Conflict of Interests

The authors do not report any conflict of interests regarding this work.

References

[1] D. Wardrop and D. Keeling, "The story of the discovery of heparin and warfarin," *British Journal of Haematology*, vol. 141, no. 6, pp. 757–763, 2008.

[2] J. Hirsh, M. O'Donnell, and J. W. Eikelboom, "Beyond unfractionated heparin and warfarin: current and future advances," *Circulation*, vol. 116, no. 5, pp. 552–560, 2007.

[3] J. van Ryn, A. Goss, N. Hauel et al., "The discovery of dabigatran etexilate," *Frontiers in Pharmacology*, vol. 4, article 12, Article ID Article 12, 2013.

[4] P. C. Wong, D. J. P. Pinto, and D. Zhang, "Preclinical discovery of apixaban, a direct and orally bioavailable factor Xa inhibitor," *Journal of Thrombosis and Thrombolysis*, vol. 31, no. 4, pp. 478–492, 2011.

[5] E. Perzborn, S. Roehrig, A. Straub, D. Kubitza, and F. Misselwitz, "The discovery and development of rivaroxaban, an oral, direct

[6] C. H. Yeh, J. C. Fredenburgh, and J. I. Weitz, "Oral direct factor Xa inhibitors," *Circulation Research*, vol. 111, no. 8, pp. 1069–1078, 2012.

[7] L. Loffredo, L. Perri, M. Del Ben, F. Angelico, and F. Violi, "New oral anticoagulants for the treatment of acute venous thromboembolism: are they safer than vitamin K antagonists? A meta-analysis of the interventional trials," *Internal and Emergency Medicine*, 2014.

[8] A. Zalpour and T. H. Oo, "Clinical utility of apixaban in the prevention and treatment of venous thromboembolism: current evidence," *Journal of Drug Design, Development and Therapy*, vol. 8, pp. 2181–2191, 2014.

[9] D. M. Monroe, "Basic principles underlying coagulation," in *Practical Hemostasis and Thrombosis*, N. Key, M. Makris, D. O'Shaughnessy, and D. Lillicrapt, Eds., pp. 1–6, Wiley-Blackwell, Oxford, UK, 2nd edition, 2009.

[10] D. Gailani and T. Renné, "Intrinsic pathway of coagulation and arterial thrombosis," *Arteriosclerosis, Thrombosis, and Vascular Biology*, vol. 27, no. 12, pp. 2507–2513, 2007.

[11] N. Mackman, R. E. Tilley, and N. S. Key, "Role of the extrinsic pathway of blood coagulation in hemostasis and thrombosis," *Arteriosclerosis, Thrombosis, and Vascular Biology*, vol. 27, no. 8, pp. 1687–1693, 2007.

[12] V. Toschi and M. Lettino, "Inhibitors of propagation of coagulation: factors V and X," *British Journal of Clinical Pharmacology*, vol. 72, no. 4, pp. 563–580, 2011.

[13] F. Scaglione, "New oral anticoagulants: comparative pharmacology with vitamin K antagonists," *Clinical Pharmacokinetics*, vol. 52, no. 2, pp. 69–82, 2013.

[14] J. Hirsh and M. N. Levine, "Low molecular weight heparins," *Blood*, vol. 79, no. 1, pp. 1–17, 1992.

[15] K. G. Mann, K. Brummel, and S. Butenas, "What is all that thrombin for?" *Journal of Thrombosis and Haemostasis*, vol. 1, no. 7, pp. 1504–1514, 2003.

[16] G. Escolar, M. Diaz-Ricart, E. Arellano-Rodrigo, and A. M. Galán, "The pharmacokinetics of edoxaban for the prevention and treatment of venous thromboembolism," *Expert Opinion on Drug Metabolism and Toxicology*, vol. 10, no. 3, pp. 445–458, 2014.

[17] Edoxaban Prescribing Information, 2015, http://www.accessdata.fda.gov/drugsatfda_docs/label/2015/206316lbl.pdf.

[18] K. Ogata, J. Mendell-Harary, M. Tachibana et al., "Clinical safety, tolerability, pharmacokinetics, and pharmacodynamics of the novel factor Xa inhibitor edoxaban in healthy volunteers," *Journal of Clinical Pharmacology*, vol. 50, no. 7, pp. 743–753, 2010.

[19] M. S. Bathala, H. Masumoto, T. Oguma, L. He, C. Lowrie, and J. Mendell, "Pharmacokinetics, biotransformation, and mass balance of edoxaban, a selective, direct factor xa inhibitor, in humans," *Drug Metabolism & Disposition*, vol. 40, no. 12, pp. 2250–2255, 2012.

[20] H. Bounameaux and A. J. Camm, "Edoxaban: an update on the new oral direct factor Xa inhibitor," *Drugs*, vol. 74, no. 11, pp. 1209–1231, 2014.

[21] O. Q. P. Yin and R. Miller, "Population pharmacokinetics and dose-exposure proportionality of edoxaban in healthy volunteers," *Clinical Drug Investigation*, vol. 34, no. 10, pp. 743–752, 2014.

factor Xa inhibitor," *Nature Reviews Drug Discovery*, vol. 10, no. 1, pp. 61–75, 2011.

[22] J. D. Wessler, L. T. Grip, J. Mendell, and R. P. Giugliano, "The P-glycoprotein transport system and cardiovascular drugs," *Journal of the American College of Cardiology*, vol. 61, no. 25, pp. 2495–2502, 2013.

[23] T. Mikkaichi, Y. Yoshigae, H. Masumoto et al., "Edoxaban transport via P-glycoprotein is a key factor for the drug's disposition," *Drug Metabolism and Disposition*, vol. 42, no. 4, pp. 520–528, 2014.

[24] O. Yousuf and D. L. Bhatt, "The evolution of antiplatelet therapy in cardiovascular disease," *Nature Reviews Cardiology*, vol. 8, no. 10, pp. 547–559, 2011.

[25] J. Yeung and M. Holinstat, "Newer agents in antiplatelet therapy: a review," *Journal of Blood Medicine*, vol. 3, pp. 33–42, 2012.

[26] E. Nutescu, I. Chuatrisorn, and E. Hellenbart, "Drug and dietary interactions of warfarin and novel oral anticoagulants: an update," *Journal of Thrombosis and Thrombolysis*, vol. 31, no. 3, pp. 326–343, 2011.

[27] J. Mendell, F. Lee, S. Chen, V. Worland, M. Shi, and M. M. Samama, "The effects of the antiplatelet agents, aspirin and naproxen, on pharmacokinetics and pharmacodynamics of the anticoagulant edoxaban, a direct factor xa inhibitor," *Journal of Cardiovascular Pharmacology*, vol. 62, no. 2, pp. 212–221, 2013.

[28] J. D. Wessler, L. T. Grip, J. Mendell, and R. P. Giugliano, "The P-glycoprotein transport system and cardiovascular drugs," *Journal of the American College of Cardiology*, vol. 61, no. 25, pp. 2495–2502, 2013.

[29] April 2015, https://www.clinicalpharmacology.com.

[30] J. D. Douketis, A. C. Spyropoulos, F. A. Spencer et al., "Perioperative management of antithrombotic therapy. Antithrombotic therapy and prevention of thrombosis, 9th ed: American College of Chest Physicians evidence-based clinical practice guidelines," *Chest*, vol. 141, no. 2, supplement, pp. e326S–e350S, 2012.

[31] A. C. Spyropoulos and J. D. Douketis, "How I treat anticoagulated patients undergoing an elective procedure or surgery," *Blood*, vol. 120, no. 15, pp. 2954–2962, 2012.

[32] T. Fuji, C.-J. Wang, S. Fujita et al., "Safety and efficacy of edoxaban, an oral factor Xa inhibitor, versus enoxaparin for thromboprophylaxis after total knee arthroplasty: the STARS E-3 trial," *Thrombosis Research*, vol. 134, no. 6, pp. 1198–1204, 2014.

[33] G. Raskob, A. T. Cohen, B. I. Eriksson et al., "Oral direct factor Xa inhibition with edoxaban for thromboprophylaxis after elective total hip replacement," *Thrombosis and Haemostasis*, vol. 104, no. 3, pp. 642–649, 2010.

[34] S. Rohatagi, J. Mendell, H. Kastrissios et al., "Characterisation of exposure versus response of edoxaban in patients undergoing total hip replacement surgery," *Thrombosis and Haemostasis*, vol. 108, no. 5, pp. 887–895, 2012.

[35] T. Fuji, S. Fujita, S. Tachibana et al., "Efficacy and safety of edoxaban versus enoxaparin for the prevention of venous thromboembolism following total hip arthroplasty: STARS J-V trial," in *Proceedings of the 52nd Annual Meeting of the American Society of Hematology*, p. 3320, Orlando, Fla, USA, December 2010.

[36] T. Fuji, S. Fujita, Y. Kawai et al., "Safety and efficacy of edoxaban in patients undergoing hip fracture surgery," *Thrombosis Research*, vol. 133, no. 6, pp. 1016–1022, 2014.

[37] The Hokusai-VTE Investigators, "Edoxaban versus warfarin for the treatment of symptomatic venous thromboembolism," *The New England Journal of Medicine*, vol. 369, pp. 1406–1415, 2013.

[38] R. P. Giugliano, C. T. Ruff, E. Braunwald et al., "Edoxaban versus warfarin in patients with atrial fibrillation," *The New England Journal of Medicine*, vol. 369, no. 22, pp. 2093–2104, 2013.

[39] R. N. H. Pugh, I. M. Murray-Lyon, and J. L. Dawson, "Transection of the oesophagus for bleeding oesophageal varices," *British Journal of Surgery*, vol. 60, no. 8, pp. 646–649, 1973.

[40] J. Graff and S. Harder, "Anticoagulant therapy with the oral direct factor Xa inhibitors rivaroxaban, apixaban and edoxaban and the thrombin inhibitor dabigatran etexilate in patients with hepatic impairment," *Clinical Pharmacokinetics*, vol. 52, no. 4, pp. 243–254, 2013.

[41] W. E. Dager and T. H. Kiser, "Systemic anticoagulation considerations in chronic kidney disease," *Advances in Chronic Kidney Disease*, vol. 17, no. 5, pp. 420–427, 2010.

[42] H. Heidbuchel, P. Verhamme, M. Alings et al., "European Heart Rhythm Association Practical Guide on the use of new oral anticoagulants in patients with non-valvular atrial fibrillation," *Europace*, vol. 15, no. 5, pp. 625–651, 2013.

[43] Y. Koretsune, T. Yamashita, and M. Yasaka, "Evaluation of edoxaban in patients with atrial fibrillation and severe renal impairment," *European Heart Journal*, vol. 34, supplement 1, 2013.

[44] D. A. Parasrampuria, T. Marbury, N. Matsushima et al., "Pharmacokinetics, safety, and tolerability of edoxaban in end-stage renal disease subjects undergoing haemodialysis," *Thrombosis and Haemostasis*, vol. 113, no. 4, pp. 719–727, 2015.

[45] P. B. Nielsen, D. A. Lane, L. H. Rasmussen, G. Y. H. Lip, and T. B. Larsen, "Renal function and non-vitamin K oral anticoagulants in comparison with warfarin on safety and efficacy outcomes in atrial fibrillation patients: a systemic review and meta-regression analysis," *Clinical Research in Cardiology*, vol. 104, no. 5, pp. 418–429, 2015.

[46] T. Fuji, S. Fujita, Y. Kawai et al., "A randomized, open-label trial of edoxaban in Japanese patients with severe renal impairment undergoing lower-limb orthopedic surgery," *Thrombosis Journal*, vol. 13, article 6, 2015.

[47] H. Kawaji, M. Ishii, Y. Tamaki, K. Sasaki, and M. Takagi, "Edoxaban for prevention of venous thromboembolism after major orthopedic surgery," *Orthopedic Research and Reviews*, vol. 4, pp. 53–64, 2012.

[48] P. Kinov, P. P. Tanchev, M. Ellis, and G. Volpin, "Antithrombotic prophylaxis in major orthopaedic surgery: an historical overview and update of current recommendations," *International Orthopaedics*, vol. 38, no. 1, pp. 169–175, 2014.

[49] Y. Falck-Ytter, C. W. Francis, N. A. Johanson et al., "Prevention of VTE in orthopedic surgery patients: Antithrombotic Therapy and Prevention of Thrombosis, 9th ed: American College of Chest Physicians Evidence-Based Clinical Practice Guidelines," *Chest*, vol. 141, supplement 2, pp. e278S–e325S, 2012.

[50] T. Fuji, S. Fujita, S. Tachibana, and Y. Kawai, "A dose-ranging study evaluating the oral factor Xa inhibitor edoxaban for the prevention of venous thromboembolism in patients undergoing total knee arthroplasty," *Journal of Thrombosis and Haemostasis*, vol. 8, no. 11, pp. 2458–2468, 2010.

[51] H. Sasaki, K. Ishida, N. Shibanuma et al., "Retrospective comparison of three thromboprophylaxis agents, edoxaban, fondaparinux, and enoxaparin, for preventing venous thromboembolism in total knee arthroplasty," *International Orthopaedics*, vol. 38, no. 3, pp. 525–529, 2014.

[52] T. Fuji, C. J. Wang, S. Fujita, Y. Kawai, T. Kimura, and S. Tachibana, "Safety and efficacy of edoxaban, an oral factor Xa

inhibitor, for thromboprophylaxis after total hip arthroplasty in Japan and Taiwan," *The Journal of Arthroplasty*, vol. 29, no. 12, pp. 2439–2436, 2014.

[53] A. C. Spyropoulos, F. A. Anderson Jr., G. FitzGerald et al., "Predictive and associative models to identify hospitalized medical patients at risk for VTE," *Chest*, vol. 140, no. 3, pp. 706–714, 2011.

[54] M. M. Samama, A. T. Cohen, J.-Y. Darmon et al., "A comparison of enoxaparin with placebo for the prevention of venous thromboembolism in acutely ill medical patients," *The New England Journal of Medicine*, vol. 341, no. 11, pp. 793–800, 1999.

[55] A. Leizorovicz, A. T. Cohen, A. G. G. Turpie, C.-G. Olsson, P. T. Vaitkus, and S. Z. Goldhaber, "Randomized, placebo-controlled trial of dalteparin for the prevention of venous thromboembolism in acutely ill medical patients," *Circulation*, vol. 110, no. 7, pp. 874–879, 2004.

[56] A. T. Cohen, B. L. Davidson, A. S. Gallus et al., "Efficacy and safety of fondaparinux for the prevention of venous thromboembolism in older acute medical patients: randomised placebo controlled trial," *British Medical Journal*, vol. 332, no. 7537, pp. 325–329, 2006.

[57] V. F. Tapson, H. Decousus, M. Pini et al., "Venous thromboembolism prophylaxis in acutely ill hospitalized medical patients: findings from the international medical prevention registry on venous thromboembolism," *Chest*, vol. 132, no. 3, pp. 936–945, 2007.

[58] C. Kearon, E. A. Akl, A. J. Comerota et al., "Antithrombotic therapy for VTE disease: antithrombotic therapy and prevention of thrombosis, 9th ed: American College of Chest Physicians evidence-based clinical practice guidelines," *Chest*, vol. 141, supplement 2, pp. e419S–e494S, 2012.

[59] S. Z. Goldhaber, A. Leizorovicz, A. K. Kakkar et al., "Apixaban versus enoxaparin for thromboprophylaxis in medically ill patients," *The New England Journal of Medicine*, vol. 365, no. 23, pp. 2167–2177, 2011.

[60] A. T. Cohen, T. E. Spiro, H. R. Buller et al., "Rivaroxaban for thromboprophylaxis in acutely ill medical patients," *The New England Journal of Medicine*, vol. 368, pp. 513–523, 2013.

[61] M. G. Beckman, W. C. Hooper, S. E. Critchley, and T. L. Ortel, "Venous thromboembolism a public health concern," *American Journal of Preventive Medicine*, vol. 38, no. 4, pp. S495–S501, 2010.

[62] C. Kearon, E. A. Akl, A. J. Comerota et al., "Antithrombotic therapy for VTE disease: antithrombotic therapy and prevention of thrombosis, 9th ed: American College of Chest Physicians evidence-based clinical practice guidelines," *Chest*, vol. 141, no. 2, supplement, pp. e419S–e494S, 2012.

[63] R. Bauersachs, S. D. Berkowitz, B. Brenner et al., "Oral rivaroxaban for symptomatic venous thromboembolism," *The New England Journal of Medicine*, vol. 363, no. 26, pp. 2499–2510, 2010.

[64] H. R. Büller, M. Prins, A. W. A. Lensing et al., "Oral rivaroxaban for the treatment of symptomatic pulmonary embolism," *The New England Journal of Medicine*, vol. 366, no. 14, pp. 1287–1297, 2012.

[65] G. Agnelli, H. R. Buller, A. Cohen et al., "Oral apixaban for the treatment of acute venous thromboembolism," *The New England Journal of Medicine*, vol. 369, no. 9, pp. 799–808, 2013.

[66] P. Prandoni, F. Noventa, A. Ghirarduzzi et al., "The risk of recurrent venous thromboembolism after discontinuing anticoagulation in patients with acute proximal deep vein thrombosis

or pulmonary embolism. A prospective cohort study in 1,626 patients," *Haematologica*, vol. 92, no. 2, pp. 199–205, 2007.

[67] M. Carrier, G. Le Gal, P. S. Wells, and M. A. Rodger, "Systematic review: case-fatality rates of recurrent venous thromboembolism and major bleeding events among patients treated for venous thromboembolism," *Annals of Internal Medicine*, vol. 152, no. 9, pp. 578–589, 2010.

[68] G. Agnelli, H. R. Buller, A. Cohen et al., "Apixaban for extended treatment of venous thromboembolism," *The New England Journal of Medicine*, vol. 368, no. 8, pp. 699–708, 2013.

[69] R. Bauersachs, S. D. Berkowitz, B. Brenner et al., "Oral rivaroxaban for symptomatic venous thromboembolism," *The New England Journal of Medicine*, vol. 363, pp. 2499–2510, 2010.

[70] A. Varki, "Trousseau's syndrome: multiple definitions and multiple mechanisms," *Blood*, vol. 110, no. 6, pp. 1723–1729, 2007.

[71] T. Wun and R. H. White, "Venous thromboembolism (VTE) in patients with cancer: epidemiology and risk factors," *Cancer Investigation*, vol. 27, no. 1, pp. 63–74, 2009.

[72] C. E. Chee, A. A. Ashrani, R. S. Marks et al., "Predictors of venous thromboembolism recurrence and bleeding among active cancer patients: a population-based cohort study," *Blood*, vol. 123, no. 25, pp. 3972–3978, 2014.

[73] J. Trujillo-Santos, J. A. Nieto, G. Tiberio et al., "Predicting recurrences or major bleeding in cancer patients with venous thromboembolism: findings from the RIETE registry," *Thrombosis & Haemostasis*, vol. 100, no. 3, pp. 435–439, 2008.

[74] A. Khorana, N. M. Kuderer, E. Culakova, G. H. Lyman, and C. W. Francis, "Development and validation of a predictive model for chemotherapy- associated thrombosis," *Blood*, vol. 111, no. 10, pp. 4902–4907, 2008.

[75] M. N. Levine, C. Gu, H. A. Liebman et al., "A randomized phase II trial of apixaban for the prevention of thromboembolism in patients with metastatic cancer," *Journal of Thrombosis and Haemostasis*, vol. 10, no. 5, pp. 807–814, 2012.

[76] M. H. Prins, A. W. A. Lensing, T. A. Brighton et al., "Oral rivaroxaban versus enoxaparin with vitamin K antagonist for the treatment of symptomatic venous thromboembolism in patients with cancer (EINSTEIN-DVT and EINSTEIN-PE): a pooled subgroup analysis of two randomised controlled trials," *The Lancet Haematology*, vol. 1, no. 1, pp. e37–e46, 2014.

[77] T. B. Larsen, P. B. Nielsen, F. Skøjoth et al., "Non-vitamin K antagonist oral anticoagulants and the treatment of venous thromboembolism in cancer patients: a systemic review and meta-analysis of safety and efficacy outcomes," *PLoS ONE*, vol. 9, no. 12, Article ID e114445, 2014.

[78] M. C. Vedovati, F. Germini, G. Agnelli, and C. Becattini, "Direct oral anticoagulants in patients With VTE and cancer," *Chest Journal*, vol. 147, no. 2, pp. 475–483, 2015.

[79] NCCN, April 2015, http://www.nccn.org/professionals/physician_gls/pdf/vte.pdf.

[80] G. H. Lyman, K. Bohlke, A. A. Khorana et al., "Venous thromboembolism prophylaxis and treatment in patients with cancer: American society of clinical oncology clinical practice guideline update 2014," *Journal of Clinical Oncology*, vol. 33, no. 6, pp. 654–656, 2015.

[81] J. L. Mega, E. Braunwald, S. D. Wiviott et al., "Rivaroxaban in patients with a recent acute coronary syndrome," *The New England Journal of Medicine*, vol. 366, no. 1, pp. 9–19, 2012.

[82] J. H. Alexander, R. D. Lopes, S. James et al., "Apixaban with antiplatelet therapy after acute coronary syndrome," *The New England Journal of Medicine*, vol. 365, no. 8, pp. 699–708, 2011.

[83] E. C. Jauch, J. L. Saver, H. P. Adams et al., "Guidelines for the early management of patients with acute ischemic stroke: a guideline for healthcare professionals from the American Heart Association/American Stroke Association," *Stroke*, vol. 44, no. 3, pp. 870–947, 2013.

[84] M. U. Zafar, D. A. Vorchheimer, J. Gaztanaga et al., "Antithrombotic effects of factor Xa inhibition with DU-176b: phase-I study of an oral, direct factor Xa inhibitor using an ex-vivo flow chamber," *Thrombosis and Haemostasis*, vol. 98, no. 4, pp. 883–888, 2007.

[85] J. I. Weitz, S. J. Connolly, I. Patel et al., "Randomised, parallel-group, multicentre, multinational phase 2 study comparing edoxaban, an oral factor Xa inhibitor, with warfarin for stroke prevention in patients with atrial fibrillation," *Thrombosis and Haemostasis*, vol. 104, no. 3, pp. 633–641, 2010.

[86] Y. Morishima and C. Kamisato, "Laboratory measurements of the oral direct factor xa inhibitor edoxaban: comparison of prothrombin time, activated partial thromboplastin time, and thrombin generation assay," *The American Journal of Clinical Pathology*, vol. 143, no. 2, pp. 241–247, 2015.

[87] T. Fukuda, Y. Honda, C. Kamisato, Y. Morishima, and T. Shibano, "Reversal of anticoagulant effects of edoxaban, an oral, direct factor Xa inhibitor, with haemostatic agents," *Thrombosis and Haemostasis*, vol. 107, no. 2, pp. 253–259, 2012.

[88] E. Herzog, F. Kaspereit, W. Krege et al., "Effective reversal of edoxaban-associated bleeding with four-factor prothrombin complex concentrate in a rabbit model of acute hemorrhage," *Anesthesiology*, vol. 122, no. 2, pp. 387–398, 2015.

[89] A.-B. Halim, M. M. Samama, and J. Mendell, "Ex vivo reversal of the anticoagulant effects of edoxaban," *Thrombosis Research*, vol. 134, no. 4, pp. 909–913, 2014.

[90] S. Kaatz, P. A. Kouides, D. A. Garcia et al., "Guidance on the emergent reversal of oral thrombin and factor Xa inhibitors," *American Journal of Hematology*, vol. 87, no. 1, pp. S141–S145, 2012.

[91] L. M. Baumann Kreuziger, J. C. Keenan, C. Morton, and D. J. Dries, "Management of bleeding patient receiving new oral anticoagulants: a role for thrombin complex concentrates," *BioMed Research International*, vol. 2014, Article ID 583794, 7 pages, 2014.

[92] H. Zahir, K. S. Brown, A. G. Vandell et al., "Edoxaban effects on bleeding following punch biopsy and reversal by a 4-FPCC prothrombin complex concentrate," *Circulation*, vol. 131, pp. 82–90, 2015.

[93] Y. Mo and F. K. Yam, "Recent advances in the development of specific antidotes for target-specific oral anticoagulants," *Pharmacotherapy*, vol. 35, no. 2, pp. 198–207, 2015.

[94] J. W. Eikelboom, M. Brueckmann, F. van de Werf et al., "Dabigatran versus warfarin in patients with mechanical heart valves," *The New England Journal of Medicine*, vol. 369, no. 13, pp. 1206–1214, 2013.

[95] M. H. Prins, L. Bamber, S. J. Cano et al., "Patient-reported treatment satisfaction with oral rivaroxaban versus standard therapy in the treatment of pulmonary embolism: results from the EINSTEIN-PE trial," *Thrombosis Research*, vol. 135, no. 2, pp. 281–288, 2015.

[96] L. Bamber, M. Y. Wang, M. H. Prins et al., "Patient-reported treatment satisfaction with oral rivaroxaban versus standard therapy in the treatment of acute symptomatic deep-vein thrombosis," *Thrombosis and Haemostasis*, vol. 110, no. 4, pp. 732–741, 2013.

[97] M. Mahmoudi and D. M. Sobieraj, "The cost-effectiveness of oral direct factor Xa inhibitors compared with low-molecular-weight heparin for the prevention of venous thromboembolism prophylaxis in total hip or knee replacement surgery," *Pharmacotherapy*, vol. 33, no. 12, pp. 1333–1340, 2013.

[98] A. Amin, A. Bruno, J. Trocio, J. Lin, and M. Lingohr-Smith, "Comparison of differences in medical costs when new oral anticoagulants are used for the treatment of patients with non-valvular atrial fibrillation and venous thromboembolism vs warfarin or placebo in the US," *Journal of Medical Economics*, vol. 18, no. 6, pp. 399–409, 2015.

34

Myeloablative Conditioning with PBSC Grafts for T Cell-Replete Haploidentical Donor Transplantation Using Posttransplant Cyclophosphamide

Scott R. Solomon, Melhem Solh, Lawrence E. Morris, H. Kent Holland, and Asad Bashey

Blood and Marrow Transplant Program at Northside Hospital, Atlanta, GA 30342, USA

Correspondence should be addressed to Scott R. Solomon; ssolomon@bmtga.com

Academic Editor: Franco Aversa

Relapse is the main cause of treatment failure after nonmyeloablative haploidentical transplant (haplo-HSCT). In an attempt to reduce relapse, we have developed a myeloablative (MA) haplo-HSCT approach utilizing posttransplant cyclophosphamide (PT/Cy) and peripheral blood stem cells as the stem cell source. We summarize the results of two consecutive clinical trials, using a busulfan-based ($n = 20$) and a TBI-based MA preparative regimen ($n = 30$), and analyze a larger cohort of 64 patients receiving MA haplo-HSCT. All patients have engrafted with full donor chimerism and no late graft failures. Grade III-IV acute GVHD and moderate-severe chronic GVHD occurred in 23% and 30%, respectively. One-year NRM was 10%. Predicted three-year overall survival, disease-free survival, and relapse were 53%, 53%, and 26%, respectively, in all patients and 79%, 74%, and 9%, respectively, in patients with a low/intermediate disease risk index (DRI). In multivariate analysis, DRI was the most significant predictor of survival and relapse. Use of TBI (versus busulfan) had no significant impact on survival but was associated with significantly less BK virus-associated hemorrhagic cystitis. We contrast our results with other published reports of MA haplo-HSCT PT/Cy in the literature and attempt to define the comparative utility of MA haplo-HSCT to other methods of transplantation.

1. Introduction

Seventy percent of patients who urgently need an allogeneic hematopoietic stem cell transplantation (HSCT) do not have an available HLA-matched sibling donor. In such patients, a search for an HLA-matched unrelated donor (MUD) can identify an 8/8 HLA-identical donor for approximately 30% to 40% of transplant recipients. The probability of finding an acceptable MUD varies by ethnic groups, ranging from 75% in the white Europeans, to 30% to 40% in the Mexican and Central/South Americans, to 15% to 20% for the African Americans and black Caribbeans [1]. In addition, MUD transplantation is also complicated by the amount of time it takes from search initiation to transplantation, causing some patients to relapse or physically deteriorate while waiting for transplantation. In contrast, a haploidentical family member (haplo) can be identified and rapidly utilized in nearly all cases.

Historically, HSCT from a partially HLA-mismatched relative has been complicated by unacceptably high incidences of graft rejection, severe graft-versus-host disease (GVHD), and nonrelapse mortality (NRM) [2, 3]. To address the risk of graft rejection and GVHD, extensive T cell depletion has been utilized in association with antithymocyte globulin (ATG) and high peripheral blood stem cell (PBSC) dose [4]; however, NRM from infectious complications remains a challenge. More recently, the investigators at Johns Hopkins University have pioneered a method to selectively deplete alloreactive cells in vivo by administering high doses of cyclophosphamide (Cy) in a narrow window after transplantation [5]. After nonmyeloablative (NMA) conditioning, this approach has resulted in low NRM (4% and 15% at 1 and 2 years, resp.), because of low rates of GVHD and infectious complications. Immune reconstitution was promising with low risk of cytomegalovirus (CMV) or invasive mold infections. Using high-dose, posttransplantation cyclophosphamide (PT/Cy), crossing the HLA barrier in HSCT is now feasible without the need for extensive T cell depletion or serotherapy.

Studies of NMA haplo-HSCT with PT/Cy show remarkable tolerability of this approach with low rates of GVHD, infection, and NRM. Relapse of malignancy remains the predominant cause of treatment failure, occurring in approximately 45% to 51% of patients [5, 6]. NMA haplo-HSCT with PT/Cy has also been associated with an approximately 10% rate of engraftment failure resulting in autologous recovery. The use of more intense/myeloablative (MA) preparative regimens and PBSC grafts may potentially reduce the rate of relapse and graft rejection following haplo-HSCT PT/Cy transplants. However, only a limited number of such studies have been reported. In this paper, we report our experience with MA conditioning and PBSC allografts for T-replete haplo-HSCT using PT/Cy. We define the major predictors of outcome following this strategy. We also describe other published reports of MA haplo-HSCT PT/Cy in the literature. Finally, we compare the outcomes of MA and NMA haplo-HSCT using PT/Cy and attempt to define the comparative utility of MA haplo-HSCT in relation to MUD transplantation.

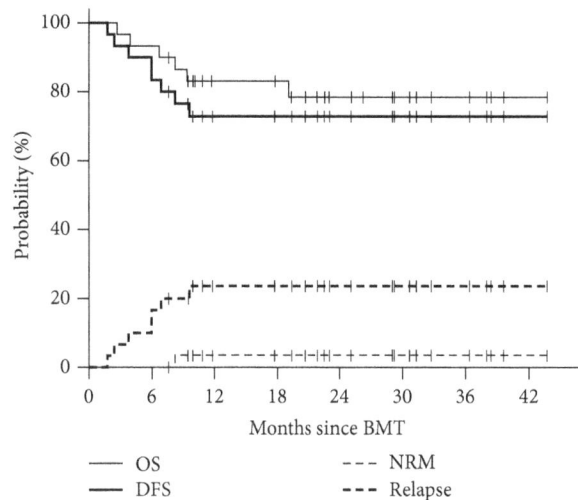

FIGURE 1: Kaplan-Meier analysis of overall survival, disease-free survival, and nonrelapse mortality and following TBI-based MA haplo-HSCT.

2. Busulfan-Based MA Haplo-HSCT (NSH 864 Protocol)

In a proof-of-principle study of MA haplo-HSCT, twenty patients with high risk hematologic malignancies were treated with a preparative regimen of fludarabine (125–180 mg/m^2), i.v. busulfan (440–520 mg/m^2) and Cy (29 mg/kg) before transplant, a G-CSF-mobilized PBSC graft, and posttransplant GVHD prophylaxis comprised of Cy 50 mg/kg/d on d +3 and +4, MMF 15 mg/kg three times daily d +5–+35, and tacrolimus (target 5–15 ng/mL) days +5 to +180 [7]. The median age of patients was 44 years (range: 25–56 years). Eleven patients (55%) underwent HSCT with relapsed/refractory disease (acute myelogenous leukemia [AML] 5, chronic myelogenous leukemia-blast crisis [CML-BC] 1, acute lymphoblastic leukemia 2, non-Hodgkin lymphoma 1, Hodgkin's disease 1, and chronic lymphocytic leukemia/Richters 1). The remaining patients had either AML CR1 with poor-risk cytogenetics and/or induction failure or chronic myelogenous leukemia resistant to all tyrosine kinase inhibitors.

All patients engrafted and demonstrated 100% donor chimerism in both peripheral blood T cell and myeloid cells from day +30. Cumulative incidence of one-year NRM was 10% and that of grade III-IV acute GVHD and severe chronic GVHD was 10% and 5%, respectively. Relapse was acceptable, occurring in 40% of patients, despite the fact that the majority had relapsed/refractory disease at time of transplant. With a median follow-up of 20 months, estimated probabilities of overall and disease-free survival (DFS) were 69% and 50%, respectively.

There were no cases of invasive mold infections or EBV-related PTLD. Only one patient had CMV disease and only one patient died of a viral infection (parainfluenza 3) suggesting that anti-infection immunity was preserved with this approach. However, nonfatal BK virus-associated hemorrhagic cystitis (HC) was seen in 75% of patients at a median of

38 days after transplant. Although it is not a life-threatening complication, it was a source of significant morbidity for some patients. We hypothesized that HC was predisposed to by the combined effect of high-dose busulfan and PT/Cy.

3. Total-Body Irradiation-Based Haplo-HSCT (NSH 922 Protocol)

In an attempt to reduce the risk of BK virus-associated HC, thirty patients were enrolled on prospective phase II trial utilizing a TBI-based myeloablative preparative regimen (fludarabine 25 mg/m^2/d × 3 d and TBI 150 cGy bid on d −4 to −1 [total dose 1200 cGy]) followed by infusion of unmanipulated peripheral blood stem cells from a haploidentical family donor [8]. Postgrafting immunosuppression again consisted of Cy 50 mg/kg/day on days 3 and 4, MMF through d 35, and tacrolimus through d 180. Median patient age was 46.5 years (range 24–60). Transplant diagnosis included AML [9], ALL [6], CML [5], MDS [1], and NHL [2]. Using the revised Dana-Farber/CIBMTR disease risk index (DRI), patients were classified as having low [4], intermediate [10], high [11], and very high [3] risk.

All patients engrafted with a median time to neutrophil and platelet recovery of 16 and 25 days, respectively. All evaluable patients achieved sustained complete donor T cell and myeloid chimerism by day +30. Acute GVHD, grades II–IV and III-IV, was seen in 43% and 23%, respectively. The cumulative incidence of moderate-to-severe chronic GVHD was 22% (severe in 10%). Nonrelapse mortality (NRM) at 2 years was 3%, which consisted of one death due to noninfectious respiratory failure/ARDS 8 months after transplant in a patient with chronic GVHD. Estimated two-year survival, DFS, and relapse were 78%, 73%, and 24%, respectively (Figure 1). Two-year DFS and relapse rate in patients with low/intermediate disease risk, determined by the DRI, were

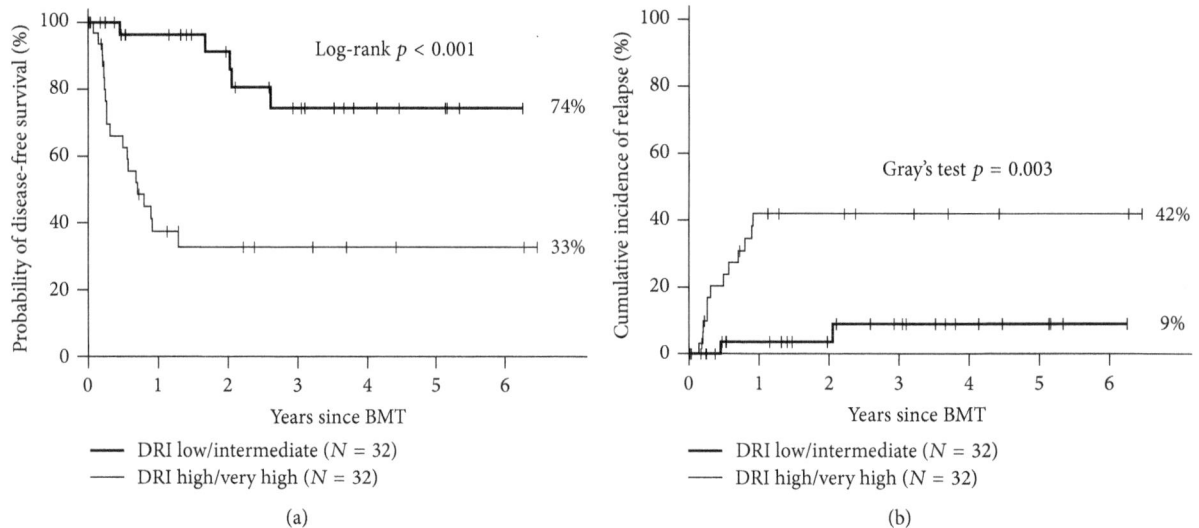

FIGURE 2: Effect of disease risk index on (a) disease-free survival and (b) relapse following MA haplo-HSCT.

100% and 0%, respectively, compared with 39% and 53% for patients with high/very high risk disease.

As noted in our prior experience with busulfan-based MA haplo-HSCT, posttransplant fever was common and occurred in the first 5 posttransplant days in nearly all patients. Fevers resolved in all patients following administration of PT/Cy. CMV reactivation ($\geq$400 copies/mL) occurred in 15/26 (58%) of at-risk patients (either donor or recipient with CMV positive serostatus) at a median of day +43 after transplant (range 11–157). CMV disease did not occur. There were no episodes of invasive mold infection or infectious death in the first 100 days after transplant. There were no cases of EBV reactivation. BK virus-associated HC of any grade occurred in 30% of patients and was severe (grade $\geq$ 3) in 7%. As compared with our previous experience with busulfan-based MA haplo-HSCT, HC occurred significantly less often following TBI-based MA haplo-HSCT (any grade: 30% versus 75%, p = 0.005; severe HC: 7% versus 30%, p = 0.037).

4. Predictors of Outcome following MA Haplo-HSCT and PT/Cy

In order to determine predictors of outcome following MA haplo-HSCT and PT/Cy, we evaluated that sixty-four consecutive patients have been transplanted following either busulfan-based (n = 20; NSH 864) or TBI-based (n = 44; including 30 patients on NSH 922 and the remaining 14 patients treated identically after completion of the trial) MA conditioning, T cell-replete PBSC infusion, PT/Cy, and tacrolimus/mycophenolate mofetil. Median age of the cohort was 43 years (range 21–60). Patient characteristics included a high/very high disease risk by the Dana-Farber/CIBMTR disease risk index (DRI) in 32 patients (50%), KPS <90 in 69%, and comorbidity index (CMI) of $\geq$2 in 58% of patients. The most common indications for transplant were AML, ALL, and advanced-phase CML in 55%, 20%, and 12% of patients,

respectively. Median follow-up for surviving patients was 24 months.

All patients engrafted with full donor chimerism and no late graft failures. Grade II–IV, III-IV acute GVHD and moderate-severe chronic GVHD occurred in 46%, 23%, and 30%, respectively. One-year NRM was 10%. Predicted three-year overall survival (OS), disease-free survival (DFS), and relapse are 53%, 53%, and 26%, respectively. In the 32 patients with standard risk disease (low/intermediate DRI), outcomes were significantly improved with one-year NRM of 0% and predicted 3-year OS, DFS, and relapse of 79%, 74%, and 9%, respectively (Figure 2).

In multivariate analysis, high/very high DRI was the most significant negative predictor of OS (HR 13.26, p < 0.001), followed by CMI $\geq$2 (HR 3.54, p = 0.01) and age (HR 1.26, p = 0.038, per 5-year increase in age). DRI was also significantly associated with DFS (HR 10.84, p < 0.001), NRM (HR 15.0, p = 0.004), and relapse (HR 8.85, p = 0.004) (Table 1). Conditioning regimen (TBI versus busulfan) had no significant impact on OS, DFS, NRM, or relapse.

5. Additional Published Experience with MA Haplo-HSCT and PT/Cy

Several other groups have published similar experiences with MA haplo-HSCT with PT/Cy. Grosso et al. [12] reported a "two-step" strategy where a defined dose of haploidentical T cells (2 × 108/kg) was infused after MA doses of TBI. Patients then received 60 mg/kg of CY on two consecutive days, followed later by infusion of highly purified CD34+ cells from the donor. All patients engrafted and the cumulative incidence of grade III-IV acute GVHD and NRM was 7.4% and 22.5%, respectively, for the 27 patients treated. With a median follow-up of 40 months, overall survival was 48%. A second study from the same group [13], which included only patients in remission at the time of transplant, demonstrated

TABLE 1: Predictors of transplant outcomes following MA haplo HSCT.

	OS		DFS		NRM		Relapse	
	HR	p	HR	p	HR	p	HR	p
DRI (high versus low/int)	**13.26**	<0.001	**10.84**	<0.001	**15.0**	0.004	**8.85**	0.004
CMI (≥2 versus <2)	**3.54**	0.010	**3.09**	0.018	**13.6**	0.007	—	—
Age (<50 versus ≥50)	**1.26**	0.038	**1.31**	0.015	**1.43**	0.055	—	—

The following variables were considered in Cox analysis: age, diagnosis, Karnofsky performance status (KPS), comorbidity index (CMI), revised Dana-Farber disease risk index (DRI), conditioning regimen (busulfan versus TBI), year of transplant, acute GVHD, and chronic GVHD. Variables were selected by 10% threshold. Acute and chronic GVHD were modeled as time-dependent variables.

a 2 yr NRM, relapse, and PFS of 4%, 19%, and 74%, respectively. The requirement for stringent ex vivo T depletion of the hematopoietic cell product differentiates this approach and may limit its widespread applicability. Furthermore, given the resistance of hematopoietic stem cells to Cy, such delayed infusion of selected CD34+ cells may be unnecessary.

Symons et al. [11] reported on 97 patients with either leukemias in complete remission or lymphoma with chemosensitive disease. Patients received MA haplo-HSCT PT/Cy utilizing bone marrow grafts. The preparative regimen consisted of IV busulfan (pharmacokinetically adjusted) on days −6 to −3 and Cy (50 mg/kg/day) on days −2 and −1, except for patients with acute lymphocytic leukemia or lymphoblastic lymphoma who received Cy (50 mg/kg/day) on days −5 and −4 and TBI (200 cGy twice daily) on days −3 to −1. Donor engraftment occurred in 73/82 (89%) patients. Estimated probabilities of NRM and grade III-IV acute GVHD at 100 days were 11% and 7%, respectively. The cumulative incidence of relapse was 44%. With a median follow-up of surviving patients of 474 days, estimated 2 yr overall and disease-free survival is 57% and 49%, respectively.

Raiola et al. [10] reported on 50 patients receiving a MA haplo-HSCT PT/Cy utilizing bone marrow grafts. The regimens used were thiotepa, busulfan, and fludarabine (n = 35) or TBI and fludarabine (n = 15). Forty-five patients (90%) engrafted with an 18-month cumulative incidence of NRM, relapse, and PFS of 18%, 22%, and 51%, respectively. PFS was 67% for patients transplanted in remission versus 37% for patients with active disease. Reported incidences of acute and chronic GVHD were low. As in our experience, HC was more common in patients receiving busulfan rather than TBI-based conditioning.

Whether PBSC or BM is the preferred stem cell source following MA haplo-HSCT remains unclear; however BM appears to be associated with a higher rate of graft failure, occurring in approximately 10% of patients in both the series by Raiola et al. [10] and the experience of Symons et al. [11]. Graft failure has not been reported with PBSC based myeloablative haplo-HSCT and PT/Cy.

6. Comparison of MA and NMA Haplo-PT/Cy

The overall risk of relapse associated with MA haplo-HSCT in the majority of studies is 20–25% [7, 8, 10, 13] and compares favorably with that reported for NMA haplo-HSCT (45–51%) [5, 6]. In our analysis of 64 patients receiving MA haplo-HSCT, relapse risk in patients with low (n = 7) or intermediate (n = 25) DRI was 9%, compared with 42% relapse rate in high (n = 24) or very high (n = 8) DRI patients. This compares favorably to that seen in the NMA setting, where relapse risk according to DRI was recently analyzed in 372 consecutive patients by the group from Johns Hopkins University [14]. In this analysis, the risk of relapse was also highly correlated with DRI, with relapse occurring in approximately 75%, 50%, and 20% of patients in the high/very high, intermediate, and low DRI groups, respectively. The finding of higher relapse following NMA conditioning parallels what has been seen following matched related or unrelated donor transplantation [9, 15–17].

7. Comparison of MA Haplo-PT/Cy with MA MUD Transplants

In order to evaluate the comparative efficacy of MA haplo-HSCT, we have compared outcomes of patients receiving TBI-based MA haplo-HSCT with PT/Cy (n = 30) with a contemporaneously treated cohort of consecutive patients at our institution receiving HLA-matched (8/8 HLA-A, HLA-B, HLA-C, and HLA-DR) MA T cell-replete MUD transplantation (n = 48) [8]. Haplo- and MUD transplant patients were well matched according to age, diagnosis, disease risk, CMV serostatus, and comorbidity index. The groups did differ in the use of PBSC as the stem cell source which was utilized in all haplotransplant recipients compared with 32 of 48 MUD transplants recipients. When compared with recipients of MA MUD transplants, outcomes after MA haplo-HSCT were statistically similar to 2 yr OS and DFS being 78% and 73%, respectively, after haplotransplant versus 71% and 64%, respectively, after MUD transplants. Grade II–IV acute GVHD was seen less often following haplotransplantation compared with MUD transplantation (43% versus 63%, p = 0.049), as was moderate-to-severe chronic GVHD (22% versus 58%, p = 0.003). The lower incidence of chronic GVHD occurred despite the greater use of PBSC in the haplo-HSCT group.

Similarly, a Center for International Blood and Marrow Transplant Research (CIBMTR) analysis [18] compared outcomes of adults with acute myeloid leukemia (AML) after haplo- (n = 192) and MUD (n = 1982) transplantation, including 104 MA haplotransplants and 1245 MA MUD transplants. In this large analysis, there were no significant differences in 1 yr NRM (12% versus 14%), 3 yr relapse (44% versus 39%), or 3 yr OS (46% versus 44%), comparing MA haplo- and MA MUD transplants, respectively. Grade II–IV acute GVHD (16% versus 33%), grade III-IV acute GVHD (7% versus 13%), and chronic GVHD (30% versus 53%) were all statistically lower in haplopatients compared with MUD patients.

8. Immune Recovery following MA Haplo-PT/Cy

Historically, MA haplotransplantation has been associated with considerable infectious morbidity and mortality. In contrast, our experience and others suggest that MA haplo-PT/Cy may significantly reduce the risk of infectious complications. In a published series of thirty patients undergoing TBI-based MA haplo-PT/Cy [8], CMV reactivation ($\geq$400 copies/mL) occurred in only 15/26 (58%) of at-risk patients (either donor or recipient with CMV positive serostatus), and CMV disease did not occur. There were no episodes of invasive mold infection or infectious death in the first 100 days after transplant. Furthermore, there were no cases of EBV, HHV6, or adenovirus infections.

The reduced risk of infectious complications following MA haplo-PT/Cy has translated into low NRM, approximately 10% in the first year after transplant. Our experience compares favorably to the results reported with T cell-depleted (TCD) MA haplo, where NRM of approximately 40% have been seen, with much of this attributable to infectious mortality [4, 19–21]. Ciurea and colleagues at the MD Anderson Cancer Center analyzed their outcomes following MA haplo-PT/Cy following a preparative regimen of fludarabine, melphalan, and thiotepa, with historical results of TCD MA haplo using the same preparative regimen [20]. In this analysis, one-year NRM favored PT/Cy (16% versus 42%) as did death directly attributable to infection (9% versus 24%), with significantly less viral and fungal infections seen in PT/Cy versus TCD patients. T cell subset analysis demonstrated significant improvements in T cell recovery in PT/Cy versus TCD patients, with more rapid reconstitution noted in multiple T cell subsets (CD4, CD8, naïve, and memory).

Immune reconstitution following haplo-PT/Cy is characterized by a diverse T cell receptor repertoire and appears dependent on T memory stem cells maturing from naïve T cells [22, 23]. These cells are adoptively transferred in the donor graft and have been shown to survive cyclophosphamide-induced deletion. Furthermore, regulatory T cells also are preferentially preserved following PT/Cy, likely due to higher aldehyde dehydrogenase in these cells [24]. Finally, murine studies have demonstrated that PT/Cy relatively spares pathogen and cancer-specific T cells [25]. The selective elimination of alloreactive donor T cells with relative preservation of non-alloreactive donor T cell clones provides a mechanistic understanding of the surprisingly low infectious mortality following MA haplo-PT/Cy.

9. Discussion

In the past decade, there has been a growing interest in the use of haplo-HSCT due to the rapid and nearly universal availability of donors, which is a critical issue in patients with advanced hematologic malignancies. A major advance in the success of haplo-HSCT is the use of properly timed PT/Cy, a technique pioneered by investigators at Johns Hopkins University [5, 26]. Using a NMA approach, this strategy has resulted in low rates of GVHD, infection, and NRM. However, relapse remains the major cause of treatment failure, occurring in approximately half of transplant recipients. One explanation for the high rate of relapse, as in other NMA HSCT trials, is that the transplantation conditioning was not intense enough to achieve sufficient tumor cytoreduction.

In order to reduce the risk of relapse in patients with high risk hematologic malignancies, our group and others have demonstrated the feasibility of performing MA haplo-HSCT utilizing PT/Cy. In 64 consecutive patients transplanted at our institution following either busulfan-based (n = 20) or TBI-based (n = 44) MA conditioning, we have noted universal engraftment with rapid donor chimerism, acceptable rates of GVHD (grade III-IV acute GVHD and moderate-severe chronic GVHD occurred in 23% and 30%, resp.), and a low one-year NRM of 10%. Predicted three-year overall survival (OS), disease-free survival (DFS), and relapse were 53%, 53%, and 26%, respectively, and in the 32 patients with standard risk disease (low/intermediate DRI), outcomes were very favorable (3-year OS, DFS, and relapse of 79%, 74%, and 9%, resp.).

Relapse appears less following MA conditioning with relapse rates in the majority of studies of 20–25% [7, 8, 10, 13], compared with that reported for NMA haplo-BMT (45–51%) [5, 6]. However, truly defining the influence of the preparative regimen intensity on relapse risk will likely require a randomized controlled trial. When comparing our results with the other published experiences of MA haplo-HSCT using PT/Cy, it becomes evident that disease risk, as defined by either the DRI or disease status at the time of transplant, is the primary driver of outcomes, with 2 yr DFS being approximately 67–74% [8, 10, 13] in patients transplanted in remission without high risk disease defined by the DRI. Whether PBSC or BM is the preferred stem cell source following myeloablative haplo-HSCT remains unclear; however BM appears to be associated with a higher rate of graft failure, occurring in approximately 10% of patients [10, 11] receiving marrow grafts, and is obviously more consequential following MA conditioning.

Although there have been no randomized studies to date, there is now compelling evidence regarding the equivalent efficacy and safety of haplo-HSCT PT/Cy and MUD transplantation, in both the NMA and MA setting [8, 18, 27–29]. When considering the optimal transplant donor type, MUD versus haplo-HSCT, one must consider the inherent advantages of haplodonors including near universal and rapid availability, as well as lower costs related to donor searching and graft acquisition, whereas as almost all patients have an available haplomatched family member, the availability of an 8/8 matched unrelated donor varies according to ethnic background, ranging from 75% for white patients of European descent to less than 20% for the African Americans. Furthermore, given the complexities inherent in registry searching, time from initiation of donor searching to transplant can be significant, averaging around 3 months.

In conclusion, our results show that MA haplo-HSCT results in favorable engraftment, acceptable rates of GVHD, and low nonrelapse mortality. Relapse rates appear lower than that reported with NMA haplo-HSCT. DRI represents the strongest predictor of outcome following MA haplo-HSCT and PT/Cy. Disease-free and overall survival is equivalent to recipients of MA MUD transplants. Therefore, in younger patients without contraindications to standard intensity conditioning, MA haplo-HSCT is a valid option for patients with advanced hematologic malignancies who lack timely access to a conventional donor.

Conflict of Interests

The authors declare that there is no conflict of interests regarding the publication of this paper.

References

[1] L. Gragert, M. Eapen, E. Williams et al., "HLA match likelihoods for hematopoietic stem-cell grafts in the U.S. registry," The New England Journal of Medicine, vol. 371, no. 4, pp. 339–348, 2014.

[2] P. G. Beatty, R. A. Clift, E. M. Mickelson et al., "Marrow transplantation from related donors other than HLA-identical siblings," The New England Journal of Medicine, vol. 313, no. 13, pp. 765–771, 1985.

[3] R. Szydlo, J. M. Goldman, J. P. Klein et al., "Results of allogeneic bone marrow transplants for leukemia using donors other than HLA-identical siblings," Journal of Clinical Oncology, vol. 15, no. 5, pp. 1767–1777, 1997.

[4] F. Aversa, A. Terenzi, A. Tabilio et al., "Full haplotype-mismatched hematopoietic stem-cell transplantation: a phase II study in patients with acute leukemia at high risk of relapse," Journal of Clinical Oncology, vol. 23, no. 15, pp. 3447–3454, 2005.

[5] L. Luznik, P. V. O'Donnell, H. J. Symons et al., "HLA-haploidentical bone marrow transplantation for hematologic malignancies using nonmyeloablative conditioning and high-dose, posttransplantation cyclophosphamide," Biology of Blood and Marrow Transplantation, vol. 14, no. 6, pp. 641–650, 2008.

[6] C. G. Brunstein, E. J. Fuchs, S. L. Carter et al., "Alternative donor transplantation after reduced intensity conditioning: results of parallel phase 2 trials using partially HLA-mismatched related bone marrow or unrelated double umbilical cord blood grafts," Blood, vol. 118, no. 2, pp. 282–288, 2011.

[7] S. R. Solomon, C. A. Sizemore, M. Sanacore et al., "Haploidentical transplantation using T cell replete peripheral blood stem cells and myeloablative conditioning in patients with high-risk hematologic malignancies who lack conventional donors is well tolerated and produces excellent relapse-free survival: results of a prospective phase II trial," Biology of Blood and Marrow Transplantation, vol. 18, no. 12, pp. 1859–1866, 2012.

[8] S. R. Solomon, C. A. Sizemore, M. Sanacore et al., "Total body irradiation-based myeloablative haploidentical stem cell transplantation is a safe and effective alternative to unrelated donor transplantation in patients without matched sibling donors," Biology of Blood and Marrow Transplantation, vol. 21, no. 7, pp. 1299–1307, 2015.

[9] O. Ringdén, M. Labopin, G. Ehninger et al., "Reduced intensity conditioning compared with myeloablative conditioning using unrelated donor transplants in patients with acute myeloid leukemia," Journal of Clinical Oncology, vol. 27, no. 27, pp. 4570–4577, 2009.

[10] A. M. Raiola, A. Dominietto, A. Ghiso et al., "Unmanipulated haploidentical bone marrow transplantation and posttransplantation cyclophosphamide for hematologic malignancies after myeloablative conditioning," Biology of Blood and Marrow Transplantation, vol. 19, no. 1, pp. 117–122, 2013.

[11] H. J. Symons, A. Chen, C. Gamper et al., "Haploidentical BMT using fully myeloablative conditioning, T cell replete bone marrow grafts, and post-transplant cyclophosphamide (PT/Cy) has limited toxicity and promising efficacy in largest reported experience with high risk hematologic malignancies," Biology of Blood and Marrow Transplantation, vol. 21, no. 2, p. S29, 2015.

[12] D. Grosso, M. Carabasi, J. Filicko-O'Hara et al., "A 2-step approach to myeloablative haploidentical stem cell transplantation: a phase 1/2 trial performed with optimized T-cell dosing," Blood, vol. 118, no. 17, pp. 4732–4739, 2011.

[13] D. Grosso, S. Gaballa, O. Alpdogan et al., "A two-step approach to myeloablative haploidentical transplantation: low nonrelapse mortality and high survival confirmed in patients with earlier stage disease," Biology of Blood and Marrow Transplantation, vol. 21, no. 4, pp. 646–652, 2015.

[14] S. R. McCurdy, J. A. Kanakry, M. M. Showel et al., "Risk-stratified outcomes of nonmyeloablative HLA-haploidentical BMT with high-dose posttransplantation cyclophosphamide," Blood, vol. 125, no. 19, pp. 3024–3031, 2015.

[15] M. Aoudjhane, M. Labopin, N. C. Gorin et al., "Comparative outcome of reduced intensity and myeloablative conditioning regimen in HLA identical sibling allogeneic haematopoietic stem cell transplantation for patients older than 50 years of age with acute myeloblastic leukaemia: a retrospective survey from the Acute Leukemia Working Party (ALWP) of the European group for Blood and Marrow Transplantation (EBMT)," Leukemia, vol. 19, no. 12, pp. 2304–2312, 2005.

[16] M. Mohty, M. Labopin, L. Volin et al., "Reduced-intensity versus conventional myeloablative conditioning allogeneic stem cell transplantation for patients with acute lymphoblastic leukemia: a retrospective study from the European Group for Blood and Marrow Transplantation," Blood, vol. 116, no. 22, pp. 4439–4443, 2010.

[17] A. Shimoni, I. Hardan, N. Shem-Tov et al., "Allogeneic hematopoietic stem-cell transplantation in AML and MDS using myeloablative versus reduced-intensity conditioning: the role of dose intensity," Leukemia, vol. 20, no. 2, pp. 322–328, 2006.

[18] S. O. Ciurea, M.-J. Zhang, A. A. Bacigalupo et al., "Haploidentical transplant with posttransplant cyclophosphamide vs matched unrelated donor transplant for acute myeloid leukemia," Blood, vol. 126, no. 8, pp. 1033–1040, 2015.

[19] F. Ciceri, M. Labopin, F. Aversa et al., "A survey of fully haploidentical hematopoietic stem cell transplantation in adults with high-risk acute leukemia: a risk factor analysis of outcomes for patients in remission at transplantation," Blood, vol. 112, no. 9, pp. 3574–3581, 2008.

[20] S. O. Ciurea, V. Mulanovich, R. M. Saliba et al., "Improved early outcomes using a T cell replete graft compared with T cell depleted haploidentical hematopoietic stem cell transplantation," Biology of Blood and Marrow Transplantation, vol. 18, no. 12, pp. 1835–1844, 2012.

[21] B. Federmann, M. Bornhauser, C. Meisner et al., "Haploidentical allogeneic hematopoietic cell transplantation in adults using CD3/CD19 depletion and reduced intensity conditioning: a

phase II study," *Haematologica*, vol. 97, no. 10, pp. 1523–1531, 2012.

[22] N. Cieri, G. Oliveira, R. Greco et al., "Generation of human memory stem T cells after haploidentical T-replete hematopoietic stem cell transplantation," *Blood*, vol. 125, no. 18, pp. 2865–2874, 2015.

[23] A. Roberto, L. Castagna, V. Zanon et al., "Role of naive-derived T memory stem cells in T-cell reconstitution following allogeneic transplantation," *Blood*, vol. 125, no. 18, pp. 2855–2864, 2015.

[24] C. G. Kanakry, S. Ganguly, M. Zahurak et al., "Aldehyde dehydrogenase expression drives human regulatory T cell resistance to posttransplantation cyclophosphamide," *Science Translational Medicine*, vol. 5, no. 211, Article ID 211ra157, 2013.

[25] D. Ross, M. Jones, K. Komanduri, and R. B. Levy, "Antigen and lymphopenia-driven donor T cells are differentially diminished by post-transplantation administration of cyclophosphamide after hematopoietic cell transplantation," *Biology of Blood and Marrow Transplantation*, vol. 19, no. 10, pp. 1430–1438, 2013.

[26] P. V. O'Donnell, L. Luznik, R. J. Jones et al., "Nonmyeloablative bone marrow transplantation from partially HLA-mismatched related donors using posttransplantation cyclophosphamide," *Biology of Blood and Marrow Transplantation*, vol. 8, no. 7, pp. 377–386, 2002.

[27] A. Bashey, X. Zhang, K. Jackson et al., "Comparison of outcomes of hematopoietic cell transplants from T-replete haploidentical donors using post-transplantation cyclophosphamide with 10 of 10 HLA-A, -B, -C, -DRB1, and -DQB1 allele-matched unrelated donors and HLA-identical sibling donors: a multivariable analysis including disease risk index," *Biology of Blood and Marrow Transplantation*, vol. 22, no. 1, pp. 125–133, 2016.

[28] A. Bashey, X. Zhang, C. A. Sizemore et al., "T-cell-replete HLA-haploidentical hematopoietic transplantation for hematologic malignancies using post-transplantation cyclophosphamide results in outcomes equivalent to those of contemporaneous HLA-matched related and unrelated donor transplantation," *Journal of Clinical Oncology*, vol. 31, no. 10, pp. 1310–1316, 2013.

[29] A. Di Stasi, D. R. Milton, L. M. Poon et al., "Similar transplantation outcomes for acute myeloid leukemia and myelodysplastic syndrome patients with haploidentical versus 10/10 human leukocyte antigen-matched unrelated and related donors," *Biology of Blood and Marrow Transplantation*, vol. 20, no. 12, pp. 1975–1981, 2014.

35

Prospects of Vitamin C as an Additive in Plasma of Stored Blood

R. Vani, R. Soumya, H. Carl, V. A. Chandni, K. Neha, B. Pankhuri, S. Trishna, and D. P. Vatsal

Center for Post Graduate Studies, Jain University, No. 18/3, 9th Main, 3rd Block, Jayanagar, Bangalore 560011, India

Correspondence should be addressed to R. Vani; tiwari.vani@gmail.com

Academic Editor: Thomas Kickler

There is a dire necessity to improve blood storage and prolong shelf-life of blood. Very few studies have focused on oxidative stress (OS) in blood and its influence on plasma with storage. This study attempts to (i) elucidate the continuous changes occurring in plasma during storage through oxidant levels and antioxidant status and (ii) evaluate the influence of vitamin C (VC) as an additive during blood storage. Blood was drawn from male *Wistar* rats and stored for 25 days at 4°C. Blood samples were divided into control and experimental groups. Plasma was isolated every 5 days and the OS markers, antioxidant enzymes, lipid peroxidation, and protein oxidation products, were studied. Catalase activity increased in all groups with storage. Lipid peroxidation decreased in VC (10) but was maintained in VC (30) and VC (60). Although there were variations in all groups, carbonyls were maintained towards the end of storage. Advanced oxidation protein products (AOPP) increased in VC (30) and were maintained in VC (10) and VC (60). Sulfhydryls were maintained in all groups. Vitamin C could not sufficiently attenuate OS and hence, this opens the possibilities for further studies on vitamin C in combination with other antioxidants, in storage solutions.

1. Introduction

Blood transfusion is an irreplaceable, lifesaving, and overall safe treatment. Continued developments in storage techniques have resulted in improved storage and blood quality. Whole blood is stored in CPDA (citrate phosphate dextrose and adenine) or ACD (acid, citrate, and dextrose) solution up to a period of 35 days at 4°C [1]. The storage of blood in *ex vivo* conditions causes biochemical and biomechanical changes (storage lesion), which in turn affect optimal functioning and survival [2–6]. Transfusions of these altered products are associated with increased morbidity and mortality [7]. However, the alterations that occur during storage appear to be partially reversible by use of improved storage conditions and additive solutions [8]. Hence, better storage will require a system that will provide critical nutrients, improve storage milieu, and reduce the stress of storage.

One of the reasons for the formation of the storage lesion is oxidative stress (OS). This was evident in our earlier study on erythrocytes of stored blood [9]. During storage, erythrocytes undergo structural and functional changes that reduce the viability of cells. These changes include variations in the levels of the endogenous and exogenous antioxidant system and oxidative modifications of (i) proteins (protein carbonyls, advanced oxidation protein products, and protein sulfhydryls) and (ii) lipids (thiobarbituric acid reactive substances) in the erythrocyte membrane which destabilize its structure [10, 11]. The lifespan of rat erythrocytes in circulation (60 days) is lower when compared to humans (120 days). Thus, rat erythrocytes undergo deterioration more rapidly than human erythrocytes. The storage lesion in rat erythrocytes stored for a week is similar to that in human erythrocytes stored for 4 weeks [12]. Hence, studying rat erythrocytes would provide an insight into the OS situation during storage.

There are many efficient antioxidants which can reduce the OS induced by storage [13–15]. For example, antioxidant effects of vitamin C (ascorbic acid) have been demonstrated in many experiments *in vitro* [16]. It is regarded as the most important water-soluble antioxidant in plasma [17], has been shown to neutralize reactive oxygen species (ROS), and reduces OS [18, 19]. In addition to scavenging ROS and reactive nitrogen species, vitamin C can regenerate other small molecule antioxidants, such as α-tocopherol, glutathione (GSH), urate, and β-carotene, from their respective radical species [20].

Studies have reported the various changes that occur in different storage solutions, the effect of curcumin on plasma [15] and the effect of vitamin C on storage in erythrocytes [21–25]. However, the utilization of plasma as a mode of assessing the changes in blood, during storage with ascorbic acid as an additive, has not been explored. Plasma is a natural environment for blood morphological components. Thus, any change occurring in the blood cells is reflected in the plasma and thereby gives an insight into the condition of stored blood.

Therefore, we aimed to study two aspects (i) the continuous changes occurring during storage and (ii) the influence of vitamin C as an additive in stored blood. The changes occurring in plasma isolated from stored blood were analyzed at regular intervals during a period of 25 days.

In this regard the following objectives were put forth:

(a) to analyze the antioxidant status of plasma through antioxidant enzymes: superoxide dismutase (SOD) and catalase (CAT),

(b) to evaluate the oxidant levels through lipid peroxidation (thiobarbituric acid reactive substances (TBARS)) and protein oxidation (protein carbonyls (PrC), advanced oxidation protein products (AOPP), and protein sulfhydryls (P-SH)),

(c) to determine the effects of ascorbic acid as an additive in storage solution.

2. Materials and Methods

2.1. Animals. Male *Wistar* rats were maintained till 4 months of age, in accordance with the ethical committee regulations. Five animals were maintained for each group. Animals were lightly anaesthetized with ether and restrained in dorsal recumbency as described earlier [26]. In brief, the syringe needle was inserted just below the xiphoid cartilage and slightly to the left of midline. 4-5 mL of blood was carefully aspirated from the heart into collecting tubes with CPDA-1 (citrate, phosphate, dextrose, and adenine).

2.2. Chemicals. Epinephrine, thiobarbituric acid, and bovine serum albumin (BSA) were purchased from Sigma-Aldrich Chemicals (St. Louis, MO, USA). All other chemicals used were of reagent grade and organic solvents were of spectral grade.

2.3. Experimental Design. Blood was drawn from male *Wistar* rats (4 months old) and stored over a period of 25 days at 4°C in CPDA-1. Blood samples were divided into two groups: controls and experimentals. Ascorbic acid of varying concentrations was added to the experimental group: 10 mM, 30 mM, and 60 mM, that is, VC (10), VC (30), and VC (60) groups. Each group consisted of samples from 5 animals. Whole blood (1 mL) was aliquoted from the stored blood every fifth day and the plasma was isolated to analyze the previously mentioned parameters.

2.4. Plasma Separation. Plasma was isolated in Eppendorf tubes by centrifuging in a fixed angle rotor for 20 min at

2000 ×g. The plasma was removed and suspended in an equal volume of isotonic phosphate buffer, pH 7.4 [27].

2.5. Superoxide Dismutase (SOD, EC 1.15.1.1). SOD was measured by the method of Misra and Fridovich [28]. Plasma was added to carbonate buffer (0.05 M). Epinephrine was added to the mixture and measured spectrophotometrically at 480 nm. SOD activity was expressed as the amount of enzyme that inhibits oxidation of epinephrine by 50%.

2.6. Catalase (CAT, EC 1.11.1.6). CAT was determined by the method of Aebi [29]. Briefly, plasma with absolute alcohol was incubated at 0°C. An aliquot was taken up with 6.6 mM H_2O_2 and decrease in absorbance was measured at 240 nm. An extinction coefficient of 43.6 $M cm^{-1}$ was used to determine enzyme activity.

2.7. Thiobarbituric Acid Reactive Substances (TBARS). TBARS was determined by the method of Bar-Or et al. [30]. Plasma with 0.9% NaCl was incubated at 37°C for 20 min. 0.8 M HCl containing 12.5% TCA and 1% TBA was added and kept in boiling water bath for 20 min and cooled at 4°C. Centrifugation was carried out at 1500 ×g and absorbance was measured at 532 nm.

2.8. Protein Carbonyls (PrC). PrC was measured as an index of protein oxidation as described by Uchida and Stadtman [31]. Protein carbonyl content was measured by forming labeled protein hydrazones derivative, using 2,4-dinitrophenyl hydrazine (DNPH), which were then quantified spectrophotometrically. Briefly after precipitation of protein with equal volume of 1% trichloroacetic acid (TCA), the pellet was resuspended in 10 mM DNPH. Samples were kept in dark for 1 h. An equal volume of 20% TCA was added and left in ice for 10 min and centrifuged at 1900 ×g and pellet was washed with ethanol-ethylacetate mixture (1 : 1) to remove the free DNPH and lipid contaminants. Final pellet was dissolved in 8 M guanidine HCl in 133 mM tris and absorbance was measured at 370 nm. The results were expressed as μmol of 2,4-DNPH incorporated/mg protein based on a molar extinction coefficient of $2.1 \times 10^4 M cm^{-1}$ for aliphatic hydrazones.

2.9. Advanced Oxidation Protein Products (AOPP). Spectrophotometric determination of AOPP levels was assayed as an index of dityrosine containing cross-linked protein products by Witko's method [32]. Plasma was diluted in phosphate buffered saline and 1.16 mol/L potassium iodide was added, followed by the addition of acetic acid. The absorbance of reaction mixture was immediately read at 340 nm. AOPP was calculated by using the extinction coefficient of 26 $mM^{-1} cm^{-1}$.

2.10. Protein Sulfhydryls (P-SH). The concentration of P-SH was measured as described by Habeeb [33]. In brief, 0.08 mol/L sodium phosphate buffer containing 0.5 mg/mL of Na_2-EDTA and 2% SDS were added to each assay tube. 0.1 mL of 5,5′-dithiobis-(2-nitrobenzoic acid) (DTNB) was added and the solution was vortexed. Color was allowed to develop at room temperature and absorbance was measured at 412 nm. P-SH was calculated from the net absorbance and molar absorptivity, 13,600 mol L^{-1} cm^{-1}.

2.11. Protein Determination.
Protein was determined in the plasma by the method of Lowry et al. [34], using bovine serum albumin as the standard.

2.12. Statistical Analyses.
Results are represented as mean ± SE. Values between the groups were analyzed by two-way ANOVA and were considered significant at $P < 0.05$. Bonferroni Post test was performed for antioxidant enzymes, SOD and CAT, lipid peroxidation product, TBARS, and protein oxidation products, PrC, AOPP, and P-SH concentrations using Graph Pad Prism 6 software.

3. Results

3.1. Superoxide Dismutase.
SOD variation was insignificant during the storage period though increments of 100%, 300%, and 200% were observed in controls on days 10, 15, and 20, respectively against day 0.

Significant differences were observed in vitamin C groups. On day 15, SOD decreased by 75% in VC (30), whereas it increased by 200% on day 25 with respect to control. In addition, increments of 100% and 300% were also observed in VC (60) against VC (10) and VC (30), respectively.

VC (10) and VC (30) showed variations in SOD activity but increased towards the end of storage. SOD in VC (60) showed an increase with storage (Figure 1).

3.2. Catalase.
Catalase varied significantly with the storage. The activity increased in controls by 13-, 41-, 42-, and 18-fold on days 5, 15, 20, and 25, respectively, when compared to day 0. Similarly, increments of 6-fold were seen on days 5, 15, 20, and 25 in VC (10) and 12-fold (day 15) and 23-fold (days 20 and 25) in VC (30). CAT increased by 20-fold on days 20 and 25 in VC (60) when compared to day 0.

Variations in CAT between different concentrations were insignificant.

Catalase activity increased in all groups with storage (Figure 2).

3.3. Thiobarbituric Acid Reactive Substances (TBARS).
Significant changes were observed in TBARS during storage. In controls, TBARS decreased by 80% and 40% on days 5 and 20, respectively, whereas they increased by 160% and 60% on days 10 and 15, respectively, when compared to day 0. TBARS also reduced on days 10, 20, and 25 by 40%, 90%, and 80%, respectively, and increased by 100% on day 5 when compared to day 0 in VC (10) samples. There were increments of 300% (day 5) and 100% (day 25) in VC (30) and decrements of 42%, 85%, and 65% on days 5, 10, and 25, respectively, in VC (60) against day 0.

TBARS elevated by 3-fold on day 0 in VC (60) with VC (30). On day 5, TBARS increased by 12-fold in VC (30)

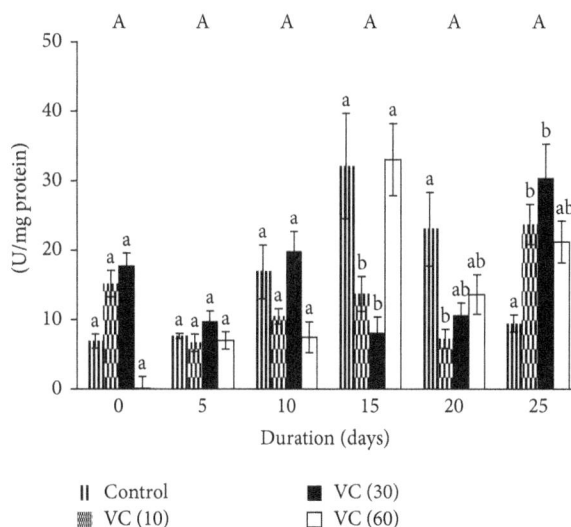

FIGURE 1: Superoxide dismutase activity in plasma isolated from stored blood. Values are mean ± SE of five animals/group. VC (10): vitamin C (10 mM); VC (30): vitamin C (30 mM); and VC (60): vitamin C (60 mM). Two-way ANOVA was performed between the groups and subgroups. Changes between the groups are insignificant. Changes within the groups are represented in lower case. Those not sharing the same letters are significantly different.

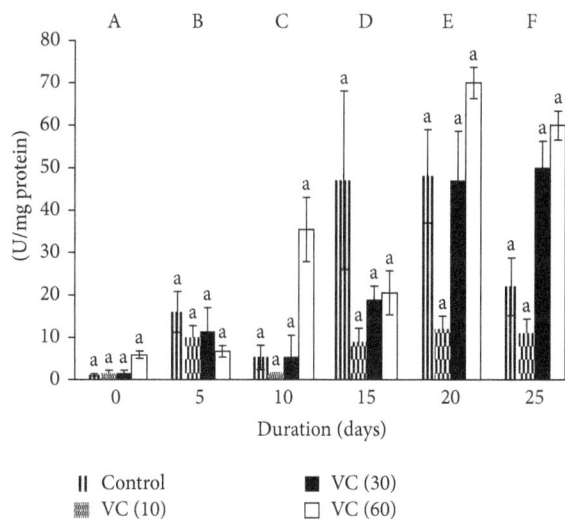

FIGURE 2: Catalase activity in stored plasma. Values are mean ± SE of five animals/group. VC (10): vitamin C (10 mM), VC (30): vitamin C (30 mM), and VC (60): vitamin C (60 mM). Two-way ANOVA was performed between the groups and subgroups. A–F values between the groups are significantly different at $P < 0.05$. Changes within the groups are represented in lower case. Those not sharing the same letters are significantly different.

whereas on day 10, it decreased by 77% in VC (10), VC (30), and VC (60) when compared to control.

TBARS decreased in VC (10) but was maintained in VC (30) and VC (60) with storage (Figure 3).

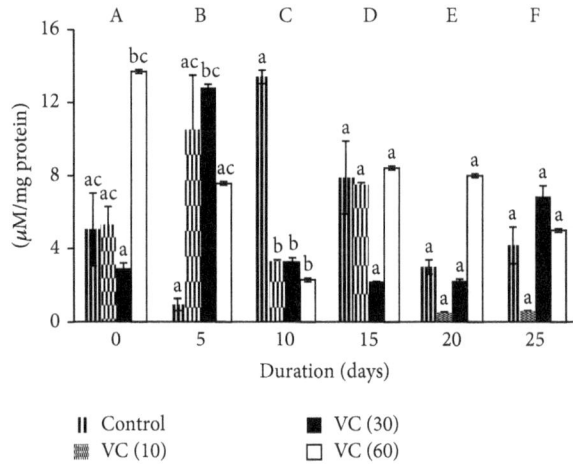

FIGURE 3: Thiobarbituric acid reactive substances in plasma isolated from stored blood. Values are mean ± SE of five animals/group. VC (10): vitamin C (10 mM), VC (30): vitamin C (30 mM), and VC (60): vitamin C (60 mM). Two-way ANOVA was performed between the groups and subgroups. A–F values between the groups are significantly different at $P < 0.05$. Changes within the groups are represented in lower case. Those not sharing the same letters are significantly different.

3.4. Protein Carbonyls (PrC).

Carbonyls of controls increased significantly by 1-, 2-, 12-, 8-, and 2-fold, respectively, from days 5 to 25 with respect to day 0. In VC (10), decrements of 43%, 89%, 42%, and 91% were observed on days 5, 15, 20, and 25, respectively, while an increment of 72% was observed on day 10 against day 0. A similar trend was noticed in VC (30) as PrC reduced by 85%, 77%, 48%, and 95% on days 5, 10, 15, and 25. But, in VC (60), PrC showed increments of 176%, 71% and 62%, and 80% on days 10, 15, and 20 and 25, respectively, with respect to control.

PrC increased by 23-fold on day 0 in VC (30) with respect to control, while it decreased by 1-fold in VC (60) against VC (30) on day 0.

Although there were variations in the levels of PrC in all groups, it was maintained towards the end of storage (Figure 4).

3.5. Advanced Oxidation Protein Products (AOPP).

AOPP increased by 300% on days 15 and 25 and by 400% on day 20 in controls. AOPP also increased by 100% (days 5, 10, and 15), 200% (day 20), and 300% (day 25) in VC (10). A similar trend was observed in VC (30) as AOPP increased by 100% on days 15 and 25, 70% on day 5, and 200% on day 20. AOPP elevated by 100% on day 10 and 200% on day 15 in VC (60) with respect to control.

AOPP reduced by 69% and 72% on days 15 and 25, respectively, in VC (10) against control. AOPP elevated by 100% and 200% on days 15 and 20, respectively, in VC (30) in comparison with VC (10). Increments of 69% and 74% were observed on days 20 and 25 when VC (30) was compared with VC (60). Decrements of 72% and 74% on days 20 and 25 were observed in VC (60) against controls.

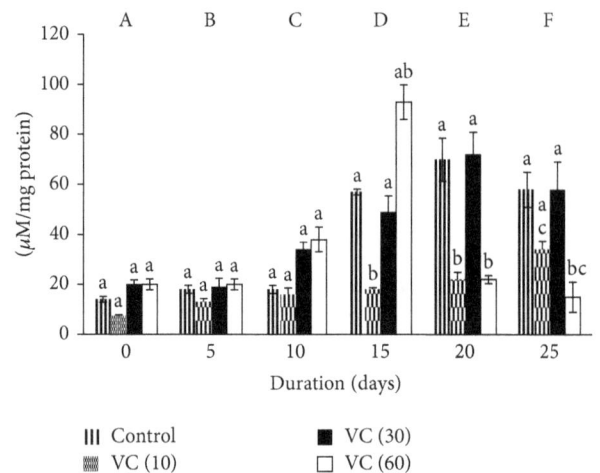

FIGURE 4: Protein carbonyls in plasma isolated from stored blood. Values are mean ± SE of five animals/group. VC (10): vitamin C (10 mM), VC (30): vitamin C (30 mM). and VC (60): vitamin C (60 mM). Two-way ANOVA was performed between the groups and subgroups. A–F values with different superscripts between groups are significantly different at $P < 0.05$. Changes within the groups are represented in lower case. Those not sharing the same letters are significantly different.

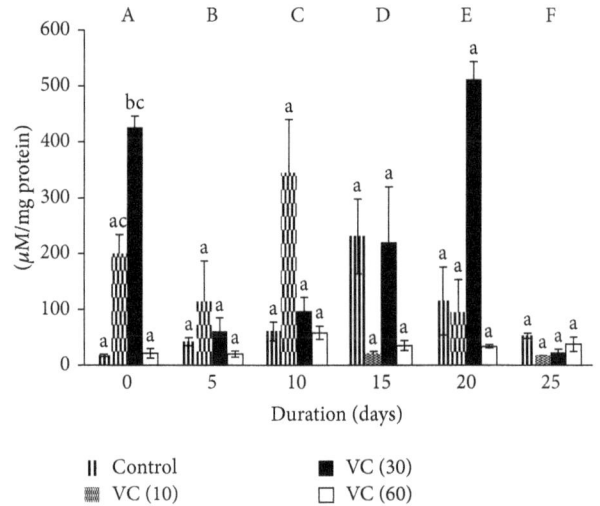

FIGURE 5: Advanced oxidation protein products in plasma isolated from stored blood. Values are mean ± SE of five animals/group. VC (10): vitamin C (10 mM), VC (30): vitamin C (30 mM), and VC (60): vitamin C (60 mM). Two-way ANOVA was performed between the groups and subgroups. A–F values between the groups are significantly different at $P < 0.05$. Changes within the groups are represented in lower case. Those not sharing the same letters are significantly different.

AOPP increased in VC (30) and was maintained in VC (10) and VC (60) (Figure 5).

3.6. Protein Sulfhydryls (P-SH).

Sulfhydryls varied significantly during storage. P-SH increased in controls by 3-, 2-, 8-, 10-, and 9-fold on days 5, 10, 15, 20, and 25, respectively, with

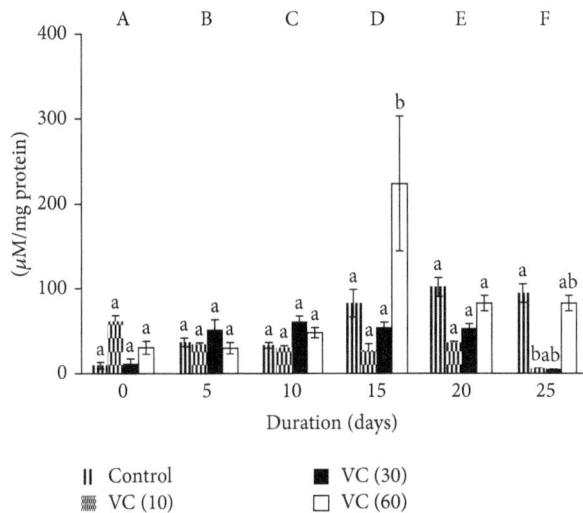

FIGURE 6: Protein sulfhydryls in plasma isolated from stored blood. Values are mean ± SE of five animals/group. VC (10): vitamin C (10 mM); VC (30): vitamin C (30 mM), and VC (60): vitamin C (60 mM). Two-way ANOVA was performed between the groups and subgroups. A–F values between the groups are significantly different at $P < 0.05$. Changes within the groups are represented in lower case. Those not sharing the same letters are significantly different.

day 0. P-SH also elevated by approximately 4-fold on days 5, 10, and 20, and 45-fold on day 15, respectively, in VC (30), when compared to day 0. An increment of 6-fold on day 15 and 1-fold on days 20 and 25 and a decrement of 54% were observed in VC (60) on day 10 against day 0.

On day 15, increases of 1-, 7-, and 3-fold were observed in VC (60) when compared with control, VC (10), and VC (30), respectively. On day 25, decrements of 1-fold were observed in VC (10) and VC (30) against controls.

Sulfhydryls were maintained in all groups throughout storage (Figure 6).

4. Discussion

The effects of vitamin C as an additive in blood during storage were evaluated through plasma. Although SOD levels were insignificant during storage, VC (10) and VC (30) decreased SOD levels on the days when ROS was found to be higher [35]. Catalase activity increased in all groups. Levels of TBARS, PrC, AOPP, and P-SH were maintained in all groups.

Blood plasma is considered well equipped with both chain-breaking and preventive antioxidants to cope with OS and prevent peroxidative damage to circulating lipids. The antioxidants do not exert their functions by merely scavenging radicals but also by inducing/activating enzymes counteracting OS or by modulating redox-sensitive metabolic pathways.

Superoxide dismutases are enzymes that convert superoxide radical to oxygen and hydrogen peroxide. These enzymes carry out catalysis via general mechanism that involves the sequential reduction and oxidation of the metals like copper,

iron, manganese, and nickel, at the active site [36]. The upregulation of SOD activity indicates an increase in free radicals during storage of blood, but a decrement in vitamin C samples (10 mM and 30 mM) may be due to the antioxidant property of ascorbic acid. Ascorbic acid is a soluble, strongly reducing agent that can react directly with free radicals, thereby resulting in decreased SOD in VC (10) and VC (30). The dismutation of superoxide radical yields hydrogen peroxide. This reaction occurs spontaneously or is catalyzed by superoxide dismutases. The high reactivity of H_2O_2 in vivo is largely explained by the Fenton reaction, where H_2O_2 reacts with partially reduced metal ions such as Fe^{2+} or Cu^+, to form the hydroxyl radical. This reaction can be sustained in vitro by the presence of mild reducing agent such as ascorbic acid that recycles the oxidized metal ions [37]. At higher concentrations, the ratio of ascorbate monoions is higher than that of the ascorbyl radical, thereby driving the Fenton reaction [38]. This may be the reason for increased SOD activity in VC (60).

Catalase rapidly catalyzes the decomposition of hydrogen peroxide to less reactive gaseous oxygen and water molecules. CAT exhibits a high K_m for H_2O_2 and can act upon H_2O_2 produced before it diffuses to other parts of the cell [39]. CAT may be uniquely suited to regulate the homeostasis of H_2O_2 in the cell. CAT activity was upregulated on all the days in the plasma of controls and vitamin C samples. This indicates that there is the formation of hydrogen peroxide, as CAT acts predominantly when H_2O_2 concentrations are enormously high. This also suggests that the endogenous antioxidants like glutathione, along with the vitamin C, could not attenuate the oxidative stress efficiently.

TBARS increased in the earlier stage of storage period but later decreased in controls. The earlier increase may be correlated to the latent phase of antioxidant activation and the decrease may be justified by the amelioration of the endogenous antioxidant system in the plasma. Vitamin C (ascorbic acid) is an important antioxidant in human plasma, where it acts as a scavenger of free radicals and protects against lipid peroxidation. Ascorbate plays a pivotal role in protecting plasma lipids from peroxidative damage initiated by aqueous peroxyl radicals [40, 41]. This was evident in our study as TBARS initially decreased in all vitamin C groups but later normalized to that of controls. This return to normalcy could be due to the unavailability of reduced ascorbate [42].

The quantification of oxidative damage to proteins has been studied almost exclusively by assessing the total carbonyl content. The oxidants responsible for carbonyl formation within the proteins in vivo are believed to be radicals, such as hydroxyl radicals. Indeed, hydroxyl radicals can be generated by metal-catalyzed oxidation systems and these systems convert several amino acid residues to carbonyl derivatives. It is known that an increase in carbonyl content reflects the oxidation of lysine, arginine, and proline residues of the proteins [43, 44].

Oxidation of proteins can lead to a whole variety of amino acid modifications. Action of chloraminated oxidants, mainly hypochlorous acid and chloramines, produced by myeloperoxidase, forms dityrosine containing cross-linked protein products known as AOPP and is also considered as one of the biomarkers to estimate the degree of oxidative modifications of proteins [36, 45].

Our results on carbonyls in controls proved that during storage period, there was production of ROS leading to oxidant damage of proteins. Ascorbyl-free radical reductase increases the ascorbic acid recycling in human plasma and is reported as a compensatory/protective mechanism that operates to maintain the ascorbic acid level in plasma and thereby minimize OS [46]. Vitamin C maintained carbonyls and AOPP as evident in our results.

Plasma is endowed with an array of antioxidant defense mechanisms. One of the important plasma antioxidants appears to be ascorbate. Protein sulfhydryl groups have also been suggested to contribute significantly to the antioxidant capacity of plasma. In particular, oxidative modification of sulfhydryl groups in proteins can be a two-faceted process: it could lead to impairment of protein function or, depending on the redox state of cysteine residues, may activate specific pathways involved in regulating key cell functions [47].

Oxidation of sulfhydryls of the membrane protein to disulfides causes reversible changes. This may be due to the disulfide exchange reactions carried out by a class of thiol-transferases that catalyze reactions between glutathione and thioredoxin to regenerate the protein sulfhydryls [48]. These may be the possible reasons for variations in sulfhydryls during the storage.

5. Conclusion

Plasma has an efficient antioxidant system and can minimize the levels of oxidants during storage of 25 days. Vitamin C at the concentrations of 10, 30, and 60 mM also enhanced the antioxidant defenses but could not protect susceptible protein groups. Our study gives an insight into the interactions of different oxidants and antioxidants (both endogenous and exogenous). Vitamin C alone could not sufficiently attenuate OS and hence this opens the possibilities for further studies on vitamin C in combination with other antioxidants, in storage solutions.

Conflict of Interests

The authors declare that there is no conflict of interests.

Acknowledgments

The authors like to thank Professor Leela Iyengar, Ms. Manasa K, and Jain University for their support.

References

[1] J. R. Hess, "Conventional blood banking and blood component storage regulation: opportunities for improvement," *Blood Transfusion*, vol. 8, no. 3, pp. s9–s15, 2010.

[2] A. Tinmouth, D. Fergusson, I. C. Yee, and P. C. Hébert, "Clinical consequences of red cell storage in the critically ill," *Transfusion*, vol. 46, no. 11, pp. 2014–2027, 2006.

[3] T. Yoshida and S. S. Shevkoplyas, "Anaerobic storage of red blood cells," *Blood Transfusion*, vol. 8, no. 4, pp. 220–236, 2010.

[4] T. Yoshida, J. P. AuBuchon, L. J. Dumont et al., "The effects of additive solution pH and metabolic rejuvenation on anaerobic storage of red cells," *Transfusion*, vol. 48, no. 10, pp. 2096–2105, 2008.

[5] G. M. D'Amici, C. Mirasole, A. D'Alessandro, T. Yoshida, L. J. Dumont, and L. Zolla, "Red blood cell storage in SAGM and AS3: a comparison through the membrane two-dimensional electrophoresis proteome," *Blood Transfusion*, vol. 10, pp. s46–s54, 2012.

[6] M. H. Antonelou, A. G. Kriebardis, K. E. Stamoulis, E. Economou-Petersen, L. H. Margaritis, and I. S. Papassideri, "Red blood cell aging markers during storage in citrate-phosphate-dextrose- saline-adenine-glucose-mannitol," *Transfusion*, vol. 50, no. 2, pp. 376–389, 2010.

[7] M. R. Kelher, T. Masuno, E. E. Moore et al., "Plasma from stored packed red blood cells and MHC class I antibodies causes acute lung injury in a 2-event *in vivo* rat model," *Blood*, vol. 113, no. 9, pp. 2079–2087, 2009.

[8] C. Hillier, L. Silberstein, P. Ness et al., *Blood Banking and Transfusion Medicine*, Elsevier, 2nd edition, 2007.

[9] V. Rajashekharaiah, A. A. Koshy, A. K. Koushik et al., "The efficacy of erythrocytes isolated from blood stored under blood bank conditions," *Transfusion and Apheresis Science*, vol. 47, no. 3, pp. 359–364, 2012.

[10] B. Kücükakin, V. Kocak, J. Lykkesfeldt et al., "Storage-induced increase in biomarkers of oxidative stress and inflammation in red blood cell components," *Scandinavian Journal of Clinical and Laboratory Investigation*, vol. 71, no. 4, pp. 299–303, 2011.

[11] D. S. Sachan, N. Hongu, and M. Johnsen, "Decreasing oxidative stress with choline and carnitine in women," *Journal of the American College of Nutrition*, vol. 24, no. 3, pp. 172–176, 2005.

[12] M. S. D'almeida, J. Jagger, M. Duggan, M. White, C. Ellis, and I. H. Chin-Yee, "A comparison of biochemical and functional alterations of rat and human erythrocytes stored in CPDA-1 for 29 days:implications for animal models of transfusion," *Transfusion Medicine*, vol. 10, no. 4, pp. 291–303, 2000.

[13] J. A. Knight and D. A. Searles, "The effects of various antioxidants on lipid peroxidation in stored whole blood," *Annals of Clinical and Laboratory Science*, vol. 24, no. 4, pp. 294–301, 1994.

[14] A. Arduini, S. Holme, J. D. Sweeney, S. Dottori, A. F. Sciarroni, and M. Calvani, "Addition of L-carnitine to additive solution-suspended red cells stored at 4°C reduces *in vitro* hemolysis and improves *in vivo* viability," *Transfusion*, vol. 37, no. 2, pp. 166–174, 1997.

[15] H. Carl, A. Chandni, K. Neha, S. Trishna, and R. Vani, "Curcumin as a modulator of oxidative stress during storage: a study on plasma," *Transfusion and Apheresis Science*, vol. 50, no. 2, pp. 288–293, 2014.

[16] C. S. Shiva Shankar Reddy, M. V. V. Subramanyam, R. Vani, and S. Asha Devi, "*In vitro* models of oxidative stress in rat erythrocytes: effect of antioxidant supplements," *Toxicology in Vitro*, vol. 21, no. 8, pp. 1355–1364, 2007.

[17] P. Møller, M. Viscovich, J. Lykkesfeldt, S. Loft, A. Jensen, and H. E. Poulsen, "Vitamin C supplementation decreases oxidative DNA damage in mononuclear blood cells of smokers," *European Journal of Nutrition*, vol. 43, no. 5, pp. 267–274, 2004.

[18] F. G. Uzun and Y. Kalender, "Protective effect of vitamins c and e on malathion-induced nephrotoxicity in male rats," *Gazi University Journal of Science*, vol. 24, no. 2, pp. 193–201, 2011.

[19] C. E. Cross, A. van der Vliet, C. A. O'Neill, S. Louie, and B. Halliwell, "Oxidants, antioxidants, and respiratory tract lining

fluids," *Environmental Health Perspectives*, vol. 102, no. 10, pp. 185–191, 1994.

[20] B. Halliwell, "Vitamin C: Antioxidant or pro-oxidant *in vivo*?" *Free Radical Research*, vol. 25, no. 5, pp. 439–454, 1996.

[21] G. L. Moore, M. E. Ledford, and M. R. Brummell, "Improved red blood cell storage using optional additive systems (OAS) containing adenine, glucose and ascorbate-2-phosphate," *Transfusion*, vol. 21, no. 6, pp. 723–731, 1981.

[22] G. L. Moore, D. H. Marks, R. A. Carmen et al., "Ascorbate-2-phosphate in red cell preservation. Clinical trials and active components," *Transfusion*, vol. 28, no. 3, pp. 221–225, 1988.

[23] L. A. Wood and E. Beutler, "The effect of periodic mixing on the preservation of 2,3 diphosphoglycerate (2,3 DPG) levels in stored blood," *Blood*, vol. 42, no. 1, pp. 17–25, 1973.

[24] V. Pallotta, F. Gevi, A. D'Alessandro, and L. Zolla, "Storing red blood cells with vitamin C and N-acetylcysteine prevents oxidative stress-related lesions: a metabolomics overview," *Blood Transfusion*, vol. 12, no. 3, pp. 376–387, 2014.

[25] S. R. Stowell, N. H. Smith, J. C. Zimring et al., "Addition of ascorbic acid solution to stored murine red blood cells increases posttransfusion recovery and decreases microparticles and alloimmunization," *Transfusion*, vol. 53, no. 10, pp. 2248–2257, 2013.

[26] R. Vani, C. S. S. S. Reddy, and S. Asha Devi, "Oxidative stress in erythrocytes: a study on the effect of antioxidant mixtures during intermittent exposures to high altitude," *International Journal of Biometeorology*, vol. 54, no. 5, pp. 553–562, 2010.

[27] J. T. Dodge, C. Mitchell, and D. J. Hanahan, "The preparation and chemical characteristics of hemoglobin-free ghosts of human erythrocytes," *Archives of Biochemistry and Biophysics*, vol. 100, no. 1, pp. 119–130, 1963.

[28] H. P. Misra and I. Fridovich, "The role of superoxide anion in the autoxidation of epinephrine and a simple assay for superoxide dismutase," *The Journal of Biological Chemistry*, vol. 247, no. 10, pp. 3170–3175, 1972.

[29] H. Aebi, "Catalase *in vitro*," *Methods in Enzymology*, vol. 105, pp. 121–126, 1984.

[30] D. Bar-Or, L. T. Rael, E. P. Lau et al., "An analog of the human albumin N-terminus (Asp-Ala-His-Lys) prevents formation of copper-induced reactive oxygen species," *Biochemical and Biophysical Research Communications*, vol. 284, no. 3, pp. 856–862, 2001.

[31] K. Uchida and E. R. Stadtman, "Covalent attachment of 4-hydroxynonenal to glyceraldehyde-3-phosphate dehydrogenase. A possible involvement of intra- and intermolecular cross-linking reaction," *The Journal of Biological Chemistry*, vol. 268, no. 9, pp. 6388–6393, 1993.

[32] V. Witko and B. Descamps-Latscha, "Microtiter plate assay for phagocyte-derived taurine-chloramines," *Journal of Clinical Laboratory Analysis*, vol. 6, no. 1, pp. 47–53, 1992.

[33] A. F. S. A. Habeeb, "Reaction of protein sulfhydryl groups with Ellman's reagent," *Methods in Enzymology*, vol. 25, pp. 457–464, 1972.

[34] O. H. Lowry, N. J. Rosenberg, A. L. Farr, and R. J. Randall, "Protein measurement with the Folin phenol reagent," *The Journal of Biological Chemistry*, vol. 193, no. 1, pp. 265–275, 1951.

[35] R. Soumya and R. Vani, "CUPRAC–BCS and antioxidant activity assays as reliable markers of antioxidant capacity in erythrocytes," *Hematology*, vol. 20, no. 3, pp. 165–174, 2015.

[36] K. B. Pandey and S. I. Rizvi, "Markers of oxidative stress in erythrocytes and plasma during aging in humans," *Oxidative Medicine and Cellular Longevity*, vol. 3, no. 1, pp. 2–12, 2010.

[37] D. Dreher and A. F. Junod, "Role of oxygen free radicals in cancer development," *European Journal of Cancer*, vol. 32, no. 1, pp. 30–38, 1996.

[38] K. Chen, J. Suh, A. C. Carr, J. D. Morrow, J. Zeind, and B. Frei, "Vitamin C suppresses oxidative lipid damage *in vivo*, even in the presence of iron overload," *The American Journal of Physiology—Endocrinology and Metabolism*, vol. 279, no. 6, pp. E1406–E1412, 2000.

[39] S. Mueller, H.-D. Riedel, and W. Stremmel, "Direct evidence for catalase as the predominant H_2O_2-removing enzyme in human erythrocytes," *Blood*, vol. 90, no. 12, pp. 4973–4978, 1997.

[40] T. L. Duarte, G. M. Almeida, and G. D. D. Jones, "Investigation of the role of extracellular H_2O_2 and transition metal ions in the genotoxic action of ascorbic acid in cell culture models," *Toxicology Letters*, vol. 170, no. 1, pp. 57–65, 2007.

[41] S. J. Padayatty, A. Katz, Y. Wang et al., "Vitamin C as an antioxidant: evaluation of its role in disease prevention," *Journal of the American College of Nutrition*, vol. 22, no. 1, pp. 18–35, 2003.

[42] J. M. May, Z.-C. Qu, and C. E. Cobb, "Human erythrocyte recycling of ascorbic acid: relative contributions from the ascorbate free radical and dehydroascorbic acid," *Journal of Biological Chemistry*, vol. 279, no. 15, pp. 14975–14982, 2004.

[43] Y. Oztas, I. Durukan, S. Unal, and N. Ozgunes, "Plasma protein oxidation is correlated positively with plasma iron levels and negatively with hemolysate zinc levels in sickle-cell anemia patients," *International Journal of Laboratory Hematology*, vol. 34, no. 2, pp. 129–135, 2012.

[44] B. S. Berlett and E. R. Stadtman, "Protein oxidation in aging, disease, and oxidative stress," *The Journal of Biological Chemistry*, vol. 272, no. 33, pp. 20313–20316, 1997.

[45] V. Witko-Sarsat, M. Friedlander, T. N. Khoa et al., "Advanced oxidation protein products as novel mediators of inflammation and monocyte activation in chronic renal failure," *Journal of Immunology*, vol. 161, no. 5, pp. 2524–2532, 1998.

[46] S. I. Rizvi, K. B. Pandey, R. Jha, and P. K. Maurya, "Ascorbate recycling by erythrocytes during aging in humans," *Rejuvenation Research*, vol. 12, no. 1, pp. 3–6, 2009.

[47] E. Herrero, J. Ros, G. Bellí, and E. Cabiscol, "Redox control and oxidative stress in yeast cells," *Biochimica et Biophysica Acta—General Subjects*, vol. 1780, no. 11, pp. 1217–1235, 2008.

[48] S. Türkes, Ö. Korkmaz, and M. Korkmaz, "Time course of the age-related alterations in stored blood," *Biophysical Chemistry*, vol. 105, no. 1, pp. 143–150, 2003.

Permissions

List of Contributors

Emma Conway O'Brien, Steven Prideaux, and Timothy Chevassut
Brighton and Sussex Medical School, University of Sussex, Falmer, Brighton BN1 9PS, UK

Giuseppe Lippi
Laboratory of Clinical Chemistry and Hematology, Academic Hospital of Parma, Via Gramsci 14, 43126 Parma, Italy

Gian Luca Salvagno, Elisa Danese and Gian Cesare Guidi
Laboratory of Clinical Biochemistry, Department of Life and Reproduction Sciences, University of Verona, Via delle Menegone, 37100 Verona, Italy

Cantor Tarperi and Federico Schena
Department of Neurological, Neuropsychological, Morphological and Movement Sciences, University of Verona, Via delle Menegone, 37100 Verona, Italy

Duni Sawadogo and Mahawa Sangaré
Department of Hematology, Faculty of Pharmacy, University Felix Houphouet Boigny, Cocody, BP 2308 Abidjan 08, Cote D'Ivoire
Unit of Hematology, Central Laboratory, Teaching Hospital of Yopougon, BP 632 Abidjan 21, Cote D'Ivoire

Aïssata Tolo-Dilkébié
Clinic Hematology Service, Teaching Hospital of Yopougon, BP 632 Abidjan 21, Cote D'Ivoire

Nelly Aguéhoundé
Department of Hematology, Faculty of Pharmacy, University Felix Houphouet Boigny, Cocody, BP 2308 Abidjan 08, Cote D'Ivoire

Hermance Kassi and Toussaint Latte
AIDS Biological Unit, Central Laboratory, Teaching Hospital of Yopougon, BP 632 Abidjan 21, Cote D'Ivoire

Linu A. Jacob, S. Aparna, K. C. Lakshmaiah, D. Lokanatha, Govind Babu, Suresh Babu and Sandhya Appachu
Department of Medical Oncology, Kidwai Memorial Institute of Oncology, Dr. M. H. Mari Gowda Road,Hombegowda Nagar, Bangalore, Karnataka 560030, India

Tayyibe Saler and Sibel KJrk
Department of Internal Medicine, Umraniye Training and Research Hospital, 34767 Istanbul, Turkey

Fakir Özgür KeGkek and Gülay OrtoLlu
Department of Internal Medicine, Numune Training and Research Hospital, Yüreğir, 01240 Adana, Turkey

Süleyman Ahbab
Department of Internal Medicine, Haseki Training and Research Hospital, 34087 Istanbul, Turkey

Ghaleb Elyamany
Department of Pathology and Blood Bank, Prince Sultan Military Medical City, P.O. Box 7897, Riyadh 11159, Saudi Arabia
Department of Hematology, Theodor Bilharz Research Institute, Egypt

Eman Al Mussaed
Hematopathology Division, Department of Basic Science, College of Medicine, Princess Nourah Bint Abdulrahman University, Riyadh, Saudi Arabia

Ali Matar Alzahrani
Department of Oncology, Prince Sultan Military Medical City, Saudi Arabia

Ilhami Berber, Mehmet Ali Erkurt, Ismet Aydogdu, Emin Kaya and Irfan Kuku
Division of Hematology, Department of Hematology, Faculty of Medicine, Medical School, Inonu University, 44280 Malatya, Turkey

Halit Diri
Department of Internal Medicine, Medical School, Inonu University, 44280 Malatya, Turkey

Han-Mou Tsai
iMAH Hematology Associates, New Hyde Park, NY 11040, USA

Elizabeth Kuo
Department of Medicine, University of Texas Southwestern School of Medicine, Dallas, TX 75235, USA

Evren Uygungül
Department of Emergency Medicine, Silifke State Hospital, Mersin, Turkey

Cuneyt Ayrik and Huseyin Narci
Department of Emergency Medicine, Faculty of Medicine, Mersin University, Mersin, Turkey

Semra ErdoLan
Department of Biostatistics, Faculty of Medicine, Mersin University, Mersin, Turkey

Ebrahim Toker
Department of Emergency Medicine, Tepecik Research Hospital, İzmir, Turkey

Filiz Demir
Department of Emergency Medicine, State Hospital, Niğde, Turkey

Ulas Karaaslan
Department of Emergency Medicine, State Hospital, Balıkesir, Turkey

Sandra Stella Lazarte, Cecilia Laura Jimenez, Miryam Emilse Ledesma Achem, Magdalena María Terán and Blanca Alicia Issé
Instituto de Bioquímica Aplicada, Facultad de Bioquímica, Química y Farmacia, Universidad Nacional de Tucumán (UNT), Balcarce 747, San Miguel de Tucumán, 4000 Tucum´an, Argentina

María Eugenia Mónaco
Instituto de Bioquímica Aplicada, Facultad de Bioquímica, Química y Farmacia, Universidad Nacional de Tucumán (UNT), Balcarce 747, San Miguel de Tucumán, 4000 Tucumán, Argentina
Instituto de Biología, Facultad de Bioquímica, Química y Farmacia, Universidad Nacional de Tucumán, Chacabuco 461, San Miguel de Tucumán, 4000 Tucumán, Argentina

Adriano Basques Fernandes, LucianaMoreira Lima, Marinez Oliveira Sousa, Vicente de Paulo Coelho Toledo and Maria das Graças Carvalho
Faculty of Pharmacy, Federal University of Minas Gerais, Avenida Antonio Carlos 6627, 31270-901 Belo Horizonte, MG, Brazil

Rashid Saeed Kazmi
Department of Haematology, University Hospital Southampton, Southampton, UK

Bashir Abdulgader Lwaleed
Faculty of Health Sciences, University of Southampton, Southampton, UK

Shannon R. McCurdy and Ephraim J. Fuchs
Sidney Kimmel Comprehensive Cancer Center at Johns Hopkins, Baltimore, MD 21287, USA

Musa A. Sani
Department of Haematology and Blood Transfusion, Kwara State Specialist Hospital, Sobi, 240001 Ilorin, Nigeria

James O. Adewuyi, Abiola S. Babatunde and Hannah O. Olawumi
Department of Haematology and Blood Transfusion, University of Ilorin Teaching Hospital, PMB 1459, 240003 Ilorin, Nigeria

Rasaki O. Shittu
Department of Family Medicine, Kwara State Specialist Hospital, Sobi, 240001 Ilorin, Nigeria

Conglei Li and June Li
Department of Laboratory Medicine and Pathobiology, University of Toronto, Toronto, ON, Canada M5S 1A8
Department of Laboratory Medicine, Keenan Research Centre, Li Ka Shing Knowledge Institute, St. Michael's Hospital, and Toronto Platelet Immunobiology Group, University of Toronto, Toronto, ON, Canada M5S 1A8

Canadian Blood Services, Toronto, ON, Canada M5G 2M1
Department of Medicine and Department of Physiology, University of Toronto, Toronto, ON, Canada M5S 1A8

Yan Li and Pingguo Chen
Department of Laboratory Medicine, Keenan Research Centre, Li Ka Shing Knowledge Institute, St. Michael's Hospital,and Toronto Platelet Immunobiology Group, University of Toronto, Toronto, ON, Canada M5S 1A8
Canadian Blood Services, Toronto, ON, Canada M5G 2M1

Sean Lang
Department of Laboratory Medicine and Pathobiology, University of Toronto, Toronto, ON, Canada M5S 1A8
Department of Laboratory Medicine, Keenan Research Centre, Li Ka Shing Knowledge Institute, St. Michael's Hospital, and Toronto Platelet Immunobiology Group, University of Toronto, Toronto, ON, Canada M5S 1A8
Canadian Blood Services, Toronto, ON, Canada M5G 2M1

Issaka Yougbare and Guangheng Zhu
Department of Laboratory Medicine, Keenan Research Centre, Li Ka Shing Knowledge Institute, St. Michael's Hospital, and Toronto Platelet Immunobiology Group, University of Toronto, Toronto, ON, Canada M5S 1A8

Heyu Ni
Department of Laboratory Medicine and Pathobiology, University of Toronto, Toronto, ON, Canada M5S 1A8
Department of Laboratory Medicine, Keenan Research Centre, Li Ka Shing Knowledge Institute, St. Michael's Hospital, and Toronto Platelet Immunobiology Group, University of Toronto, Toronto, ON, Canada M5S 1A8
Canadian Blood Services, Toronto, ON, Canada M5G 2M1
Department of Medicine and Department of Physiology, University of Toronto, Toronto, ON, Canada M5S 1A8

Thomas J. Humphries and Prasad Mathew
Bayer HealthCare, 100 Bayer Boulevard, P.O. Box 915, Whippany, NJ 08981-0915, USA

Stephan Rauchensteiner
Bayer Pharma AG, Global Medical Affairs Therapeutic Areas (GMA), Muellerstrasse 178, 13353 Berlin, Germany

Claudia Tückmantel
Bayer Pharma AG, Aprather Weg 18a, Building 470, 42096Wuppertal, Germany

Alexander Pieper
M.A.R.C.O. GmbH&Co. KG, Moskauer Strasse 25, 40227Düsseldorf, Germany

Monika Maas Enriquez
Bayer Pharma AG, Global Clinical Development Therapeutic Area NOHI, Aprather Weg, 42096Wuppertal, Germany

Ghaleb Elyamany
Department of Hematology and Blood Bank, Theodor Bilharz Research Institute, Giza 12411, Egypt, Egypt
Department of Central Military Laboratory, Prince Sultan Military Medical City, P.O. Box 7897, Riyadh 11159, Saudi Arabia

Mohammad Awad
Department of Central Military Laboratory, Prince Sultan Military Medical City, P.O. Box 7897, Riyadh 11159, Saudi Arabia

Kamal Fadalla, Mohamed Albalawi and Abdulaziz Al Abdulaaly
Department of Adult Clinical Hematology and Stem Cell Therapy, Prince Sultan Military Medical City, Riyadh, Saudi Arabia

Mohammad Al Shahrani
Department of Pediatric Hematology/Oncology, Prince Sultan Military Medical City, P.O. Box 7897, Riyadh 11159, Saudi Arabia
Agata Sobczy Nska-Malefora, Dominic J. Harrington, Kieran Voong, and Martin J. Shearer
The Nutristasis Unit, The Centre for Haemostasis and Thrombosis, GSTS Pathology (Part of King's Healthcare Partners), St.Thomas' Hospital, London SE1 7EH, UK

Sarawut Saichanma, Sucha Chulsomlee, Nonthaya Thangrua, Pornsuri Pongsuchart and Duangmanee Sanmun
Division of Clinical Microscopy, Faculty of Medical Technology, Huachiew Chalermprakiet University,Samut Prakan 10540,Thailand

Pairaya Rujirojindakul and Pornprot Limprasert
Department of Pathology, Faculty of Medicine, Prince of Songkla University, Hat Yai, Songkhla 90110, Thailand

Virasakdi Chongsuvivatwong
Epidemiology Unit, Faculty of Medicine, Prince of Songkla University, Hat Yai, Songkhla 90110, Thailand

Cemil Bilir, Hüseyin Engin, and Yasemin Bakkal Temi
Bülent Ecevit University School of Medicine, Department of Internal Medicine, Division of Medical Oncology, 67100 Zonguldak, Turkey

Donna Reece
Princess Margaret Hospital, University Health Network, 610 University Avenue, Toronto, ON, Canada M5G 2M9

C. TomKouroukis
Department of Oncology, Juravinski Cancer Centre, 699 Concession Street, Hamilton, ON, Canada L8V 5C2

Richard LeBlanc
Hôpital Maisonneuve-Rosemont, University of Montreal, Montreal, QC, Canada H1T 2M4

Michael Sebag
McGill University Health Centre, McGill University, Montreal, QC, Canada H3A 1A1

Kevin Song
Leukemia/BMT Program of British Columbia, Vancouver General Hospital, Vancouver, BC, Canada V5Z 1M9

John Ashkenas
SCRIPT, Toronto, ON, Canada M4S 1Z9

Suvro Sankha Datta
Department of Transfusion Medicine, The Mission Hospital, Durgapur, West Bengal 713212, India

Somnath Mukherjee
Department of Transfusion Medicine, AIIMS, Bhubaneswar 751019, India

Biplabendu Talukder, Prasun Bhattacharya and Krishnendu Mukherjee
Department of Immunohematology & Blood Transfusion, MCH, Kolkata 700073, India

Alice Charwudzi
Department of Chemical Pathology, University of Cape Coast School of Medical Sciences, Cape Coast, Ghana

Edeghonghon E. Olayemi and Ivy Ekem
Department of Haematology, University of Ghana Medical School, Accra, Ghana

Olufunmilayo Olopade and Mariann Coyle
Department of Medicine, University of Chicago, 929 East 57th Street, Chicago, IL 60637, USA

Amma Anima Benneh
Department of Haematology, Korle-Bu Teaching Hospital, Accra, Ghana

Emmanuel Alote Allotey
Haematology Unit, Tamale Teaching Hospital, Tamale, Ghana

Patrick Van Dreden
Diagnostica Stago, 125 Avenue Louis Roche, 92635 Gennevilliers Cedex, France

Guy Hue
Biochemistry Department, IBC, Rouen University Hospital, 76031 Rouen Cedex, France

Jean-François Dreyfus
Clinical Research Unit, Hôpital Foch, University of Versailles, 92151 Suresnes Cedex, France

Barry Woodhams
HaemaCon Ltd, Bromley, Kent CT18 7TW, UK

Marc Vasse
Clinical Biology Department & EA 4531, Hospital Foch, 40 rue Worth, 92151 Suresnes Cedex, France

Ravindra Kumar
Central Research Laboratory, Sri Aurobindo Medical College and PG Institute, Indore, Madhya Pradesh 453111, India

Vandana Arya
Department of Molecular Hematology, Sir Ganga Ram Hospital, New Delhi 110060, India

Sarita Agarwal
Department of Genetics, Sanjay Gandhi Post Graduate Institute of Medical Sciences, Lucknow, Uttar Pradesh 226014, India

Alessandro Morotti, Giovanna Carrà, Cristina Panuzzo, Sabrina Crivellaro, Angelo Guerrasio and Giuseppe Saglio
Department of Clinical and Biological Sciences, University of Turin, 10043 Orbassano, Italy

Riccardo Taulli
Department of Oncology, University of Turin, 10043 Orbassano, Italy

A. Schmidt-Tanguy and M.-P. Moles-Moreau
Hematology Department of the University of Angers, Angers, France

R. Houot and T. Lamy
Hematology Department of the University of Rennes, Rennes, France

S. Lissandre
Hematology Department of the University of Tours, Tours, France

J. F. Abgrall
Hematology Department of the University of Brest, Brest, France

P. Casassus
Hematology Department of the University of Bobigny, Bobigny, France

P. Rodon
Hematology Department of the Hospital of Blois, Blois, France

B. Desablens and J. P. Marolleau
Hematology Department of the University of Amiens, Amiens, France

R. Garidi
Hematology Department, St. Quentin General Hospital, St. Quentin, France

G. Damaj
University Hospital of Amiens, Department of Clinical Haematology, Avenue Laennec, 80054 Amiens, France

Marc Gregory Y. Yu, Ralph Elvi M. Villalobos, Ma. Jasmin Marinela C. Juan-Bartolome, and Regina P. Berba
Department of Medicine, Philippine General Hospital, Taft Avenue, Ermita, 1000 Manila, Philippines

Keith L. Davis
RTI Health Solutions, Research Triangle Park, NC 27709, USA

Isabelle Côté, Estella Mendelson and Haitao Gao
Novartis Pharmaceuticals Corporation, East Hanover, NJ 07936, USA

James A. Kaye
RTI Health Solutions, Waltham, MA 02451, USA

Julian Perez Ronco
Novartis Pharma AG, 4056 Basel, Switzerland

Mahesh ChandMeena, Alok Hemal, Mukul Satija and Shilpa Khanna Arora
Department of Pediatrics, PGIMER and Dr. RML Hospital, New Delhi 110001, India

Shahina Bano
Department of Radiology, PGIMER and Dr. RML Hospital, New Delhi 110001, India

Anthony A. Oyekunle, Rahman A. Bolarinwa,Lateef Salawu and Muheez A. Durosinmi
Department of Hematology and Immunology, Obafemi Awolowo University, Ile-Ife 234-220005, Nigeria
Department of Hematology and Blood Transfusion, Obafemi Awolowo University Teaching Hospital Complex, Ile-Ife 234-220005, Nigeria

Adesola T. Oyelese
Department of Hematology and Blood Transfusion, Obafemi Awolowo University Teaching Hospital Complex, Ile-Ife 234-220005, Nigeria

Lidice Bernardo
The Canadian Blood Services, Canada
Department of Laboratory Medicine and the Keenan Research Centre in the Li Ka Shing Knowledge Institute of St. Michael's Hospital,

Gregory A. Denomme
Immunohematology Reference Laboratory, Blood Center of Wisconsin, Milwaukee, WI 53226, USA

Kunjlata Shah
Department of Transfusion Medicine, St. Michael's Hospital, Toronto, ON, Canada M5B 1W8

Alan H. Lazarus
The Canadian Blood Services, Canada
Department of Laboratory Medicine and the Keenan Research Centre in the Li Ka Shing Knowledge Institute of St. Michael's Hospital, 30 Bond Street, Toronto, ON, Canada M5B 1W8
Departments of Medicine and Laboratory Medicine & Pathobiology, University of Toronto, Toronto, ON, Canada

Ali Zalpou
University of Texas MD Anderson Cancer Center, 1400 Pressler Avenue, Unit 1465, FCT 13.5021, Houston, TX 77030, USA

Thein Hlaing Oo
Section of Thrombosis & Benign Hematology, The University of Texas MD Anderson Cancer Center, Houston, TX, USA
Scott R. Solomon, Melhem Solh, Lawrence E. Morris, H. Kent Holland, and Asad Bashey
Blood and Marrow Transplant Program at Northside Hospital, Atlanta, GA 30342, USA

R. Vani, R. Soumya, H. Carl, V. A. Chandni, K. Neha, B. Pankhuri, S. Trishna and D. P. Vatsal
Center for Post Graduate Studies, Jain University, No. 18/3, 9th Main, 3rd Block, Jayanagar, Bangalore 560011, India

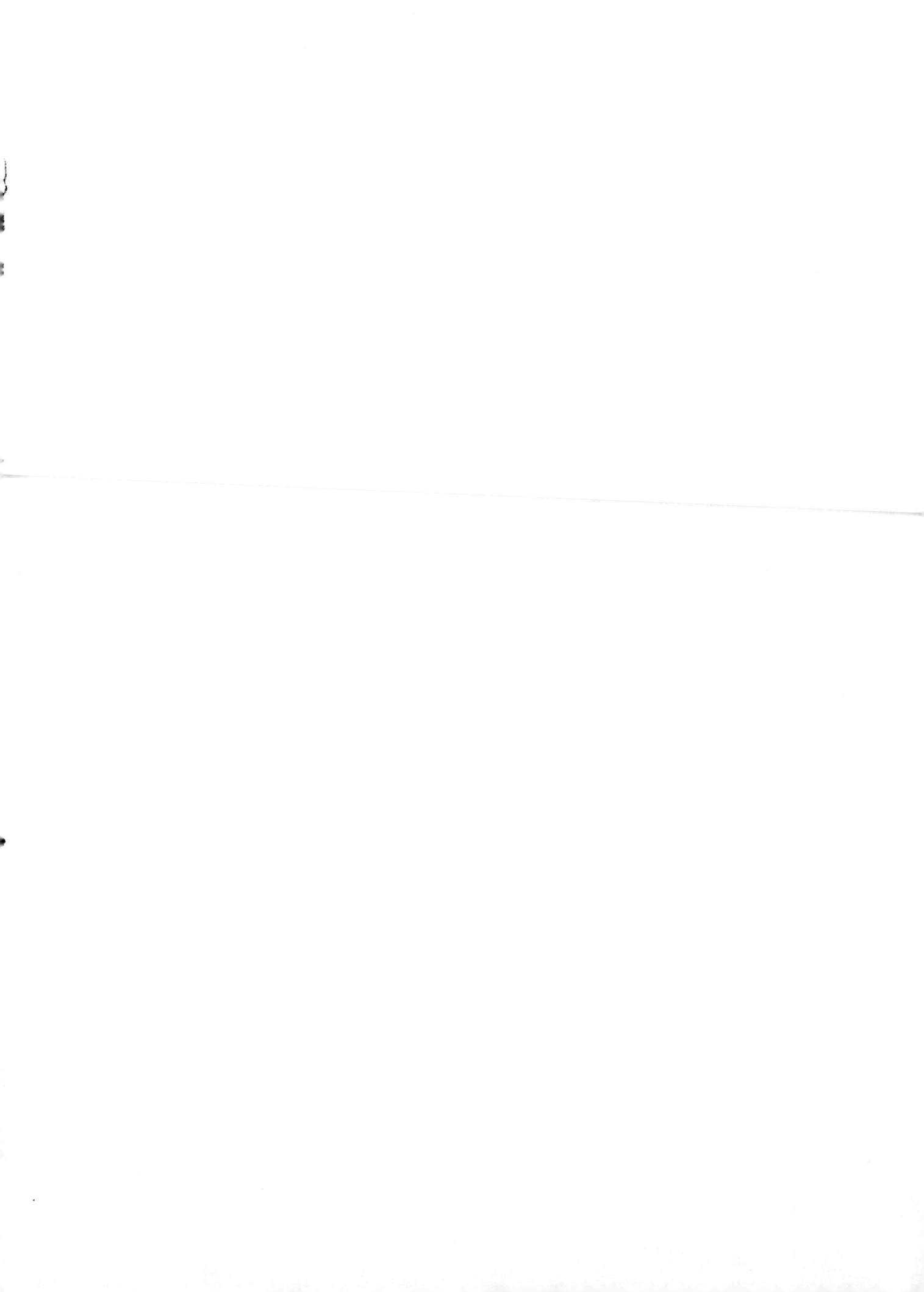

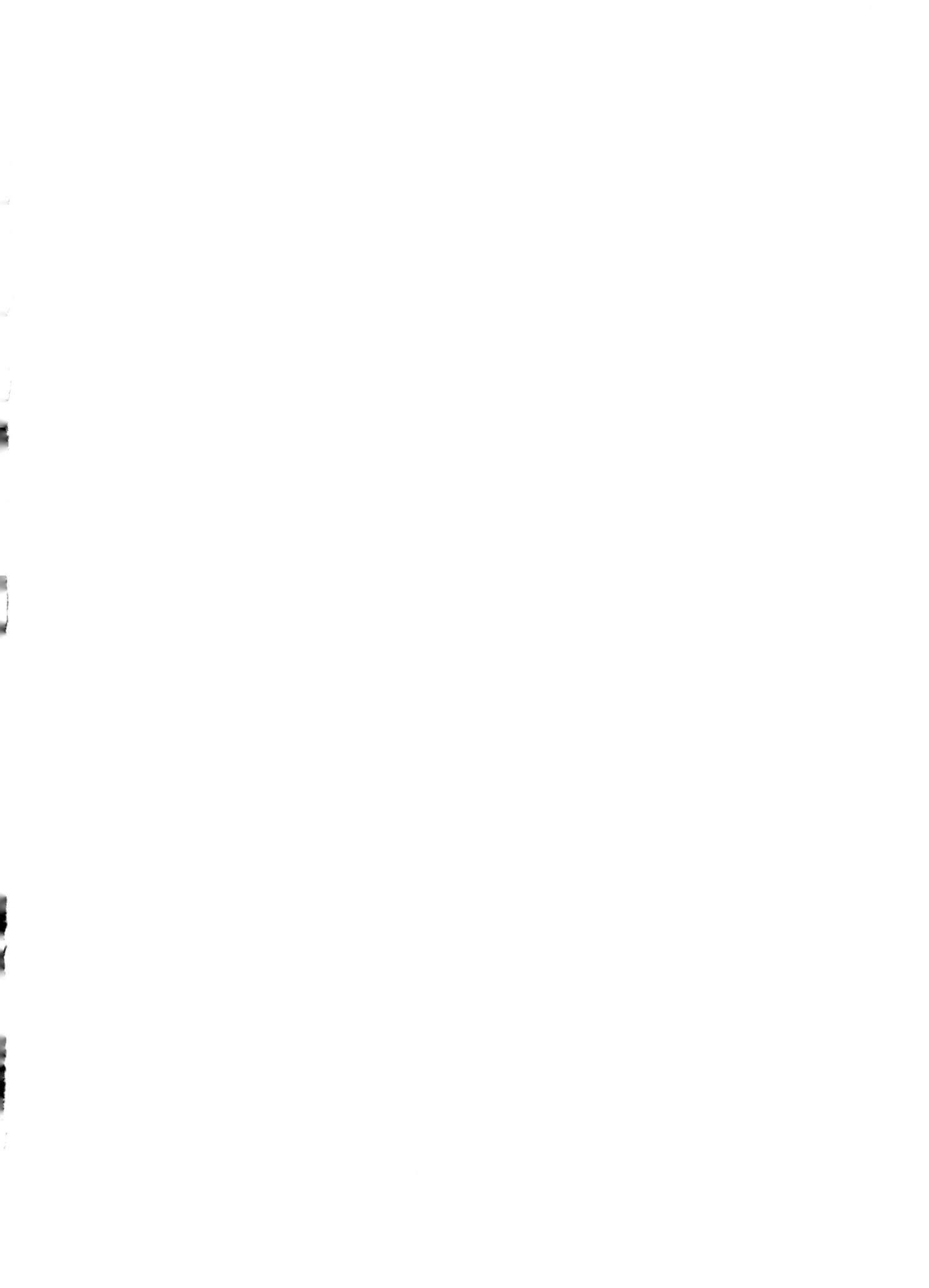